Disclaimers
"This publication is designed to provide accurate and authoritative information in regard to the subject matter covered. It is sold or distributed with the understanding that the publisher is not engaged in rendering legal, accounting, or other professional service. If legal advice or other expert assistance is required, the services of a competent professional person should be sought."
—From the Declaration of Principles jointly adopted by the American Bar Association and a Committee of Publishers and Associations

The author, A. Lee Dellon, MD, has a proprietary interest in the Disk-Criminator™, the Pressure-Specified Sensory Device™, Digit-Grip™, and the Skin Compliance Device™.

ISBN 1-56900-049-2

Printed in the United States of America

Director of the Institute for Peripheral Nerve Surgery:
A. Lee Dellon, MD

Editor: Diane Stamm

Cover Design: Glenn G. Dellon, Swirly Ink,
529 N. Charles St., Apt 102, Baltimore, MD 21201.

THIS BOOK
IS DEDICATED TO
MY SENSATIONAL TEACHERS,
Raymond M. Curtis, MD,
Erik Moberg, MD,
AND
Nebojsa Kovacevic

ACKNOWLEDGEMENT

The presentation of crucial concepts in this book has relied upon the insights and artistry of its illustrator. The artist was carefully chosen. I have known him, and observed his work develop over the past 22 years. That artist, Glenn George Dellon, my son, did his illustrations for this book during his senior year in high school, and the cover design for this hard cover edition while at the Maryland Institute College of Art, in graduate studies. The illustrations have been prepared in the style of a cartoonist to convey the spirit of joy and enthusiasm that has always surrounded the subject of the peripheral nerve for me. Seeing Glenn's unique perspective transform neuroscience has added immeasurably to the thrill of preparing this book.

I want to thank those who took the time to review portions of the text during the stages of its preparation for the soft cover edition: Pegge Carter-Wilson, OTR, CHT; Beth Wojiciechowski-Roros, OTR; Patsy L. Tassler, Ph.D.; John (Jack) E. Barham, MEd; David Seiler, MBA; Stephanie Hollenback, BSN, RNFA; Oskar C. Aszmann, MD; and Jennifer R. Berman, MD. Their time and understanding enabled me to believe that the text was both readable and relevant to its intended audience.

A special thanks goes to Luiann O. Greer, whose infectious enthusiasm for Quantitative Sensory Testing generated the interest that resulted in this hard cover edition.

Finally, I wish to express appreciation to Steve Hammet's group at Kirby Lithographic for this excellent production.

table of
contents

• FOREWORD •

• PREFACE •

• SECTION ONE BASIC PRINCIPLES

CHAPTER 1. THE NEURON

CHAPTER 2. CUTANEOUS SENSORY RECEPTORS

CHAPTER 3. PROPRIOCEPTION

CHAPTER 4. NERVE RECONSTRUCTION

SECTION TWO
QUANTITATIVE SENSORY TESTING

SECTION THREE
SENSORY REHABILITATION

CHAPTER 9. GRADING PERIPHERAL NERVE FUNCTION

CHAPTER 10. CORTICAL PLASTICITY

CHAPTER 11. SENSORY REEDUCATION

SECTION FOUR
SPECIFIC APPLICATIONS & NORMATIVE DATA

CHAPTER 12. UPPER EXTREMITY

CHAPTER 17. THE PENIS

CHAPTER 18. CUMULATIVE TRAUMA DISORDERS

CHAPTER 19. PLEGIA

SECTION FIVE
THERAPIST AS RESEARCHER AND TEACHER

CHAPTER 20. THERAPIST AS RESEARCHER

SECTION SIX
REFERENCES & INDEX

foreword

foreword

• • •

At the 26th Annual Meeting of the American Society for Surgery of the Hand, held in San Francisco in March 1971, Lee Dellon presented a paper, coauthored by Raymond Curtis and Milton Edgerton entitled, "Re-education of Sensation in the Hand After Nerve Injury and Repair." His presentation was published as an abstract in the *Journal of Bone and Joint Surgery,* followed by publication of the full version in 1974 in the *Journal of Plastic and Reconstructive Surgery.* That original "little paper" changed forever the course of clinical care of the patient with an upper extremity injury to the peripheral nerve.

The purpose of the paper was to present the most recent neurophysiological findings on cutaneous sensation, set a specific reeducation program, and give an appropriate timetable for that reeducation. Lee Dellon was just beginning his career as a hand surgeon, and hand therapy was in its very infancy. The only other published work describing a specific sensory reeducation program of the peripheral nerves in the upper extremity was contained in Wynn Parry's 1966 edition of *Rehabilitation of the Hand.* Lee's publication was unique in that it was the first time someone had attempted to increase the understanding of clinical testing by correlating the methods directly with the latest findings of neurophysiological research.

On a personal note, I was just starting my career in hand therapy in 1974. Lee's first article on peripheral nerve evaluation and reeducation had a profound impact on me, creating an interest in sensibility that continues to this day. I was very fortunate in those early years to be able to teach with Lee at various hand symposiums across the country. He was tireless in trying to encourage therapists to expand their knowledge base in neurophysiology and their testing skills as clinicians. Throughout the years, we have collaborated, discussed, and even disagreed. Lee has always been a very patient teacher. My hope is that through his latest effort, a new generation of students and clinicians will become as fascinated with sensibility as I did over twenty years ago.

Since that modest beginning in 1971, Lee Dellon has never wavered from his concept of incorporating the basic sciences with clinical skills. In 1981, he published *Evaluation of Sensibility and Re-education of Sensation in the Hand,* an entire text dedicated to increasing understanding of nerve physiology, evaluation of sensibility, and nerve rehabilitation. True to his nature as a teacher, Lee approached the subject in a highly personal fashion, making it accessible to the clinician. His approach created some con-troversy, but also provided the impetus that helped to increase interest in, and study of, the evaluation and reeducation of the peripheral nerve, both nationally and internationally. As a direct result of his publications, Lee provided the tools that enabled the therapist not only to evaluate the status of the peripheral nerve, but also to interpret the physiological meaning of the test results.

Somatosensory Testing and Rehabilitation, Lee Dellon's most recent endeavor, brings us up-to-date on both the latest findings of neurophysiological research and the technological changes in evaluation. Advances in surgical techniques, particularly in plastic surgery, create a very apparent expansion from the author's previous work. His latest contribution is a Herculean effort that encompasses not only evaluation and reeducation of the upper extremity, but also includes the entire body extending beyond the peripheral nerve to include all aspects of plegias and cortical plasticity. Once more, he has approached his subject as a teacher, offering basic neurophysiology and anatomy, methods of quantitative testing and techniques of sensory reeducation, fol-lowed by specific applications for each area of the body. He ends by challenging the therapist to become both a researcher and a teacher by being an integral member of the research team, publishing results, and presenting those results to peers in a teaching environment. The final section of the text is an excellent teaching tool, consisting of self-administered questions and answers to help the student of somatosensory rehabilitation test his or her level of comprehension of the material.

When Lee authored his first text, he stated that his purpose "was to bridge the potential, if not actual, gap between those involved with the neurosciences and those involved with the care of the peripheral nerve." He did that. With this latest effort, he goes beyond that to bring us abreast of not only neurophysiological research and its application in the clinic, but also the implications of changing technology. I doubt he is finished. I'm sure he will continue his journey to keep the student and the clinician current with the wealth of research knowledge and technology that in the end will give the patient the benefit of the highest quality of care both now and in the future.

Margaret S. Carter, OTR, CHT
August 6, 1995
Past President, American Society for Hand Therapy

• • •

preface

preface

• • •

Tube, or not tube...........that is the question:
   Whether 'tis nobler in the mind to suffer
The stings and shooting pains of neuroma formation,
   Or to take our nerve after a divisive injury,
And oppose its ends within a tube?....To frustrate,
   No more, and by entubulation will end
The pain and the thousand natural shocks
   That nerve is heir to....'tis a consummation
Devoutly to be wish'd. To regenerate,
   To rehabilitate! perchance to discriminate....ay,
There's the sense.

HamLeet,
Act III, Scene I*

• • •

We all come into the world virtually devoid of sensory experience. Virtually, because perhaps, during the 9 or so months of life *in utero,* the physical interface between the skin and the temperature-controlled surrounding liquid environment imparts the first stimuli to the nerve fibers that subserve the transmission of sensory information to the brain. It may well

....
* A. Lee Dellon, MD, Editorial, *Journal of Hand Surgery, 19B:* 271, 1994.

be that the stimuli also have reached the brain through acoustic mechanisms, through the transmission of vibratory stimuli. Yet, certainly, these vibrations have been cushioned by their passage across the maternal body and the water interface with the tympanic membrane. And so, we all come into the world virtually devoid of sensory experience.

Then, BANG!, an explosion of sensory stimuli, and the awareness of the central nervous system that it must deal with this new torrential rain of information from the periphery. Understanding the mechanisms that let us process this information in health and disease, understanding the techniques to quantitate sensibility in health and disease, and developing approaches to rehabilitate these systems constitute the subject of this book.

There was a prophet, Raymond M. Curtis, originally from Columbus, Missouri, who preached of the need to do meticulous surgery to reconstruct the injured hand, and to spend at least an equal amount of attention on the rehabilitation of that hand. In 1969, during the summer between my second and third years at the Johns Hopkins University School of Medicine, I received permission to observe Dr. Curtis in surgery at the Children's Hospital in Baltimore on Tuesday after-

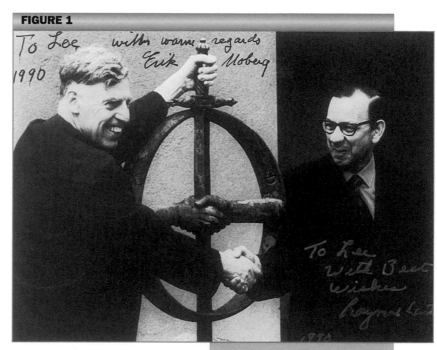

FIGURE 1

Erik Moberg, left, shakes hands with Raymond M. Curtis, at a Hand Surgery Club meeting in Scandinavia, circa 1980.

noons. He operated in Room 2. It was the contrast between the precision I observed in his work with nerves and the inability clinically to be able to quantitate the function of those nerves that led to my first research with the peripheral nerve.

Part of my job as Dr. Curtis's first Hand Fellow in 1977, in his new Hand Center, was to establish research models in his lab, a converted labor and delivery room at Union Memorial Hospital. From that lab, during the academic year 1981-1982, the last year of his active practice, were initiated the basic science models that led to our understanding of chronic nerve compression, the double crush syndrome, neuroma formation, and neural regeneration through bioabsorbable conduits.

When I last visited Dr. Curtis in 1992, at his home on Gibson Island, Maryland, he was still reading the *Journal of Hand Surgery* and asking provocative questions about current research activities. His wife, Anne, was able to make him aware of this book's dedication to him prior to his death. He died on October 9, 1994 in Seattle, Washington. He left with us the Curtis Hand Center, whose Surgery and Rehabilitation Departments radiate his preachings to the world.

There was another prophet in the surgical community, Erik Moberg of

Gotteborg, Sweden, who preached of the essential need to quantitate sensibility. He visited Baltimore in 1969, to go sailing with Dr. Curtis. I was in my third year of medical school and, having been inspired by Dr. Curtis to study the pattern of recovery of sensation after nerve injury, was given the opportunity to present my research to Dr. Moberg. It was the beginning of a long association. I last had dinner with him in Seattle in 1989, at the meeting of American Society for Surgery of the Hand. At the last lecture I heard him give, which was in Vienna, Austria, in November 1991, he was still intent on creating a device to make better two-point discrimination measurements. Dr. Moberg died on February 14, 1993. He was single-handedly responsible for awakening the spirit necessary to make sensibility testing available worldwide.

A third prophet has formed a bridge from the scientific community to the medical community. Born Nebojsa Kovacevic, in the village of Kovacevic, Slavonia, Yugoslavia, this survivor of World War II, and the only survivor of my Three Wise Men, helped his brother and sister become physicians, while he became an aviator. He began, in 1944 at the age of 17, by flying a homemade glider from a cliff, and later sus-

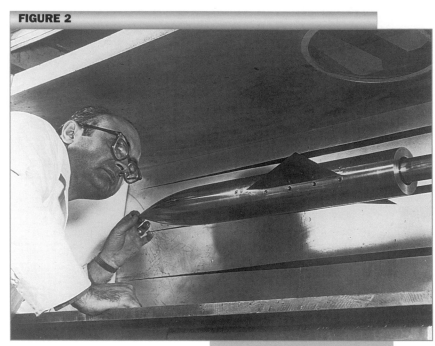

FIGURE 2

Nebojsa Kovacevic setting a laboratory test on a reentry vehicle, 1975. Photo courtesy of Nebojsa Kovacevic and Karen Gotfredson.

pending it over the Danube River. From this he learned to measure the force of the wind against his wings. Perhaps as a memorial to those early experiences, he recently developed a desktop, computerized wind tunnel to teach aeronautical engineering students.

He came to the United States in 1959, and since then his professional life has been devoted to the challenges of theoretical aerodynamics, especially astronautics, including a fellowship at the University of Maryland where he was involved with several NASA research projects. In 1970, Nebs began to expand his aeronautical engineering measurement horizons into medical applications and computer technology.

Nebs and I met in 1987 in

his laboratory outside Minneapolis, where he developed state-of-the-art, computer-assisted sensorimotor testing equipment that will bring us into the 21st century.

It is in recognition of the influence on me of these three prophets that I dedicate this book to Raymond M. Curtis, Erik Moberg, and Nebojsa Kovacevic (see Figures 1 & 2).

S *omatosensory Testing and Rehabilitation* must fill the void of texts needed to educate the new generation of therapists who will provide the essential service of quantitating sensibility and reeducating sensation. And these services will be provided not just for the hand, and not even just for the limbs, but for the entire body surface, including its mucocutaneous and mucous membrane-lined surfaces. And these services will be provided not just for hand injuries, but also for people with peripheral neuropathy, and for people who have developed the side effects of many of the modern chemotherapy agents, sensory loss in the hands and feet.

Somatosensory Testing and Rehabilitation comes at a time when the United States federal government, through Medicare, has agreed to pay for the costs of protective footwear if the referring doctor documents the need for such protection, and at a time when the American Peripheral Neuropathy Association (neurologists) has recognized that electrodiagnostic testing has limitations that can be overcome by quantitative sensory testing. This book comes at a time when the American Diabetes Association (internists, endocrinologists), through its 1988, 1993, and most recently its 1996 consensus statement, has mandated periodic testing of cutaneous vibratory and pressure thresholds to follow the sensory changes characteristic of the neuropathy that affects approximately 5 million Americans. Plastic surgeons have begun to quantitate the sensation recovered in women following breast re-

construction, and in men after penile reconstruction. Plastic surgeons, as well as ear nose and throat surgeons, have begun to quantitate the sensation in the oral cavity after reconstruction for cancer of the oral cavity and pharynx, and in the face after craniofacial trauma. Urologists have become increasingly aware of the sensory deficits present in men with impotence. And in 1991, the American Society for the Peripheral Nerve was founded.

Yes, *Somatosensory Testing and Rehabilitation* is a book whose time has finally come. It is for these reasons that this book is not a second edition of *Evaluation of Sensibility and Re-education of Sensation in the Hand,* my first book, published in 1981, reprinted in 1984 and 1987, and translated into Japanese in 1993. The title of this new book reflects the emergence of technology for sensibility testing that will carry us into the 21st century, and the expansion of my original concepts from the hand to the entire body.

To accomplish its function as a textbook, this book is written in a user-friendly style. The language is factual yet straightforward, with an emphasis on understanding the physiology and pathophysiology. This textbook does not assume the reader has extensive basic science knowledge. This book contains information on areas of sensibility not covered in my

first book. For example, there are extensive discussions of the diagnosis and treatment of pain problems (Chapter 7), as well as an entire chapter on cortical plasticity (Chapter 10), which is now understood to be the basis for the success of sensory reeducation. This new book also explains the theoretical and practical reasons that allow a unification of threshold and innervation density testing. There are no footnotes and the text is without numbered references; however, at the end of each chapter are sections of references and additional readings for those students who wish to pursue their interests further. Names that should at least become familiar to the student are included as part of the text, with some clarifying biographical comments to broaden the subject. A series of self-administered questions, keyed to each chapter, is included in Chapter 21. They may be used by the teacher of the course or by the student for testing or continuing education purposes.

The book is organized anatomically by functional region to facilitate special interests in education, therapy, or research. Each of these anatomic regions is introduced with a review of the pertinent neuroanatomy, and contains tables that record the known normal and abnormal values for quantitative sensitivity testing for that anatomic area. To the extent that specific protocols for sensory rehabilitation exist, they are included in the pertinent regions. Where these do not already exist, techniques for rehabilitation are suggested based on general principles learned from the other areas. Clinical examples are introduced into each area to establish the relevance of the more didactic points. Application of the newest, state-of-the-art, computer-assisted sensibility testing is also included, both as a subject in its own right and as it applies to each anatomical region.

A. Lee Dellon, MD
Baltimore, Maryland
July 23, 1995

• • •

SECTION

basic principles

the neuron

• ANATOMY •

The *neuron* is the cell that is the most basic unit of the nervous system. In the central nervous system (CNS), the neuron is contained completely within the brain or the spinal cord. In the peripheral nervous system (PNS), the neuron is located in such a way that it communicates between the CNS (the brain and spinal cord) and the rest of the body. In the PNS, therefore, the neuron has its cell body located either within the spinal cord, for the *motor neuron,* or next to it in the *dorsal root ganglion,* for the *sensory neuron.* The cell process that extends from the cell body to the periphery is called the *axon* for both the motor neuron and the sensory neuron. The motor neuron's distal part, the axon, is located outside the CNS, enabling the motor neuron to send an effector message from within the CNS to a motor end-organ in the periphery, like a muscle in the hand. The sensory neuron's distal part, the axon, is also located outside the CNS, enabling the sensory neuron to transmit toward the brain a message from a sensory receptor in the periphery, like the *Meissner corpuscle* in a fingertip. The process that extends from the cell body into the spinal cord is called the *dendrite* for both the motor and the sensory neuron. The cell body for the motor neuron is located in the ventral horn of the spinal cord. The cell body for the sensory neuron is located in the dorsal root ganglion (see Figure 1.1). A *ganglion* is a collection of cell bodies.

Sympathetic and parasympathetic neurons are specialized forms of motor neurons. Instead of going from the CNS to a skeletal muscle, these effector cells go to such end-organs as the sweat glands, the erector pillae muscles at the base of hair follicles, and the muscles in the walls of the arteries. The difference in function between the sympathetic and the parasympathetic neurons is exemplified by penile function. In general, the parasympathetic neuron causes a relaxation or inhibition. This activity, with respect to penile function, causes vasodilatation, resulting in an increase in blood flow into the corpora cavernosa, creating an erection. In general, the sympathetic neuron causes increased activity. With respect to penile function, this causes contraction of the muscles in the prostatic urethra, resulting in ejaculation. (See Chapter 17, "The Penis," for more information on this subject.) The cell bodies for these neurons are located just lateral to the ventral horn in the intermediate or lateral grey region of the spinal cord, or in ganglia that lie along the spinal cord

(paraspinal ganglia), like the stellate ganglion in the neck or the lumbar ganglia in the back.

There are other neurons that lie within the brain that control functions outside the brain but are still considered part of the CNS. For example, the autonomic nervous system is primarily controlled by neurons that give rise to the vagus nerve, the 10th cranial nerve. These neurons are located in the brain stem, travel through the

base of the skull to enter the neck, and then innervate the heart and the gastrointestinal system. Overactivity of the autonomic neurons of the vagus nerve can cause fainting (syncope) by causing an inhibition of the heart muscle. Two of the cranial nerves are contained totally within the CNS. These are (a) the olfactory nerve (smell), the first cranial nerve, and (b) the optic nerve (vision), the second cranial nerve. Even the end-

FIGURE 1.1

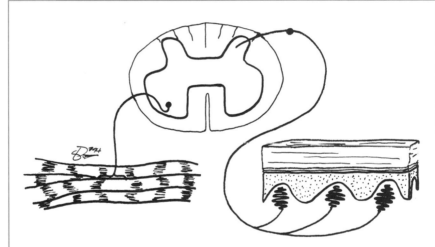

The motor neuron (top) has its cell body in the ventral horn of the spinal cord, and its axon extends to a skeletal muscle. Its central process, the dendrite, communicates with the central nervous system by receiving messages that have been transmitted along the pyramidal tract directly from the motor cortex in the precentral gyrus of the brain. The sensory neuron (bottom) has its cell body in the dorsal root ganglion, and its axon extends to a sensory receptor in the fingertip. Its central process, the dendrite, communicates with the central nervous system through a series of relay stations that modify the series of neural impulses in anatomic regions such as the thalamus before the final input reaches the sensory cortex in the post-central gyrus of the brain.

organs of these two cranial nerves, the retina of the eye and the olfactory lobes, are embryologically part of the CNS. Although the neurons of the rest of the cranial nerves are located within the CNS, their axons travel outside the CNS; therefore, with regard to neural regenera-tion, they behave like peripheral nerves and can regenerate. Thus, division of the optic nerve results in blindness which, so far, cannot be restored by nerve repair, whereas division of the facial nerve results in facial paralysis, which can be restored by nerve repair.

The neuron does not exist alone, but rather functions in conjunction with a host of supporting cells which, in the CNS are called *glial cells*. Examples of glial cells are the *astrocyte* and *oligodendrocyte*. The analogous cell in the PNS is called the *Schwann cell*. The axon is always ensheathed by a glial cell process. In the PNS, every axon is ensheathed by Schwann cells. The axons that conduct impulses the fastest require a form of insulation, which is *myelin,* a lipoprotein. One Schwann cell relates to each myelinated axon at any given site along its length. Many Schwann cells are required to ensheathe an axon along its entire length. The slower conducting axons of the PNS are not myelinated. One Schwann cell ensheathes more than one unmyelinated axon (see Figure 1.2). In the CNS, the oligodendrocyte makes a myelin protein, too, but it differs in its chemical composition.

Schwann cells, in addition to making myelin, serve another critical support function for the peripheral nerve, which is to make nerve growth factor. It is this critical support function that the Schwann cell performs for the peripheral nerve, that the oligodendrocyte does not perform for the

FIGURE 1.2

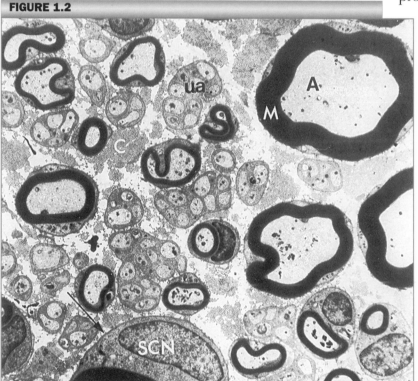

Electron micrograph from the rat sciatic nerve, demonstrating large and small myelinated axons (MA), each of which is ensheathed by a single Schwann cell (SCN), and unmyelinated axons (ua), a cluster of which is ensheathed by a single Schwann cell (osmium stain, magnified 2000x). The large myelinated axon may range from 15 to 20 microns in diameter, the small myelinated axons may range from 2 to 4 microns in diameter, and the unmyelinated axons may range from 0.5 to 1.5 microns in diameter. The large myelinated axons subserve both muscle function and the perception of touch. The small myelinated fibers subserve the perception of pain. The unmyelinated fibers subserve the perception of hot and cold, as well as burning pain. Photo courtesy of A. Lee Dellon, M.D.

TABLE 1.1 CLASSIFICATION OF NERVE FIBERS

Group	Myelination	Size	Function
Aα	myelinated	15-20 microns	motor
Aβ	myelinated	10-15 microns	touch
Aδ	myelinated	2-5 microns	sticking pain & temperature
C	unmyelinated	0.5-1.5 microns	burning pain

Note: From *Evaluation of Sensibility and Re-education of Sensation of the Hand,* by A. L. Dellon, 1981. Baltimore: Williams & Wilkins. Reprinted with permission of the author.

CNS, that enables the peripheral nerve to regenerate. Furthermore, it is likely that certain supporting cells of the CNS, perhaps the astrocytes, make a glycoprotein that actually inhibits the efforts of injured CNS neurons to regenerate. We know this because if a peripheral nerve is placed into the spinal cord, the neurons of the CNS will regenerate into the peripheral nerve, where the Schwann cells create an environment hospitable for neural regeneration, whereas those same CNS neurons will not regenerate sufficiently to reestablish function in the spinal cord.

The word *nerve* is usually not meant to imply a neuron, but rather a peripheral or cranial nerve. A nerve is composed of hundreds, and more commonly tens of thousands, of nerve fibers, which are the axons of the neuron. A neuron is microscopic. Table 1.1 lists a classification of neurons that is based on their size and myelination. This classification by Erlanger and Gasser (1937) of Johns Hopkins University was awarded the Nobel Prize in physiology and medicine. In contrast, a nerve is composed of a longitudinal array of neurons. The word *fascicle,* which is commonly used to refer to such a collection, is derived from the Latin word fasciculus, meaning bundle. Each fascicle is surrounded by a serial coating or layers of connective tissue called the *perineurium,* which creates a unique environment for the individual neurons, which are also called nerve fibers. The space within the fascicle also contains elastic fibers and collagen fibers, and is called the *endoneurium.* The small blood vessels within this space are therefore called the *endoneurial micro-vessels.*

The collection of fascicles surrounded by connective tissue is called the nerve, the peripheral nerve, or the cranial nerve. The connective tissue uniting these fascicles is called the *epineurium.* The epineurium between the fascicles is called the *interfascicular epineurium,* and the epineurium that surrounds the circumference of the nerve is termed the *external epineurium* (see Figure 1.3). The epineurium and the perineurium each contain elastin fibers (see Figure 1.4). These terms are important to define because they will be used to describe both the normal and the pathophysiologic condition of the nerve, and to describe surgical strategies to repair and reconstruct the nerve.

• PHYSIOLOGY •

The most critical function a nerve fiber must be capable of performing is the transmission of an impulse that will conduct a message from one location to another. To do this, the cell membrane of the neuron is specialized to permit the

FIGURE 1.3

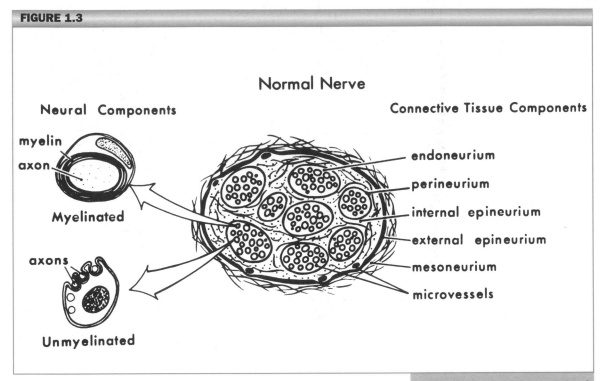

Normal Nerve

Neural Components

myelin
axon

Myelinated

axons

Unmyelinated

Connective Tissue Components

endoneurium
perineurium
internal epineurium
external epineurium
mesoneurium
microvessels

passage of sodium and potassium ions through regions of its lipoprotein structure. These regions are often called *channels*. Energy is required to maintain the integrity of these channels which, at a biochemical level, use the energy-rich phosphate bond of adenine triphosphate (ATP) to power the so-called sodium/potassium pump. When this pump is functioning, there exists an electrical difference between the outside and the inside of the neuron's membrane. A particular stimulus will destabilize this system, permitting potassium to flow into the neuron, initiating the chain of molecular events that results in the conduction or propagation of an electrical impulse

along the axon. The speed with which this impulse travels is about 1 to 2 m/s along an unmyelinated axon.

The speed of propagation is increased by having the Schwann cells arrange themselves along the length of the axon, forming myelinated rings around the axon and leaving small unmyelinated regions between one Schwann cell and the next. These regions are called the *nodes of Ranvier,* and the distance between them is the *internodal length*. If the impulse jumps from one node to the other, the conduction is called *saltatory conduction,* and is much faster than if the impulse moves linearly along the axon. If the myelin is thicker, this insulation layer further increases

The nerve is composed of groups of nerve fibers bound together into bundles, or fascicles. The connective tissue layers that surround the fascicle are called the perineurium. Within the fascicle, the space is termed the endoneurium and contains, in addition to the nerve fibers, elastic and collagen fibers, and microvessels. The connective tissue that lies between the fascicles is called the interfascicular epineurium, and the connective tissue that surrounds the entire nerve is called the external epineurium. From Surgery of the Peripheral Nerve, *by S. E. Mackinnon & A. L. Dellon, 1988, New York: Thieme Publishing. Reprinted with permission of the authors.*

FIGURE 1.4

The physiological environment established by the fascicle is due to the blood/nerve barrier that is created by the tight junctions of the endothelial cells lining the perineurial arterioles. When the blood/ nerve barrier is intact (A), the fluorescent dye (reddish color) remains within the blood vessels, and the endoneurial environment (green is color) is protected. When the blood nerve barrier is damaged as, for example, after 8 hours of ischemia (B), or after local pressure of 400 mm Hg for 2 hours (C), then the blood vessel wall becomes permeable,

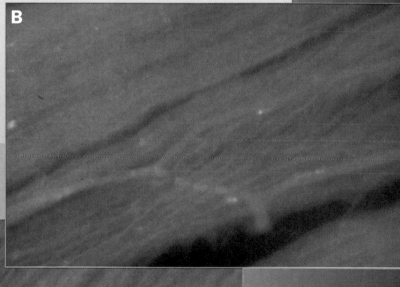

and the fluorescent dye escapes into the endoneurium. The ability of the nerve to glide with adjacent joint movements, and for fascicles to glide with respect to other fascicles and respond within limits to stretch and traction injuries, is due to the viscoelastic properties of the structural proteins elastin and collagen. These structural proteins are denoted by their histochemical and ultrastructural properties. From Nerve Injury and Repair, by G. Lundborg, 1988, Edinburgh: Churchill Livingstone. Reprinted with permission of the authors.

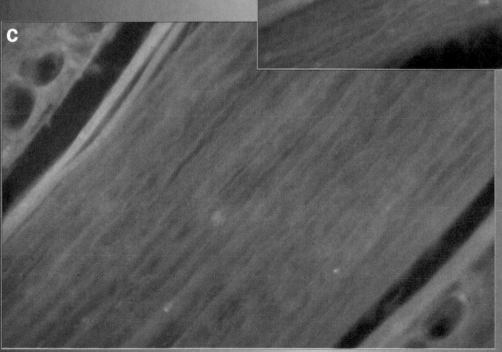

the speed of impulse conduction. Thus, a greater internode distance and thicker myelin will permit conduction velocities greater than 60 m/s, such as is found in the Group A-alpha (motor) and Group A-beta (touch) fibers. This is in contrast to the thinner Group A-delta (pain) fibers which conduct at about 20 m/s, and the unmyelinated C-fibers, which conduct at about 2 m/s. Electrodiagnostic testing uses these properties of the peripheral nerve.

An individual nerve fiber must maintain communication between its end in the spinal cord and its end in the extremity. This distance can be more than 3 feet long for the sensory nerve fibers to the big toe. Communication is achieved by means of *axoplasmic flow*. Despite the stationary appearance given to the nerve by histologic sections, the axon is a dynamic environment. The microtubules within the axoplasm are composed of the protein tubulin, which acts as a transit system, using energy to transport structural proteins. These are necessary to maintain the integrity of the cell membrane and for neural regeneration, where they form the growth cone. This system is called the *slow component of anterograde axoplasmic transport*, and may move these macromolecules at speeds of 2-30 m/s. The fast component of axoplasmic transport moves at speed of 40-400

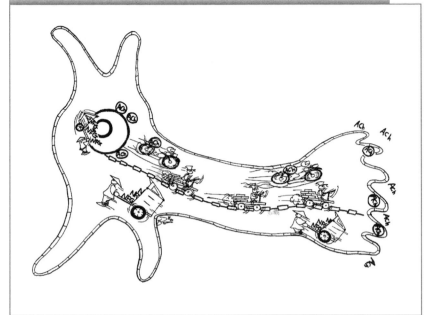

FIGURE 1.5

The relationship of the nucleus to the distant structures of the peripheral nerve is maintained by the transportation of molecules through the cell. This process is called axoplasmic transport. The transport that goes from the nucleus is anterograde, and has slow and fast components. The fast component (motorcycle) transports smaller molecules, like the neurotransmitter acetylcholine (ACh). The slow component (railroad hand cart) transports macromolecules (blocks) required for maintaining the cell membrane. These structural proteins are moved along the system of microtubules within the axoplasm. The transport that goes from the cell's most peripheral end toward the nucleus is retrograde transport, slowly transporting (rickshaw) molecules like nerve growth factor (NGF) from the Schwann cell. Drawing by Glenn George Dellon. Reprinted with permission.

m/s, and moves smaller chemicals like the neurotransmitters. Information from the periphery, such as growth factors, can be transmitted backward to the nucleus by retrograde axoplasmic transport, also at speeds of 2-30 m/s (see Figure 1.5). Many pathologic conditions, like the neuropathy of dia-

betes or the neurotoxic complications of chemotherapy (vincristine, cisplatin, taxol), manifest themselves through interruption of axoplasmic transport (see Chapter 14).

The group A-beta class of nerve fibers have special physiologic properties of adaptation that are useful in understanding the percep-

FIGURE 1.6

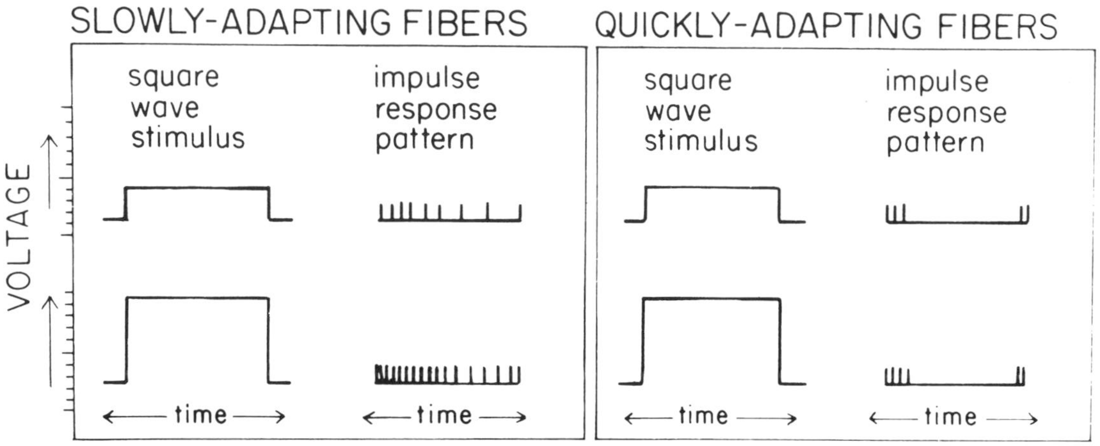

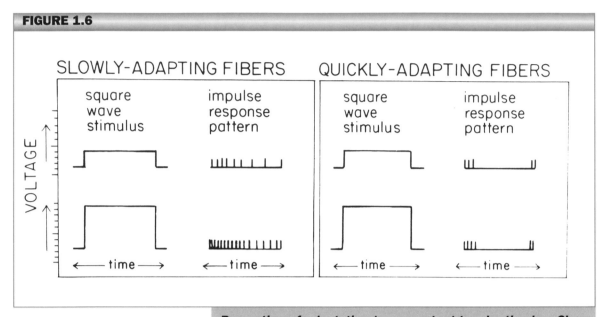

Properties of adaptation to a constant-touch stimulus. Slowly-adapting fibers continue to discharge impulses throughout duration of stimulus and increase impulse frequency in response to increased stimulus intensity. Quickly-adapting fibers fire very briefly after stimulation and then cease. There may be an "off" response. There is no change in impulse pattern with intensity change for this stimulus. From **Evaluation of Sensibility and Re-education of Sensation in the Hand,** ***by A. L. Dellon, 1981, Baltimore: Williams & Wilkins. Reprinted with permission of the authors.***

tion of touch. These nerve fibers are related to the skin by specialized mechanoreceptors and are, therefore, also called *mechanoreceptive afferents.* If these nerve fibers are isolated and individually recorded, their electrophysiology may be studied under conditions in which the fingertip is given well-defined sensory stimuli. This type of research work led Vernon B. Mountcastle, Professor of Neurophysiology at Johns Hopkins University School of Medicine, to classify these group A-beta fibers into slowly- and quickly-adapting fibers (Mountcastle, 1968). The slowly-adapting fibers begin to transmit impulses as soon as the fingertip is touched, and will continue to generate impulses for the entire time the stimulus remains in contact with the skin surface. During this time of stimulus contact only the rate of impulse generation decreases; that is, it adapts slowly to the stimulus. This stimulus would be perceived as constant- or static-touch. If the force applied to this constant-touch stimulus increases, which would be perceived as increased pressure, the slowly-adapting fiber will increase its rate of firing. The sensory receptor associated with this type of fiber is the *Merkel cell neurite complex* in the glabrous (non-hairy) skin, and the *Ruffini end-organ* in hairy skin (see Figure 1.6).

Two subtypes of slowly-adapting fibers can be distinguished electrophysiologically. Type I does all that has just been described. Type II, in addition, has a regular spontaneous discharge and responds to lateral stretching of the skin. While Type II is called a Ruffini-type, the Ruffini end-organ has not been identified in glabrous skin, and for glabrous skin the identity of the exact receptor ending remains undefined. In contrast, the quickly-adapting fibers generate just one or two impulses and then stop firing during a constant-touch stimulus. The quickly-adapting fiber will generate another impulse when the constant-touch stimulus stops, giving rise to an "on/off" type response; that is, it adapts quickly to the stimulus. The quickly-adapting fiber will not increase its rate of firing in response to an increase in stimulus intensity and, therefore, cannot transmit information about perception of pressure. The *Pacinian* and *Meissner corpuscles* are both quickly-adapting receptors associated with the quickly-adapting fibers in glabrous skin, while the hair follicle is the corresponding receptor in hairy skin (see Figure 1.6 and Table 1.2).

The quickly-adapting group A-beta fibers are also responsible for the perception of movement and vibration. The quick response to any touch stimuli permits a series of different quickly-adapting fibers to respond to a horizontally moving touch in a sequence that corresponds to the direction of movement (see Figure 1.7B). This same physiologic property permits any given group of quickly-adapting fibers in the vicinity of a vertically varying touch stimulus, such as the oscillating end of a tuning fork, to mediate the perception of vibration. While any quickly-adapting fiber will respond to any frequency vibration, provided that the stimulus intensity is sufficiently strong, there are two major subdivisions with response to frequency. Those quickly-adapting fibers that are associated with Pacinian corpuscles are most sensitive to high-frequency stimuli, at about 256 Hz (cycles per second). Those quickly-adapting fibers that are associated with Meissner corpuscles are most sensitive to low-frequency stimuli, at about 30 Hz. As will be discussed in detail in Chapter 4, regarding neural regeneration, it is easier to reinnervate a Meissner corpuscle than a Pacinian corpuscle. Therefore, these two subpopulations of fibers/receptors recover at different rates during nerve recovery. These physiologic properties have application to sensibility testing in that tuning forks of different frequencies can be used to evaluate these different subpopulations of nerve fibers (see Table 1.2).

This overview of sensory fiber/receptor correlations is

TABLE 1.2 CORRELATION OF GROUP A-BETA FIBER ADAPTATION PROPERTIES, SENSORY RECEPTORS, AND PERCEPTION

Nerve Fiber Type	Receptor	Perception
Slowly-Adapting I	Merkel cell	constant-touch pressure
Slowly-Adapting II	Ruffini end-organ	constant-touch pressure lateral stretch
Quickly-Adapting	Meissner corpuscle	movement vibration (30 Hz)
Quickly-Adapting	Pacinian corpuscle	movement vibration (256 Hz)

Note: From *Evaluation of Sensibility and Re-education of Sensation of the Hand*, by A. L. Dellon, 1981. Baltimore: Williams & Wilkins. Reprinted with permission of the author.

FIGURE 1.7

A

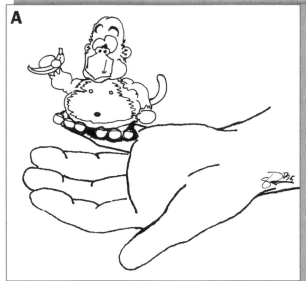

B

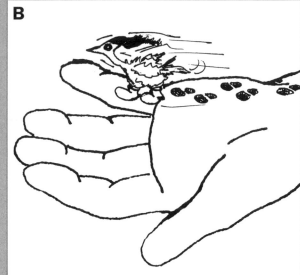

Slowly and quickly-adapting nerve fibers. (A) The slowly-adapting fibers detect the presence of stimuli of varying pressure. The heavier the weight of the stimulus, the greater the pressure, and the more frequent the neural impulses generated. (B) The quickly-adapting fibers detect the presence of movement. These fibers send an impulse after each is stimulated. Patterns of impulses result in movement perception. Drawing by Glenn George Dellon. Reprinted with permission.

simplified to present a theoretical framework for sensibility testing that has been clinically useful for the past 25 years. For example, because the examiner's hand has small but real intrinsic oscillations, as does a patient's, even a constant-touch stimulus will set off some quickly-adapting fibers. However, as will be discussed in detail in the section on reliability and validity of sensibility testing (see Chapters 5, 6, and 7), the perception by the patient is that the test stimulus is stationary, that is, not moving, at the spot being tested. This perception is due to the signal processing that occurs of the impulses generated at the periphery as they travel to the post-central gyrus through the second and third order sensory ganglia and the thalamus. An analogy would be the way the signal processing in the auditory system enables you to hear radio music by filtering out the static.

TABLE 1.3 STAGING NERVE INJURY

Seddon/Sunderland		Pathophysiology	Type of Regeneration
Neurapraxia	1st degree	metabolic block or demyelination	complete in 3 to 6 weeks
Axonotmesis	2nd degree	loss of axonal continuity	complete at 1 mm/day
	3rd degree	loss of epineurium	incomplete at 1 mm/day
	4th degree	neuroma-in-continuity	none
Neurotmesis	5th degree	loss of continuity	none

FIGURE 1.8

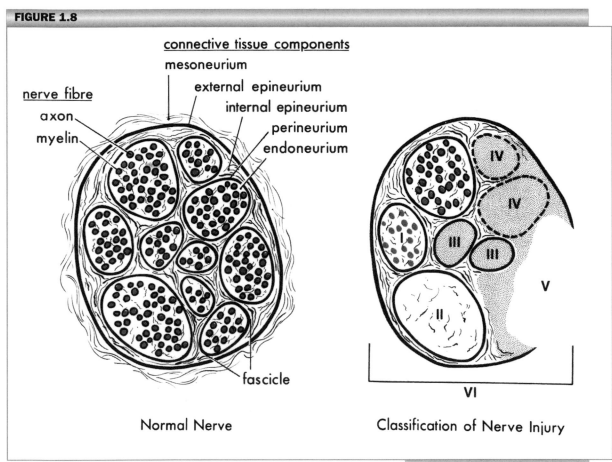

connective tissue components
mesoneurium
external epineurium
internal epineurium
perineurium
endoneurium

nerve fibre
axon
myelin

fascicle

Normal Nerve

Classification of Nerve Injury

• RESPONSE TO INJURY •

The neuron's response to injury depends on the nature of the injury. While it is true that if the neuron dies there will be no function of that nerve fiber, an injury may be such that the nerve fiber stops transmitting or generating impulses even though the neuron is still biologically alive. The function of a given peripheral nerve, like the median nerve, is the sum of all the individual nerve fibers it contains. The ability to evaluate the sensibility of skin supplied by the median nerve will depend, therefore, on understanding the effect on the neuron of various degrees of injury, and on the connective tissues that support the tens of thousands of nerve fibers within the peripheral nerve. *The ability to understand the basis for a patient's symptoms and signs, and the ability to devise an appropriate rehabilitation plan, also will depend on understanding the peripheral nerve's response to injury.*

At the neuron level, it is well documented that the response to complete transection of the axon is for the distal portion of the nerve to die. These observations were made

Response of the peripheral nerve to injury depends on the mechanism of injury and on the pathophysiologic processes that result from that mechanism. The degree of structural changes within the peripheral nerve can be categorized as illustrated here. The numerical values correspond to those in Table 1.3, which correlates the clinical manifestations of these histologic features. From Surgery of the Peripheral Nerve, *by S. E. Mackinnon & A. L. Dellon, 1988, New York: Thieme Publishing. Reprinted with permission of the authors.*

by August Waller in 1850 in the glossopharyngeal and hypoglossal nerves of the frog, and are still referred to as *Wallerian degeneration*. The axoplasm degenerates and the Schwann cell ingests the myelin. The basement membrane that surrounds the Schwann cell, and which is elaborated by the Schwann cell, remains because the Schwann cell is still alive. These basement membrane profiles surrounding the Schwann cell processes appear as bands or tubes depending on the histologic section, and remain indefinitely in the degenerated peripheral nerve. The perineurium remains after the nerve is divided, as does the connective tissue of the epineurium and the endoneurium; therefore, the degenerated peripheral nerve remains unchanged in its clinical appearance from a normal nerve. As will be discussed in Chapter 4 on neural regeneration, this condition of the distal nerve is ideal because there is no fibrosis or scarring within the nerve distally to impede the regenerating axon. If the nerve division is repaired, peripheral nerve function can be recovered to some degree once the nerve fibers have regenerated to the periphery (at about 1 mm/day or 1 in./month).

In contrast, if the peripheral nerve is injured by a stretch/traction type of injury, or a severe crush, then the nerve fibers can also be completely disrupted, and Wallerian degeneration will occur just the same as if the nerve had been sharply divided. However, in the case of stretch/traction or crush mechanisms of injury, the connective tissue components of the nerve are injured over a given length, and respond to that injury with varying degrees of increased collagen formation. This collagen creates a scar blockade that may completely prevent axonal regeneration through the injured region if the divided ends of the nerve are repaired. In another mechanism, the nerve fibers may remain anatomically completely intact, but cease to function. This can occur from lack of oxygen (ischemia) or chemical mechanisms (ionic block, like a local anesthetic). In this situation, no Wallerian degeneration occurs because the connection of the distal axon to the nucleus (and axoplasmic flow) remains intact, and complete nerve function can be recovered quickly when this temporary biochemical situation is reversed biochemically. These concepts regarding the mechanism of injury, response to injury, and clinical recovery have been described by both Seddon (1975) and Sunderland (1978). These concepts remain conceptually valid and clinically useful and are correlated in Table 1.3 and Figure 1.8.

The response of the central portion of the neuron to injury is to prepare for repair. This occurs within the nucleus by changes that reflect increased amounts of messenger RNA activity designed to produce the structural proteins and meet the energy requirements for axonal sprouting and elongation. However, if the level of nerve fiber transection is sufficiently close to the cell body in the spinal cord or dorsal root ganglia, then the loss of cell volume resulting from Wallerian degeneration appears to be too severe, and a percentage of the neurons will die. In those neurons that survive, the portion of the axon just proximal to the site of transection will have axonal loss for just the first internode length. The portion of the axon just proximal to this will be the site of growth cone formation within the first 12 to 18 hours after injury.

The response of the sensory receptors to injury is described in Chapter 2.

• • •

● REFERENCES ●

Dellon, A. L. *Evaluation of Sensibility and Re-education of Sensation in the Hand.* Baltimore: Williams & Wilkins, 1981.

Erlanger, J., & Gasser, H. S. *Electrical Signs of Nervous Activity.* Philadelphia: University of Pennsylvania Press, 1937.

Lundborg, G. *Nerve Injury and Repair.* Edinburgh: Churchill Livingstone, 1988.

Mackinnon, S. E., & Dellon, A. L. *Surgery of the Peripheral Nerve.* New York: Thieme, 1988.

Mountcastle, V. B. *Medical Physiology* 12th edition. St. Louis: Mosby, 1968.

Seddon, H. J. *Surgical Disorders of the Peripheral Nerves.* Edinburgh: Churchill Livingstone, 1975.

Sunderland, S. *Nerves and Nerve Injuries* 2nd edition. Edinburgh: Churchill Livingstone, 1978.

Tassler, P. L., Dellon, A. L., & Canoun, C. Identification of elastic fibers in the peripheral nerve. *Journal of Hand Surgery 19B:*48-54, 1994.

Waller, A. Experiments on the section of the glossopharyngeal and hypoglossal nerves of the frog, and observations of the alterations produced thereby in the structure of their primitive fibers. *Philosophical Transactions of the Royal Society of London 140:*423-429, 1850.

trauma, edema formation and nerve function. *Journal of Bone Joint Surgery 57A:*938-948, 1975.

Mountcastle, V. B., Talbot, W. H., Darian-Smith, I., & Kornhuber, H. H. Neural basis for the sense of flutter-vibration. *Science 155:*597-600, 1967.

Rydevik, B., & Lundborg, G. Permeability of intraneural microvessels in perineurium following acute graded experimental nerve compression. *Plastic Reconstructive Surgery (Scandinavia) 11:*179, 1977.

Seddon, H. J. Three types of nerve injury. *Brain 66:* 237, 1943.

Sunderland, S. The connective tissues of peripheral nerves. *Brain 88:*841, 1956.

Talbot, W. H., Darian-Smith, I., Kornhuber, H. H., & Mountcastle, V. B. The sense of flutter-vibration: Comparison of the human capacity with response patterns of mechanoreceptive afferents from the monkey hand. *Journal of Neurophysiology 31:*301-334, 1968.

Werner, G., & Mountcastle, V. B. Neural activity in mechanoreceptive afferents: Stimulus-response relations, Weber functions, and information transmission. *Journal of Neurophysiology 28:*359-397, 1965.

● ● ●

● ADDITIONAL READINGS ●

Chambers, M. R., Andres, K. H., & von Duering, M. The structure and function of the slowly-adapting type II mechanorecptors in hairy skin. *Quarterly Journal of Experimental Physiology 57:*417-445, 1972.

Dellon, A. L., Dellon, E. S., & Seiler, W. A. IV. The effect of tarsal tunnel decompression in the streptozotocin-induced diabetic rat. Microsurgery 15:265-268, 1994.

Lundborg, G. Structure and function of the intraneural microvessels as related to

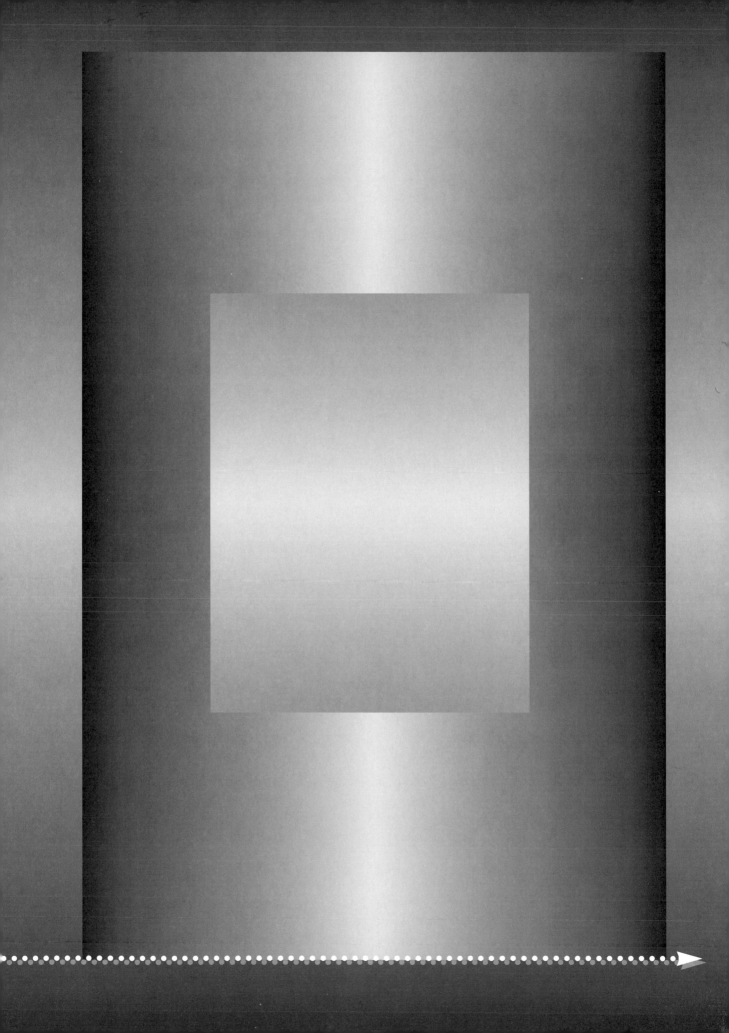

cutaneous sensory receptors

• CRETACEOUS PARK • AND GLABROUS SKIN

The *cutaneous sensory receptors*, the "encapsulated" structures in the dermis, the Meissner corpuscles, Pacinian corpuscles, and the Merkel cell neurite complexes, must be organized to transmit stimuli from the skin to the central nervous system. The stimulus is presented to the skin as some form of energy which must be transduced into a neural impulse. For example, the perception of heat occurs because the energy that is transferred from the hot stimulus through the skin initiates a neural impulse. This impulse travels to the dorsal column of the spinal cord, and is then relayed through specific pathways to the opposite side of the brain that enable the sensory cortex to interpret those impulse patterns as being due to a stimulus whose temperature is greater than that of the skin it stimulated.

Because skin all over the body must be able to perform this particular protective sensory function, no unique skin modification and no unique sensory end-organ developed. Furthermore, the earliest forms of life needed to detect temperature changes. Therefore, the sensory receptor that mediates the perception of temperature is the simplest: the *"free" nerve ending.* (Free nerve endings do not relate to specific receptors.) The same general considerations apply to the perception of pain, which is also mediated by free nerve endings, or *terminals.* The diffuse layer of thinly myelinated and unmyelinated nerve networks in the dermis, and the free nerve endings in the base of the epidermis, are the physical manifestations of these *receptors,* and they are uniformly represented throughout the body surface area. These neural nets were surely present in the vertebrates that existed in the Jurassic period of geologic time, about 135-180 million years ago.

In the Cretaceous period, which was the most recent period of the Mesozoic era, from 70-135 million years ago, the dinosaurs were gone. Animals like the duck and the goose, with more specialized skin regions, such as the bill, originated. These animals did not have fingers and toes, but rather used their bills to search beneath the water for food. The neural network is still present in the animals of this time period, but now their bills contain an encapsulated end-organ, the *Herbst corpuscle,* which is analogous to the Pacinian corpuscle and the quickly-adapting fiber/receptor system. Their bills also contain an expanded-tip ending of the nerve in close approximation to an epithelial cell, originally described by Grandy (1869), which is

analogous to the Merkel cell neurite complex and the slowly-adapting fiber/receptor system.

Mammals of the Cretaceous period had other unique nasal skin modifications that helped their survival. The mole, for example, is blind and must rely on the sensory apparatus in its snout. This snout sensory organ was described by Eimer (1871), and contains an encapsulated end-organ and an expanded tip-ending in conjunction with an epithelial cell. The opossum, in the geologic transition time between the Cretaceous and the more recent Eocene period, has Pacinian and Merkel cell neurite complexes in its snout. It is not, however, until we reach the mouse, one of the earliest rodents, that we find the forerunner of the first Meissner corpuscle, an encapsulated sensory end-organ with more than one nerve entering it, and a lobulated appearance, quite different from the Herbst corpuscle of the birds. Finally, all suborders of primates, including humans, have the specialized skin at the fingertips that contain the definitive arrangement for transduction of mechanical stimuli. This arrangement, as depicted in Figure 2.1, arose between 35 and 55 million years ago.

The specialized relationship between the Merkel cell neurite complex and the

papillary ridge maximizes the transduction of vertical forces against the skin into impulses to mediate the perception of constant-touch of varying intensity, or pressure. So, too, does the location of the Meissner corpuscle on either side of the intermediate ridge in the *dermal papillae.* A movement across the fingertip will transfer its horizontal component of force to the papillary ridge, causing it to move within the space bounded by the limiting ridges (see Figure 2.1), much like a pendulum. The movement of the intermediate ridge causes direct stimulation of the Meissner corpuscle. This is similar to what you experience when you ride across railroad tracks in your car; your horizontal motion is transformed into a vertical, oscillatory motion by the tracks. This low-frequency perturbation, or vibration, is what the Meissner afferents, quickly-adapting group A-beta fibers (see Chapter 1) are best at mediating.

Electron microscopy has clarified the fact that the "encapsulated" end-organ, like the Meissner corpuscle, is not really bounded by a capsule. The myelinated nerve fiber loses its myelin upon entering the corpuscle. The Schwann cell processes continue to ensheathe the axons, and the Schwann cell nucleus represents the supporting cell and its nucleus of the corpuscle. The space between the cell processes is contiguous with the extracellular space of the dermal papillae. In contrast, the Pacinian corpuscle represents one axon that is completely bounded by *concentric lamellae* of supporting structures. This large corpuscle is exquisitely sensitive to mechanical stimuli. For example, it is the Pacinian corpuscle that mediates the perception of the very gentle stimulus of a breeze blowing against the skin. The Merkel cell is a clear cell histologically, which ultrastructurally contains granules that contain an as yet unidentified neurotransmitter.

The relationship between the sensory end-organs and the myelinated nerve fiber is critical to understanding the order of sensory recovery during neural regeneration (see Chapter 4). Table 2.1 lists the ratio of nerve fibers innervating the end-organ to the end-organ. From this calculation it is clear that the Meissner corpuscle will be the easiest to reinnervate because any of 9 different nerves may innervate it, and

from any direction. In contrast, the football-shaped Pacinian corpuscle may only be reinnervated by a single nerve fiber entering it at precisely one of its tapered ends. The Merkel cell neurite complex is also hard to reinnervate, in that one nerve must make contact with more than one Merkel cell. Since transduction of constant-touch probably still occurs even if all the Merkel cells are not reinnervated, achieving function of the high-frequency, quickly-adapting fiber/receptor system is the most difficult. For the reinnervated Merkel cell neurite complex, recovered function will be with a lower than normal innervation

density and a higher than normal threshold for stimulation. For the Pacinian, reinnervation may not occur at all. The Meissner afferents have the potential to achieve near-normal innervation density with close to a normal threshold for stimulation. These theoretical formulations have been observed during single-unit nerve fiber recordings in baboons following median nerve repair by Terzis, Dykes, and Hakstian (1976), and by many clinicians in observing patients following nerve repair if they test their patients with 30 and 256 Hz tuning forks, and with two-point discrimination testing.

● NON-GLABROUS SKIN ●

The sensory receptor of the hairy skin is the hair follicle. The same four types of group A-beta fibers that exist in *glabrous* skin are present in hairy skin. When these fiber types grow toward the skin from their *dermal plexus* they encounter, instead of various epidermal ridges, hair follicles. The quickly-adapting fibers form *lanceolate endings* around the base of the hair follicles. The slowly-adapting fibers form expanded-tip endings in relationship to the hair follicle, as well as the Ruffini end-organ (see Figure 2.2). Similar structures have been identified in animals, and direct recordings

TABLE 2.1 NUMERICAL RELATIONSHIP OF A-BETA FIBERS TO THEIR SENSORY RECEPTORS

Receptor	Number of Fibers	Number of Receptors	Ratio (fibers/receptors)
Pacinian	1	1	1
Meissner	1-9	1	>1
Merkel cell	1	4–5	<1

FIGURE 2.1

The fingertip is hairless skin that has been modified by the presence of papillary ridges, or fingerprints. Directly beneath this is the intermediate ridge of dermis into which sweat glands (SG) send their ducts (SD). The Merkel cells are located about the intermediate ridge in proximity to the sweat ducts (MD), and are innervated by a slowly-adapting nerve fiber to form the Merkel cell neurite complex. The Pacinian corpuscle is located in the subcutaneous layer (PC), and is innervated by a single, quickly-adapting fiber. The Meissner corpuscles (MC) line the dermal papillae on either side of the intermediate ridge, and are each innervated by more than one quickly-adapting fiber. In this view, a portion of the epidermis has been removed to demonstrate the array of sensory corpuscles organized with respect to the papillary ridges. Note that the intermediate ridge is free to swing pendulum-like in the dermis within the space bounded by the limiting ridge's collagen attachment to the deeper tissues. From Evaluation of Sensibility and Re-education of Sensation in the Hand, *by A. L. Dellon, 1981, Baltimore: Williams & Wilkins. Reprinted with permission of the author.*

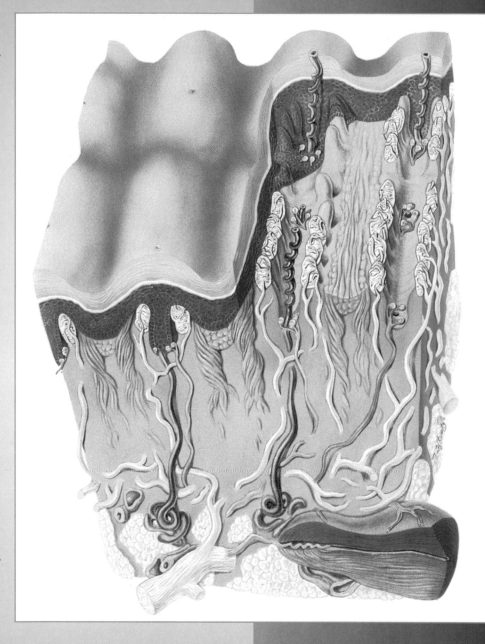

FIGURE 2.2

Hairy skin sensory receptors are the hair follicles. The lanceolate ending about the hair follicle base and shaft, as shown here, is a quickly-adapting fiber/receptor system similar to the Meissner corpuscle. The expanded tip-ending in conjunction with epithelial cells at the base of certain hair follicles (not shown) is a slowly-adapting fiber/receptor system similar to the Merkel cell neurite complex. In the hairy skin, this is the Ruffini end-organ. Photo courtesy of Bryce Munger, PhD, Department of Anatomy, University of Tasmania, Australia.

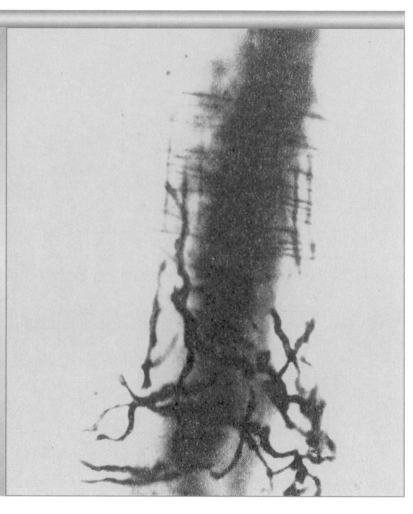

of them made. It is clear that while the number of nerve fibers in a given area of hairy skin is less than in a given area of glabrous skin, hairy skin is able to transduce all the same stimuli as nonhairy skin.

• OTHER SENSORY RECEPTORS RELATED TO THE SKIN •

There are regions of the skin surface that are best considered as transition zones. The vermillion of the lip is one such zone, being a transition between skin and mucous membrane. This zone was observed by Krause (1866) to contain a rounded sensory end-organ innervated by a large myelinated fiber that became known as the *Krause end-bulb.* Krause end-bulbs were identified by Krause in the conjunctiva of the eye and in the tip of the penis. No one has identified them in the glabrous skin. Von Fry (1896) assigned the Krause end-bulb to be the sensory receptor for the perception of cold. This is now known to be incorrect; as described in Chapter 1, the free nerve ending of the thinly myelinated fibers subserve the perception of cold. Krause end-bulbs are best considered as quickly-adapting receptors whose supporting cells differ from those of the Meissner corpuscle due to the nature of the skin covering itself. These are best termed the mucocutaneous end-organ, and should be considered in the series midway between the Meissner corpuscle of glabrous skin and the lanceolate ending of the hairy skin. A histologic example of the *mucocutaneous end-organ* from the penis is given in Figure 17.3.

The sensory receptors re-lated to muscles and joints will be discussed in Chapter 3. Among these are the *Ruffini spray endings*. As indicated above for the Krause end-bulb, von Fry (1896) ascribed the perception of heat to the Ruffini ending.

This, too, is now known to be incorrect. The Ruffini end-organ is a slowly-adapting, large, myelinated fiber/receptor which mediates information regarding stretching for the joints, as it does for the skin.

FIGURE 2.3 A

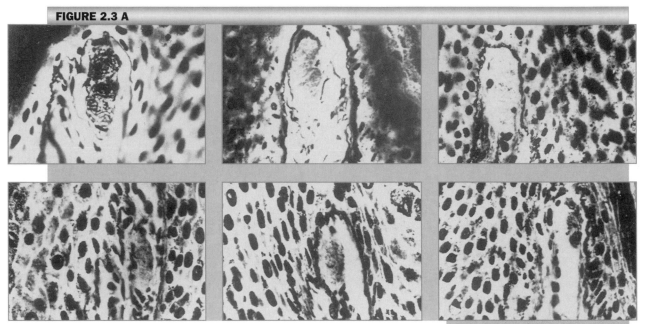

Response of Meissner corpuscle to progressive denervation and reinnervation over 9 months. The Meissner corpuscles in the fingertip skin of the monkey are located in the dermal papilla and are surrounded by the normal dermis (photomicrographs [160 x]). Silver stain stains axons black.

• DENERVATION AND REINNERVATION •

The transection of the nerve to cutaneous sensory receptors initiates a predictable and well-documented series of events that has critical clinical importance. Wallerian degeneration (see Chapter 1) occurs in the axon. For the thinly myelinated A-delta fibers and the unmyelinated C-fibers that mediate the perception of temperature and pain, this is the whole story because they have free nerve endings; that is, they do not relate to specific receptors. At any length of time after the nerve division, the nerve fibers can (a) be reconstructed by any known and accepted technique (see Chapter 4), (b) be expected to regenerate distally, (c) reinnervate skin, and (d) reestablish perception of temperature and pain. For the large, myelinated A-beta fibers that mediate the perception of touch, the response of their specialized end-organs to denervation is to undergo various degrees of degeneration

based on their unique connective tissue components.

The onion-bulb-like concentric layers of the Pacinian corpuscle are most resistant to change following dener-

FIGURE 2.3B

(A) is the normal appearance of the corpuscle. After division of the median nerve, the complete loss of axons is noted in (B) at 48 hours after nerve division, and (C) after 6 weeks, when Wallerian degeneration has been completed.

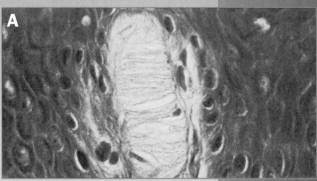

Note the progressive decrease in size of the corpuscle's connective tissue components following Wallerian degeneration. The median nerve was primarily repaired at the wrist level in this monkey, and the earliest axons to reinnervate the corpuscle are apparent with silver stain at (D) 3 months after repair. There is progressive reinnervation during the (E) 6- and (F) 9-month observation periods, with return of the multilobulated appearance of the corpuscle. Mallory trichrome stain stains connective tissue components blue and axoplasm pink. From "Reinnervation of Denervated Meissner Corpuscles: A Sequential Histologic Study in Primates Following Interfascicular Nerve Repair," by A. L. Dellon, 1976, Journal of Hand Surgery 1:98-109. Reprinted with permission of the author.

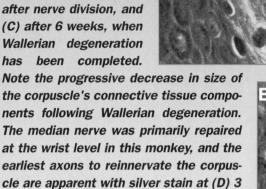

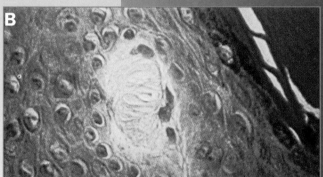

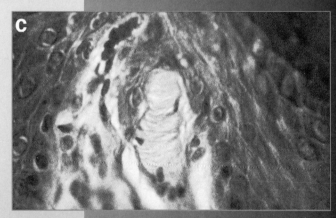

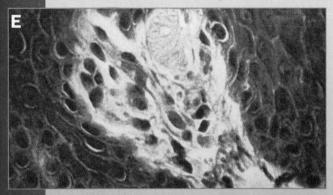

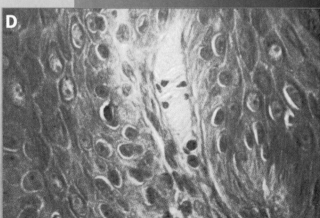

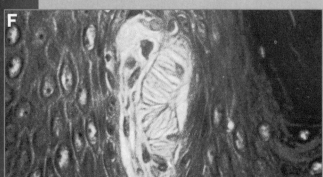

vation. Examples of virtually unchanged, although axonless, Pacinian corpuscles have been documented years after proximal nerve injury. The reason it is difficult to reinnervate the Pacinian afferents after nerve reconstruction is not because the end-organ is no longer present, but because, as was discussed above, it is difficult for a regenerating axon to directly contact the opening at one end of this large (up to 4 mm in size) structure.

The response of the more loosely knit lobular structure of the Meissner corpuscle to denervation also has been well documented (see Figures 2.3 A and 2.3 B). There is progressive shrinkage of the connective tissue components following denervation, but the *lamellar cells*, which are modified Schwann cells, remain alive, and can form relationships again with regenerating axons, giving the appearance that the Meissner corpuscle can be reinnervated. The same sequence is expected for the Merkel cell neurite complex as for the Meissner corpuscle. Studies similar to those illustrated in Figure 2.3 for the Meissner have been done for a Merkel cell-related structure in the cat, the *touch dome*, which is a slowly-adapting fiber/receptor system. These studies, by Burgess and Horch (1973), demonstrate complete disappearance of the touch dome after denervation, but

FIGURE 2.4

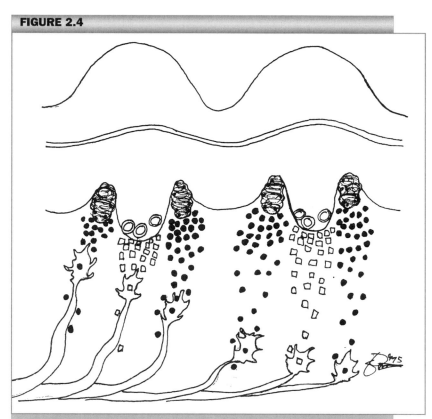

The regenerating sensory axons leave the subdermal plexus and begin their approach to the dermis, most likely following the chemical gradient of neurotrophic substances, like nerve growth factor (NGF, symbolized by filled circles and hollow squares). The NGF is probably synthesized and released by the former connective tissue components of the Meissner corpuscle (filled circles) or the former epithelial cell component of the Merkel cell neurite complex (hollow squares) at precise locations along the base of the epidermis (see Figure 2.1). It is likely that a degree of misconnection will still occur, such that the quickly-adapting fiber that formerly innervated a Meissner corpuscle or a Pacinian corpuscle will now enter the complex of Merkel cells. The resulting abnormalities in threshold and innervation density provide the need for sensory rehabilitation. Drawn by Glenn George Dellon. Reprinted with permission.

reappearance of it in the same location after reinnervation. This is predictable, given that the Merkel cell is an epithelial cell not dependent on the axon for survival, but only for some

trophic interaction that may result in its size and appearance. The epithelial cell will remain in its unique position in the dermis, and be available for reestablishing the expanded-tip/epithelial cell

FIGURE 2.5

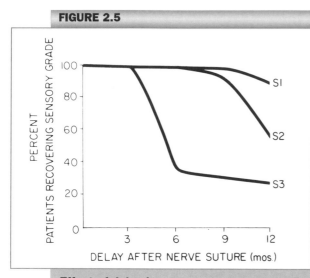
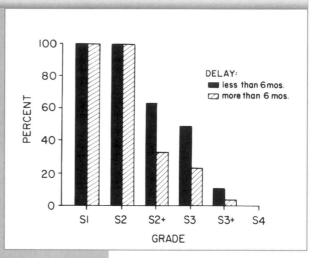

Effect of delay in nerve suture upon the final degree of sensory recovery. Using the British classification system, S4 is a normal degree of sensation, S3+ has "some" two-point discrimination, S3 has touch perception without hyperalgesia, and S1 and S2 are of just sufficient sensibility to provide protective function. These studies, published in the late 1950s on patients with median nerve injuries, demonstrate that if more than 6 months elapse after nerve injury, protective sensation can always be recovered, but functional sensibility may not be recovered. It should be noted that in interpreting these graphs, none of the patients in the early studies had the benefit of sensory reeducation. From Evaluation of Sensibility and Re-education of Sensation in the Hand, *by A. L. Dellon, 1981, Baltimore: Williams & Wilkins. Adapted with permission of the author.*

interaction that creates the unique slowly-adapting mechanoreceptor properties.

It may be hypothesized that the denervated lamellar cells of the Meissner corpuscle, and the denervated Merkel cell, being Schwann cell analogues, have the capacity to respond to loss of neurotrophic interaction with the axon following denervation by upregulating the genes that produce nerve growth factor. It may be the release of *nerve growth factor* by these supporting cells in the dermis that permits the regenerating axon sprouts to find their way back to these potential end-organ sites (see Figure 2.4). This implies that at any time following nerve injury, it is possible to recover some degree of touch sensation by nerve reconstruction (see Figure 2.5).

This is clearly different from the situation with muscle in which, if the regenerating axon does not reach the muscle by about 1 year following denervation, the muscle cell, though still alive, no longer produces the acetylcholinesterase (AChE) receptor necessary to reestablish the motor endplate and, therefore, cannot be reinnervated. The reinnervation of the Meissner corpuscle in Figure 2.3 appears normal; however, it is not clear that after a prolonged period of time the reinnervated corpuscle or the reestablished Merkel cell neurite complex is capable of achieving normal thresholds, and it is unlikely that the complex events of regeneration will permit normal innervation density (see Figures 2.3 & 2.4). Furthermore, the nerve growth factor may attract a slowly-adapting fiber that used to relate to a Merkel cell to reinnervate a dermal papilla and interact with the lamellar cells of a former Meissner corpuscle. The net effect of this inappropriate reinnervation is unclear. These types of abnormal reinnervation patterns among the cutaneous sensory receptors create the need for sensory rehabilitation, which will be described in Chapter 12.

Finally, it is appropriate now to consider a study that correlates much of the information in these first two chapters. Because the innervation density in normal skin is high, biopsy of normally innervated fingertip skin would yield too many receptors to correlate with any measurements of sensibility. However, fingertip biopsy of the middle finger of a patient about 6 months after median nerve repair at the wrist permitted careful sensibility testing of this small region of skin, which then could be biopsied. Serial sections of this specimen permitted a correlation of the reinnervated sensory receptors with the clinical measurements (Dellon & Munger, 1983). The results of that study confirmed in humans the electrophysiological studies done in animals, and the theoretical considerations that went into the correlations in Table 1.2. This type of clinical research has provided the basis for the approach to evaluating sensibility that will be described in Chapters 6 and 7.

• • •

• REFERENCES •

Burgess, P. R., & Horch, K. W. Specific regeneration of cutaneous fibers in the cat. *Journal of Neurophysiology 36:*101-114, 1973.

Dellon, A. L. *Evaluation of Sensibility and Re-education of Sensation in the Hand.* Baltimore: Williams & Wilkins, 1981.

Dellon, A. L. Reinnervation of denervated Meissner corpuscles: A sequential histologic study in primates following interfascicular nerve repair. *Journal of Hand Surgery 1:*98-109, 1976.

Dellon, A. L., & Munger, B. L. Correlation of histology and sensibility after nerve repair. *Journal of Hand Surgery 8:*871-878, 1983.

Dellon, A. L., Witebsky, F. G., & Terrill, R. E. The denervated Meissner corpuscle: A sequential histologic study following nerve division in the Rhesus monkey. *Plastic and Reconstructive Surgery 56:*182-193, 1975.

Terzis, J. K., Dykes, R. W., & Hakstian, R. W. Electrophysiologic recordings in peripheral nerve surgery — A review. *Journal of Hand Surgery 1:*52-66, 1976.

Winkelman, R. K. *Nerve Endings in Normal and Pathologic Skin. Contributions to the Anatomy of Sensation.* Springfield, IL: Charles C. Thomas, Publishers, 1960.

• ADDITIONAL READINGS •

Biemesderfer, D., Munger, B. L., & Binck, J. The Pilo-Ruffini complex: A non-sinus hair and associated slowly-adapting mechanoreceptor in primate facial skin. *Experimental Brain Research 142:*197-222, 1978.

Cauna, N. Nature and functions of the papillary ridges of the digital skin. *Anatomical Record 119:*449-468, 1954.

Cauna, N. Nerve supply and nerve endings in Meissner's corpuscles. *American Journal of Anatomy 99:*315-350, 1956.

Dykes, R. W., & Terzis, J. K. Reinnervation of glabrous skin in baboons: Properties of cutaneous mechanoreceptors subsequent to nerve crush. *Journal of Neurophysiology 42:*1461-1478, 1979.

Halata, Z. The sensory innervation of the glans penis and the prepuce in man (an ultrastructural study). In *Sensory Receptor Mechanisms,* W. Hamann & A. Iggo, Editors. Singapore: World Scientific Publishing Co., 1984.

Halata, Z., & Munger, B. L. The neuroanatomical basis for the protopathic sensibility of the human glans penis. *Brain Research 371:*205-230, 1986.

Iggo, A. New specific sensory structures in hairy skin. *Acta Neurosurgery 24:*175-180, 1963.

Iggo, A., & Muir, A. R. The structure and function of a slowly adapting touch corpuscle in hairy skin. *Journal of Physiology 200:*763-796, 1969.

Munger, B. L., & Pubols, L. M. The sensorineural organization of the digital skin of the raccoon. *Brain, Behavior and Evolution 5:*367-393, 1972.

Munger, B. L., Pubols, L. M., & Pubols, B. H., Jr. The Merkel rete papilla — A slowly-adapting sensory receptor in mammalian glabrous skin. *Brain Research 29:*47-61, 1971.

Pubols, L. M., Pubols, B. H., Jr., & Munger, B. L. Functional properties of mechanoreceptors in glabrous skin of the raccoon's forepaw. E*xperimental Neurology 31:*165-182, 1971.

Sunderland, S. Capacity of reinnervated muscles to function efficiently after prolonged denervation. *Archives of Neurology and Psychology 64:*755-771, 1950.

• • •

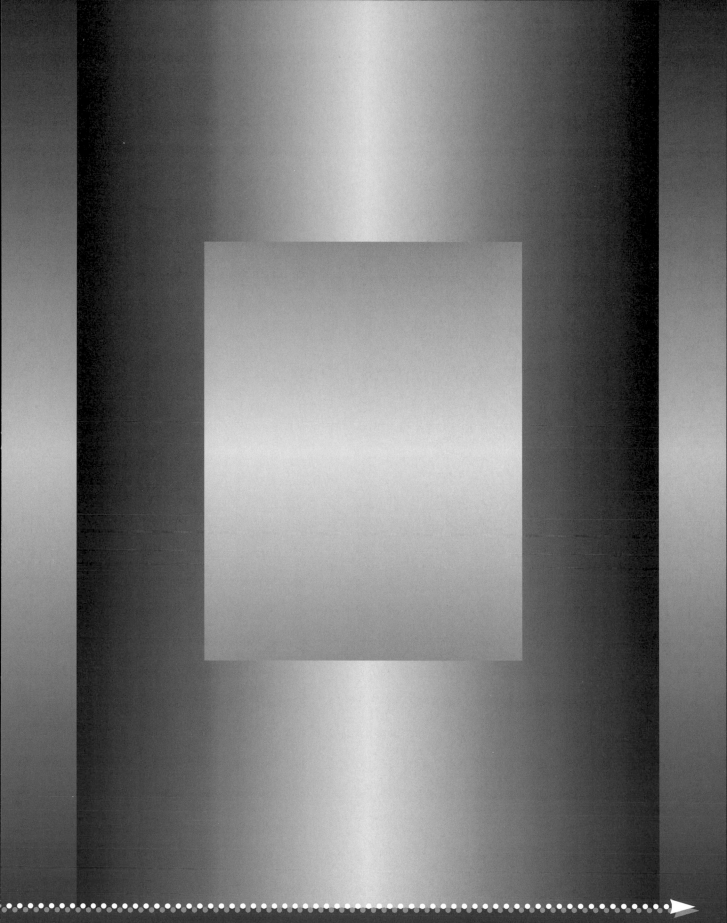

3

proprioception

• CONTRIBUTION • FROM JOINTS

Proprioception is our awareness of the position of our joints. If you have a person shut their eyes and then move their finger so it is either flexed or extended, the person can you tell you correctly whether it is flexed or extended. In fact, a person can usually tell correctly within a few degrees the position of the extremity of a joint. It seems only reasonable that this should be a function of the joint receptors. And there are, without any doubt, well-documented Pacinian corpuscles and Ruffini end-organs within joints. They are located within the ligaments and within the capsules of joints. These two sensory receptors are related to the same quickly- and slowly-adapting fibers as their counterparts in the fingertips and in hairy skin. Classical neurology teaches that an injury to the posterior columns of the spinal cord causes loss of proprioception. It seems perfectly straightforward, then, that proprioception is due to the sensory afferents coming from the joint structures. However, this is not clinically true.

Moberg (1984) made observations that argued against proprioception being due primarily to joint receptors. These observations have been confirmed by direct basic and clinical research by others, and should be taken as true. These observations include:

1. Injection of local anesthetic into a joint, which anesthetizes the joint receptors, does not cause loss of position sense.
2. Following a surgical procedure to replace a joint, like the hip, with an artificial joint, the patient can still identify the position of the joint within 5-10° (Grigg, Finerman, & Riley, 1973).
3. Direct recording of the afferent nerves from a joint in the cat demonstrated few if any impulses during the normal range of motion of that joint, but showed rapid impulse generation as the extremes of joint range of motion are reached (Clark & Burgess, 1975; Grigg & Greenspan, 1977).
4. Direct recording of the afferent impulses from the human in whom the finger was taken through a range of motion, demonstrated almost no activity from nerve fibers that had no cutaneous receptive field (Clark, Horch, & Bach, 1979).

• CONTRIBUTION FROM MUSCLE •

A *muscle sense* has been described in humans (Gelfan & Carter, 1967). This implies that humans are conscious of the movement of the muscles themselves and, therefore, that the movement of the muscles that cause movement of a joint may be responsible for proprioception.

This premise has been directly tested and found not to be true. For example, during surgery to decompress the carpal tunnel in humans, just the skin for the incision can be anesthetized. With the patient's eyes covered, all the flexor tendons at the wrist level can be pulled, simulating what would occur if the muscle contracted. Similarly, the tendons can be pulled distally, as they would be if the finger were extended. When this is done, the patient is not aware that the finger has moved at all, until the muscle is stretched sufficiently to cause movement of the overlying skin.

There are an enormous number of sensory receptors within the *musculotendinous system*. The names for these are the *muscle spindle,* located within the muscle, and the *Golgi tendon-organ* (see Figure 3.1 on next page). These sensory receptors, which will not be the subject of much discussion in this textbook, are organized so that their impulses travel to the cerebellum, not to the cerebral cortex. Thus, all the sensory input from the muscle and tendon goes to a subconscious level. Imagine if we were aware of all the different tensions within every muscle of our body every second of the day! It is safe to conclude that muscle sense is not related to proprioception.

It is likely that in the future, as we begin to appreciate the availability of sensory receptors within muscle, a cutaneous sensory nerve may be sutured to a motor nerve in the hope of restoring sensibility to areas difficult to reconstruct by traditional techniques. Up to one-third of the fibers in a so-called *pure motor nerve* are sensory and not motor, representing the sensory nerve fibers from the muscle spindles and tendon-organs. Chang, DeArmond, and Buncke (1986) observed, for example, that if the sural nerve was sutured to the motor branch (thoracodorsal nerve) of the latissimus dorsi muscle being transferred to a microvascular free flap for heel coverage, the patient appeared to recover the ability to perceive sensation through the skin-grafted muscle. These motor afferents previously reported to the cerebral cortex. However, I hypothesized in 1991 that with regeneration of the cutaneous afferents into the muscle sensory receptors, so that they innervate the muscle spindles or Golgi tendon-organs, touching the muscle would transmit sensory impulses to the conscious level, permitting perception of sensation in a reconstructed foot (see Figure 3.2).

FIGURE 3.1

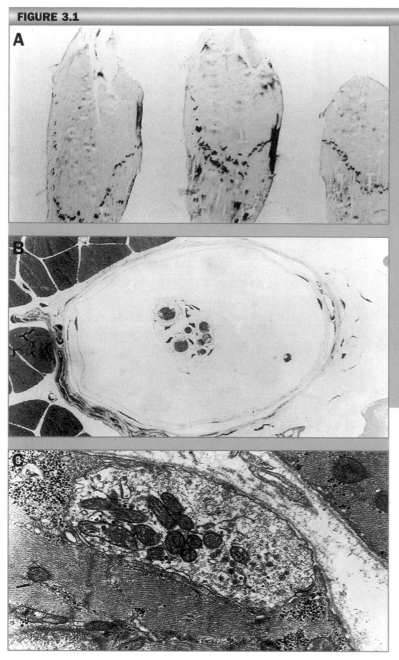

The normal muscle spindle. (A) Pattern of toluidine blue-stained muscle spindles (dark spots) in three sections of a hamstring muscle from the cat, at 10x magnification. (B) Transection of a muscle spindle at its widest zone lying next to muscle fibers, at 400x magnification. (C) Electron microscope image of the mitochondria-filled sensory axon within the muscle spindle, immediately adjacent to the intrafusal actin/myosin muscle filaments, at 10,000x magnification. Photos reproduced with permission from Mark DeSantis (1990), University of Idaho.

● CONTRIBUTION FROM SKIN ●

There were some very early observations that suggested a relationship between cutaneous sensibility and proprioception. For example, Fox and Klemperer (1942) noted that among a series of patients they were testing, there were some who had lost proprioception and who also had lost vibratory perception. Moberg (1972) carried out a series of anesthetic blocks to areas of skin, and tested proprioception in patients who had lost sensibility in various areas of skin due to nerve injuries. He noted that if the patient had lost cutaneous sensibility in the area of skin that would be stretched by movement of the underlying joint, then the patient also lost proprioception for that joint. Moberg also directly noted that proprioception for the proximal interphalangeal joint of the finger was most directly related to static two-point discrimination in the fingertip of that finger (Moberg, 1976).

These observations, taken in conjunction with the observations given above for joint receptors and for muscle sense, lead me to con-

FIGURE 3.2

A

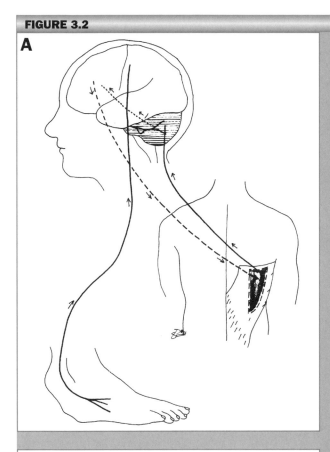

B

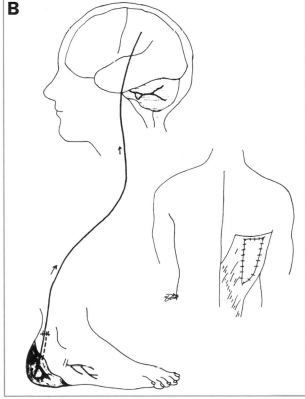

Muscle spindles and Golgi tendon-organs are the sensory receptors within muscle. The sensory nerve fibers from these sensory receptors report to the cerebellum, which is not part of our consciousness. We are not aware of the various strains upon our muscles on a moment-to-moment basis. It is possible, theoretically, to connect a cutaneous nerve, like the sural, which normally directly reports to our consciousness, to a motor nerve. This will not restore motor function, but, if the regenerating sensory nerves reinnervate the muscle spindles, then movement of this muscle, or perhaps directly touching this muscle, may stimulate the spindles to fire, sending impulses to the conscious level. Such a strategy may be employed to reconstruct the heel of the foot by a microvascular free muscle transfer and, at the same time, achieve some degree of sensibility in that part of the foot, as illustrated here. (A) Sural nerve afferents report to the conscious level in the post-central gyrus, while the afferents from the latissimus muscle report to the subconscious level, the cerebellum. From the cerebellum, this information in muscle tension can pass to the precentral gyrus, from which voluntary commands can cause muscle contraction. (B) After free muscle transfer, and connection of the sural nerve to the thoracodorsal (motor) nerve of the muscle, the reinnervated muscle spindles provide sensory information to the conscious level by the new sural nerve pathways, leaving the normal sural nerve cutaneous territory denervated. From "Muscle Sense or Non-Sense," by A. L. Dellon, 1991, Annals of Plastic Surgery 26:444-448. Reprinted with permission of the author and by permission of Little, Brown and Co., Inc.

clude, as did Moberg, that:

1. The musculotendinous afferents which affect primarily synergistic/antagonistic muscle balances and report to the subconscious are not responsible for proprioception.

2. The joint receptors, which appear to begin entering the conscious level only as potentially injurious joint activity (extremes) is approached, are not responsible for proprioception.

3. The large myelinated nerves subserving cutaneous sensibility are responsible primarily for our awareness of joint position (proprioception) in the normal range of motion.

• • •

• REFERENCES •

Chang, K. N., DeArmond, S. J., & Buncke, H. J., Jr. Sensory reinnervation in microsurgical reconstruction of the heel. *Plastic and Reconstructive Surgery 78:*652-663, 1986.

Clark, F. J., & Burgess, P. R. Slowly-adapting receptors in cat knee joint: Can they signal joint angle? *Journal of Neurophysiology 38:*1448-1463, 1975.

Clark, F. J., Horch, K. W., & Bach, S. M. Contributions of cutaneous and joint receptors to static knee-position sense in man. *Journal of Neurophysiology 42:*877-888, 1979.

Dellon, A. L. Muscle sense or non-sense. *Annals of Plastic Surgery 26:*444-448, 1991.

Fox, J. C., & Klemperer, W. W. Vibratory sensibility. *Archives of Neurology and Psychology 48:*622-645, 1942.

Gelfan, S., & Carter, S. Muscle sense in man. *Experimental Neurology 18:*469-473, 1967.

Grigg, P., Finerman, G. A., & Riley, L. H. Joint-position sense after total hip replacement. *Journal of Bone and Joint Surgery 5 5A:*1061-1025, 1973.

Grigg, P., & Greenspan, B. J. Response of primate joint afferent neurons to mechanical stimulation of knee joint. *Journal of Neurophysiology 40:*1-8, 1977.

Moberg, E. Fingers were made before forks. *Hand 4:*201-206, 1972.

Moberg, E. Reconstructive hand surgery in tetraplegia, stroke and cerebral palsy: Some basic concepts on physiology and neurology. *Journal of Hand Surgery 1:*29-34, 1976.

Moberg, E. The role of cutaneous afferents in position sense, kinaesthesia and motor function of the hand. *Brain 106:*1-12, 1984.

• ADDITIONAL READINGS •

Boyd, I. A., & Smith, R. S. The muscle spindle. In *Peripheral Neuropathy,* 2nd edition, P. J. Dyck, P. K. Thomas, E. H. Lambert, & R. Bunge, Editors. Philadelphia: Saunders, 171-202, 1984.

Dellon, A. L. *Evaluation of Sensibility and Re-education of Sensation in the Hand.* Baltimore: Williams & Wilkins, 1981.

DeSantis, M., & Norman, W. P. An ultrastructural study of nerve terminal degeneration in muscle spindles of the tenuissimus muscle of the cat. *Journal of Neurocytology 8:*67-71, 1979.

Hulliger, M., Nordh, E., & Thelin, A. E. The response of afferent fibers from the glabrous skin of the hand during voluntary finger movements in man. *Journal of Physiology 291:*233-249, 1979.

• • •

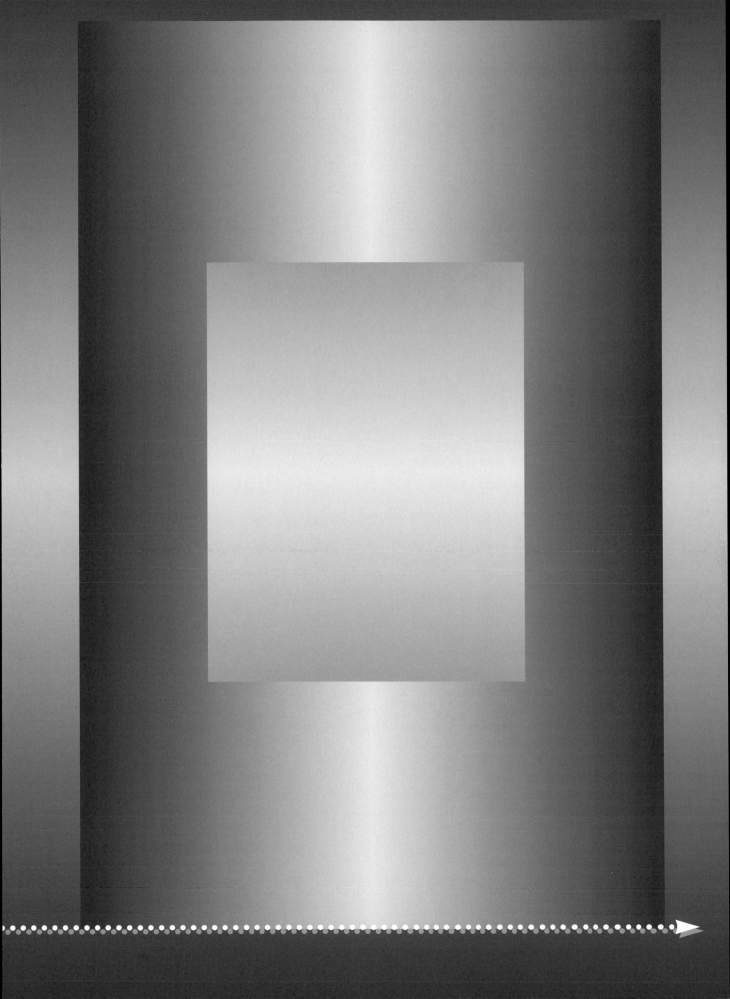

nerve reconstruction

• NEURAL REGENERATION •

An injured peripheral nerve will attempt to repair itself through the process of *neural regeneration*. Individual neurons have their nucleus in the dorsal root ganglion or in the ventral horn of the spinal cord, and most of these nuclei survive an injury as long as it occurs within the extremity. As discussed in Chapter 1, if the injury to the nerve is quite proximal, for example, within the brachial plexus, many more of the nuclei die as a direct result of the mechanism of injury itself. This greatly reduces the ultimate possibilities for functional recovery because there are fewer neurons to regenerate.

The process of neural regeneration begins with receipt by the nucleus of an injury message. While it is not clear what the exact mechanism is, it is most likely that an influx of extracellular calcium into the damaged nerve initiates a series of molecular events that alerts the nucleus to the injury. For example, a calcium influx causes certain protein complexes to alter their function. The nucleus, geared to receiving certain trophic messages from the periphery by *retrograde axoplasmic transport,* recognizes that something has changed distally. The nucleus responds by preparing to rebuild its damaged cell membranes and to extend its axon toward the periphery in an attempt to reestablish communication with its motor and sensory end-organs. Within 12 to 18 hours after disruption of the axon, the nucleus has responded sufficiently to its changed message pattern that the injured distal end of the axon has been transformed into a growth cone. Each injured axon will produce up to 15 axon sprouts, each of which will have its own growth cone (see Figure 4.1).

FIGURE 4.1

(A) Neural regeneration may be visualized by observing the events that occur proximally to the end of the individual nerve fiber after nerve transection. (B) There is a retrograde loss of at least the first node of Ranvier, and perhaps more if the mechanism of injury is more forceful. From the internode just proximal to this, the axon will form up to 15 sprouts. (C) Each of these will regenerate distally, spearheaded by its growth cone. The growth cone has numerous filopodia that seek out trophic factor and contact guidance cues from the environment. The basement membrane serves as the most important contact guidance cue. Schwann cells will migrate distally with the regenerating axon. (D) Finally, a regenerating unit is formed containing many sprouts from the same axon, ensheathed by the same Schwann cell. Once one growth cone makes the appropriate contact with its target organ, the remaining sprouts will be recalled, or pruned. From Surgery of the Peripheral Nerve, by S. E. Mackinnon & A. L. Dellon, 1988, New York: Thieme Publishing. Reprinted with permission of the authors.

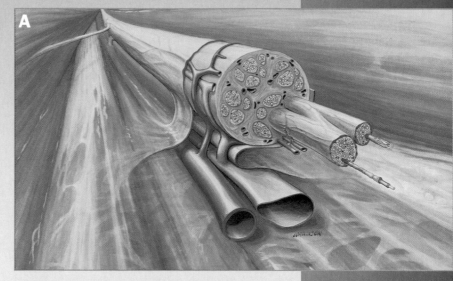

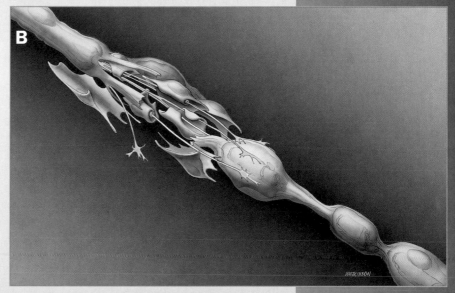

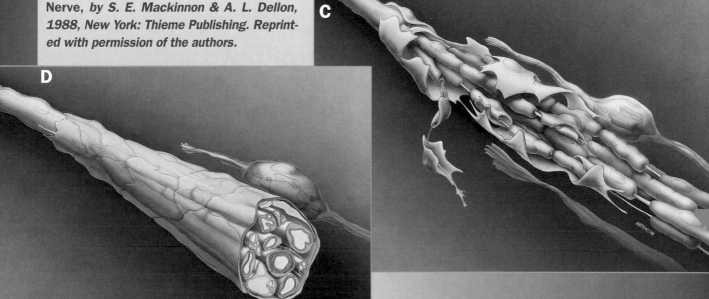

The growth cone is a highly active site for exploration of the environment. The goal of that exploration is to regenerate distally toward the appropriate site, that site being the previously innervated skin or muscle. This goal is achieved by the active extension of small, feet-like projections called *filopodia* into the adjacent environment. The membrane of these feelers responds to chemical gradients that might signal an appropriate distal target. Such chemicals have been called *neurotrophic factors*. The first to be identified was *nerve growth factor* (NGF). Rita Levi-Montalcini was awarded the Nobel Prize for the discovery of NGF in 1952. Many *trophic factors* have since been isolated, each of which has its own unique set of nerve fiber types that it will stimulate, as well as other cells that it can stimulate.

Trophic factors are proteins that are regulated by genes. They are probably all expressed, or upregulated, in a particular sequence during embryonic development and growth, and then are downregulated once that growth has been achieved. Nerve injury appears to resequence embryonic events, causing upregulation of these growth factors. It is clear now that Schwann cells in the distal portion of the injured nerve, in response to Wallerian degeneration, undergo changes that permit them to phagocytose myelin, and to upregulate the pro-

duction of NGF. Thus, the growth cone, as it extends distally into its new environment, has an increasingly strong gradient of NGF it can follow in an attempt to find its former distal end. It is possible that the end-organs themselves, the muscle cell, or the supporting cells of the sensory corpuscles also make certain neurotrophic factors that become significant once the growth cone has reached the end of its journey.

The growth cone can also respond to directional cues given by proteins in its immediate environment. The growth cone is attracted particularly to negatively charged proteins. The basement membrane is composed of three proteins that have the highest ability to attract the growth cone. These proteins are *laminen, fibronectin,* and *type IV collagen*. Researchers such as Letourneau (1983) have spread a trail of laminen onto a culture dish and observed the growth cone to track only along its surface. Once the growth cone touches basement membrane, its filopodia attaches based on the charged molecules. The growth cone contains the contractile protein *actin*, the same protein present in muscle. Upon attaching to basement membrane, the filopodia contract in response to the actin, pulling the proximal end of the nerve distally. This is the process known as axonal elongation. This process re-

quires a great deal of energy and transport of structural proteins. Time-lapse movies of the regenerating nerve demonstrate the growth cone to be highly active (see Figure 4.2). The net result of all this activity is the regeneration of the injured nerve at the rate of about 1 mm/day.

The concepts of neural regeneration just reviewed will

FIGURE 4.2

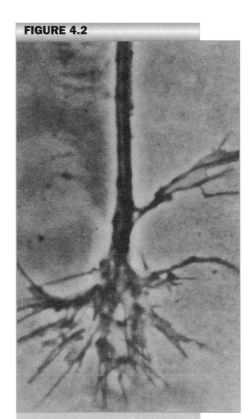

Growth cone and contact guidance from tissue culture. From "Neurite Extension by Peripheral and Central Nervous System Neurons in Response to Substratum Bound Fibronectin and Laminin," by P. C. LeTourneau, 1983, Developmental Biology 98:*212-215.*

FIGURE 4.3

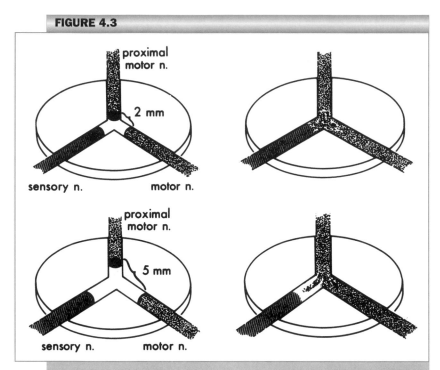

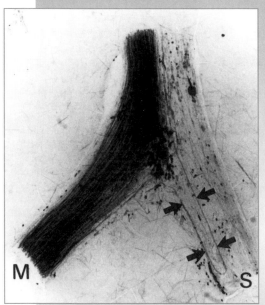

Nerve fibers regenerate distally along a single path and then, at a crossroad, will diverge. This is now understood to occur largely at random, so that if the axons are examined early in the process of regeneration there will be a large number of axon sprouts down each tube. Axon sprouts will regenerate distally until they meet their distal target end-organ, which is either a muscle (M) or sensory receptor (S). Once they reach this digital goal, the still wandering axons along the other pathway are called back, or "pruned," so that later it will appear as if the axons all regenerated properly down the correct limb of the "y." From "Selective Reinnervation of Distal Motor Stumps by Peripheral Motor Axons," by T. M. Brushart, & W. A. Seiler, 1987, Experimental Neurology 97:289-300. Reprinted with permission of the authors.

clarify one traditional teaching that is incorrect, and will resolve two traditional controversies. The traditional teaching was that regenerating axons take about 3 weeks to cross the suture line, and another 3 weeks at the distal end, once they reached the skin or muscle, to reestablish function with their end-organs. It is clear from the above discussion, however, that such a set of delay periods does not occur. This has direct application for the length of time required for postoperative immobilization of the reconstructed nerve.

The first controversy was whether any segment of nerve could be the source for neural regeneration (Dellon & Dellon, 1993). This led to studies in which fragments of sensory nerve were placed between ends of motor nerves, and vice versa. That 19th century controversy was resolved with the realization that neural regeneration had to proceed from the central neuron distally, regardless of whether it was a motor or sensory nerve. The second controversy was between neurotropism and contact guidance. This led to studies in which various substances were plated in tissue culture to evaluate contact guidance, and to studies in which various straight and y-shaped tubes were placed between two ends of nerves. That 20th century controversy was resolved with the realization that both neurotropism and contact guidance occur during neural regeneration.

Lundborg's group, in Malmo, Sweden, have been leaders in elucidating the process of neural regeneration in silicone chambers (Lundborg, 1988). Brushart and Seiler (1987) conduct research to study whether the specificity of the regenerating nerve is controlled by unique molecules in the basement membrane of motor fibers that are not present in sensory fibers, and to study central mechanisms by which axons that have regenerated to an inappropriate place are recalled, or pruned back, once one of their sibling sprouts reaches the appropriate target end-organ (see Figure 4.3). These strategies are of value in choosing surgical techniques for nerve reconstruction: for example, whether to use a bioabsorbable nerve conduit to reconstruct nerve gaps of up to 3 cm.

The events related to neural regeneration described above occur without exception and for all nerve fiber types. The thinly myelinated, large myelinated, and unmyelinated nerve fibers all develop growth cones and axon sprouts, respond to neurotrophic factors, and have contact guidance. The rate of axonal regeneration is enzymatically controlled, and theoretically all these fiber types should regenerate at the same rate. However, it has been observed clinically

that this is not the case (Dellon, 1981). The perception of pain and temperature occurs before that of the touch submodalities. It may be that this is related to the size of the volume of the axoplasm that must be regenerated for each of these fibers. The unmyelinated and thinly myelinated fibers would require much less volume of axoplasm than would the much larger diameter

touch fibers. If a given nucleus can produce axoplasm at a given rate, then the larger diameter touch fibers would be the last to recover function if their thin axon sprouts were to arrive at a point similar in time to the pain and temperature fibers (see Figure 4.4). This clinical finding is important in devising a strategy for testing sensibility in the nerve following reconstruction.

FIGURE 4.4

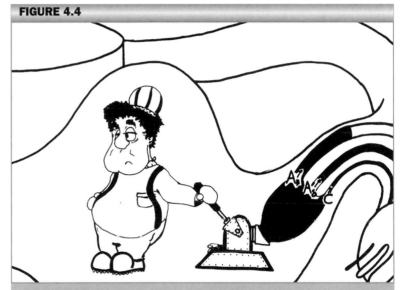

During regeneration the nucleus of the neuron must assemble the building materials necessary for axonal elongation. The rate for this is fixed biochemically. The nucleus for the thin fibers must produce axoplasm and cell membrane components at the same rate as the nucleus for the large myelinated fibers. Regardless of their ultimate nerve fiber diameter, all regenerating sprouts are about the same size, which is thin. Clinically, however, regeneration is observed to occur first for those nerve fibers which ultimately will have small diameters, that is, those that detect pain and temperature, whereas those with large diameter nerve fibers, that is, those that detect touch, are the last to recover. It is as if there were a pump in the nucleus producing at a fixed rate; therefore, it is easier to fill the volume required for the smaller fibers than it is for the larger ones. Drawing by Glenn George Dellon. Reprinted with permission.

FIGURE 4.5

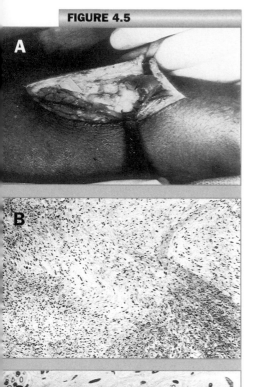

Histologic appearance of a neuroma (A) from the radial sensory nerve. Disorganized axon sprouts and regenerating units are enmeshed in dense collagen (B) at 153x magnitude. Histology cannot distinguish a painful from a nonpainful neuroma (C) at 614x magnitude. From Surgery of the Peripheral Nerve, *by S. E. Mackinnon & A. L. Dellon, 1988, New York: Thieme Publishing. Reprinted with permission of the authors.*

• NEUROMA •

When neural regeneration is proceeding without interference, there are often sensations perceived by the patient that are disturbing. They may feel sharp shooting pains, hot or cold flashes, water running down their arm, buzzing, tingling, numbness, or sometimes nothing at all. During regeneration, these perceptions are expected, and the patient should be made aware prior to nerve reconstruction that they will occur. The treatment for the patient who is uncomfortable during this time is discussed in Chapter 12 under desensitization. However, when the expected course of regeneration is blocked by scar, by disruption of nerve reconstruction, or by some other misfortune, the result is that regenerating sprouts become trapped in the wrong environment and are thwarted in their attempt to regenerate distally.

These sprouts become surrounded by connective tissue and are, by definition, therefore, termed a *neuroma* (see Figure 4.5). However, a neuroma is not by definition painful. If the neuroma is in an environment related to tendon movement or joint motion, then the entrapped distal end of failed regenerating units will signal painful messages whenever the neuroma is stimulated by movement of the adjacent soft tissues. Clearly, direct pressure on the neuroma will stimulate it, too. Often, these neuromas are in an environment in which adjacent nerve fibers that would not normally communicate with each other do communicate with each other. This cross talk is the result of an abnormal or *ephaptic conduction,* which is an interneuron communication without a normal synapse. This has been documented between the various A-delta and C-fibers in neuromas in rats as well as in monkeys, and may represent the pain generator site within the neuroma (Meyer et al., 1985).

If the neuroma is on a motor nerve, like the posterior interosseous nerve, the sensory fibers within that nerve that carry impulses from the joints that are also innervated by that nerve, can signal aching or pain from that joint. This, for example, can be the source of wrist pain from wrist sprains, from healed distal radius fractures, or even from a fused wrist (Dellon & Horner, 1993). The best technique to demonstrate that pain is due to a neuroma of a particular nerve is to block that nerve with a local anesthetic (see Figure 4.6). If the patient's perceived pain is relieved by the injection of xylocaine or marcaine into the tissues adjacent to the nerve, the source of the pain signal has been confirmed. The nerve itself should never be directly injected with anything, since this interfascicular injection, in and of itself, could injure the nerve and create another source of pain. The nonsurgical techniques to treat a painful neuroma include desensitization and splinting by the therapist, injection of steroids into the vicinity of the neuroma by the physician, steroid iontophoresis by the therapist and, ultimately, resection of the neuroma by the surgeon.

The treatment of neuroma pain by the surgeon requires (a) the ability to determine precisely which nerve or nerves are the source of pain, and (b) a strategy to treat the end of the nerve from which the neuroma has been resected, so that another painful neuroma does not develop as the nerve again goes through the natural sequence of neural regeneration. Nerve blocks are the most sure technique to prove the source of the pain. A nerve should not be resected for the treatment of pain unless such a block relieves the pain and the patient agrees to accept the degree of sensory loss that will inevitably follow such a resection.

More than one nerve may be involved in the pain problem. For example, about 75% of patients have both the lateral antebrachial and the radial sensory nerve overlap in providing axons to the dorsoradial aspect of the wrist. A very small percentage may even have a third nerve, the *palmar cutaneous branch* of the median nerve, supply fibers to this area at its volar border, or the dorsal cutaneous branch of the ulnar nerve of the posterior cutaneous nerve of the forearm may

FIGURE 4.6

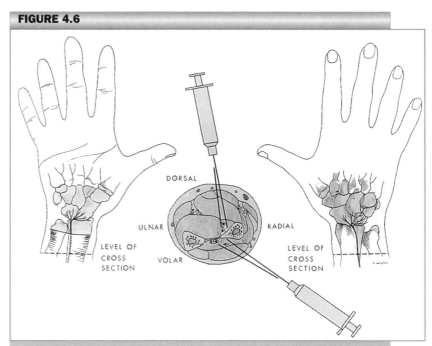

Nerve blocks with a local anesthetic are the best technique to demonstrate that a particular nerve is the source of pain. This is illustrated here by the technique to block the anterior and posterior interosseous nerves just proximal to the wrist in evaluating the source of wrist pain. From "Partial Wrist Denervation," by G. Horner & A. L. Dellon, 1993, in Problems in Plastic and Reconstructive Surgery: The Wrist, *S. Levin, Editor, Philadelphia: Lippincott. Reprinted with permission of the authors.*

supply fibers to this area at its dorsal border.

This emphasizes the importance of diagnostic nerve blocks. The surgical strategy for treatment of a painful neuroma must include resection of the neuroma to remove the pain-generating source, and then relocating the proximal end of the nerve into a site away from movement, direct pressure, and sensory neurotrophic stimuli (see Figure 4.7). These requirements for the new location are best met by

implanting the end of the nerve into a large muscle which has relatively little excursion. The commonest neuromas that cause pain in the upper extremity are those over the dorsum of the hand, and the usual approach requires resection of both the lateral antebrachial cutaneous nerve and the radial sensory nerve, and implantation of both of these nerves into the brachioradialis muscle (see Figure 4.7) (Dellon & Mackinnon, 1986; Mackinnon & Dellon, 1987).

● **REFLEX SYMPATHETIC** ●
DYSTROPHY

Reflex sympathetic dystrophy, or RSD, is a well-defined, if still poorly understood, clinical problem. Because the patient's complaints are those of diffuse pain, many clinically painful conditions are misdiagnosed as RSD. Today, the diagnosis of RSD should be given for a clinical pain problem only when the following criteria are satisfied (Mackinnon & Holder, 1984):

1. There is a region of diffuse pain not in the distribution of a single peripheral nerve;
2. There is swelling and/or stiffness of the region that is affected by the pain;
3. There are signs of sympathetic overactivity, for example, sweating, coldness, or color change;
4. There is impaired function of the affected part.

It should be clear from the above criteria that RSD can be applied to parts of the body other than the hand, such as the foot. While the region affected by RSD can be extensive, it almost always begins distally, and extends proximally. This means that a part of the body affected with RSD is not in the middle of two uninvolved areas; that is, if there is a problem with the elbow, but the hand and shoulder are normal, the criteria for RSD have not been met. RSD also is not burning pain in the distribution of a single peripheral nerve, for example, in the index finger and thumb. This type of pain was described by Silas Weir Mitchell (1872), a neurologist, during the Civil War. He observed soldiers injured by musket ball fire, and called this pain "causalgia."

The best conceptual framework in which to understand diagnosis and treatment strategies for RSD is one in which a normal reflex continues to occur. The most well-known reflexes are the knee-jerk and the blink. With a blink, a sensory stimulus, which is visual, occurs, is processed in the brain, and a motor response, the rapid closure of the eyelid, occurs. With the knee-jerk, a sensory stimulus, which is the perception that the quadriceps tendon has been stretched, occurs, is processed in the spinal cord, and a motor response, knee extension, occurs (see Figure 4.8). With any pain stimulus, there is normally a response mediated through the spinal cord that prepares the body for emergency. The sympathetic nervous system is the motor system (see Chapter 1) for this normal response to pain. Thus, the normal reflex is for a sensory stimulus, pain, to occur, for this to be processed in the spinal cord and, finally, for the motor response (hair stands up, sweating occurs, blood vessels constrict) to occur. Note that normally a sympathetic response is not painful.

FIGURE 4.7

A

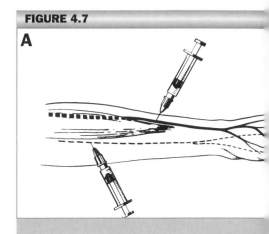

B

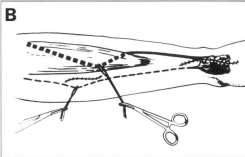

C

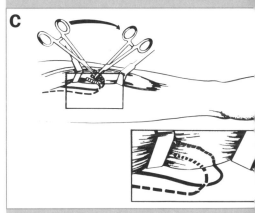

Example of the treatment of a painful neuroma of the dorsoradial aspect of the hand. (A) Nerve blocks identify the appropriate nerves. (B) Both the lateral antebrachial cutaneous nerve and the radial sensory nerve have had their neuroma resected. (C) The proximal end of each nerve is implanted into the deep surface of the brachioradialis. (D) Clinical example of

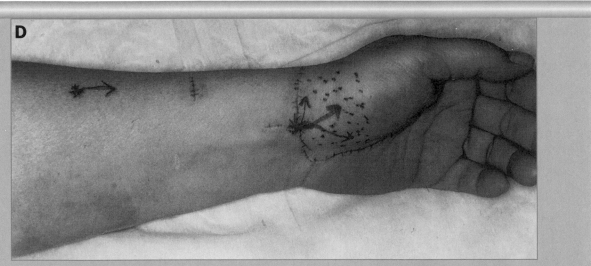

D

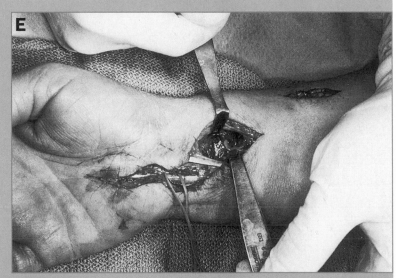

E

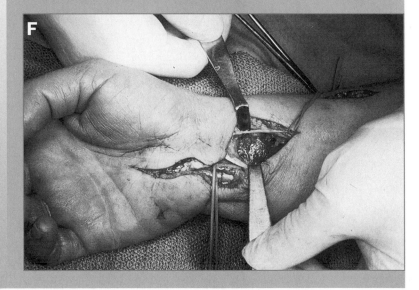

F

painful neuroma of palmar cutaneous branch of median nerve, identified by nerve block. A block in the forearm, at the radial sensory nerve, did not relieve pain. (E) This patient also had a neurolysis of the median nerve for recurrent carpal tunnel syndrome. Note the palmar cutaneous nerve between the retractor which, in (F), is implanted into the pronator quadratus muscle. (A), (B), (C), from "Results of Treatment of Recurrent Dorsoradial Wrist Neuromas," by S. E. Mackinnon & A. L. Dellon, 1987, Annals of Plastic Surgery 19:54-61. With permission of Lippincott-Raven Publishers. (D), (E), (F), from "Implantation of Palmar Cutaneous Branch of the Median Nerve into the Pronator Quadratus for Treatment of Painful Neuroma," by G. R. D. Evans & A. L. Dellon, 1994, Churchhill Livingston Journal of Hand Surgery 19A: 204-205. Reprinted with permission of the authors.

A hypothesis that seems plausible to explain pain associated with sympathetic activity is that the pain reflex continues to occur because there is a continuing source of pain, for example, an injured intact nerve, such as a neuroma-in-continuity, or one or more disrupted nerves. The spinal cord, then, in response to a continuous input of pain impulses, alters its usual firing pattern in the dorsal root entry zone. Intermediary neurons begin continually to relay and stim- ulate the sympathetic neurons to fire. This much has been demonstrated in animal experiments. The mechanism by which the release of the normally nonpain-producing norepinephrine neurotransmitter from the sympathetic ending elicits the perception of pain is still conjectural. It is possible that the C- and A-delta fibers upregulate norepinephrine receptors as a response to pain or persistent pain, that these transmitters are transported to the periphery, and in that location the norepinephrine released by the sympathetic nerve endings can give rise to a pain stimulus. What is clear from this conceptual framework is that RSD must be approached by strategies that attempt to eliminate the continuing source of pain impulses arising from injured peripheral nerves, as well as by strategies that attempt to block sympathetic activity (see Figure 4.9).

The therapist is often the first person involved in the patient's care to note the onset of RSD. RSD evolves from an acute stage, when it can be most successfully treated, to more chronic stages, when secondary problems, such as joint stiffness and drug dependence, greatly diminish the chances for a successful outcome. In the earliest stage, the therapist will note that the hand is cool, sweating, and swollen even at the start of therapy. If these signs develop during therapy, the therapist must carefully note this and inform the referring physician. For reasons that are unclear, too much activity appears to set off RSD. This may be due to chemical mediators of the inflammatory process, like prostaglandins and interleukins, that are released into the soft tissues by the already inflamed and/or damaged connective tissues and ligaments from the original injury.

The therapist must learn to gauge the capacity of each individual hand for therapy.

FIGURE 4.8

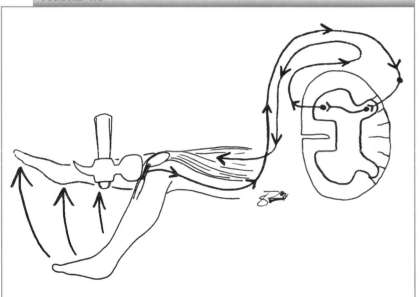

The classic reflex involves a sensory stimulus that is transmitted through the spinal cord and causes a motor response in the periphery. This is typified by the knee-jerk. The response of the stretch receptors to the quadriceps tendon being percussed is to generate neural impulses that are processed through the dorsal root entry zone of the spinal cord. Through an intermediary neuron, the motor neuron in the ventral horn of the spinal cord causes a contraction of the quadriceps muscle, resulting in the knee jerk. Drawing by Glenn George Dellon. Reprinted with permission.

FIGURE 4.9

(A) Hypothetical reflex arc of reflex sympathetic dystrophy (RSD). The response of the C- and A-delta pain fibers to a pain stimulus, such as a crush injury, is to generate neural impulses that are processed through the dorsal root entry zone of the spinal cord. Through a relay neuron, the sympathetic neuron in the intermediate grey of the spinal cord is stimulated, and generates a sympathetic response in the periphery. This is due to release of the neurotransmitter, norepinephrine, whose alpha-adrenergic stimulation causes hair follicle erection, sweat production, and arterial vasoconstriction. None of these normal sympathetic responses is painful. In RSD, the entire hand or foot (B and C), not just the injured part, will be painful, swollen, and stiff. It is possible that in response to persistent pain, C- and A-delta fibers develop a norepinephrine receptor, or else they always have such a receptor but it is inactive. In RSD, this norepinephrine receptor on the C- and A-delta fibers can respond to the norepinephrine released during the sympathetic stimulation. This conceptual framework suggests that strategies to treat RSD should include plans to eliminate the source of the pain signal from the original injury, as well as to eliminate the sympathetic discharge. Illustration (A) by Glenn George Dellon. Illustrations (B) and (C) copyright A. Lee Dellon. Reprinted with permission.

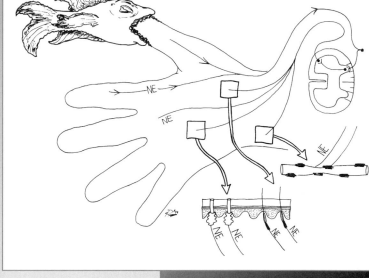

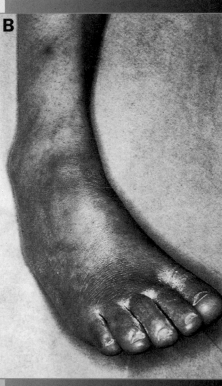

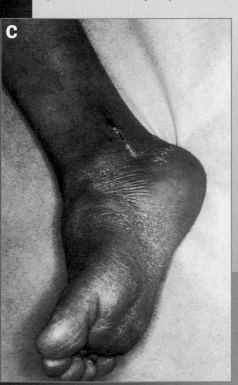

Measurement of hand volume with the traditional water displacement methods should occur before and after each treatment session. Measurement of skin compliance at selected sites of the hand may be found to give another aspect of quantitation of edema, hardness, or stiffness that is either complimentary to, or may replace, the volumetric measurement. Skin compliance may be checked easily during therapy, and if the measurements demonstrate increased hardness (decreased compliance), therapy may be altered or the session curtailed for that day (see Chapter 21, "Potential Research Projects for Therapists").

At this earliest stage, the most appropriate diagnostic test is a 3-phase flow study. This radiographic imaging is often called a bone scan, uses Technetium 99, and in the third, or 3-hour phase of the scan will demonstrate increased uptake of nucleotide diffusely throughout all the joints of the fingers and wrist. If the 3-hour, or delayed phase, of the bone scan is normal, it is highly unlikely that the patient has RSD. The delayed phase of the bone scan is almost always positive in a patient with the acute stage of RSD.

The initial treatment of RSD by the physician should include referral for a stellate ganglion block for the upper extremity, and for a lumbar sympathetic block for RSD of the lower extremity. A series of blocks is often required. For a block to be successful, there must be a decrease in the patient's pain without loss of sensation in the limb that is blocked. If the anesthetic agent spills over from the sympathetic ganglia to the roots of the brachial plexus, then the patient might experience pain relief in the hand because the pain impulses from the periphery were blocked on their way to the cortex, and not because of the decreased sympathetic activity.

During a successful sympathetic block, the extremity becomes more pink, and warmer. Associated with the stellate ganglion block is *Horner's syndrome,* during which the patient will experience on the same side as the block narrowing of the pupil (*miosis*), drooping of the upper lid (*ptosis*), and dryness of the eye (*anhydrosis*). This is due to disruption of the sympathetic fibers to the eye. For the upper extremity, a more distal blockade of the sympathetic nervous system may be tried, such as an axillary block. Another regional anesthetic technique useful for treating RSD is a Bier block. A Bier block replaces all the blood in the extremity with a local anesthetic agent, with or without a drug to inhibit the sympathetic nervous system, like reserpine (which depletes the terminals of norepineph-

rine), or guanethidine (which blocks the transmitter). If there is stiffness in the extremity, steroid may be added to the solution that is infused into it.

The duration of pain relief from a successful initial sympathetic block may range from hours to permanent relief. If there is only brief relief, it is appropriate to repeat the block. If the hand is quite stiff, but has been too painful for therapy, the therapist should be called in during the time of the block to begin active and passive range of motion as soon as possible. This may be started even in the anesthesia induction room, where the Bier block is often done. This therapy may even be required on an inpatient basis. Sometimes an indwelling axillary block catheter can be placed for the upper extremity, or an indwelling catheter left in the epidural space for the lower extremity. This technique permits daily inpatient therapy with good pain control.

Once interruption of the pain generating nerve(s) has occurred, it is appropriate to institute rehabilitation at a pace geared to each individual. We have no way to measure the degree of therapy that will be tolerated for any given individual. Unfortunately, this means that at some point in therapy, even if geared to the individual's level of discomfort and with monitoring of extremity swelling, there may come a time when there will be a flare-up of the dystrophy. If this occurs too frequently, repeated stellate or lumbar blocks may be required, and if so, this may identify the individual who will require a sympathectomy in addition to the interruption of peripheral pain pathways. Prior to a surgical sympathectomy, it is reasonable to test the patient's response to an intravenous sympatholytic agent, like propranolol. Pain relief, in response to this chemical sympathectomy, as described by Raja, Treede, Davis, and Campbell (1991), identifies a patient with sympathetically maintained pain.

If the patient fails to achieve pain relief from sympathetic blocks, whether intravenous or regional, then the possibility of a central nervous system pain-generating mechanism must be considered. Such individuals become candidates for implantation by neurosurgeons of dorsal column stimulators. While implantation of such stimulators along more proximal aspects of the peripheral nervous system have been suggested for pain control, such a peripheral source of pain control can be confirmed by regional anesthetic blocks of these peripheral nerves. Interruption of nerve function at such a location is probably more predictable than implantation of peripheral nerve stimulators, since the silicone sheaths that attach even the most sophisticated implantable neural stimulators can themselves become a source of chronic nerve compression and pain.

Although reflex sympathetic dystrophy can be a devastating problem, cautious optimism may be displayed by those involved in the patient's care. Appropriate use of radiographic imaging, local anesthetic, and intravenous sympatholytic agents for diagnosis will assure all those involved that the diagnosis is correct. Specific therapy can be determined again by local and regional anesthetic blocks for therapy, leading to strategies to interrupt peripheral nerve pain generating signals, to regain control of the sympathetic overactivity. Rehabilitation efforts must be an integral part of the overall treatment plan from the very beginning. This approach can salvage many patients with RSD, returning them to productive lives (see Figures 4.9 & 11.10)

• NERVE REPAIR •

Nerve repair is the appropriate terminology for the surgical technique that joins two nerve ends together. These two ends can be from the same nerve, such as in repairing a divided digital nerve, or from two different nerves, such as in reinnervating the tip of the median nerve-supplied index finger by rerouting a digital nerve from the ulnar-supplied ring finger (see Chapter 13). When a segment of one nerve is interposed between two ends of another nerve, and the ends of the interposed nerve segment are joined to the ends of the other nerve, the interposed segment is termed a *nerve graft.* The technique of joining the ends of the nerve in a nerve graft may be the same as those used for a nerve repair, but traditionally a nerve repair does not refer to a nerve graft. When nerve ends are joined it is correct to speak of repairing them, connecting them, reconstructing them, or of a nerve juncture, but the term *anastomoses* is not correct. Anastomoses refers to the joining of two hollow structures, like blood vessels.

Suturing is not the only technique for repairing a nerve. Because it requires time for the surgeon to do a nerve repair by placing sutures, and because the suture material itself may serve as a source of scarring, techniques other than suturing have been developed. The two ends of a nerve may be safely connected by the means of a glue. Fibrin, a natural protein contained in blood, has been separated from blood, then separated from possible blood-born infectious agents, such as HIV virus. It is available, at least in Europe, for use in the operating room to place between the ends of nerve.

Neural regeneration proceeds normally through a fibrin interface. Laser has been used to weld together two ends of a nerve by forming a heat-induced coagulum between the nerve ends, and this, too, does not impede neural regeneration.

The two ends of a nerve can be brought together by wrapping something around the nerve, again using a strategy that is designed to remove any suture material from within the nerve. Nerve wrapping, or *entubulation,* also offers the theoretical advantage of confining the regenerating axon sprouts to prevent them from growing into surrounding tissues. This provides the benefit of guiding the axons distally and minimizing the extent of a suture line, in-continuity neuroma. Such neuromas, which form in some degree at most nerve repair sites, may be a source of postoperative pain. The wrapping technique has a disadvantage, which is that if the wrapping material is nonabsorbable, such as silicone, it will remain around the regenerated nerve and may become a site of chronic nerve compression or irritation.

A final variation on nerve repair is related to techniques that minimize tension at the repair site and minimize damage to the neural tissue itself. A technique employing freezing the ends of the nerve prior to trimming them, bathing the nerve

ends in a chemical solution that minimizes calcium ion shifts, and suturing the nerve to a background sheet of material at a distance from the actual nerve repair site has been investigated by deMedinacelli, Wyatt, and Freed (1983).

The exact connective tissue site within the nerve, and the timing of the nerve repair with respect to the time of injury, are two other classic points for discussion about nerve repair technique. In general, if the nerve subserves a single function, such as sensory to the index finger, simply placing two 8-0 or 10-0 nylon sutures through the epineurium is sufficient for the nerve repair. In a nerve with multiple fascicles, which subserve many different functions, such as the median nerve at the wrist, it is ideal to do an interfascicular dissection proximally, identify the different fascicles distally, and do individual fascicular repairs, with two 8-0 or 10-0 nylon sutures for the motor fascicle to the thenar muscles, the common volar digital nerve to the middle/ring web space, the common volar digital nerve to the index/middle web space, and the sensory fascicles to the thumb and the radial side of the index finger. These sutures may be placed into the perineurium. Care to avoid too much intraneural scarring due to dissection is required. In a multifascicular

nerve in which the function subserved by each fascicle is not known with any degree of certainty, such as in the median nerve in the upper arm, the best strategy is to do an epineural repair of the entire nerve. If several groups of fascicles are readily identified, a grouped-fascicular repair should be done, in which case the sutures may actually go through both the interfascicular epineurium and the perineurium.

With respect to the timing of a nerve repair, it is best to repair the nerve as soon after it is injured as possible, as long as certain other considerations are met. These considerations include the wound being clean, the nerve injury being relatively sharp, the patient's physical condition permitting, and the availability of appropriate operating facilities and a surgeon trained in microsurgery.

A nerve repair performed soon after the injury occurs is called a *primary nerve repair.* If the nerve cannot be repaired for the first few days, the repair is termed a *delayed primary.* If the repair is done after about 3 weeks, it is best to call this a *secondary nerve repair.* After 3 weeks, the injured ends of the nerve will have formed thickened, rounded ends, called the *proximal neuroma* and the *distal glioma.* These will require resection back to normal, nonscarred nerve for the nerve repair to be successful. Usually, such a resection creates a gap between the nerve ends that cannot be closed without creating too much tension at the nerve repair site. This tension would prevent good neural regeneration and, in this situation, a nerve graft would become the preferred technique for nerve reconstruction, rather than a nerve repair.

The results of nerve repair for various nerves are given in Chapter 11.

• NERVE GRAFT •

A nerve graft is a technique which places a nerve segment from one nerve into a nerve defect in another nerve. The simple division of a peripheral nerve creates a gap between the two ends of the nerve due to the nerve's inherent elastic properties. While there is some tension placed on a suture line that reconnects the two ends of such a divided nerve, this tension has little effect on the amount of scar tissue formed by the fibroblasts in the nerve during neural regeneration. However, if a piece of nerve is removed, either by the injury itself or by the surgeon excising scarring from the injured nerve, then there is a true deficiency of nerve tissue, called a *nerve defect*. If the ends of the divided nerve are united by a suture when there is a nerve defect, then there is sufficient tension at the suture line to cause an increase in the amount of collagen deposited at the site of nerve healing. This collagen is type I collagen and creates a barrier for the regenerating axon, as opposed to the type IV collagen normally present in basement membrane, which is useful for contact guidance neural regeneration (see above). Thus, tension is to be avoided at the nerve repair site. For this reason, the results of repairing a nerve defect by direct nerve repair have been unsuccessful. Indeed, it is because the results of repairing a nerve defect by flexing adjacent joints and hauling the ends of the nerve together with large sutures has been so unsuccessful that surgeons, under the leadership of Hano Millesi, began in the mid 1970s to return to nerve grafting as a technique for nerve reconstruction (Millesi, 1972).

The practical objection to nerve grafting was that the nerve grafts that were used during World War I simply did not work. Reevaluation of that technique by Millesi (1974) led to the realization that the nerves used for the graft were large diameter, or trunk grafts (see Figure 4.10). These grafts required revascularization for survival as a tissue, as do all nonvascularized tissue transfers. The centers of these large diameter nerves became poorly vascularized and,

therefore, fibrosed. These internally scarred nerves were then a poor conduit for neural regeneration. In addition to recognizing and then proving that nerve repair under tension resulted in increased scar at the suture line, Millesi realized using small diameter nerves as a graft would correct this problem. Finally, Millesi employed the concept of *internal neurolysis* to divide a large nerve into its component functional groups, as described above by the terms *grouped fascicular repair* or *perineurial repair*, and applied this to nerve grafting.

Thus came the currently accepted technique of using small diameter cutaneous nerves to reconstruct a nerve defect by placing them as interfascicular interposition nerve grafts. These grafts are laid side by side to encourage vascularization, rather than intertwining them to produce what was termed a cable graft, which would place portions of nerve centrally and discourage vascularization. The theoretical disadvantages to nerve grafting are that time must be spent harvesting the donor nerve, there is scarring at the nerve graft donor site, and there is a sensory loss at the donor site with the potential for a painful neuroma proximally at the site of nerve transection. A further theoretical disadvantage is that the regenerating nerve must cross two sites of

FIGURE 4.10

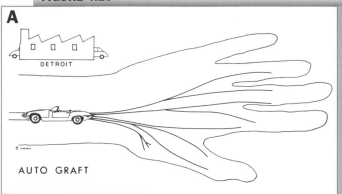

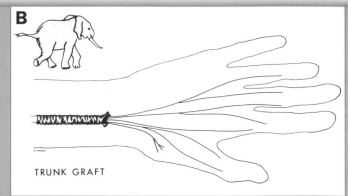

Nerve graft nomenclature. (A) An autograft is a nerve from one person put into that same person, in contrast to an allograft, which is a nerve from one person placed into another person, or a xenograft, which is a graft from one species placed into another species. (B) A trunk graft was an entire large diameter nerve used as the graft. These are poorly vascularized and result in poor nerve function. (C) The cable graft referred to several nerves twisted together. This also results in poor vascularization. (D) The best nerve graft results are obtained with the Millessi's approach, that is, several small diameter grafts placed alongside each other to obtain optimal vascularization. From "Management of Peripheral Nerve Injuries: Basic Principles of Microneurosurgical Repair," by A. L. Dellon, 1992, Oral Maxilofacial Surgery Clinics—North America 4:393-403. *Reprinted with permission of the author.*

nerve repair, giving the potential for two sites of nerve disruption and two sites for a painful incontinuity neuroma. Table 4.1 lists the commonest sites for nerve graft harvesting and the potential areas of sensory loss.

Despite the practical and theoretical disadvantages of nerve grafting, the overall results of reconstructing nerve injuries would be improved without question if more nerve grafting were done. Even when it is clear to the surgeon at the time of injury that the mechanism of injury will require a large amount of nerve to be resected due to the ensuing fibrosis that will surely occur over the next 3 weeks, the surgeon more often than not will carry out a primary nerve repair rather than close the wound and return in 3 weeks to do a secondary nerve graft. The results of neural regeneration through this scarred nerve repair site are often accepted as the final result, rather than returning to the operating room in 6 months, when it is clear that functional sensibility will not be recovered. It is not surprising, then, that there has been a search to replace autogenous nerve grafting with some substitute.

The patient's own muscle and vein have been used instead of nerve to reconstruct a nerve defect. The vein is used as a nerve conduit, simply placing one end of the nerve into each end of the vein. The nerve will regenerate through this vein, although with functional results that are not as good as those achieved with bioabsorbable conduits (see Chapter 12). Muscle must first be frozen and thawed through several cycles with liquid nitrogen. This treatment kills the muscle cells, but leaves intact the basement membrane that surrounds each muscle cell (Glasby, Gschmeissner, Hitchcock, & Huang, 1986). Remember that it is the basement membrane (plus the Schwann cells) that survive in the

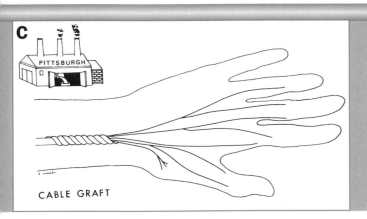

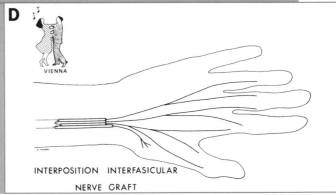

Nerve	Region of Sensory Loss
TABLE 4.1 NERVE DONOR SITES FOR GRAFTING	
Upper Extremity	
Medial anterbrachial cutaneous	volar and medial forearm
Lateral anterbrachial cutaneous	volar and lateral forearm
Posterior interosseous, terminal branch	dorsal wrist capsule
Radial sensory[+]	dorsal radial forearm/hand
Ulnar nerve[+]	ulnar border of hand, 4 & 5 digits
Common volar digital to index/middle	web of index/middle fingers
Lower extremity	
Posterior femoral cutaneous	posterior thigh
Sural	dorsolateral foot
Superficial peroneal[*]	dorsum of foot
Deep peroneal[*]	web space 1st/2nd toe
Head & Neck	
Greater auricular	ear lobe

Note:

[+] Especially if grafting to restore radial nerve motor function.

[+] Especially if grafting to reconstruct a total brachial plexus palsy; may also be taken as a vascularized nerve graft.

[*] Especially if grafting to reconstruct deep peroneal nerve at knee level.

[*] As a vascularized nerve graft for digital nerve reconstruction.

nerve graft. Thus, acellular muscle is essentially a basement membrane scaffolding through or along which the nerve can regenerate. Clinical trials with freeze/thawed muscle interposition grafting have been done in England, where this technique originated. Unfortunately, however, they do not result in as good functional recovery for sensibility when used to reconstruct a mixed motor/sensory nerve as do conventional nerve grafts (see Chapter 12).

Nerve grafts that are obtained from one person and put back into that same person are called *autografts*. As with all transplant surgery, if the nerve graft donor tissue comes from one person and is put into another person, it is called an *allograft* or *homograft*. If it is transferred from one species into another species, for example, from a dog to a monkey, it is called a *xenograft* or *heterograft*. The closer the genetic match between the transferred tissues, the less is the immune response generated by the host. Thus, there is essentially only a mild inflammatory response at the site of nerve repair, with some further reaction directed to the suture material. However, with an allograft, there is an immune response at both the humoral and cellular level that will lead to a rejection of the graft. Thus, as with kidney, heart, or liver transplants, a nerve transplant will be rejected (Fish, Bain, McKee, & Mackinnon, 1992).

There are times when the need for donor nerves is so great that there would be a value to being able to do a nerve transplant. At present, doing such a nerve reconstruction with nerve taken from another person requires immunosuppression. In contrast to the transplantation of a kidney, heart, or liver, without which life is not possible, the side effects

of immunosuppression are usually considered to be too great for the potential benefit conferred by nerve reconstruction. However, in 1992 Mackinnon and Hudson reported the first successful human nerve allograft. It was used to reconstruct a 23 cm sciatic nerve defect in an 8-year-old boy providing, ultimately, sensibility to the plantar aspect of the foot. The cyclosporin A immunosuppression was stopped at the 26th postoperative month. It was possible to do this because of two unique attributes of peripheral nerve.

First, nerve is much less antigenic than skin, kidney, heart, or liver. Second, once neural regeneration has proceeded across the nerve graft and has entered regions in which it is supported by host Schwann cells, immunosuppression can be discontinued. Once immunosuppression is discontinued, even if

the donor graft is rejected, the host axons transitting through the graft survive. In time, the host Schwann cells, which are the component of the nerve graft most required for regeneration across large gaps, are replaced by host Schwann cells that migrate from the proximal and distal ends of the host nerve across the region of the graft. It is possible that techniques now being developed in Mackinnon's research laboratory, such as prolonged cold storage preservation, and specific antibodies against adhesion molecules, may sufficiently reduce the immunogenicity of nerve allografts to the point that they may be used with little or no systemic immunosuppression, opening the door to clinically practical nerve tissue banking and transplantation.

The results of nerve grafting for various nerves are given in Chapter 11.

● NERVE CONDUITS ●

It has become clear over the past two decades of microsurgical nerve reconstruction that increasing manipulation of the nerve repair site by the surgeon has not significantly improved the results of nerve repair over and above that achieved by using small diameter cutaneous nerve grafts to minimize tension at the repair site. The ideal nerve reconstruction technique would be one that (a) eliminates tension at the nerve repair site, (b) permits immediate reconstruction at the time of injury, (c) does not require sacrifice of another functioning nerve, (d) does not create a scar at a site not already injured, (e) does not add appreciable intraoperative time, (f) does not place a foreign material permanently into the body, (g) does not create the potential for chronic nerve entrapment, and (h) permits neurobiology to enhance neural regeneration.

While the nerve allograft, described above, will meet most of these requirements if the need for immunosuppression can be overcome, it has become increasingly clear that endogenous growth factors and molecular biology, each already available to us, can be harnessed to aid neural regeneration. These trends have set the intellectual framework for the development of *nerve conduits*, tubes through which neural regeneration can proceed (Mackinnon & Dellon, 1988).

The following statements have been proven experimentally with regard to neural regeneration through nerve conduits: Both nonabsorbable and absorbable conduits permit neural regeneration and minimize suture line neuromas (see Figure 4.11). A silicone tube will not permit regeneration beyond 10 mm, probably because of lack of oxygen. A silicone tube can cause chronic nerve compression, and if used for a nerve conduit, clinically should probably be removed at a second operation (Soteranos & Dellon, 1995; Dellon, 1994). Bioabsorbable porous tubes will sustain neural regeneration across a 3 cm gap with the quality of that regenera-

tion being at least as good as, and possibly superior to, that obtained by interposition interfascicular nerve grafting. Beyond 3 cm, the regenerating nerve will cross a conduit, but the number of nerve fibers reaching the distal nerve is few. If neural regeneration is to produce a good result across a gap greater than 3 cm, some support, such as cultured Schwann cells, a neurotrophic factor, or contact guidance substance like laminin, will be required (Dellon & Mackinnon, 1988).

The most successful bioabsorbable conduit has been one made of polyglycolic acid (PGA). The PGA material has been in use for two decades as an absorbable suture material. This PGA bioabsorbable nerve conduit, called the Neurotube™, was approved by the Food and Drug Administration (FDA) for clinical field trials within the United States in 1994. This tube has been demonstrated to be successful in reconstructing a 3 cm ulnar nerve defect at the elbow level in the monkey. In these animals, the degree of nerve regeneration 1 year after the use of the Neurotube™ was compared with the results 1 year after microsurgical interfascicular interposition nerve grafting of the same defect in the opposite arm (see Figure 4.11). The Neurotube™ results were the

same or better than those of nerve grafting, with the number of myelinated axons and degree of myelination being the same, electrodiagnostic testing being the same, and with reinnervation of intrinsic muscles being better in the PGA bioabsorbable nerve conduit compared to nerve grafting. Following the success of the Neurotube™ in subhuman primates, a preliminary study investigated the results of this conduit for digital nerve defects in humans. The results are given in detail in Chapter 12, but the demonstrated results were as good or better than the historic results of digital nerve repair or grafts. The availability of a Neurotube™ in the operating room will permit the surgeon, at the time of the initial injury, to resect as much damaged nerve as is deemed appropriate based on the mechanism of injury (up to 3 cm), and to still carry out a primary reconstruction without the concerns of doing a primary nerve graft. It is anticipated that the 21st century will witness the extensive use of bioabsorbable conduits to reconstruct short nerve defects, to permit neurobiology to be effective in nerve injuries without significant loss of neural tissue and, in combination with additives to the tubes, such as growth factors or laminin, to reconstruct even long nerve defects.

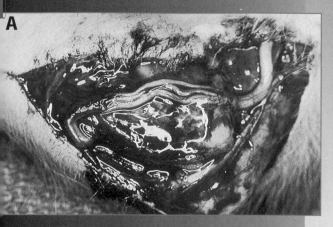

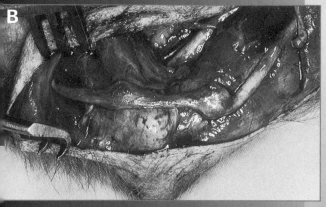

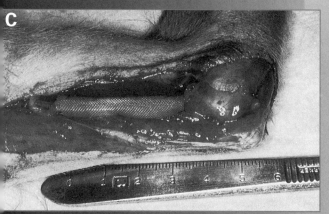

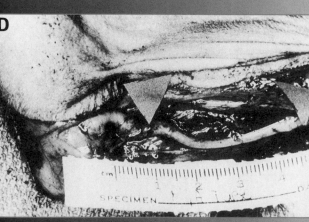

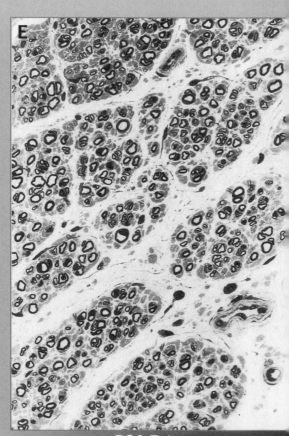

FIGURE 4.11

Nerve Conduit. In this series of intraoperative photos, a 3 cm segment of the monkey ulnar nerve at the elbow has been reconstructed with a bioabsorbable, polyglycolic acid (PGA) Neurotube™. Photos (A) and (C) are at the time of surgery, and photos (B) and (D) are 1 year later, at the time specimens were obtained for histologic assessment (E) of the results of neural regeneration. In (A) and (B), the control group used traditional interposition interfascicular sural nerve grafts. In (C) and (D) are the Neurotube™ group. Note that in (B), even with a microneurosurgical repair, there are still incontinuity suture line neuromas formed at both repair sites. Note that in (D), after the Neurotube™, has been absorbed, there is what appears to be a normal nerve bridging the original 3 cm defect. From "An Alternative to the Classical Nerve Graft for the Management of the Short Nerve Gap," by A. L. Dellon & S. E. Mackinnon, 1988, Plastic and Reconstructive Surgery 82:849-856. Reprinted with permission of the authors.

PGA Tube

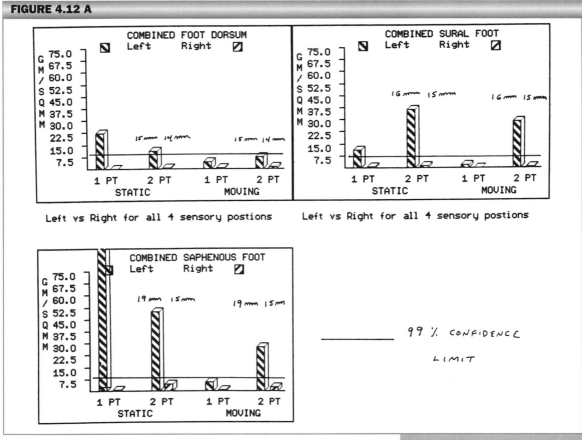

FIGURE 4.12 A

Collateral sprouting. (A) This patient is 3 years after harvesting the left sural nerve for median nerve reconstruction. Theoretically, there should be no sensory function of the left sural nerve, yet there is, including two-point discrimination. The assumption that the reinnervation of the foot came from the adjacent territories of the saphenous nerve and the peroneal nerve is suggested by the elevated thresholds of these nerves, and confirmed when an anesthetic block of these nerves caused loss of sensation in the sural nerve territory. (See Figure 4.12 B on next page.)

• COLLATERAL SPROUTING •

The patient must be made aware that following resection of the neuroma, the adjacent normal nerves, whose territories overlap that of the resected nerve, will attempt to send axons into the newly denervated region. This phenomenon is called *collateral sprouting*. Most likely the nerve growth factor released from the distal end of the resected nerve can stimulate uninjured adjacent C-fibers and A-delta fibers to grow into the denervated region (Jackson & Diamond, 1977). It is also possible that the adjacent normal nerves detect the absence of some trophic factor from the resected nerve, and that this absence may contribute to the mechanism of collateral sprouting. Proof of collateral sprouting is easily obtained, although very little has been written about it clinically (see Figures 4.12A & 4.12B).

Examination of the forearm of a patient after the harvesting of a sensory nerve, like the medial antebrachial cutaneous or the lateral antebrachial cutaneous, for a nerve graft donor, or examination of the lateral aspect of the foot after the harvesting of the sural nerve for a nerve graft donor, will

FIGURE 4.12 B

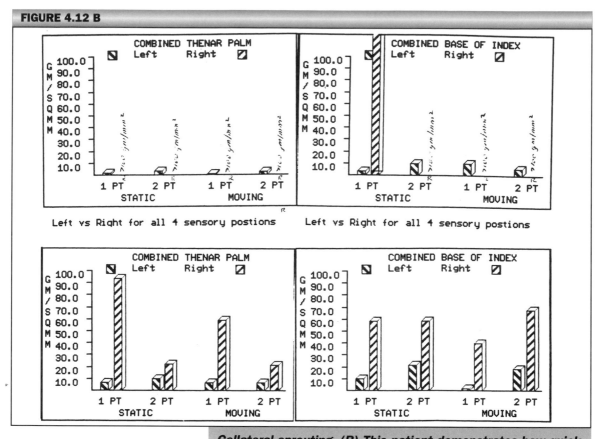

Collatoral sprouting. (B) This patient demonstrates how quickly the collateral sprouting occurs. The top two panels are 8 days after resection of the palmar cutaneous branch of the median nerve and document the expected sensory loss. The bottom two panels are measurements made on the 22nd postoperation day, and demonstrate recovery of sensation. At this time the patient had no pain, but felt a "crawling" or "tingling" in the skin. Note the recovered though elevated thresholds obtained with the Pressure Specified Sensory Device™.

reveal a very small residual area of diminished sensation by 1 year after the nerve graft harvesting. This reduction in size of the area from the original large area of anesthesia to the small area of hypesthesia is the result of collateral sprouting, and is due to peripheral nerve changes.

The central nervous system changes that accompany peripheral denervation will be described in Chapter 10, under cortical plasticity, but these central changes are not responsible for collateral sprouting. Collateral sprouting, in and of itself, can generate disturbing sensations such as the feeling of crawling of the skin, tingling, or itching. If a painful neuroma has been resected, the therapist must be able to reassure the patient that the perceptions related to collateral sprouting, a normal, compensatory mechanism, are short-lived (about 3 weeks to 3 months), can be helped by reeducation techniques (see Chapter 12), and are not the original neuroma pain returning. The desensitization techniques that the therapist will employ to treat the disturbing sensations associated with collateral sprouting help the cortical reorganization that occurs following peripheral denervation.

• • •

• REFERENCES •

Brushart, T. M., & Seiler, W. A. Selective reinnervation of distal motor stumps by peripheral motor axons. *Experimental Neurology* 97:289-300, 1987.

Dellon, A. L. *Evaluation of Sensibility and Re-education of Sensation in the Hand.* Baltimore: Williams & Wilkins, 1981.

Dellon, A. L. Management of peripheral nerve injuries: Basic principles of microneurosurgical repair. *Oral Maxilofacial Surgery Clinics — North America 4:*393-403, 1992.

Dellon, A. L. Tube, or not tube.... (Editorial) *Journal of Hand Surgery 19B:*271-272, 1994.

Dellon, A. L., & Horner, G. Partial wrist denervation. In *Problems in Plastic and Reconstruction Surgery: The Wrist,* S. Levin, Editor. Philadelphia: Lippincott, 1993.

Dellon, A. L., & Mackinnon, S. E. An alternative to the classical nerve graft for the management of the short nerve gap, *Plastic and Reconstructive Surgery 82:*849-856, 1988.

DeMedinacelli, L., Wyatt, R. J., & Freed, W. J. Peripheral nerve reconnection: Mechanical, thermal and ionic conditions that promote the return of function. *Experimental Neurology 81:*469-474, 1983.

Evans, G. R. D., & Dellon, A. L. Implantation of palmar cutaneous branch of the median nerve into the pronator quadratus for treatment of painful neuroma. *Journal of Hand Surgery 19A:*203-206, 1944.

Fish, J. S., Bain, J. R., McKee, N., & Mackinnon, S. E. The peripheral nerve allograft in the primate immunosuppressed with cyclosporin A: II. Functional evaluation of reinnervated muscle. *Plastic and Reconstructive Surgery 90:*1047-1052, 1992.

Glasby, M. A., Gschmeissner, S. E., Hitchcock, R. J. I., & Huang, C. L. H. The dependence of nerve regeneration through muscle grafts in the rat on the availability and orientation of basement membrane. *Journal of Neurocytology 15:*497-510, 1986.

Letourneau, P. C. Neurite extension by peripheral and central nervous system neurons in response to substratum bound fibronectin and laminin. *Developmental Biology 98:*212-215, 1983.

Lundborg, G. *Nerve Injury and Repair.* Edinburgh: Churchill Livingston, 1988.

Mackinnon, S. E., & Dellon, A. L. Results of treatment of recurrent dorsoradial wrist neuromas. *Annals of Plastic Surgery 19:*54-61, 1987.

Mackinnon, S. E., & Dellon, A. L. *Surgery of the Peripheral Nerve.* New York: Thieme, 1988.

Mackinnon, S. E., & Hudson, A. R. Clinical application of peripheral nerve transplantation. *Plastic and Reconstructive Surgery 90:*695-699, 1992.

Meyer, R. A., Raja, S. N., Campbell, J. N., Mackinnon, S. E., & Dellon, A. L. Neural activity originating from a neuroma in the baboon. *Brain Research 325:*255-260, 1985.

Millesi, H., Meisse, G., & Berger, A. The interfascicular nerve grafting of the median and ulnar nerves. *Journal of Bone and Joint Surgery 54A:*727-750, 1972.

Mitchell, S. W. *Injuries of Nerves and their Consequences.* American Academy of Neurology Reprint Series. New York: Dover, 1965.

Raja, S. N., Treede, R., Davis, K. D., & Campbell, J. N. Systemic alpha-adrenergic blockade with phentolamine: A diagnostic test for sympathetically maintained pain. *Anesthesiology 74:*691-698, 1991.

Soteranos, D. G., & Dellon, A. L. Chronic ulnar nerve compression caused by an implantable silastic neural stimulator. *Journal of Neurosurgery,* submitted: 1995.

• ADDITIONAL READINGS •

Altissimi, M., Mancini, G. B., & Azzara, A. Results of primary repair of digital nerves. *Journal of Hand Surgery 16B:*546-547, 1991.

Dellon, A. L. Interruption of nerve function. In *Current Therapy in Plastic and Reconstructive Surgery*, J. Marsh, Editor. Toronto: BC Becke, 1988.

Dellon, A. L. Wound healing in nerve. *Clinics in Plastic Surgery 17:*545-570, 1990.

Dellon, A. L., & Mackinnon, S. E. Treatment of the painful neuroma by neuroma resection and muscle implantation. *Plastic and Reconstructive Surgery 77:*427-436, 1986.

Dellon, E. S., & Dellon, A. L. The first nerve graft, Vulpian and the 19th Century neural regeneration controversy. *Journal of Hand Surgery 4:*1993.

Diao, E., & Peimer, C. A. Sutureless methods of nerve repair. In *Operative Nerve Repair and Reconstruction,* R. H. Gelberman, Editor. Philadelphia: Lippincott, 1991, pp. 305-314.

Hammarback, J. A., Palm, S. L., Furct, L. T., & Letourneau, P. C. Guidance of neurite growth by pathways of substra absorbed lamini. *Journal of Neuroscience Research 13:*213-222, 1985.

Ide, C. Nerve regeneration through the basal lamina scaffold of the skeletal muscle. *Journal of Neurosciece Research 1:*379-391, 1984.

Jackson, P., & Diamond, J. Colchicine block of cholinesterase transport in rabbit sensory nerves without interference with the long-term viability of the axons. *Brain 130:*579-584, 1977.

Laquerriere, A., Peulve, P., & Jin, O. Effect of basic fibroblast growth factor and alpha-melanocytic stimulating hormone on nerve regeneration through a collagen channel. *Microsurgery 15:*203-210, 1994.

Mackinnon, S. E., & Dellon, A. L. Clinical nerve reconstruction with a bioabsorbable polyglycolic acid tube. *Plastic and Reconstructive Surgery 85:*419-424, 1990.

Mackinnon, S. E., Dellon, A. L., Hudson, A. R., & Hunter, D. A. Alteration of neuroma formation by manipulation of neural microenvironment. *Plastic and Reconstructive Surgery 76:*345-352, 1985.

Mackinnon, S. E., Dellon, A. L., Lundborg, G., Hudson, A. R. & Hunter, D. A. A study of neurotropism in a primate model. *Journal of Hand Surgery 11:*888-894, 1986.

Mackinnon, S. E., & Holder, L. E. Use of three-phase radionuclide bone scanning in the diagnosis of reflex sympathetic dystrophy. *Journal of Hand Surgery 9:*556-563, 1984.

Millesi, H. Nerve grafting. *Clinics in Plastic Surgery 11:*105-120, 1984.

Millesi, H., & Terzis, J. K. Nomenclature in peripheral nerve surgery. *Clinics in Plastic Surgery 11:*3-8, 1984.

Raja, S. N., Davis, K. D., & Campbell, J. N. The adrenergic pharmacology of sympathetically-maintained pain. *Journal of Reconstructive Microsurgery 8:*63-69, 1989.

Schwartzman, R. J., & McLellan, T. L. Reflex sympathetic dystrophy: A review. *Archives of Neurology 44:*554-561, 1987.

Vergara, J., Medina, L., Maulen, J., Inestrosa, N. C., & Alvarez, J. Nerve regeneration is improved by insulin-like growth factor I (IGF-I) and basic fibroblast growth factor (bFGF). *Restorative Neurology Neuroscience 5:*181-189, 1993.

Zachary, L. S., Dellon, E. S., Nicholas, E. M., & Dellon, A. L. The structural basis of Felice Fontana's spiral bands and their relationship to nerve injury. *Journal of Reconstructive Microsurgery 9:*March, 1993.

• • •

quantitative sensory testing

5

goals

• • •

*A*s clinicians, we are prepared with a body of knowledge, and throughout our careers we acquire new knowledge, to help individuals overcome the problems associated with disabling conditions. The best solution, and, of course our goal, is to resolve problems that would create disabling conditions. But in many cases this is not totally possible, because disability takes many forms: it occurs when a person is unable to carry out the activities, tasks, and roles that are important to them in their own environment. What then is our goal? I worry that I see so many "hand" therapists focusing primarily upon the hand's impairment, and not looking at what that impairment means in the lives of the people they are serving. Our goal must be to remember that we are working with people who have lives, and that any major trauma to that life, for example from a hand injury, has consequences far beyond that injury. As we learn how to deliver the most effective hand care, it remains basic that we **consider the person** who needs assistance in the context of their environment and in what it is they need and want to do with their life. We must look at people's lives and what injury means to those lives plays a big part in their recovery and acceptance of that which cannot be fixed. I think that occupational therapists and physical therapists who choose a specialization in hands must go to that specialization with the body of knowledge and a commitment to the rehabilitation process of an individual whose tools for living are impaired and **the most important thing is their living,** not their hands.*

Carolyn M. Baum, PhD, OTR/C
Elias Michael Director and Associate Professor
of Occupational Therapy and Neurology
Washington University School of Medicine
St. Louis, May 4, 1995

....

* See Figure 5.1.

FIGURE 5.1
(A) The goal of rehabilitation must be beyond the impaired body part to focus on the improvement of the individual's life. (B) Interplay of categories affecting the goal of rehabilitation, with measures to evaluate and document progress. (A) From "Creating the Future: A Joint Effort," by M. Law & C. M. Baum, 1994, Health Care Brochure. (B) From "From ICV to Community: A Model for Determining effectiveness," by C. M. Baum & D. F. Edwards, presented at the American Occupational Therapy Association Annual Meeting, Denver, 1995. Reprinted with permission of the authors.

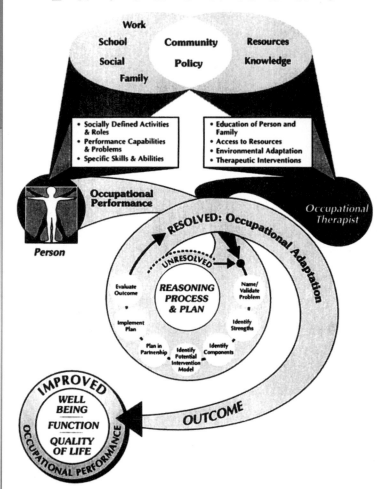

A

ENVIRONMENT

Work
School · Community · Resources
Social · Policy · Knowledge
Family

- Socially Defined Activities & Roles
- Performance Capabilities & Problems
- Specific Skills & Abilities

- Education of Person and Family
- Access to Resources
- Environmental Adaptation
- Therapeutic Interventions

Occupational Performance

Occupational Therapist

Person

RESOLVED: Occupational Adaptation

UNRESOLVED

REASONING PROCESS & PLAN

Evaluate Outcome
Implement Plan
Plan in Partnership
Identify Potential Intervention Model
Identify Components
Identify Strengths
Name/Validate Problem

IMPROVED
WELL BEING
FUNCTION
QUALITY OF LIFE
OCCUPATIONAL PERFORMANCE

OUTCOME

B

Societal Limitation	Disability	Functional Limitation	Impairment	Pathophysiology
Restriction attributable to social policy or barriers (structural or attitudinal) which limits fullfilment of roles or denies access to services or opportunities	Inability or limitation in performing socially defined activities and roles within a social and physical environment as a result of internal or external factors and their interplay	Restriction or lack of ability to perform an action or activity in the manner or range considered normal that results from impairment.	Loss and/or abnormality of mental, emotional, physiological, or anatomical structure or function; including secondary losses and pain.	Interuption or interference of normal physiological and developmental processes or structures
Performance of Roles by Person in Societal Context	Task Performance of Person in Physical and Social Context	Performance of Action or Activity	Organs and Organ Systems	Cells and Tissue
Accessibilty, Inclusion, and Accomodation and Health Promotion	Performance of Self-Care, Instrumental, Work and Educational Tasks with Consideration of the Physical, Cognitive, and Social Environment.	Physical, and Mental Aspects of Performance i.e. Sit, Stand, Reach, Walk, Grasp, Initiate, Organize, Interact, Control	Cognitive, Sensory, Motor, Physiological, and Psychological Function	• Neurological Deficit • Physiological Deficit • Immunological Deficit
Measures: Cost of Care Length of Stay Carer Burden Rankin Scale Community Re-Integration SF 36	Measures: IWJ Functional Assessment FIM/FAM/Executive Activity Card Sort Functional Behavior Profile Kitchen Task Assessment	Measures: IWJ Functional Assessment (Feeding, Grooming, Hygiene, UE Dressing) FIM/FAM/Executive William's Latch Board Nine Hole Peg Test Grip, Pinch ARA	Measures: Stroke Scales Mini Mental State Visual Perception Motor Planning	Measures: NIH Stroke Scale Glasgow Coma Scale APACHE

Venues of Care
- - - Community Health Maintenance & Promotion - - - - - - - - - Home Health - - - - - - - - - Acute and SubAcute Care
- - - - - - - - - - - - - Rehabilitation/Skilled Nursing Facility - - - - - - - - -
- - - - - - - - - - Out-Patient - - - - - - - - - -

• DOCUMENTATION •

The measurement of hand function remains elusive. Much of what we do with our hands every day is so automatic and effortless that when we stop to divide the hand's function into its component parts, we are confounded. The ability of the hand to perform precise skills, such as crafting a violin, requires the integration of sensory and motor function (see Figure 5.2). While much of what we do with our hands goes on as if guided by an "automatic pilot," the function is not truly subconscious, but is the result of practiced rhythms or patterns that require little control. These hand functions, nevertheless, rely on a continuous stream of afferent neural impulses originating from cutaneous sensory receptors, as well as on truly subconscious motor afferents. These inputs are then modified by our desired outcomes and result in a stream of efferent, or motor, impulses that yield the desired hand activity. The goal of quantitative sensorimotor testing is to document the level of sensory and motor function that are present. Although we are using the hand as an example, quantitative sensory testing can be applied to any body surface.

Documentation implies measurement. Documentation of sensorimotor function is more than just a research necessity—it is essential to patient care. It is critical to be able to document the physical manifestations of neuromuscular disease. Such documentation establishes a baseline necessary for diagnosis, and against which the results of treatment can be measured. Documentation of sensorimotor function over time provides the basis for prognostication and determination of impairment. Without documentation of sensorimotor function much of the science is lost from our ability to provide 21st-century medical care.

Motor function, with the exception of pinch and grasp, remains an area in which quantitative testing has lagged behind sensory testing. This is ironic because it has always been easier to observe deficits in motor function, so motor func-

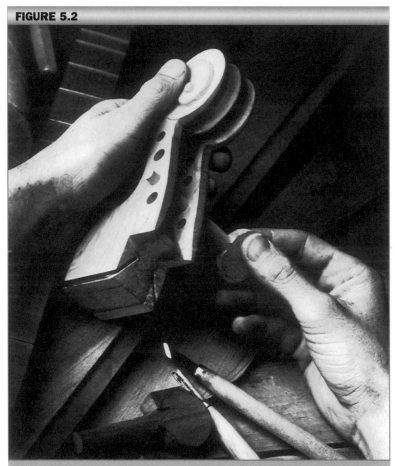

FIGURE 5.2

Hand function requires the integration of sensory and motor function. Even when performing skills requiring extreme precision, such as crafting a violin, much of what the hand does is almost effortless, and is accomplished at an almost subconscious level. Documenting the sensory and motor function of the hand requires instruments that are reliable and valid. Photo reprinted with permission of Robert Shenk, MD, Chicago.

tion has always preceded sensory function in our descriptive attempts. Most motor testing, however, has been descriptive; that is, muscle atrophy is described qualitatively (minimal, moderate, or severe), because few instruments exist to permit quantitative testing of anything except pinch and grip strength. Alternatively, motor function has been described as the ability of the muscle to act against a force like gravity or some other form of resistance, with these observations being given some numerical value, such as 1 out of 5. Instruments that are capable of quantitative motor testing are few, and are discussed in Chapter 7. It is clear that these attempts to document motor function are, for most of the muscles of the body, primarily qualitative.

While lack of motor function is obvious, lack of sensory function may not be. Moberg (1958) was the first to introduce quantitative sensory testing into the practice of hand surgery, demonstrating that classic, static (Weber, 1835), two-point discrimination was the only one of the existing neurologic tests that could predict static grip. The list of tests that purport to document sensory function in a quantitative manner is long, and continues to grow (see Table 5.1).

Quantitation of sensation did not begin to be applied universally until the last two decades, primarily through the efforts of Moberg (1958, 1966, 1972, & 1976) in hand surgery, and Bell-Krotoski and Buford (1988) and Bell-Krotoski (1990) in hand therapy. The very nature of sensibility lent itself to quantitative neurophysiologically-based tests; however, the basic scientists were generally unaware of the clinician's needs, and the clinicians were generally unaware of the advances in basic science that might pertain to documentation of sensorimotor function. The book, *Evaluation of Sensibility and Re-education of Sensation in the Hand,* (Dellon, 1981) was the first to bridge these two extremes, presenting a unified approach to understanding

TABLE 5.1	TESTS OF SENSIBILITY	
1835	Weber	static two-point discrimination
1894	von Frey	graded sensory hairs
1906	von Frey	vibratory hairs
1909	Trotter & Davie	localization
1915	Tinel	tingling sign
1934	Wartenberg	cogwheel
1943	Seddon	digit writing
1958	Moberg	ninhydrin test
1962	Semmes & Weinstein	nylon monofilaments
1966	Porter	letter recognition
1966	Wynn Parry	timed recognition test
1972	Dellon	constant- and moving-touch
1973	O'Rain	skin wrinkling
1977	Daniel & Bower	120 Hz vibrometer
1978	Dellon	moving two-point discrimination
1978	Dellon	30 and 256 Hz tuning forks
1979	Poppen	Ridge Device
1985	Mackinnon & Dellon	Disk-Criminator™
1990	Brunelli	Gnostic Rings
1992	Dellon & Dellon	Pressure-Specified Sensory Device™
1994	Novak & Mackinnon	Braille dot cell
1994	Weinstein	WEST™
1995	Dellon & Dellon	Force-Defined Vibrometer

the basis for a functionally relevant examination of sensibility, and presenting an approach to rehabilitation.

The National Institute of Standards and Technology (NIST) in Washington, DC, has the responsibility of defining a measurement. It has the standard weight for an ounce and the standard length for a meter. Whereas these defined measures are physical, they can nevertheless be represented by a standardized electrical signal. The comparison of a given electrical signal with that from NIST to calibrate a device is called *metrology*, the science of measurement. If a testing device is sufficiently accurate that it can be calibrated to meet NIST's requirements, the device is said to be traceable. At present, the only measurement devices that are *traceable* are the computer-assisted Pressure-Specified Sensory Device™, the Digit-Grip™, and the Pinch Sensor, available from the NK Biotechnical Corporation (see Chapter 7).

• VALIDITY •

Moberg (1958) emphasized that a sensory test should relate to what the hand does, that is, to its function, similar to the way a test of visual acuity tests eye function. In that respect, Moberg may have been among the first to emphasize that a quantitative test of sensation should be valid; that is, static two-point discrimination should be correlated with the ability to perform different grips with the hand. For a test to be valid, it must measure what it is supposed to measure. If a test of sensibility is to be clinically useful it must, therefore, measure a quality of sensation that will correlate with hand function. Thus, for a test of sensibility to be considered valid, it is necessary to have a test of hand function. Table 5.2 provides a list of hand function tests.

This discussion assumes that there is an accepted definition of hand function, which, of course, there is not. For example, whereas Moberg (1958) defined hand function in terms of static grips, that is, precision sensory grip and gross grip, it appears more reasonable today to define hand function in terms of object recognition. This realization came about because as more and more hand surgeons began to measure static two-point discrimination, they found increasing numbers of patients who had static two-point values greater than 15 mm who could still perform well on the pick-up test. These observations led to the description of the moving two-point discrimination test in 1978, which was subsequently demonstrated to correlate extremely well with object recognition (Dellon & Kallman, 1983). We are, therefore, at the point where it is necessary first to decide what attributes of hand function, or for that matter, of foot, breast, or mouth function we are trying to measure, reconstruct, or modify. It will then be necessary to select the test of sensibility that will measure that aspect of sensation correlating well with that function. Clearly, a different test of sensibility may be necessary to evaluate the ability of the skin of the foot to protect itself against being burned by hot pavement or water, from that necessary to evaluate whether a blind person can read Braille, and from that necessary to evaluate the origin of male impotence.

Another aspect of the validity of a test of sensibility is whether that test of hand function requires motor function to be performed. If motor function is required, then a coexisting motor impairment would be reflected in a poor sensibility test result, thereby overestimating the degree of impairment. Conversely, if the test of hand function permits the use of vision, then sight may be substituted for tactile sensibility, in which case the degree of impairment would be underestimated. Table 5.2 identifies the tests of hand function that do not require sight or normal motor function.

A valid measuring device should have the ability to record throughout the range of the variable being measured and, ideally, to record

TABLE 5.2   TESTS OF HAND FUNCTION

1930	Baxter & Ballard	Minnesota Rate of Manipulation
1948	Tiffin & Asher	Purdue Pegboard
1958	Moberg	Timed Pick-Up
1966	Wynn Parry	Timed Object Recognition✢
1969	Jebsen et al	Timed Activities of Daily Living
1981	Dellon	Modified Timed Object Recognition✢
1989	Chao et al.	Mayo Dexterity Test
1991	Imai & Tajima	Modified Object Recognition✦

Notes:
✢ Eliminates visual cues.
✦ Eliminates motor function.

those measurements continuously. A variable intensity vibrometer is an example of such a device, recording the entire range of the vibration perception threshold within the limits of power input to the vibrating tactor or stimulating head. In contrast, the Semmes-Weinstein nylon monofilament does not meet this requirement. Even the full set of 20 filaments can only give an estimate of the range at 20 intervals. Because there is an overlap and discontinuity within the set of 20 filaments, for practical clinical use the nylon monofilament set that is usually sold contains just 5 filaments. Clearly this restricts the "measurement" to an estimate of 1 of 5 different intervals. (Table 6.1 gives these ranges.) The Semmes-Weinstein nylon monofilaments, therefore, are best thought of as recording a range for the perception of pressure, and

not a true measurement of the pressure perception threshold (see Figure 7.19D). Furthermore, the nylon monofilaments are not traceable. Even the new, improved WEST™ device is not traceable, even though for this device each filament is at least tested in the factory to determine if it records within the given range it estimates. Only the computer-assisted Pressure-Specified Sensory Device™ has the ability to record a continuous measurement of the pressure threshold from 0.1 g/mm^2 to 100 g/mm^2.

A final variation would be if the test correlated with hand function, but had inherent measurement inaccuracies. The Jamar dynamometer is a good example of this. This device, designed in the 1950s, is hydraulic and has a curved handle. It was designed to record the force averaged at the center of the

curved handle. If a patient has an ulnar nerve injury, clearly the center of the patient's grip strength will shift toward the index finger and away from the center of the curved handle. Strength measurements will be discussed further in Chapter 7, but it is clear from this one example that even though there may be a correlation between Jamar-measured grip strength and the ability to perform a strength-requiring task, the Jamar has an inherent design flaw that renders it essentially invalid. Until the development of the Computer-Assisted Digit-Grip™, there was no alternative for the measurement of grip strength. Furthermore, the measurements made with the Jamar are not traceable to NIST. A recording of 31 kg made with a Jamar may or may not really be 31 kg.

Once a test is valid, it must be standardized to be applied meaningfully clinically, or for research. *Standardization* means that a description exists as to how exactly to do the test, that is, how the patient is positioned, what the instructions are, and what the testing paradigm or protocol is. Standardization implies that there will be normative data, and this implies further that variables such as sex, handedness, age, height, and weight have been evaluated to determine if they impact the measurement. Vibratory perception threshold, for example, has been shown to be related significantly to age, frequency, body site tested, and the force of application of the vibrating stimulus, but not to sex, handedness, or anthropomorphic factors. In contrast, strength testing has been shown to be related significantly to anthropomorphic measurements, sex, and handedness.

There has been a challenge to the entire concept of doing sensory testing with hand-held instruments. The challenge was raised because of the observation that the subject's hand and the examiner's hand have some movement associated with them that may alter the measurement. There is a natural frequency in the human body that is created by the biological consequences of the heart beating, by the force of gravity, and by the earth's magnetic field. We will never be able to eliminate these factors. The challenge by Bell-Krotoski and Buford (1988) to doing sensory testing with hand-held instruments took the form of oscilloscope tracings that depicted the variation in force exerted by the tester against a stationary object. Movement of the examiner's hand must certainly be considered a legitimate theoretical objection.

An appropriate response to this challenge must look at the scientific question being asked by the testing situation. If the question is one of basic science in a labora-tory, where each condition of the measurement can be controlled, then the reality of movement of the testing instrument must be minimized as completely as possible unless, of course, the stimulus is one that involves movement, like vibration or moving touch. For single-unit nerve fiber recordings, a stimulator such as the Chubik, which is computer-controlled, can be used. Such a six-degree of freedom, computer-driven holder for quantitative sensory testing has been developed for testing humans by the NK Biotechnical Corporation of Minneapolis, Minnesota.

At the other extreme are rapid clinical decisions that require a good approximation of the true sensibility. For this type of information qualitative screening with a tuning fork, the Semmes-Weinstein monofilaments, WEST™, or the Disk-Criminator™ can give sufficiently accurate information. For the motor system there is the stand-alone version of the Digit-Grip™. The fact remains that if the examiner holds a testing instrument in constant touch with the subject's fingertip, the subject will not perceive the slight movement that is discernable on the oscilloscope screen. The explanation for this must be that as the sensory impulses travel to the sensory cortex, they pass through one or more filtering stations, for example, the thalamus. Careful analysis by Novak, Mackinnon, Williams, and Kelly (1993) of the results of many different types of hand-held sensory testing instruments has demonstrated that hand-held instruments are capable of giving valid information. The examiner, however, must always be mindful of the need to be precise and steady in the application of the stimulus, and to position the subject so that the part being tested is firmly supported. Finally, damping devices can be added to hand-held, computer-assisted instruments, such as that supplied with the Pressure-Specified Sensory Device™, that minimize the inherent oscillations superimposed on the measured force-transducer signal (see Chapter 7).

• RELIABILITY •

Reliability has to do with the concept that the measuring device will perform as you expect it to perform. If you believe you are measuring temperature perception, you expect the end of the probe to deliver a temperature that changes, and you expect that if the dial indicates the probe tip is 45°C, it is 45°C.

Reliability has to do with the concept that each time you

use the device it is doing the same thing, exactly as it did it before. If the same examiner measures the same area of a subject several times, at the same session or at two different sessions, reliability implies that the examiner will get a result for each measurement that is acceptably close to the other measurements each time the measurement is made. This is *intratest* or *intertest correlation*. Reliability also has to do with the concept that if different examiners use the device to measure the same area of the same subject, each examiner will get a result that is acceptably close to the measurement made by the other examiner. This is *intertester correlation*. These correlations are determined statistically by the intraclass correlation coefficient.

Reliability of the device is an engineering concept and as such is the responsibility of the manufacturer. The relationship between reliability and validity may be illustrated by the grouping of data on the x–axis (see Figure 5.3).

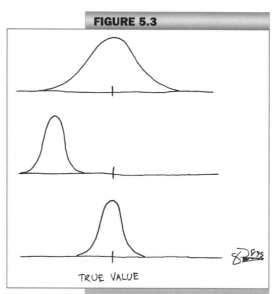

FIGURE 5.3

TRUE VALUE

Validity versus reliability. A statistical illustration is useful to depict the difference between these two concepts. The true value is represented by the short vertical bar along the x–axis. In the top graph is a test that gives values (results) that center on the true value in a valid test, but if there is a large spread in those values, even though the values are centered, the test is not reliable. In the center graph is a test that has very little spread in its values and is, therefore, reliable. But, since the central value of this test's results is away from the true value, the test is not valid. In the bottom graph, the test results are centered on the true value with little spread, and therefore the test is both valid and reliable. Courtesy of Patsy L. Tassler, BA, PhD candidate, Johns Hopkins University School of Hygiene and Public Health.

• COMPUTER-ASSISTED TESTING •

The value of placing a computer between the patient and the examiner is that the computer can be related to testing instruments which expand sensorimotor testing to a height previously unobtainable. Computer-assisted sensorimotor testing still requires an examiner, who may be a therapist, nurse, physician, or certified technician, as long as he or she is compulsive about the testing methodology. Computer-assisted sensorimotor testing still requires an appropriate subject, in that the subject must be able to communicate with the examiner at least to the extent of being able to either push a button with the opposite hand or press on a foot pedal, or give a verbal response to the stimulus. For some computer-assisted devices the patient must actually interact with the device (see Chapter 7, "Automated Tactile Tester"). In all instances, computer-assisted testing makes the assumption that the patient is telling the truth and is, therefore, not objective in the way that electrodiagnostic testing or somatosensory-evoked potentials are (see Chapter 8).

Signals generated by the testing or measurement devices can be analyzed through sophisticated techniques by the computer that are simply not possible by the examiner who gets one look at the dial of a traditional testing instrument. For example, a hydraulic grip meter will record just the peak strength. The Digit-Grip™, in contrast, will record the rate of rise of the force until the peak is reached and, if the patient is asked to maintain that grip for a timed period, as denoted by a beep from the computer, the stored data over time will display a curve. The area under that curve can be calculated by the computer and will be found to be related to endurance or to neuromuscular function. Fluctuations in that curve may be related to voluntary effort and may be used, therefore, to detect malingering (see Impairment Rating, below).

With regard to the sensory system, traditionally there was the choice of estimating the cutaneous pressure threshold and/or the distance at which one from two points could be distinguished. By placing a force transducer between each of two stimulating prongs and the computer, a signal is generated that can be converted into a measurement of the pressure threshold required for that two-point discrimination to occur. Thus, computer-assisted sensory testing permits a solution to criticism of two-point discrimination testing: How hard was the examiner pressing the two ends of the paper clip or Disk-Criminator™ against the skin?

The first computer-assisted sensorimotor testing available was the Hand Assessment System from the NK Biotechnical Corporation. This system has state-of-the-art pinch and grip strength testing equipment (designed in conjunction with Ed Chao, PhD, a biomedical engineer, and William Cooney, MD) and a pressure perception threshold measuring device (designed in conjunction with A. Lee Dellon, MD). These devices are fully described in Chapter 7. They make measurements so accurate that they are traceable to NIST.

The Pressure-Specified Sensory Device™ can measure sensibility on any body surface. The Hand Assessment System is modular in design, meaning that you can get just motor or just sensory devices, and they can be connected to any IBM-compatible computer. Additional modular components may be added to measure skin compliance, rapid exchange grip (to detect malingering), goniometers, and anthropomorphic measurements.

The unique feature of the NK or Hand Assessment System's devices is that they make traceable measurements. The NK software does not at present transfer these measurements into a word processor program for an impairment rating report, nor does it incorporate video photos of a patient's hand. These are expensive software features that are available on other systems (see Table 5.3). The Hand Assessment System also does not measure temperature perception. It does have a separate variable frequency (16, 32, 64, 128, 256, 500, 1000 Hz), variable intensity vibrometer. This vibrometer is force-defined, indicating that it contacts the skin with a force set to match the skin compliance and maintain the vibrating tactor probe in contact with the skin.

The most recent computer-assisted sensory testing device, the Automated Tactile Tester™, designed by neurophysiologist Ken Horch, PhD, was reported on in 1992 (Horch, Hardy, Jimenez, & Jabaley). The Automated Tactile Tester™ (see Chapter 7) permits measurement of vibration threshold at 120 Hz, temperature perception, one-point touch threshold (reported in microns of skin displacement, not pressure), and two-point discrimination, recorded in millimeters. Its software does not put this data into an impairment rating report. Its measurements are not traceable. It cannot measure joint range of motion, or make anthropomorphic measurements (see Table 5.3). It is a single unit applicable only to the hand, and cannot record pinch or grip strength.

There are currently commercially available four computer-assisted devices that are similar to each other in that their main feature is software that can report an

TABLE 5.3   COMPUTER-ASSISTED SYSTEMS

Computer-Assisted System	Devices Available on this System				
	Sensory	Pinch/Grip	Joint	Vibro	Temp
NK Hand Assessment	X	X	X	X	
Greanleaf		X	X		
Dexter		X	X		
Henley					
ATT	X			X	X

impairment rating. The software varies among the four, but results may be reported in color, may incorporate photos of the hand itself, and one of the systems may be voice actuated.

All of these systems rely on the therapist to measure by hand the cutaneous pressure threshold using Semmes-Weinstein monofilaments and/or two-point discrimination using a Disk-Criminator™. The therapist must then enter the values into the computer by means of a mouse and keyboard. The measurement itself is not computer-assisted. The pinch/grip strength measurements are essentially electronic dynamometers whose measurements are recorded by a device connected to the computer but whose measurement is not traceable. None of these four have a vibrometer. All have range of motion and

anthropomorphic measurement devices. The Data-Glove™ manufactured by Greenleaf, is a unique device that is computer-assisted to measure range of motion of

hand joints. The Greenleaf EVAL™ system is the only system that is not IBM-compatible.

• IMPAIRMENT RATING •

Impairment rating is most often required to resolve the claim of an injured worker. Either the insurance carrier for the employer or the lawyer for the injured worker, or both, will require an impairment rating. Theoretically, an impairment rating is done by an impartial party and is based on anatomic loss or deficits observed and recorded by that party during the evaluation. The combination of findings is summarized and reported as a percent permanent partial impairment of the finger, the hand, the whole extremity, or the whole body. The calculation of that percentage is given very specifically in the American Medical Association's *Guides to Impairment*. The table for the upper extremity spinal nerves is given in Table 5.4. All of this is designed so that a fair evaluation of the patient is possible based on anatomic findings that should be recorded equally by any two examiners.

The exam is often based by the physician, at least in part, on measurements made by the therapist during a recent evaluation. Because the impairment rating can be lengthy if inclusion of joint range of motion, grip and pinch strength, and sensibility must each be measured for several anatomic

TABLE 5.4 IMPAIRMENT OF UPPER EXTREMITY SPINAL NERVES

Nerve	Maximum % Loss of Function due to *Sensory*	Maximum % Loss of Function due to *Motor*	% Upper Extremity *Impairment*
Axillary	5	35	0–38
Long Thoracic	0	15	0–15
Medial Antebrach Cut.	5	0	0–5
Median			
above mid-forearm	40	55	0–73
below mid-forearm			
br. thumb, radial	7	0	0–7
br. thumb, ulnar	0	0–11	
br. index, radial	0	0–5	
br. ring, radial	3	0	0–3
Musculocutaneous	5	25	0–29
Radial			
proximal to triceps	5	55	0–57
distal to triceps	5	40	0–43
Ulnar			
above mid-forearm	10	35	0–42
below mid-forearm	10	25	0–33
br. little, radial	2	0	0–2
br. little ulnar	3	0	0–3

Note: Table adapted by A. Lee Dellon, M.D., from *Guides to Impairment, 3rd Edition,* Table 14, p. 46, of the American Medical Association.

areas (wrist and elbow) or parts (3 fingers), the physician again is often relying on measurements made by the therapist. If the therapist has available a computer-assisted software program, a report is more easily generated. Such a report may or may not allow for adjustments to the basic percentage figure, adjustments due to pain, or the patient's perceived lack of cooperation with the testing procedure.

Impairment based on anatomic findings does not correlate with disability or, necessarily, with hand function. For example, if a professional violinist had the distal phalanx of the left index finger amputated, the *impairment* rating might be 25% of the index finger, 5% of the hand, and 1% of the entire left upper extremity. However, the violinist is 100% *disabled* in his own occupation. Yet, the violinist could carry out virtually every hand *function* required for activities of daily living, and could function in some occupation other than that of violinist (Tarlov, 1991).

The result of an impairment rating, percent impairment, is a value of great economic importance. Insurance carriers will base their monetary award on that percentage. It is, therefore, critical that the instruments used to make the measurements of the degree of anatomic loss be valid and reliable and, if possible, traceable. For example, if a grip strength measurement is 25 kg instead of 35 kg, the degree of ulnar nerve motor function is much more impaired. An instrument such as the dynamometer, which is not self-calibrating and which measures the grip strength at the center of the curved handle instead of across the entire handle, has a good chance of making a major error in measurement.

An attempt to combine anatomic loss with hand function is Millesi's global assessment approach (Deutinger, Girsh, & Burgasser, 1993). His approach gives a numerical score to areas of anatomic loss, such as range of motion and digital length, and combines this with a numerical score for pinch and grip strength, for sensation (two-point discrimination and cutaneous pressure threshold), and for a pick-up test. Individual scores are multiplied by a factor to normalize them. Finally, the global hand assessment score is given a value of up to 10,000 points by multipliers for each subgroup, weighting them. While extremely intensive in terms of measurements and mathematical calculations required, this approach does provide a global picture of

hand function. This technique has been reported on by Deutinger, Girsh, and Burgasser (1933) for patients with median and ulnar nerve injuries, and provided a score sufficiently different for these two different nerve functions that the patients could be distinguished, one group from the other.

An impairment rating is often called a *disability* rating. As defined for the hand, impairment is not disability. In a civil lawsuit, the lawyer for the injured party, the plaintiff's lawyer, may require an impairment rating. He or she may then request

a work analysis, or work-capacity evaluation, for information relating to whether the injured party can, for example, be a motorcycle mechanic. The expert witness testifying must rely on the known correlation of two-point discrimination and threshold testing to know whether the hand is capable of that function. If it is not, then based on valid measurements, the expert can suggest vocational rehabilitation and retraining, and the lawyer or actuary can construct a wage loss estimate related to job description (disability).

• MALINGERING •

Malingering implies that a patient's complaints or symptoms are magnified or exaggerated beyond reality for the purpose of achieving economic gain. This definition would exclude patients with a hysterical personality trait who, by nature, tend to exaggerate. The hysteric has an exaggerated pain response, which must be understood as being distinct from an intention, during an impairment rating, for example, to exaggerate symptoms and minimize voluntary effort during the examination. Of course, the most difficult situation would be attempting to evaluate objectively an injured hysteric at the time of an impairment rating.

Identifying an individual who is malingering can be difficult. After a median nerve injury a patient may state that they have no feeling in their hand. Questioning specifically about the little finger may reveal a real complaint about it not previously identified, requiring further work up, evaluation, and treatment. Or, it may be that the median-innervated side of the hand has such intense discomfort that it just feels as if the whole hand is a problem. A medically knowledgeable malingerer, however, will present a series of complaints that are appropriate. This is one of the rare occasions in which it is necessary to use a sterile #25 needle as a testing instrument. After swabbing the patient's finger

FIGURE 5.4

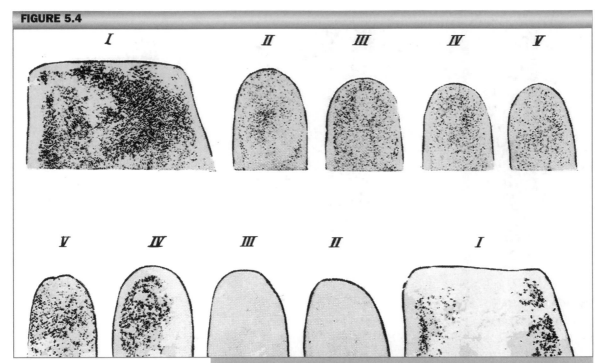

Use of the ninhydrin test to detect malingering. This objective test demonstrates innervation by staining the amino acids present in sweat. Where there are no colored dots, there is no innervation. Conversely, however, the presence of sweating does not correlate with degree of innervation or hand function. The top row of fingerprints is from the noninjured, normal hand. Note that all fingers have black dots, indicating sweat stained with ninhydrin. In contrast, the bottom row shows the fingerprints from a person who has the median nerve cut. The edges of the thumb stain positively because of overlap from the radial sensory nerve. Note that there are no dots in the center of the thumb, on the index and middle fingers, or on the radial half of the ring finger, consistent with the commonest pattern of median nerve innervation of the fingers. From "Methods for Examining Sensibility of the Hand," by E. Moberg, 1966, in Hand Surgery, J. E. Flynn, Editor, Baltimore: Williams & Wilkins. Reprinted with permission of the author.

with alcohol, the proclaimed insensitive finger should be held gently by one of the examiner's hands, while the examiner with the other hand strikes the needle with sufficient force to draw blood into the indicated "anesthetic" finger. The examiner will feel the finger pull back or withdraw when stuck, despite the patient's outward attempt to remain peaceful.

A claim of complete loss of feeling can be objectively examined in three ways. They are: (a) The O'Rain finger wrinkling test. To administer this test, place the anesthetic finger into a bowl of water for 10 minutes. Innervated fingers will wrinkle. (The mechanism for this nonwrinkling is unknown.) (b) Moberg's ninhydrin test.

The patient's fingerprints are placed onto a prepared piece of paper, revealing a pattern reflecting innervated sweat glands. The amino acids in the sweat are absorbed into the paper. The paper is then sprayed with

ninhydrin, which reacts with the amino acids to give colored spots in all areas in which there is innervation. Absence of colored spots occurs where there is denervation (see Figure 5.4). Ninhydrin test results do not correlate with hand function or with the degree of reinnervation following nerve repair. (c) Electrodiagnostic studies. If these show no electrical response from the sensory nerve going to the indicated finger(s), there is support for denervation.

Malingering also can be identified during the motor examination. This is the best way to identify the malingerer because it will be rare for the person being tested to claim complete loss of sensation of the finger. The assumption during motor testing is that the patient consciously will be attempting to give less than the maximal effort during strength testing, that is, during the measurement of grip strength. Lister (1977) observed that while attempting to grip the Jamar dynamometer at its five different positions, a curve results that approximates a bell-shaped curve. If a patient gives maximal effort, the grip strength increases from position 1 (smallest grip) to about position 3 or 4. Thereafter, the strength reduces in positions 4 and 5. In a patient who is malingering the curve is more likely to be flat rather than bell-shaped.

A more detailed analysis of this effect of malingering was done comparing the difference between the dominant and nondominant hand when the dynamometer was alternatively gripped by one hand and then the other. The analysis was complicated and yielded results which were counterintuitive; that is, if the test demonstrated malingering, it was because the difference was positive, meaning a stronger than expected result in the injured hand. Intuitively, the test should show the injured hand of a malingerer to be weaker. A psychophysical explanation of attention paying was used to explain this result. Recently, rapid exchange grip was again suggested to identify malingerers (Joughin et al., 1993). The rapid-exchange grip test can be done now with computer-assisted analysis in real time, giving a printout of the difference between the two hands that enables identification of a malingerer to be more convincingly achieved. I do not believe, however, that a study has been published validating this particular computer-assisted technique with evidence of malingering.

If you do not have rapid-exchange grip software for your computer, but do have a computer-assisted Digit-Grip™ device, malingering also may be detected (see Figure 5.5 A). This demonstration uses the observation that if a person voluntarily tries to grip with a maximum effort with this device, there is a constant relationship between the force generated by the index/middle finger pair and the ring/little finger pair. The relationship is that the force generated by the index/middle finger pair is a little stronger. Therefore, in a hand that is weak, the total force of all fingers will be less than for the opposite hand, and less than predicted for that person's sex/hand dominance, but the relationship between the index/middle finger pair and the ring/little finger pair should still have a constant relationship to each other.

In the malingerer, there will be a reversal of the pattern between the index/middle finger pair and the ring/little finger pair of measurements, and an increase in the variability between the measurements obtained in one hand compared with the other. That is, in the person giving a maximum effort, there should be less than 15% variation between individual grasp measurements, and less than 5% difference between the variability of the left versus the right hand. While this theory also has not been validated, this pattern is easy to detect on the computer printout (see Figure 5.5 B), and should raise the suspicion of malingering if the pattern is detected (Dellon & Muse, unpublished observations). A suggestion for a research protocol to test this hypothesis with the Digit-Grip™ is given in Chapter 20.

FIGURE 5.5

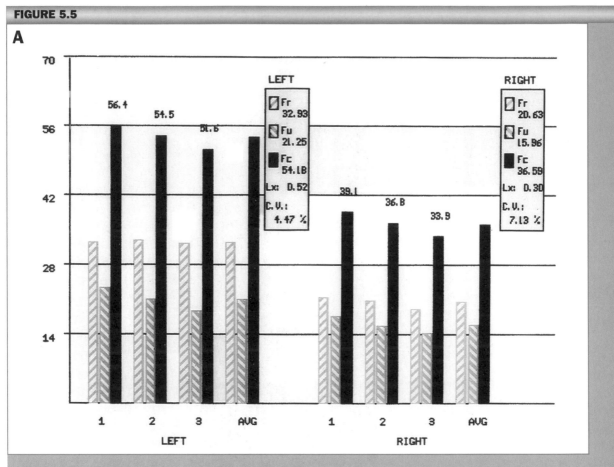

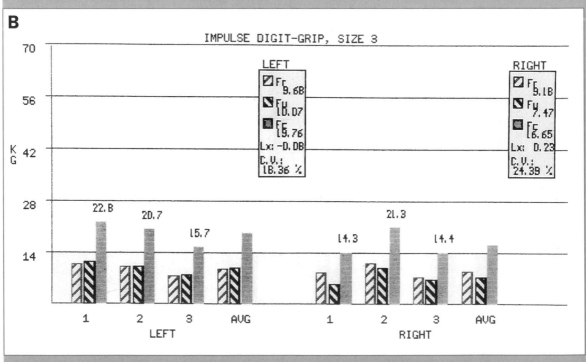

Use of the Impulse Analysis mode of the Digit-Grip™ on the NK Biotechnical computer-assisted testing device to detect malingering. (A) Normal set of measurements. Each grip is represented by three bars. The first bar is the grip from the radial two fingers, the second bar is the grip from the ulnar two fingers, and the third bar, always the tallest, is the summation of the first two bars. Each set of three bars is one grasp. The three grasps are then averaged to give the fourth set of bars. The coefficient of variation for each of the three bars is calculated by the computer. There is usually less than 15% variation within grasps for a given hand, and about 5% difference between the variance of the left versus the right hand when honest effort is made to do the test. Note that the bar height for the radial two fingers is always higher than that for the ulnar two fingers. (B) In a person giving less than their best effort to produce a strong grip, there will be a larger coefficient of variation (> 15.0%) with the height of the bar for the radial two fingers not always being higher than the bar for the ulnar two fingers. When this pattern is present, there is a statistically significant chance (p < .001) that the patient is giving a submaximal effort. Unpublished material with permission from Mitterhauser, Dellon, Muse and Jetzer, 1996.

• REFERENCES •

Baum, C. M., & Edwards, D. F. *From ICV to community: A model for determining effectiveness.* Presented at the American Occupational Therapy Association Annual Meeting, Denver, 1995.

Bell-Krotoski, J. A., & Buford, W. L. The force/time relationships of clinically used sensory testing instruments. *Journal of Hand Therapy 1:*76-81, 1988.

Dellon, A. L. *Evaluation of Sensibility and Re-Education of Sensation in the Hand.* Baltimore: Williams & Wilkins, 1981.

Deutinger, M., Girsh, W., & Burgasser, G. Clinical application of motorsensory differentiated nerve repair. *Microsurgery 14:*297-303, 1993.

Guides to Impairment, 3rd Edition, American Medical Association, Chicago, 1990.

Hardy, M., Jimenez, S., Jabaley, M., & Horch, K. Evaluation of nerve compression with the automated tactile tester. *Journal of Hand Surgery 17A:*838-842, 1992.

Horch, K., Hardy, M., Jimenez, S., & Jabaley, M. An automated tactile tester for evaluation of cutaneous sensibility. *Journal of Hand Surgery 17A:*829-837, 1992.

Joughin, K., Gulati, P. Mackinnon, S. E., McCabe, S., Murray, J. F., Griffiths, S., & Richards, R. An evaluation of rapid exchange and simultaneous grip tests. *Journal of Hand Surgery 18A:*245-252, 1993.

Law, M., & Baum, C. M. *Creating the future: A joint effort.* Health Care Brochure, 1994.

Lister, G. *The Hand: Diagnosis and Indications.* Edinburgh: Churchill Livingstone, 1977.

Moberg, E. Fingers were made before forks. *Hand 4:*201-206, 1972.

Moberg, E. Methods for examining sensibility of the hand. In *Hand Surgery,* J. E. Flynn, Editor. Baltimore: Williams & Wilkins, 1966.

Moberg, E. Objective methods of determining functional value of sensibility in the hand. *Journal of Bone and Joint Surgery (British) 40:*454-466, 1958.

Moberg, E. Reconstructive hand surgery in tetraplegia, stroke and cerebral palsy: Some basic concepts on physiology and neurology. *Journal of Hand Surgery 1:*29-34, 1976.

Novak, C. B., Mackinnon, S. E., & Kelly, L. Correlation of two-point discrimination and hand function following median nerve injury. *Annals of Plastic Surgery 31:*495-498, 1993.

Novak, C. B., Mackinnon, S. E., Williams, J. I., & Kelly, L. Establishment of reliability in the evaluation of hand sensibility. *Plastic and Reconstructive Surgery 92:*312-322, 1993.

Tarlov, A. R. *Disability in America: Towards a National Agenda for Prevention.* Washington, DC: National Academy Press, 1991.

• ADDITIONAL READINGS •

Bell-Krotoski, J. A. Light touch-deep pressure testing using Semmes-Weinstein monofilaments. In *Rehabilitation of the Hand: Surgery and Therapy,* J. M. Hunter, L. H. Schneider, E. J. Mackin, & A. D. Callahan, Editors. St. Louis: Mosby, 1990.

Bell-Krotoski, J. A., & Tomancik, E. The repeatability of testing with Semmes-Weinstein monofilaments. *Journal of Hand Surgery 12A:*155-161, 1987.

Dellon, A. L. A numerical grading scale for peripheral nerve function. *Journal of Hand Therapy 6:*152-160, 1993.

Dellon, A. L., & Kallman, C. H. Evaluation of functional sensation in the hand. *Journal of Hand Surgery 8:*865-870, 1983.

Dellon, A. L., & Muse, V. Detection of malingering using the impulse mode of the NK Digit-Grip. *Journal of Hand Surgery,* submitted: 1995.

Dellon, E. S., Crone, S., Mourey, R., & Dellon, A. L. Comparison of the Semmes-Weinstein monofilaments with the Pressure-Specified Sensory Device. *Restorative Neurology Neuroscience 5:*323-326, 1993.

Dellon, E. S., & Dellon, A. L. Quantitative sensory testing with the force-defined vibrometer. *Journal of Reconstructive Microsurgery,* in press: 1995.

Dellon, E. S., Keller, K., Moratz, V., & Dellon, A. L., Validation of cutaneous pressure threshold measurements for the evaluation of hand function. *Plastic and Reconstructive Surgery,* in press: 1995.

Dellon, E. S., Mourey, R., & Dellon, A. L. Human pressure perception values for constant and moving one- and two-point discrimination. *Plastic and Reconstructive Surgery 90:*112-117, 1992.

Fess, E. E. Documentation: Essential elements of an upper extremity assessment battery. In *Rehabilitation of the Hand: Surgery and Therapy,* J. M. Hunter, L. H. Schneider, E. J. Mackin, & A. D. Callahan, Editors. St. Louis: Mosby, 1985.

Kendall, H. O., & Kendall, F. P. *Muscles: Testing and Function.* Baltimore: Williams & Wilkins, 1949.

Levin, S., Pearsall, G., & Ruderman, R. J. von Frey's method of measuring pressure sensibility in the hand: An engineering analysis of the Weinstein-Semmes pressure aesthesiometer. *Journal of Hand Surgery 3:*211-216, 1978.

MacDermid, J. C., Kramer, J. F., Woodbury, M. G., McFarlane, R. M., & Roth, J. H. Interrater reliability of pinch and grip strength measurements in patients with cumulative trauma disorders. *Journal of Hand Therapy 7:*10-14, 1994.

Mackinnon, S. E., & Dellon, A. L. Two-point discrimination tester. *Journal of Hand Surgery 10:*906-907, 1985.

Mathiowetz, V., Weber, K., & Volland, G. Reliability and validity of grip and pinch strength evaluations. *Journal of Hand Surgery 9:*222-226, 1984.

Research Plan for the National Center for Medical Rehabilitation on Research. National Institutes of Health Publication #93-3509, 1993.

Seddon, H. J. Peripheral nerve injuries. *Medical Research Council, Special Report Series 282.* London: Her Majesty's Stationery Office, 1954.

Shrout, P. E., & Fleiss, J. L. Intraclass correlation coefficient: Uses in assessing rater reliability. *Psychology Bulletin 86:*420-428, 1979.

• • •

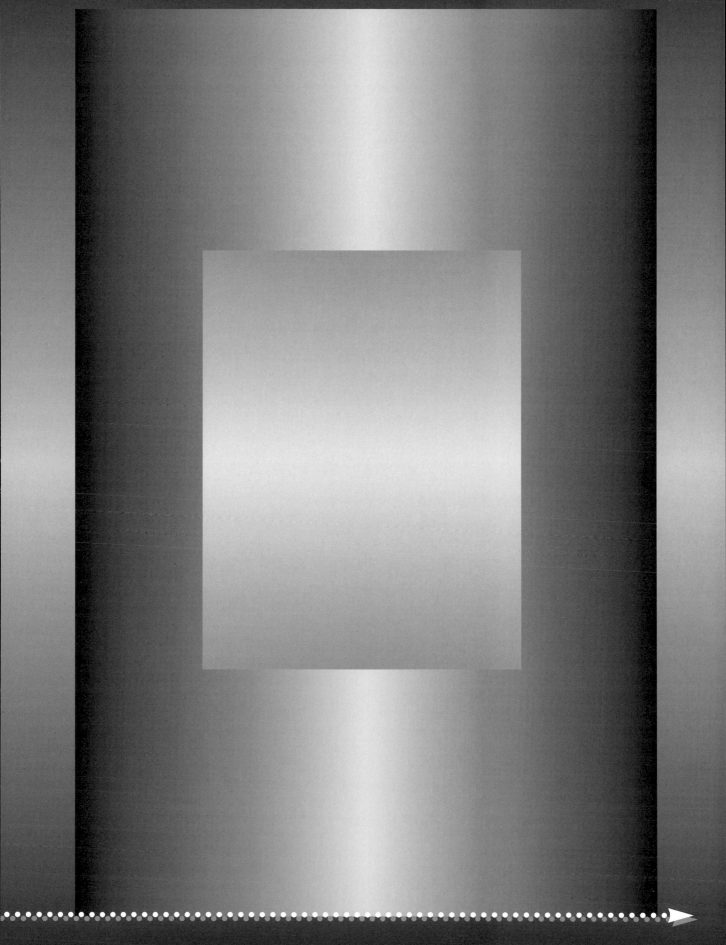

6

threshold versus innervation density

• HISTORICAL PERSPECTIVE •

Around 1905, the widespread concept of sensibility testing concerned examination of the skin as if it were composed of individual spots or points, each of which had its own unique quality of sensation. This concept is evident even in words chosen by the German researcher von Frey, who called the touch spots *Druckepuncte,* or pressure points (see Figure 6.1). This led him to develop touch hairs. To quantitate the ability to perceive touch, he chose hairs of different sizes. The finest hair that could be perceived by the subject being tested was the one chosen to define that area of the skin's touch threshold. Von Frey noted that a thicker hair was no longer perceived as touch but as pain, and he developed a series of graded pain hairs.

In contrast was the histological observation that there were nets of nerves in the dermis, and scattered sensory corpuscles throughout the dermis. The nerve networks were thought to be responsible for so-called *protopathic,* or diffuse, sensation. The fine nerve terminals and their receptors were thought to be responsible for so-called *epicritic* sensation, the ability to make distinctions or to discriminate. *Threshold* was considered to be the relationship of a nerve fiber to its *receptor,* or mechanical transduction system. About 70 years earlier, in 1835, Weber had described the ability to distinguish

FIGURE 6.1

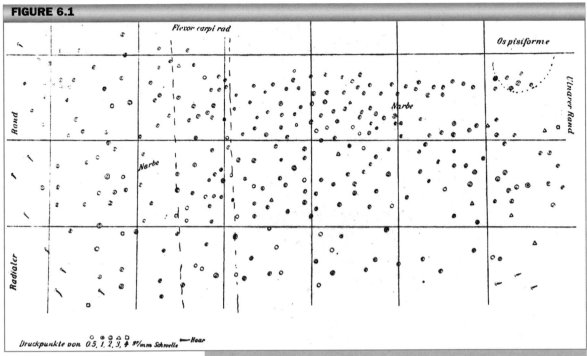

Pattern of skin touch spots as mapped by von Frey. This concept gave use to our present-day threshold testing. Historically the instrumentation has gone from human hairs glued to a candle, to hairs glued to wood, to nylon filaments of varying diameters, to single-diameter metal probes linked by a force transducer to a computer. *From* Evaluation of Sensibility and Re-education of Sensation in the Hand, *by A. L. Dellon, 1981, Baltimore: Williams & Wilkins. Reprinted with permission of the author.*

one point from two points touching the skin, but this observation was not incorporated into von Frey's theory of sensibility testing. Indeed, neurologists tended to think that two-point discrimination was a central processing function related to the cerebral cortex. Even today, neurologists often equate this function with *stereognosis*, the ability to identify a shape just by touching it.

The distance at which two points are distinguished as one traditionally has not been considered a threshold. As the area of skin innervated by a single nerve fiber was defined by electrophysiological studies, it became evident that the individual nerve fibers innervate a specific territory that overlaps the territory of the adjacent

nerve. Mountcastle (1968) called this the concept of partially shifted, overlapping, peripheral receptive fields (see Figure 6.2). It was thought that this overlap of nerve territories could be the basis for two-point discrimination, rather than for a relationship between a nerve fiber and its receptor. The number of nerve fibers innervating a given area of skin was called the *innervation density*. It was observed that two-point discrimination was best; that is, two points

could be distinguished as two points at a smaller distance between the points in places where innervation density was highest, like the lip and the fingertip, and was poorest where innervation density was lowest, like the back.

I found it convenient to distinguish the concept of threshold from that of innervation density, and did so in my first book, *Evaluation of Sensibility and Re-education of Sensation in the Hand* (1981). The separation of threshold and innervation density fa-

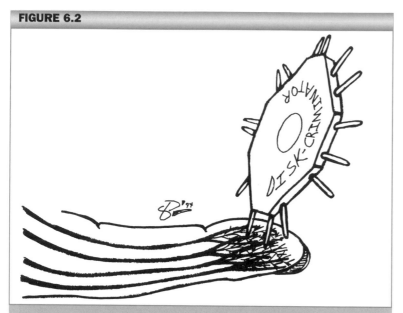

FIGURE 6.2

Pattern of skin territories innervated by individual nerves in a fingertip. This pattern has been defined by electrophysiologic testing. Note that the territories are overlapping. The interplay of impulses stimulated by two simultaneous touch stimuli can be distinguished from a one-touch stimulus. This requires both an intact peripheral nerve and cortical interpretation. Two-point discrimination is better in an area like the fingertip than the back and is, therefore, also related to the number of nerve fibers innervating a given area, or innervation density. Drawing by Glenn George Dellon. Reprinted with permission.

cilitated teaching clinical neurophysiology, and facilitated dividing tests into those clinically useful for early stages of disease and those useful for advanced stages. The correlation of sensory receptors with a neurophysiologically defined subgroup of nerve fibers yielded a nerve fiber/receptor combination, like the Meissner corpuscle/quickly-adapting fiber group, which could be defined for threshold by vibratory perception and innervation density by the moving two-point dis-

crimination test. Similarly, there was the Merkel cell neurite complex/slowly-adapting fiber group, which could be defined for threshold by the cutaneous pressure perception and for in-

nervation density by the static two-point discrimination test. The phrase "two-point discrimination" was never described in the literature as a threshold test. The utility of this dualization for teaching is apparent in Figure 6.3.

A disadvantage of the dualization of testing terminology is that it has permitted confusion, if not actual controversy. It is debated, for example, whether it is more appropriate to evaluate the patient with a chronic nerve compression, like carpal tunnel syndrome, with threshold testing or with a test of innervation density. It is clear today, especially with the advent of new instrumentation like the Pressure-Specified Sensory Device™, that it is most appropriate to use both tests. That is because it is understood that the pathophysiology of chronic nerve compression causes a continuum of symptoms and changing physical findings, depending on how severe the compression has become. Furthermore, as will be made clear at the end of this chapter, two-point discrimination is also a threshold test.

● INNERVATION DENSITY ●

It has been clear since Moberg's work in 1958 that abnormal static two-point discrimination correlates with hand function. Moberg defined hand function as static grips, and static two-point discrimination less than 6 mm correlated with the ability to do a precision sensory grip, such as holding a sewing needle. A static two-point discrimination greater than 30 mm correlated only with the ability to grasp

FIGURE 6.3

The relationship between threshold and innervation density can be conceived as a classroom situation in which the student (sensory receptor) has a relationship with the chair (nerve fiber). (A) Normally this relationship is a happy one, all receptors are functioning perfectly, and all nerve fibers are present, resulting in normal innervation density. (B) After listening to the lecture for a period of time, some students are losing interest and falling asleep, but all are still present in the classroom, resulting in abnormal cutaneous threshold with a normal innervation density. With the threshold higher, the teacher must speak in a louder voice to stimulate the student. If a new student tries to sit anywhere in the room, that student will be Immediately detected, because there are no empty seats. (C) By the end of the lecture, not only have students fallen asleep, some are angry at the teacher's comments and some have left the room, resulting in abnormal cutaneous threshold and abnormal innervation density. The teacher must speak very loudly or in a different manner to stimulate the students now. If a new student enters the room, that student's presence might go totally unnoticed because there are so many empty seats. From "Double and Multiple 'Crush' Syndromes," by S.E. Mackinnon, 1992, Hand Clinics 8:369-390. Reprinted with permission of the author.

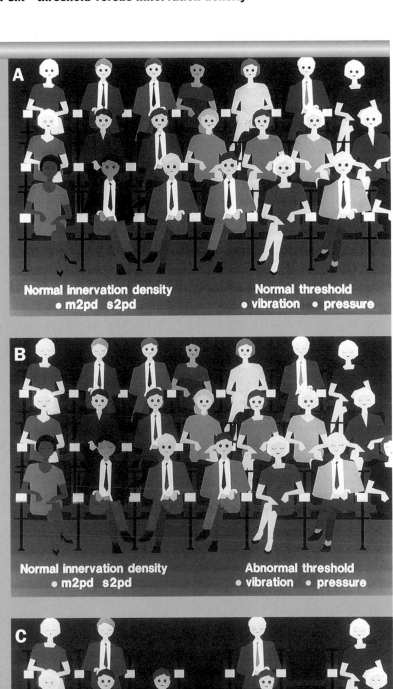
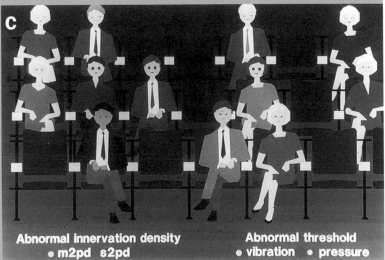

FIGURE 6.4

Correlation of moving two-point discrimination with hand function. Hand function, as measured with a timed object recognition test, best correlated with moving two-point discrimination (p < .001). From "Evaluation of Functional Sensation in the Hand," by A. L. Dellon & C. H. Kallman, 1983, Journal of Hand Surgery 8:865-870, Churchill Livingstone, New York. Reprinted with permission of the authors.

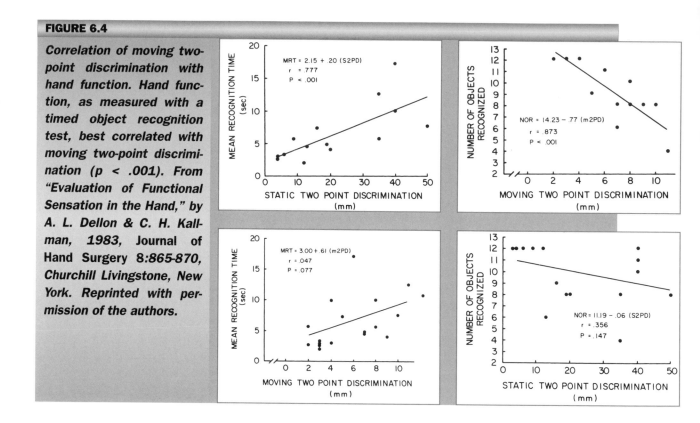

a bottle for pouring, or an ax handle for chopping wood. Moberg found that only Weber's (1835) classic, static two-point discrimination test could predict the patient's ability to do a blindfolded pick-up test successfully. Moberg used no statistical analysis, and his number of patients was small, about 10. But his observations have withstood the test of time, requiring only some modification as our understanding of neurophysiology improved. In 1972, A. L. Dellon attempted a rationalization for Moberg's neurological testing observations by suggesting that static two-point discrimination was mediated by slowly-adapting nerve fibers,

which subserve the perception of static-touch and pressure, the qualities necessary for precision sensory grip.

As two-point discrimination testing spread in popularity it was natural for exceptions to be identified; that is, individuals were tested who, while having little, if any, static two-point discrimination, could still do the pick-up test. This paradox was resolved in 1978 by Dellon's description of the moving two-point discrimination test. In this test, the two points are moved longitudinally and apart from each other toward the fingertip. This stimulates the quickly-adapting fiber/receptors, which in the finger outnumber the slowly-adapting

group by 2 or 3 to 1. If patients recovered the ability to distinguish two points moving before they could distinguish two static points, then static two-point discrimination would underestimate the level of sensibility and, therefore, underestimate the true ability of the hand to function.

In fact, moving two-point discrimination recovers earlier than static two-point discrimination, probably because of the increased ease of reinnervation of the Meissner corpuscle than of the Merkel cell neurite complex. This observation has been observed consistently by many investigators since 1978, and moving two-point discrimination testing has

FIGURE 6.5

Correlation of Ridge Device with hand function. (A) The Ridge Device most closely resembles the measurement of moving two-point discrimination and is, therefore, expected to correlate with hand function. Here, static two-point discrimination is correlated with the Ridge Device (see Figure 6.4). (B) Lack of correlation of hand function with Semmes-Weinstein monofilament testing. From "Recovery of Sensibility After Suture of Digital Nerves," by N. K. Poppen, H. K. McCarroll, Jr., & J. Doyle, 1979, Journal of Hand Surgery 4:212-226, Churchill Livingstone, New York. Reprinted with permission of the authors.

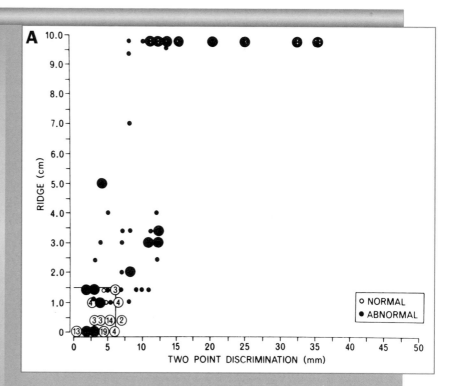

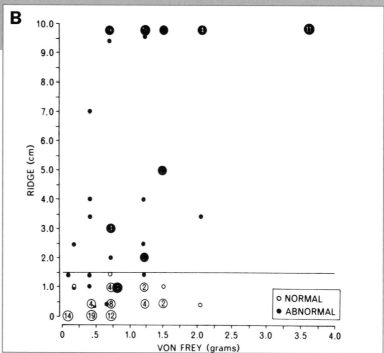

become required as the standard for end-result assessment after nerve repair, nerve grafting, or reconstruction with innervated soft tissue flaps.

With regard to hand function, in 1983 Dellon and Kallman repeated Moberg's 1958 study, but this time statistically correlated a timed object identification test with measurements of cutaneous pressure threshold (Semmes-Weinstein monofilaments), vibratory threshold (Biothesiometer, 120 Hz), and static and moving two-point discrimination. Only the measurements of innervation density correlated with hand function (see Figure 6.4).

This observation has been confirmed by other investigators (see Figures 6.5 and 6.6). I am unaware of any

published study that demonstrates that cutaneous pressure threshold testing with the Semmes-Weinstein

FIGURE 6.6

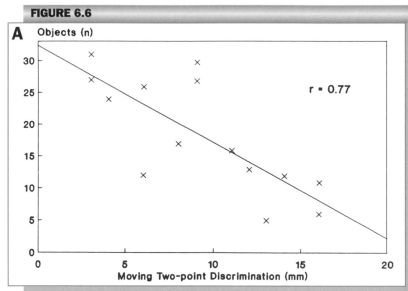

A. Objects (n) vs. Moving Two-point Discrimination (mm). r = 0.77

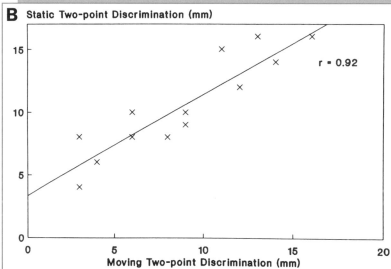

B. Static Two-point Discrimination (mm) vs. Moving Two-point Discrimination (mm). r = 0.92

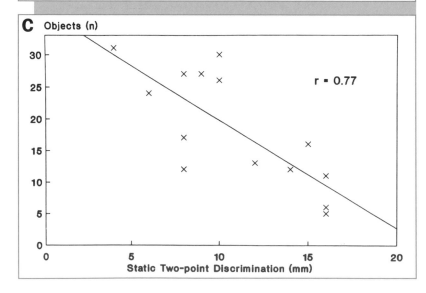

C. Objects (n) vs. Static Two-point Discrimination (mm). r = 0.77

Correlation of two-point discrimination with hand function after median nerve grafting. (A) Moving two-point discrimination. (B) Static two-point discrimination. (C) Correlation of moving and static two-point discrimination measurements. The r value is the Spearman rank correlation, and for r = .77 the p < .005, and for r = .92 the p < .0001. From "Sensory Recovery After Median Nerve Grafting," by C. B. Novak, L. Kelly, & S. E. Mackinnon, 1992, Journal of Hand Surgery 17A:59-66, Churchill Livingstone, New York. Reprinted with permission of the authors.

monofilaments correlates with hand function.

As our concepts of chronic nerve compression have evolved from basic science models, histology, and close clinical observation, it has become clear that early in nerve compression there are only physiologic changes, such as changes in the blood nerve barrier, creating endoneurial edema. With more time, there are changes in myelination; that is, there is thinning. It is not until late in chronic nerve compression that there is loss of nerve fibers. This provides the basis for classifying some of the observations on sensibility testing in clinical conditions like the carpal, cubital, or tarsal tunnel syndromes.

Clearly, if two-point discrimination (as measured in mm) is related to number of nerve fibers, and nerve fibers are not lost until late in the natural history of nerve compression, then measuring two-point discrimination with a paper clip or a Disk-Criminator™ will not be found to be abnormal until late in the disease process. Measuring changes in pressure perception or vibratory perception should identify the problem earlier. This was demonstrated in the first report of the use of the Biothesiometer for vibratory testing in patients with carpal and cubital tunnel syndrome by Dellon in 1983. Using traditional instruments for two-point discrimination testing as a screening test for chronic nerve compression would, therefore, only identify patients with advanced disease, that is, those who could not be helped by job modification or splinting, but who required surgical decompression. In my everyday office practice, tuning fork stimulation has been a reliable test to screen for early nerve compression. However, tuning fork testing is qualitative. Cutaneous pressure threshold testing theoretically would become abnormal before the traditional measurement of two-point discrimination; that is, Semmes-Weinstein monofilaments should detect a carpal tunnel syndrome patient before a Disk-Criminator™ would. As

will be seen later in this chapter, the Pressure-Specified Sensory Device™ combines the unique qualities required to resolve this problem. The first parameter to become abnormal with chronic nerve compression is the pressure required to discriminate one from two point static touch.

The theoretical and practical objection to innervation density is that there has been no way to define either how hard the examiner should press the instrument against the skin, or how hard the examiner in fact pressed the instrument against the skin to obtain the distance in millimeters that two points could be distinguished as two. Moberg's (1958, 1962) recommendation was to press only hard enough to cause the skin to blanch. It has never been determined what pressure is required to do this. Should that degree of pressure vary based on skin thickness, sympathetic

tone to the blood vessels, alcohol usage, or ambient room temperature, all of which may theoretically alter the amount of pressure necessary for skin blanching?

Moberg also was concerned that pressure greater than that required for skin blanching causes a depression of the skin, extending the stimulus to other areas of the fingertip beyond the two points. Yet our goal, as Moberg himself wrote, is to learn "what does the finger feel?" In his last writings, Moberg constructed a small device with a weight on it that would apply the two points at a given pressure (Moberg, 1990). Clearly the goal is to have an instrument capable of specifying the pressure at which two-point discrimination occurs. This instrument, the Pressure-Specified Sensory Device™, exists and permits unification of the threshold versus innervation density controversy.

• THRESHOLD •

A threshold separates two different regions, a region of perception from a region of lack of perception. A threshold is a physical property that can be measured in response to a defined stimulus. In general, the threshold is a point along a continuum or physical spectrum below which there is no detection of an event's existence, and above which there is awareness of the event's existence. The threshold may not always be the same for each person experiencing the stimulus. Consider, for example, selecting the wavelength of light that defines the color called red. If a color chart from white to black were shown, and the chart contained 20 regions of color separation defined by a different wavelength, for example, yellow, yellow-orange, orange, orange-red, red, red-purple, purple, and so forth, then different observers might choose as "red" slightly different shades.

The more separates we could give them from which to choose, the closer together the wavelength choices of the different observers would be, even though there would always be some range of wavelengths they would call red. Therefore, a strategy must be used for presenting the color choices to the subjects, and then statistical analysis must be applied to describe the threshold. For the color spectrum, again as an example, the colors might be presented in sequence going from white *up to* red, and then passing red after the selection had been made and going, thereafter, in the reverse fashion *down from* blue to purple to red. This type of strategy, approaching the threshold from both extremes, is termed the *method of limits*. For the method of limits, the process might be repeated 5 times and the high and low wavelengths given by the subject discarded, and then the middle three values averaged to give a mean wavelength as the threshold for red for that individual.

If this were done for a group of individuals of varying ages, an age-related set of thresholds would be determined. As eyes "get weaker" as one gets older, it is conceivable that the thresh-

old might change for red. Certainly, this is the situation for the vibratory threshold. It has been demonstrated repeatedly that the vibratory threshold goes up with age. It is also known that the number of Meissner corpuscles decreases with age, and this may be the basis for that age-related cutaneous vibratory threshold observation.

Another definition of threshold defines the threshold for a physical stimulus as the point at which the subject can detect the event 50% of the time. In this strategy, the wavelength would be presented in ascending grade with the subject being given only two choices—to say that the wavelength being presented is or is not red. Such a strategy is termed a *forced choice*. In forced-choice testing, the stimulus intensity is increased until it is detected, then reverses, and the subject indicates again when it is detected, then it reverses going up, then down, etcetera, for a total usually of 7 times. The values at the turning points are then averaged, and the mean is taken to be the threshold value. In general, forced-choice alternatives require greater time for the testing procedure, and usually a computer-driven stimulus intensity device. The numerical value given as the threshold may never be any of the values given by the subject because the threshold is the value at

which the subject will detect the event 50% of the time.

Detection of an event, such as perception of a constant-touch stimulus, should be measured, ideally, by a device that can record continuous values for the given stimulus. That is, a probe of a *single* defined shape would be brought into contact with the skin surface with the least possible force, and that force gradually would be increased until the stimulus is perceived. An increasing constant-touch stimulus is perceived as increasing pressure. The threshold value could be expressed as the distance the skin was indented, that is, microns of skin displacement (as is measured by the Automated Tactile Tester™), as the force applied to the skin, that is, milligrams (as is done by the Semmes-Weinstein monofilaments and the WEST™), or as the pressure applied, that is, gm/mm^2 (as is measured with the Pressure-Specified Sensory Device™) (see Chapter 7 for a description of these instruments).

The Automated Tactile Tester™ and the Pressure-Specified Sensory Device™ each measure the variable continuously through the desired range of pressure. In contrast, the Semmes-Weinstein monofilaments and the WEST™ do not measure the variable continuously. Rather, each filament in the set applies a stimulus force that ranges from 0 to the upper limit determined by the filament's thickness, that is, its

TABLE 6.1   MONOFILAMENT TESTING OF CUTANEOUS PRESSURE-PERCEPTION: ESTIMATE OF A RANGE, NOT A THRESHOLD MEASUREMENT

Semmes-Weinstein Filament Number Marking	Calculated Upper Limit of Pressure[+]	Estimate of Range[*]
2.83	4.9	
		5.0 to 17.7
3.61	17.7	
		17.8 to 33.1
4.31	33.1	
		33.2 to 107
5.46	107	
		107.1 to 337
6.45	337	

Note:

[+] In g/mm^2.

[*] Range of pressures possible for detection if this filament is the lowest numbered filament the patient is able to detect in g/mm^2.

From "von Frye's Method of Measuring Pressure Sensibilities in the Hand: An Engineering Analysis of the Semmes-Weinstein Pressure Aesthesiometer," by S. Levin, G. Pearsall, & R. J. Ruderman, 1978, *Journal of Hand Surgery 3:*211-216.

cross-sectional area. The actual threshold may be anywhere less than the stimulus value, but not greater. By using a series of filaments, each of a different thickness, intervals or ranges are created between the filament values. Thus, the correct statement is that the Semmes-Weinstein monofilaments and the WEST™ do not measure, but rather give an estimate of, a range for the cutaneous pressure threshold for static-touch (see Table 6.1 and Figure 7.19 D).

A further theoretical prob-lem for the Semmes-Wein-stein monofilaments is that each filament has a *different* cross-sectional area and, therefore, each filament pre-sents two different stimuli to the subject each time he or she is tested; that is, there is a difference in force and a difference in surface area stimulated. A different sur-face area implies a different number of sensory receptors. Thus, the Semmes-Weinstein monofilaments do not fit the definition of a test of thresh-old, as stated in the opening paragraph of this section.

In contrast to the Semmes-Weinstein monofilaments, the Pressure-Specified Senso-ry Device™ has a single, shaped, constant probe stim-ulating tip so that only the force variable is changed throughout the stimulus pe-riod. In contrast to both the Semmes-Weinstein monofila-ments and the WEST™, this new device measures the threshold continuously from 0.1-100 g/mm^2. Furthermore, the threshold for both con-stant-touch and moving-touch stimuli can be measured. This ability is necessary for evaluating neural regeneration, in which the Meissner corpuscles are the first to be reinnervated, providing the perception of movement and low frequency vibration, that is, one-point moving-touch threshold.

• UNIFICATION •

It is time for a clinically comprehensive approach to sensibility testing to incorporate both threshold and innervation density tests in a conceptually inclusive, noncompetitive theory. It is time for *unification*. For politicians, unification hopes to bring a better situation to both halves of a divided country, or a settlement of differences between two warring factions. It is hoped that both sides of a political settlement feel they have been treated equally, each gaining some advantage for the concessions they must make. Similarly, unification of sensibility testing will provide a conceptual framework within which the proponents of threshold and the proponents of innervation density testing will each make a concession, gain an advantage, and hopefully do peaceful sensibility testing and teaching evermore.

The first phase of unification is to appreciate that the traditional test of innervation density, two-point discrimination is, in reality, a threshold measurement. The distance given in millimeters for either static or moving two-point discrimination is the threshold for detecting that two discrete points are being distinguished from one point. When two points are very close together, below the threshold for detecting two discrete points, they are perceived as just one point. As the two points are spread apart a little and approach the threshold, they may be perceived as a wide bar. Then, at the threshold, two points can clearly be perceived as two points. Thereafter, regardless of how far apart they are, they are always perceived as two points. Furthermore, traditionally, a wide distance is chosen and the distance progressively decreased, with the stimulus alternating between one or two points and the patient being given only a choice of answering 1 or 2. As the detection distance is passed, progressing toward a smaller distance between the points, the test is repeated again in this range until the patient gives the correct answer. At this distance of detection, the patient must give correct answers 3 out of 5 or 7 out of 10 times, depending on the degree of certainty required for this information.

There is no reason why two-point discrimination testing should not be considered threshold testing. The early literature referred to the *two-point limen*, where limen is a word

suitable to substitute for threshold. However, it never entered common usage. I have always written and taught about two-point discrimination as being related to innervation density, not as a threshold. It was convenient to consider testing devices with a single probe, like the Semmes-Weinstein monofilaments for pressure and the Biothesiometer for vibration, as instruments that measured threshold, in contrast to those with two probes that measured innervation density. It is time for me to change my writing and teaching. The availability, in 1989, of the Pressure-Specified Sensory Device™ brought the realization that the pressure required to measure the distance at which one from two points is distinguished was possible.

On careful consideration, I had always pressed sufficiently hard for the patient to perceive that two points were being used, although previously I was unable to record that pressure. In fact, it was noted as early as 1865, in the writings of Silas Weir Mitchell, the Civil War neurologist, that the soldiers with a nerve injury might move the finger or press it harder into the testing device for the Weber two-point discrimination test. The clinical implication of this activity on the patient's part was that, given the chance to obtain more information pertinent to the brain's task of detecting two points, the patient

FIGURE 6.7

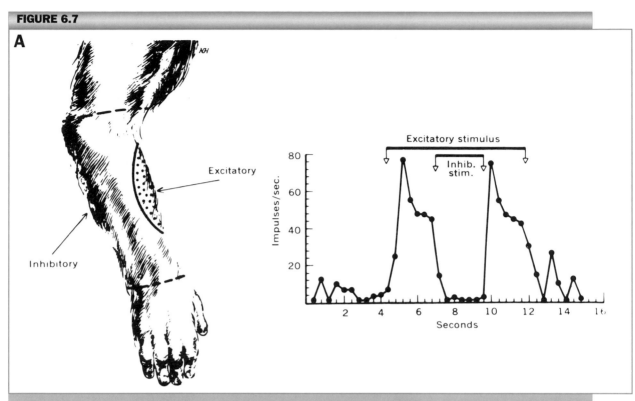

A

Excitatory

Inhibitory

Excitatory stimulus

Inhib. stim.

80

60

40

20

Impulses/sec.

2   4   6   8   10   12   14   16

Seconds

Theoretical model for two-point discrimination in which (A) stimulation of an area of skin inhibits impulses generated in surrounding skin. (B) This inhibition clarifies what otherwise would have been a large mound of data into two separate peaks. From "Neural Mechanisms Subserving Cutaneous Sensibility with Special Reference to the Role of Afferent Inhibition in Sensory Perception and Discrimination," by V. B. Mountcastle and T. P. S. Powell, 1959, Bulletin of Johns Hopkins Hospital 105:201-232. Reprinted with permission of the authors.

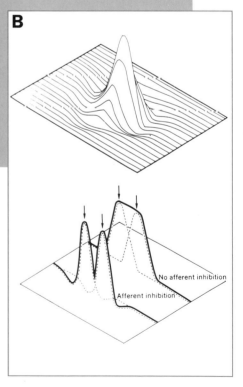

B

No afferent inhibition

Afferent inhibition

sought information from movement and from increased pressure. In other words, the information related to distinguishing one point from two points required input related to distance *and* pressure. The testing strategy for the use of the Pressure-Specified Sensory Device™ is given in Chapter 7.

The neurophysiologic basis for two-point discrimination is still unclear. The observation remains valid that where two-point discrimination is best, there are more nerve fibers. Another insight into the neurophysiologic mechanism comes from the observation that stimulation of one area of skin can cause a central (cortical) inhibition of impulses. This was described by Mountcastle (1968) (see Figure 6.7) to explain the transformation of a huge amount of information into peaks and a trough or, if you will, two points. It is conceivable, today, that greater clarification of the impulse signal is given by increasing the firing rate of the nerve fibers in the area by increasing stimulus intensity, that is, by pressing harder. It is probably best understood that innervation density is the necessary, but not sufficient, variable required for two-point discrimination.

In addition to innervation density, the stimulus intensity is required, as well as cortical processing and interpretation, to have two-point discrimination. Chapter 20 will discuss research projects designed to elucidate these mechanisms, and the relationship between pressure and distance in two-point discrimination testing. It is interesting that being able to describe two-point discrimination now in terms of distance and pressure permits three-dimensional graphing, an example of which is given in Figure 7.20 (C) and (D). Such graphing may permit further analysis of the information available through the Pressure- Specified Sensory Device™.

The second phase of unification of threshold and innervation density concerns the traditional description of the pathophysiologic process of chronic nerve compression. Our current understanding of chronic nerve compression is based on basic science models, histologic

examination of animal and human peripheral nerves that have been compressed, and clinical examination of the nerves that are compressed (Mackinnon, Dellon, Hudson, & Hunter, 1984, 1985; Mackinnon & Dellon, 1986; Dellon & Mackinnon, 1987). There exists a continuum beginning with symptoms without signs. These include intermittent numbness and a normal examination, with the exception of positive Tinel's sign, a positive pressure provocative test, positive Phalen's sign, or positive elbow flexion sign.

The next degree of compression gives symptoms plus signs of threshold change. These include intermittent numbness with increased threshold for pressure and vibration, and weakness of the profundus to the little finger, in the case of the cubital tunnel syndrome. The final degree of compression will have symptoms plus signs of abnormal innervation density. These include persistent numbness, abnormal two-point discrimination, and muscle atrophy. These categories would correspond to minimal, moderate, and severe degrees of nerve compression (see Chapter 9 on numerical grading scales).

Traditional teaching would state that two-point discrimination testing is only abnormal in the advanced degree of nerve compression. I hypothesized, there-

fore, that when the Pressure-Specified Sensory Device™ was used to evaluate patients with chronic nerve compression, the first variable (of the ones this device could measure) to become abnormal was going to be the one-point static or one-point moving touch. I theorized, further, that the next variable to change would be the pressure required to distinguish one from two points and that, finally, when nerve fibers had died, the two-point discrimination distance would change. A study of 125 carpal tunnel syndrome and 71 cubital tunnel syndrome patients who had quantitative sensory testing was analyzed for the sequence in which the four parameters measurable with the Pressure-Specified Sensory Device™ changed (Dellon & Keller, 1995). The study demonstrated, contrary to my hypothesis, that the first parameter to become abnormal with chronic nerve compression was the *pressure* threshold (g/mm^2) for static two-point discrimination. This occurred while the *distance* for discriminating one from two points remained normal, that is, 3-4 mm. The cutaneous pressure thresholds for one-point static and one-point moving touch stimuli were often normal when the pressure threshold for distinguishing one from two static points was already abnormal.

An independent study

(Tassler & Dellon, 1995) found that this same order of touch submodality thresholds became abnormal in patients with tarsal tunnel syndrome and compression of the peroneal nerve at the fibular head. Therefore, the unification of the traditional description of sensory testing must be restated now: The earliest change that can be detected in chronic nerve compression is the pressure required to distinguish one from two static points touching the skin.

The third phase of unification of traditional testing is to recognize that of all available devices to measure cutaneous pressure threshold, the one that is best is reliable, valid, and capable of measuring all aspects of the perception of cutaneous pressure perception. This one is the Pressure-Specified Sensory Device™. Under unification, independent measurement of cutaneous pressure threshold with the Semmes-Weinstein monofilaments or the WEST™ or the Disk-Criminator™ are clearly inferior to computer-assisted sensorimotor testing with the Pressure-Specified Sensory Device™.

• • •

• REFERENCES •

Dellon, A. L. *Evaluation of Sensibility and Re-education of Sensation in the Hand.* Baltimore: Williams and Wilkins, 1981.

Dellon, A. L. The vibrometer. *Plastic and Reconstructive Surgery 71:*427-431, 1983.

Dellon, A. L., & Kallman, C. H. Evaluation of functional sensation in the hand. *Journal of Hand Surgery 8:*865-870, 1983.

Dellon, A. L., & Keller, K. Cutaneous pressure threshold measurement in carpal and cubital tunnel syndrome. *Annals of Plastic Surgery 38:* 493-502, 1997.

Dellon, A. L., Mackinnon, S. E., & Crosby, P. M. Reliability of two-point discrimination measurements. *Journal of Hand Surgery 12A:*693-696, 1987.

Dellon, E. S., Mourey, R., & Dellon, A. L. Human pressure perception values for constant and moving one- and two-point discrimination. *Plastic and Reconstructive Surgery 90:*112-117, 1992.

Levin, S., Pearsall, G., Ruderman, R. J. von Frye's method of measuring pressure sensibility in the hand: An engineering analysis of the Weinstein-Semmes pressure aesthesiometer. *Journal of Hand Surgery 3:*211-216, 1978.

Mackinnon, S. E. Double and multiple "crush" syndromes. *Hand Clinics 8:*369-390, 1992.

Mackinnon, S. E., & Dellon, A. L. Experimental study of chronic nerve compression: Clinical implications. *Clinics of Hand Surgery 2:*639-650, 1986.

Mackinnon, S. E., Dellon, A. L., Hudson, A. R., & Hunter, D. A. A primate model for chronic nerve compression. *Journal of Reconstructive Microsurgery 1:*185-194, 1985.

Mackinnon, S. E., Dellon, A. L., Hudson, A. R., & Hunter, D. A. Chronic nerve compression—An experimental model in the rat. *Annals of Plastic Surgery 13:*112-120, 1984.

Mitchell, S. W. *Injuries of Nerves and their Consequences.* American Academy of Neurology Reprint Series. New York: Dover, 1965.

Moberg, E. Criticism in study of methods for examining sensibility in the hand. *Neurology (Minneapolis) 12:*8-19, 1962.

Moberg, E. Objective methods of determining functional value of sensibility in the skin. *Journal of Bone and Joint Surgery (British) 40B:*454-466, 1958.

Moberg, E. Two-point discrimination test. *Scandinavian Journal of Rehabilitation Medicine 22:*127-134, 1990.

Mountcastle, V. B. *Medical Physiology.* St. Louis: C. V. Mosby Company, chapters 61-63, 1968.

Mountcastle, V. B., & Powell, T. P. S. Neural mechanisms subserving cutaneous sensibility with special reference to the role of afferent inhibition in sensory perception and discrimination. *Bulletin of Johns Hopkins Hospital 105*:201-232, 1959.

Novak, C. B., Kelly, L., & Mackinnon, S. E. Sensory recovery after median nerve grafting. *Journal of Hand Surgery 17A*:59-66, 1992.

Poppen, N. K., McCarroll, H. K., Jr., & Doyle, J. Recovery of sensibility after suture of digital nerves. *Journal of Hand Surgery 4*:212-226, 1979.

Tassler, P. L., & Dellon, A. L. Lower extremity cutaneous pressure thresholds: Normative data and tarsal tunnel syndrome. *Muscle and Nerve,* in press: 1996.

von Frey, M. The distribution of afferent nerves in the skin. *Journal of the American Medical Association 47*:645-648, 1906.

Weber, E. Ueber den Tatsinn. Archive fur Anatomy und Physiology. *Wissenshaft Medical Muller's Archives 1*:152-159, 1835.

crosurgery *4:*179-187, 1988.

Dellon, E. S., Keller, K. M., Moratz, V., & Dellon, A. L. Validation of cutaneous pressure threshold measurement with the Pressure-Specified Sensory Device. *Annals of Plastic Surgery, 38:* 485-492, 1997.

LaMotte, R. H., & Mountcastle, V. B. Disorders in somesthesia following lesions of parietal lobe. *Journal of Neurophysiology 42*:400-419, 1979.

Moberg, E. Aspects of sensation in reconstructive surgery of the upper extremity. *Journal of Bone and Joint Surgery 46A*:817-825, 1964.

Novak, C. B., Mackinnon, S. E., & Kelly, L. Correlation of two-point discrimination and hand function following median nerve injury. *Annals of Plastic Surgery 31*:495-498, 1993.

Rydevik, B., & Lundborg, G. Permeability of intraneural microvessels in perineurium following acute graded experimental nerve compression. *Plastic and Reconstructive Surgery (Scandinavia) 11*:179, 1977.

• • •

• ADDITIONAL READINGS •

Bell, J. A. Sensibility evaluation. In *Rehabilitation of the Hand: Surgery and Therapy,* J. M. Hunter, L. H. Schneider, E. J. Mackin & A. D. Callahan, Editors. St. Louis: C. V. Mosby Company, 1978.

Bell-Krotoski, J. A. Light touch-deep pressure testing using Semmes-Weinstein monofilaments. In *Rehabilitation of the Hand: Surgery and Therapy,* J. M. Hunter, L. H. Schneider, E. J. Mackin & A. D. Callahan, Editors. St. Louis: C. V. Mosby Company, 1990.

Dellon, A. L. Clinical use of vibratory stimuli to evaluate peripheral nerve injury and compression neuropathy. *Plastic and Reconstructive Surgery 65:*466-476, 1980.

Dellon, A. L., & Mackinnon, S. E. Human ulnar nerve compression at the elbow: Clinical, histologic and electrodiagnostic correlations. *Journal of Reconstructive Mi-*

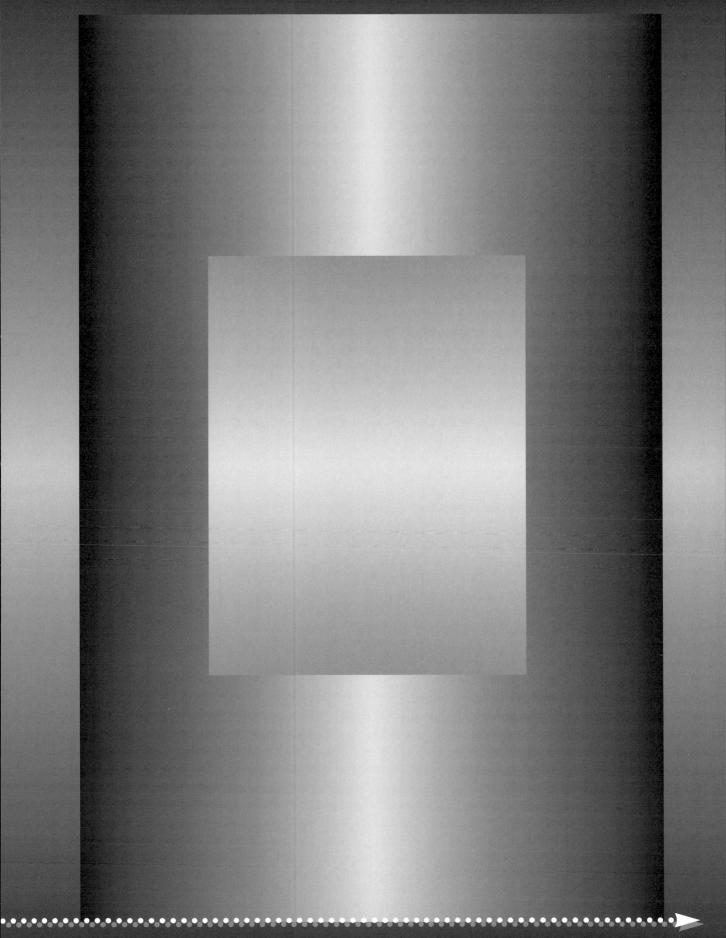

instrumentation

Since the early 1970s, the Department of Neurology at the Mayo Clinic, under the direction of Peter J. Dyck, MD, has pioneered the concept of quantitative sensory testing. This emphasis has led to the development of testing strategies and instrumentation, and to the development of the Mayo Clinic's own computer-assisted sensory testing device, the CASE IV System, which is described below. Despite the widespread recognition of the need for the level of reliability and validity that computer-assisted quantitative sensorimotor testing might provide, the overwhelming majority of sensory and motor testing is currently done manually by the patient's treating physician or therapist.

Such a clinical approach, using a wisp of cotton, a pin, a tuning fork, or a Whartenberg wheel (pizza pie cutter) can provide a quick survey of the body surface that is useful in a wide range of circumstances. But it must be realized that such qualitative testing is useful primarily to screen for gross sensory loss, especially if this is well demarcated. Hand-held devices that give quantitative information, such as hand-held vibrometers, two-point discrimination testers, and filament testing of pressure threshold provide a bridge to the more defined stimulation of computer-assisted technology. A computer's microprocessor provides the ability to control stimulus intervals, frequency or intensity, and sequencing of stimuli, all of which lead to more precise measurement.

This chapter will review the different computer-assisted sensorimotor testing devices that are commercially available, and their strengths and weaknesses. Normative data and data from selected clinical studies with each device are included as they pertain to the understanding of each instrument. Clinical data related to specific regions of the body are reviewed in detail in subsequent chapters. A few of the classic testing instruments are reviewed as well, since they provide a historic counterpoint to computer-assisted sensorimotor testing.

Computer-assisted sensory testing, as envisioned by Dyck et al. (1978), will perform the following roles in the future:

1. Assess the anatomic variability of detection thresholds with age and sex.
2. Study the physiology of sensation, such as spatial and temporal summation, and cutaneous distribution of receptor types.
3. Characterize sensory abnormality in varieties of neurologic disease.
4. Infer the class of sensory fibers that are dysfunctional in disease.
5. Detect subclinical involvement in a specific population, such as genetic kindreds, industrial workers, and geographic isolates.
6. Assess various modes of therapy in controlled clinical trials.
7. Relate abnormalities of sensation to measured attributes of the peripheral nerve, such as nerve conduction, axonal flow, and numbers of myelinated and unmyelinated fibers.

• PERCEPTION OF PAIN •

The sensation of pain, perhaps more than any other sensation, is uniquely subjective. The measurement of pain, therefore, remains a challenge. Textbooks on pain often concentrate more on descriptions of clinical problems that are associated with it and the medical and surgical techniques to treat it, than on the difficult problem of pain measurement.

In the broadest conceptualization, there are two related problems for pain measurement. The first is physiological—the ability to measure the threshold for the stimulation of the nociceptors, or pain fibers (unmyelinated C-fibers and thinly myelinated A-delta fibers). The second is psychological—the ability to measure the intensity of the perceived pain. The instrumentation required for the physiological measurements of pain generally consists of devices that apply a graded pain stimulus to the surface of the skin. The instrumentation required for the psychological measurements generally consists of some form of questionnaire or use of a visual analog scale.

THE VITAPULP™

The Vitapulp™ is a device that generates an electrical stimulus. It was developed for use in dentistry to determine the viability of the nerves that innervate the tooth. Dental pain is a form of pain with which most of us who grew up in the age prior to fluorination are, unfortunately, very familiar. For persistent tooth pain, the root canal procedure "kills" the branch of the inferior or superior alveolar nerve to that tooth. The electrical stimulus applied to the alveolus is adjusted by increasing the intensity of the current, and the point at which the stimulus is perceived as painful is considered the threshold. The units of threshold measurement are, therefore, electrical, being either in amps or volts. This instrument has been used once, as far as I am aware, outside the dental field, and is discussed in Chapter 16, "The Breast."

THE AUTOMATED TACTILE TESTER™

This device contains a computer-driven stimulus that propels a 20- or 22-gauge needle into the skin at a known ramp speed. At low intensity, the stimulus is perceived as dull. As the stimulus is increased, there will come a point at which the stimulus is perceived as painful. The depth to which the needle had to go to be perceived as pain is determined by the force applied; therefore, the unit of measurement for this stimulus is grams. (See a more comprehensive description of this computer-assisted device under the section on Perception of Touch, below, and Figure 7.1 for its normative data and Table 7.1 for clinical applications.)

TABLE 7.1   INDICATIONS FOR TESTING CLINICAL DEFICITS
Related to Small Diameter Nerve Fibers
Peripheral neuropathy . . . . Chapter 14
Syringomyelia . . . . .Chapter 19
Collateral sprouting . . . . .Chapter 4
Nerve regeneration .Chapter 4
Hypersensitivity states . . . . .Chapter 4

THE NEUROMETER™

By measuring the threshold for the perception of a constant, low-frequency, electrical current, this device may give insight into the functioning of the small fiber population that mediates the perception of pain. The 5 Hz sinusoid wave form is supposed to be neuroselective for the C-fiber population, and the 250 Hz sinusoid is supposed to be neuroselective for the A-delta fiber population (see description below.)

HEAT AS A PAIN STIMULUS

One of the methodological problems of delivering a pain stimulus is that

FIGURE 7.1

Automated Tactile Tester™. Normative data for pinprick (pain, sharp/dull) and temperature. The 99% confidence limit is shown as a line whose equation is given at the top of the graph. The correlation coefficient with age is .280 for pinprick and .432 for temperature. From "An Automated Tactile Tester for Evaluation of Cutaneous Sensibility," by K. Horch, M. Hardy, S. Jimenez, & M. Jabaley, 1992, Journal of Hand Surgery 17A:829-837, Churchill Livingstone, New York. Reprinted with permission of the authors.

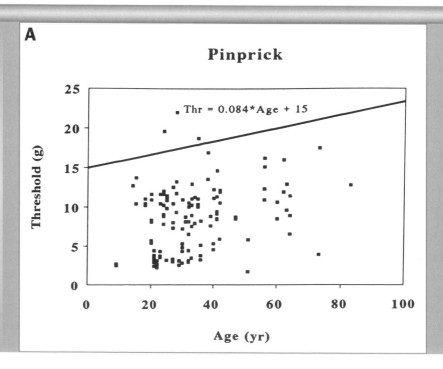

the stimulus must touch the skin, and that physical act of touching may, in and of itself, produce a perception. A solution to this problem was developed in the mid-1970s by Vernon Mountcastle, MD, Emeritus Professor of Neurophysiology, and James N. Campbell, MD, Professor of Neurosurgery at the Johns Hopkins University School of Medicine. They used a laser beam to deliver a heat stimulus to the skin. From this work, Campbell's group has gone on to study pain in great detail.

Because the same unmyelinated nerve fibers are responsible for both mechanical and heat perception, they may be called *C-fiber mechano-heat nociceptors* (CMHs). These can be studied in humans by inserting a needle directly through the skin and recording the results intraneurally while a heat stimulus is being given. Alternatively, they can be studied by applying a laser beam of known intensity and described in degrees Centigrade, or the stimulus can be delivered by a warming probe or warmed air convection currents, with the subject reporting or grading the intensity of the heat on a numerical scale. These observations can be correlated with measurements made in anesthetized monkeys of the thermal threshold required to stimulate this same population of nerve fibers. Such a psychophysical correlation study for the heat-stimulated perception of pain is given in Figure 7.2.

This as well as other lines of evidence demonstrate that the C-fibers mediating the perception of heat also mediate the perception of pain. For example, a selective block of A-fibers by ischemia demonstrates that the subject will perceive heat-stimulated pain. (A tourniquet applied to the arm will create a relative lack of oxygen, and the thicker, myelinated fibers are more susceptible to a decrease in oxygen concentration than are the thin unmyelinated C-fibers.) In contrast, a selective block of C-fibers by local anesthetic will eliminate the perception of heat-stimulated pain. (Local anesthetic diffuses into the nerve and will block the function of the thin unmyelinated C-fibers before it blocks the function of the thicker myelinated fibers.)

When a heat stimulus is applied to the hairy skin sufficient to produce pain, the pain usually is experienced in two phases. At first, the perception is that there is an initial stinging pain, followed by a burning pain. This is because the A-delta fibers, with their myelin sheath, conduct neural impulses faster. Therefore, the "first pain," or stinging pain perception is mediated through the A-delta fibers. The burning second pain is mediated by the slower-conducting C-fibers (see Table 7.2).

Devices for delivering graded thermal stimuli are considered below.

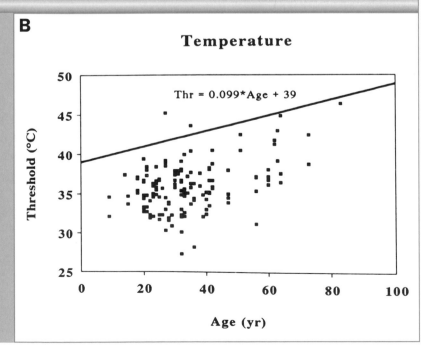

Temperature

$$Thr = 0.099*Age + 39$$

Threshold (°C) vs Age (yr)

FIGURE 7.2

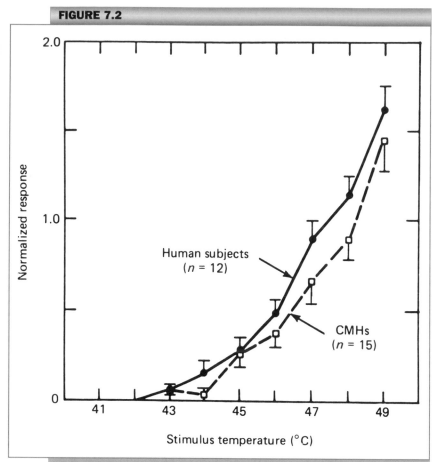

C-fiber mechano-heat nociceptors (CMHs) code for pain from heat stimuli applied to the skin. Normalized responses of human subjects and CMHs in monkey exposed to identical heat stimuli on glabrous skin. Human judgments of pain were measured by the magnitude estimation technique. Subjects assigned an arbitrary number to the intensity of pain evoked by the first 45°C stimulus and judged the painfulness of all subsequent stimuli relative to this number. From "Peripheral Neural Coding of Pain Sensation," by R. A. Meyer & J. N. Campbell, 1981, Johns Hopkins APL Technical Digest 2:164-171. Reprinted with permission of the authors.

VISUAL ANALOG SCALES

The need to record degree of pain is essential to many aspects of medicine. To accomplish this goal, rating scales have become probably the most widespread instrument or tool. The scale can be visual or verbal, with definitions supplied by the examiner. However, since pain is multidimensional, each person's experience with it is unique. Therefore, permitting each patient to scale their own pain experience gives a form of normalization that in its simplicity has proven to be valid.

Several studies, including those by, for example, Revill, Robinson, Rosen, and Hogg (1976), and Price, McGrath, Rafii, and Buckingham (1974), have carefully scrutinized the visual analog scale (VAS) and have found it to be both reliable and valid. Subjects can report a pain experience based on a memory that is distant in time, and report it with a similar rating on different occasions thereafter. The method of recording the rating is to draw a 10 cm line in the patient's chart, or on a specifically prepared pain rating form, and to label one end "0" and the other end "10." This distance has been tested against a 5 cm and a 20 cm distance and has been found to be the most reliable.

Tell the patient that the 0 end of the scale represents no pain, and that the 10 end represents the worst pain the patient has ever experienced. The patient is then given a pen and asked to draw a vertical line across the horizontal line somewhere between 0 and 10, representing the level of their pain. Alternatively, for a verbal response scale (VRS), the patient is given the same instruction and asked to state the number that corresponds to their pain level. This numerical value would then be recorded on the chart. In general, the correlation between the VAS and VRS is 0.6, which is quite good.

These scales are very useful for the therapist managing patients with pain. At the start of therapy, whether it is formal desensitization or management of a stiff hand, ask the patient to indicate their pain level. At the midpoint of therapy ask them to rate it again. Clearly, if pain level is increasing during therapy, you many wish to alter your modalities. If you are doing *phonophoresis*, or application of a 10s unit, recording the pain level before and after will be "objective" in terms of documenting an assess-

ment of the value of the therapy session. An example of an actual chart recording for a patient with knee pain is given as it was used to assess the value of a local anesthetic block of knee joint afferents to determine the potential effectiveness of a partial knee denervation procedure (see Figure 7.3).

THE MCGILL PAIN QUESTIONNAIRE

In 1975, Ron Melzak, MD, Professor of Psychology at McGill University in Montreal, Canada, created a questionnaire from the observations that patients, students, and physicians had a high level of agreement on concerning the meaning of

adjectives that describe pain (Melzak, 1975). He arranged 78 adjectives into 20 groups, reflecting similar pain qualities (see Figure 7.4). Patients were given the opportunity to describe their pain on a number of dimensions, permitting the multidimensional aspects of pain to be described. For example, there are both emotional and sensory descriptors.

The McGill Pain Questionnaire is an attempt to quantify the language of pain. It has been used in clinical and laboratory trials of pain management. The questionnaire is supposed to provide information on three dimensions of pain: groups 1-10 are supposed to

TABLE 7.2   PHYSIOLOGIC PROPERTIES OF NOCICEPTORS

Property	C-fiber	A-delta fiber Type I	Type II
Receptive field	19 mm²	37 mm²	2 mm²
Skin type	glabrous & hairy	glabrous & hairy	only hairy
Heat threshold	44°C	> 49°C	43°C
Time to respond	> 50 msec	> 600 msec	< 200 msec
Adaptation	both	slowly	quickly
Conduction velocity	0.8 m/sec	31 m/sec	15 m/sec
Presumed role	burning pain & hyperalgesia in hairy skin	hyperalg esia in glabrous skin	pricking pain

Note: Adapted from "Hyperalgesia and Sensitization of Primary Afferent Fibers," by S. N. Raja, R. A. Meyer, & J. N. Campbell, 1990, in *Pain Syndromes in Neurology*, H. L. Fields, Editor, London: Butterworths.

FIGURE 7.3

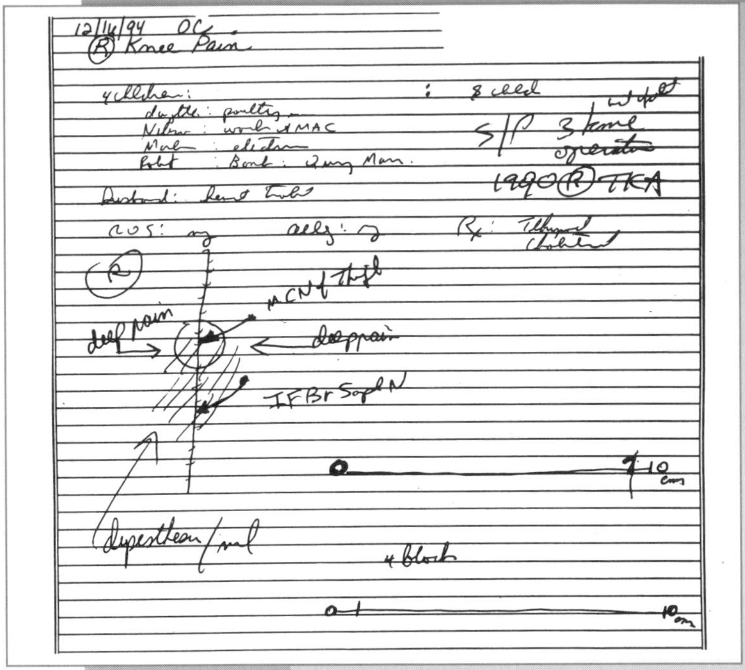

Example of a Visual Analog Scale (VAS) used to document in a patient's chart the effect of a nerve block with a local anesthetic. In this case, the patient has persistent knee pain 1 year after a total knee arthroplasty. The diagram (left, with arrows) indicates the location of an area of dysesthesia in the distribution of the infrapatellar branch of the saphenous nerve (IFBrSaphN) and the medial cutaneous nerve of the thigh (MCN of thigh), with arrows indicating location of deep pain related to the medial and lateral retinacular nerves, which innervate those regions of the knee joint. Note that prior to the blocks, the patient had marked that the pain level was near the 10 end of the rating scale (horizontal lines, lower right), the end at which 10 indicates the worst pain the patient had ever experienced. The infrapatellar branch of the saphenous nerve, the medial cutaneous nerve of the thigh, and both the medial and lateral knee innervations were blocked with xylocaine and marcaine. Note that 20 minutes after the blocks, as indicated in the 0 to 10 scale below the 4 ("4 block"), the patient has now indicated that the pain level was toward the 0 end of the scale (vertical bar near 0 end of the lower of the two horizontal lines), with some pain remaining about the distal lateral knee (this region is the proximal tibiofibular joint, and was not denervated by these blocks). VASs are a reliable and valid method to document and record the patient's level of pain. Reprinted with permission of A. L. Dellon, Johns Hopkins University School of Medicine, Baltimore, Maryland.

reflect the sensory aspects of the pain, groups 11-15, and 20 are supposed to reflect the affective aspects of the pain, and group 16 is supposed to reflect the valuative aspect of pain. There have been many studies of the reliability and validity of the McGill Pain Questionnaire. In general, these have demonstrated that there is a linear hierarchy within the subgroups, and that there is a difference between the sensory and affective groups. The McGill Pain Questionnaire is considered to be both reliable and valid for documenting the character and intensity of the pain experience.

THE MENSANA CLINIC BACK PAIN TEST

The relationship of chronic pain to the presence of preexisting or coexisting psychiatric disorders is addressed by the Mensana Clinic Back Pain Test. The Mensana Clinic was founded, and is still run, by Nelson Hendler, MD, a psychiatrist on the faculty of Neurosurgery at the Johns Hopkins University School of Medicine. The test, described in 1979, is a questionnaire that deals with the thoughts and activities of the patient experiencing

FIGURE 7.4

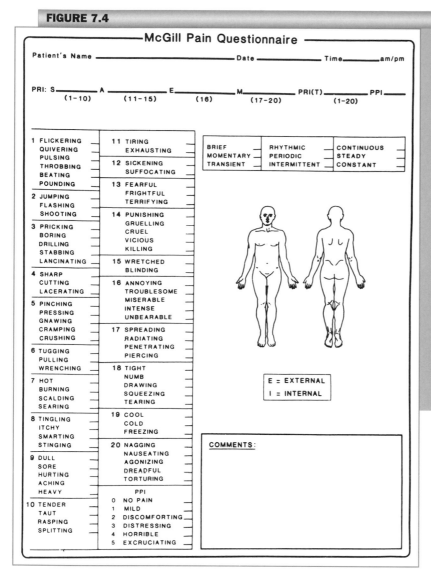

──────── McGill Pain Questionnaire ────────

Patient's Name _____ Date _____ Time_____am/pm

PRI: S_____ A_____ E_____ M_____ PRI(T)_____ PPI_____
(1–10)   (11–15)   (16)   (17–20)   (1–20)

1 FLICKERING QUIVERING PULSING THROBBING BEATING POUNDING	11 TIRING EXHAUSTING		
2 JUMPING FLASHING SHOOTING	12 SICKENING SUFFOCATING		
3 PRICKING BORING DRILLING STABBING LANCINATING	13 FEARFUL FRIGHTFUL TERRIFYING		
4 SHARP CUTTING LACERATING	14 PUNISHING GRUELLING CRUEL VICIOUS KILLING		
5 PINCHING PRESSING GNAWING CRAMPING CRUSHING	15 WRETCHED BLINDING		
6 TUGGING PULLING WRENCHING	16 ANNOYING TROUBLESOME MISERABLE INTENSE UNBEARABLE		
7 HOT BURNING SCALDING SEARING	17 SPREADING RADIATING PENETRATING PIERCING		
8 TINGLING ITCHY SMARTING STINGING	18 TIGHT NUMB DRAWING SQUEEZING TEARING		
9 DULL SORE HURTING ACHING HEAVY	19 COOL COLD FREEZING		
10 TENDER TAUT RASPING SPLITTING	20 NAGGING NAUSEATING AGONIZING DREADFUL TORTURING		

BRIEF / MOMENTARY / TRANSIENT
RHYTHMIC / PERIODIC / INTERMITTENT
CONTINUOUS / STEADY / CONSTANT

E = EXTERNAL
I = INTERNAL

PPI
0 NO PAIN
1 MILD
2 DISCOMFORTING
3 DISTRESSING
4 HORRIBLE
5 EXCRUCIATING

COMMENTS:

The McGill Pain Questionnaire. Pain may be described by many adjectives. This questionnaire subgroups 78 adjectives that can describe pain into 20 categories, within which the patient is asked to assign a numerical value from 0 to 5. This questionnaire is a reliable and valid method to describe the character and intensity of a patient's pain experience. From Textbook of Pain, *by P. D. Wall & R. Melzak, 1984, Edinburgh: Churchill Livingstone, Inc. Reprinted with permission of the authors.*

chronic pain (Hendler, Mollett, Talo, & Levin, 1988). The answers receive a numerical grade. Based on this numerical grade, a categorization is made as to the relationship between the patient's pain and likelihood of major associated psychiatric problems. The Mensana Clinic Back Pain Test takes about 10 minutes to administer. It has been correlated with the Minnesota Multiphasic Personality Inventory (MMPI) and with the results of electrodiagnostic testing, thermography, and radiologic imaging.

The results of that study of 83 chronic pain patients demonstrated that the MMPI cannot be considered a valid test for predicting the presence of physical abnormalities in these patients. In contrast, the Mensana Clinic Back Pain Test correlated highly with the presence of physical abnormalities. By evaluating the effect of chronic pain on the functional aspects of life, the Mensana Clinic Back Pain Test is considered a valid and reliable test of the presence of an organic basis for chronic pain, regardless of underlying psychiatric problems. Furthermore, this test gives the clinician an insight into the presence of those associated psychiatric conditions which may require consultation and care during the pre- and postoperative phases of rehabilitation. This test can be administered and interpreted by a therapist.

PERCEPTION OF TEMPERATURE

The perception of temperature changes through the skin is mediated by unmyelinated fibers, by C-fibers for warmth, and by thinly myelinated A-delta fibers for cold. Table 7.2 gives properties for the fibers related to the perception of heat, which are also characteristic of nociceptors (pain receptors).

THERMOGRAPHY

From advertisements to movies, we have all seen the beautiful computer images that can be colored based on the degrees of heat intensity of whatever image has been captured. Application of that technology to the skin produces a colored picture with the colors related to the temperature of the skin. Such a measurement is called *thermography*. It can be done with paper coated with thermosensitive chemicals, or these chemicals can be directly placed on the skin. Images can be directly captured on film, or the treated paper can be photographed. The photo images can be directly input into a computer and then digitized for statistical analysis. While thermography does not give a measurement of the temperature threshold, it can give an overview of the temperature pattern in the skin in an area of injury, disease, or pain.

Thermography can be qualitative or quantitative. In this regard, thermography has been used to assess the sympathetic response of the skin in such conditions as vasospastic disorders, reflex sympathetic dystrophy, and thoracic outlet syndrome. For example, Uematsu, Hendler, Hungerford, Long, and Ono (1981) reported that thermography was positive, that is, abnormal, in 89% of patients with clinical and electrodiagnostic support for the presence of reflex sympathetic dystrophy or causalgia.

THE AUTOMATED TACTILE TESTER™

Perception of temperature is measured by using an aluminum disk which is heated. If it is heated sufficiently high, this can also test pain (nociception), although the device is programmed not to heat above 52°C, thereby theoretically preventing skin damage. The interval between successive stimuli is 10 seconds. The cold threshold is not measured by this instrument. Figure 7.1 presents the normative data for this device for the warming threshold related to age of the normal subjects. Other aspects of this device are presented below.

THE CASE IV SYSTEM

The CASE IV (Computer-Assisted Sensory Examination, Model IV) System is the computer-assisted sensory testing device designed by Peter Dyck, MD at the Mayo Clinic, mentioned at the beginning of this chapter. Extensive normative data is available on this device, which is described in greater detail below under the section on Perception of Touch. This device can detect the threshold for both warming and cooling. The results of the *thermode*, the module that tests temperature perception, are illustrated in Figure 7.5. The thermode can have its surface area for stimulation varied by use of different size probes. It is water cooled, permitting steeper ramps of change in temperature (0 to 4°C/sec) and greater stimulus magnitudes. Temperature range is 10 to 50°C. The initial skin temperature is measured by an infrared thermometer, and the temperature of the aluminum block is adjusted to this temperature. This is the baseline temperature. The detection strategies can be either a linear ramp or a forced-choice algorithm. The delivered temperature is calibrated to be within 0.5°C. The normative data for 8 subjects is given in Figure 7.5.

THE NEUROMETER™

By measuring the threshold for the perception of a constant, low-frequency, electrical current, this device may give insight into the functioning of the small fiber population that mediates the perception of temperature. The 5 Hz sinusoid wave form is supposed to be neuroselective for the C-fiber population, and the 250 Hz sinusoid wave form is supposed to be selective for the A-delta fiber population (see description below, and Figures 7.28 & 7.29).

OTHERS

There are other thermal testing systems available. Among them are the Minnesota Thermal Disks (Dyck, Curtis, Bushek, & Litchy, 1974) which uses heat transfer differences between materials, such as glass, plastic, steel, and copper; the Marstock stimulator (Guy, Clark, Malcolm, & Watkins, 1985); and the Thermal Sensitivity Tester (Arezzo, Schaumberg, & Laudadio, 1986). The latter two use two different probes that can be set at different temperatures. The temperature perception threshold is defined by these instruments as the smallest difference in temperature that can be distinguished between the two probes.

The probes are made of nickel-coated copper

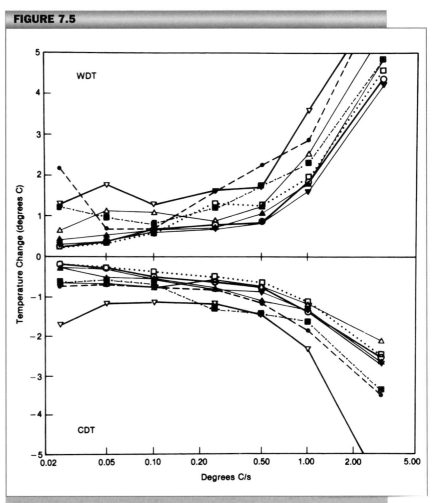

FIGURE 7.5

A CASE IV system measurement of the threshold for warming (WDT) and cooling (CDT) in 8 healthy subjects. From "Detection Thresholds of Cutaneous Sensation in Humans," by P. J. Dyck, J. L. Karnes, P. C. O'Brien, & I. Zimmerman, 1993, Peripheral Neuropathy, 3rd Edition, P. J. Dyck, P. K. Thomas, J. W. Griffin, P. A. Low, & J. F. Poduslo, Editors, Philadelphia: W. B. Saunders Company. Reprinted with permission of the authors.

plates. They differ from the single probe that is heated to a known temperature, such as with the Automated Tactile Tester™, described above. For a more comprehensive description of these thermal testing devices, please see the appropriate reference in this chapter.

Another computer-controlled temperature stimulus device is the TSA-2001, Thermal Sensory Analyzer, available from Compass Medical Technologies (see Chapter 7 Appendix). This is a relatively new instrument, about which I have no knowledge.

• PERCEPTION OF TOUCH •

SEMMES-WEINSTEIN NYLON MONOFILAMENTS

The Semmes-Weinstein nylon monofilaments have been used universally since they were introduced in 1960, for the evaluation of the perception of light touch-deep pressure. To appreciate the impact of this set of filaments (see Figures 7.6, 7.7, & 7.8), it is important to realize that von Frey in 1905 used hair of varying diameters to quantify the human touch threshold, thereby preparing subsequent investigators for the concept that such a system was reliable. The introduction of the nylon monofilaments into clinical use in the U.S. military by George Omer, with the assistance of his therapists, von Prince and Werner, led to the accumulation of a great deal of experience. The nylon monofilaments became the sensory testing instrument used by Evelyn Mackin's therapists at the Jefferson Hand Center in Philadelphia (Callahan, 1984; Bell-Krotoski, 1990). The subsequent efforts of Judy Bell, now Judy Bell-Krotoski (see Chapter 20), have created an environment in which pressure threshold testing is part of the evaluation of any peripheral nerve problem (see Chapter 6).

The background of the development of these filaments is critical to understanding what they can and cannot tell us, and what they are capable and incapable of measuring. This background is described in a book by Josephine Semmes, PhD, Sidney Weinstein, PhD, Lila Ghent, PhD, and Hans-Lukas Teuber, PhD, entitled *Somatosensory Changes After Penetrating Brain Injuries in Man* (1960). These authors were working in the Psychobiology Laboratory of the New York University-Bellevue Medical Center, directed by Teuber. Semmes, whose PhD was from Yale, joined the Bellevue group after completing a postdoctoral fellowship in the U.S. Public Health Service from 1952-1954. She had studied somatosensory function following experimental ablations in monkeys, and wished to study this area in humans. She ultimately became Director of the Laboratory of Psychology at the National Institute of Mental Health. Weinstein brought to the group experience in evaluating weight judgment in humans. Ghent's interest lay in tactile-pattern learning after brain injury.

The group studied 350 World War II and Korean War veterans who had documented penetrating brain injuries (232) or peripheral nerve injuries (118). Their purpose was to learn from studying the sensory thresholds in these men the relationship between cerebral localization and object-quality discrimination, and to learn whether it was possible to predict performance on certain perceptual tasks from the presence or absence of abnormal sensory thresholds. They reported their results as it applied to groups of patients. They needed quantitative tests so that they could "define abnormal performance in terms of the degree to

FIGURE 7.6

Semmes-Weinstein nylon monofilaments. (A) The full set of 20 filaments with close-up view of different cross-sectional areas of representative filaments. (B) The correct use of the filaments. With the fingertip supported, the filament first touched to the skin surface and then over a period of about 3 seconds the examiner increases pressure until the filament is bent, at which time the theoretical calculated force is applied to the skin surface. Errors are related to uneven surface area, the edge of the tip instead of the full surface being in contact with the skin when the filament is bent, variation in actual force applied by the filaments, application too quickly or with movement, and misinterpretation of the meaning of the marking on the filament. From "Sensibility Testing: Clinical Methods," by A. D. Callahan, 1984, in Rehabilitation of the Hand: Surgery and Therapy, *2nd edition, J. M. Hunter, L. H. Schneider, E. J. Mackin, & A. D. Callahan, Editors. St. Louis: C. V. Mosby Company, Chapter 36. Reprinted with permission of the author.*

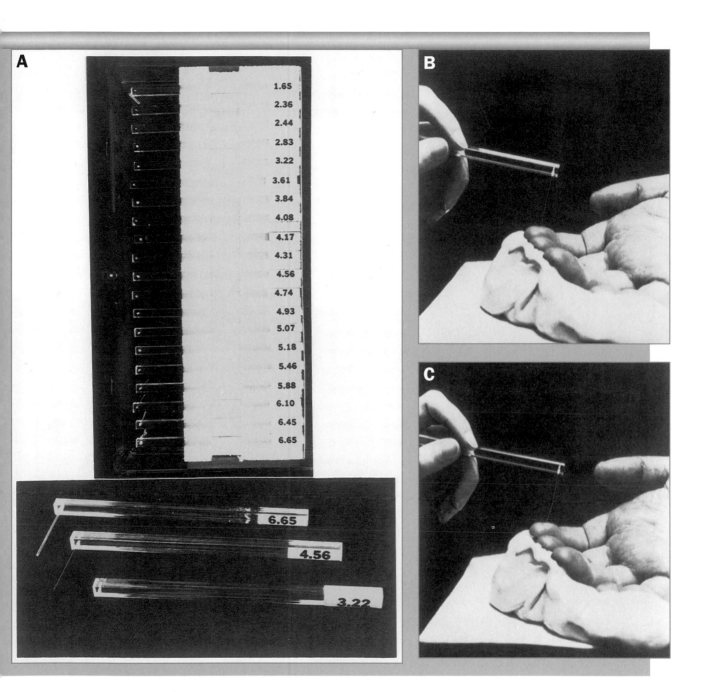

which a given score deviated from the average score of a closely matched group of control subjects." Their tests were "pressure sensitivity, two-point discrimination, and point localization" (Semmes, Weinstein, Ghent, & Teuber, 1960).

• • •

*T*he response to punctate stimuli was measured on the center of the palm and the ball of the thumb of each hand. Twenty nylon monofilaments were used, which ranged in diameter from .06 to 1.14 mm. Each filament was embedded at one end in a plastic rod handle. The free end of each filament was 38 mm in length. The force required to bend each filament by pressing against the tip was measured on a chemical balance....[T]hey were bent maximally. The

FIGURE 7.7

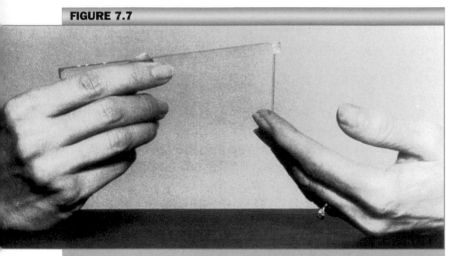

*Semmes-Weinstein nylon monofilaments. A large diameter filament being used to test the cutaneous pressure threshold for constant-touch, that is, one-point static touch, on the index finger. This filament is sufficiently thick that it in fact does not bend until a force sufficient to generate pain is created. The filament has a marking on its handle that represents the log to the base 10 of the force in 10ths of milligrams required to bend the filament. The pressure threshold is then calculated by dividing that force by the cross-sectional area of the filament's tip. The values for the pressures generated by the different filaments is given in Table 7.3. From **Surgery of the Peripheral Nerve**, by S. E. Mackinnon & A. L. Dellon, 1988, New York: Thieme Publishing. Reprinted with permission of the authors.*

common logarithm of the force was used in computation of thresholds. This measure was related to the serial order of the filaments (based upon their diameters) in an approximately linear fashion, and, therefore, a scale of stimuli with roughly equal intervals resulted...subject was instructed to close his eyes, and to "Touch" whenever he felt anything....Each contact was applied for about 1 second with intervals of about 3 to 8 seconds between applications. Six determinations were made for each part, three in ascending and three in descending order. Record was made of the first filament perceived in each ascending determination, and of the last filament perceived in each descending determination. The arithmetic mean of the values of these filaments was taken as the threshold.

(Semmes et al., 1960)

● ● ●

The values recorded for force by Semmes et al. are given in Table 7.3, along with values recorded by Levin et al.

(1978) in a separate analysis of these filaments.

The normative data obtained by Semmes et al. is interesting in that it is one of the few places in which Semmes-Weinstein monofilament data is described statistically, rather than as a simple table with definitions (see Table 7.4). Their normative population consisted of 33 veterans with nerve injuries in the legs, with a mean age of 34.7 years, + 4.8 years. They found that the mean pressure threshold for the right thumb was 3.26 (the log value of the force in 10ths of milligrams), with a standard deviation of .38 log units. The 99% upper confidence limit for normal was 4.02 log units. This is of special interest considering that the usual tables of color coded normal have normal end with the 2.83 nylon filament. A separate test/retest paradigm was used to determine reliability of their filament testing on 30 normal subjects, with an interval of 1 to 4 days between tests. The Pearson product-moment correlation coefficient was .78 for the right hand and .89 for the left hand, indicating excellent reliability.

CRITICAL ANALYSIS OF MONOFILAMENTS

It is important to emphasize that the sensory threshold evaluations that Semmes et al. (1960) chose were specifically to *screen for*

FIGURE 7.8

Example of mapping the sensibility of the hand with the Semmes-Weinstein nylon monofilaments. (A) The numbers obtained during the examination are the markings on the filament handles. (B) The colored representation of the examination, with a color corresponding to a given marking number, these correlations are listed in Table 7.4. Note that since the markings are log values, the difference in force required to perceive touch between the little finger and the index finger is not a difference of about 2 but a difference of 10^2, or one hundred times! (C and D) Mapping can demonstrate clinical change. This patient has an untreated median nerve compression at the wrist, and in the four-month interval between (C) and (D) she has been downgraded from diminished light-touch to untestable with monofilaments. (A) and (B) from "Sensibility Testing: Clinical Methods," by A. D. Callahan, 1984, Chapter 36; (C) and (D) from "Light Touch-Deep Pressure Testing Using Semmes-Weinstein Monofilaments," by J. A. Bell-Krotoski, 1984, Chapter 35; in Rehabilitation of the Hand: Surgery and Therapy, 2nd Edition, J. M. Hunter, L. H. Schneider, E. J. Mackin, & A. D. Callahan, Editors. St. Louis: C. V. Mosby Company. Reprinted with permission of the authors.

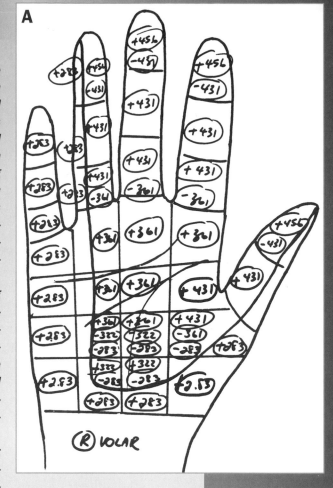

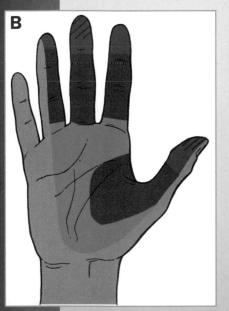

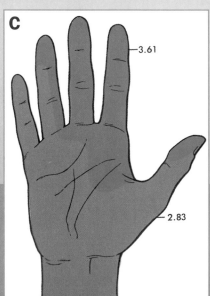

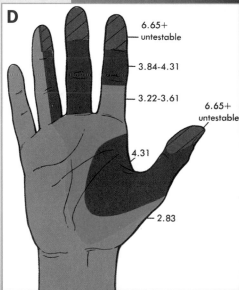

gross sensory defects in the hand following penetrating brain injury. This population did not have peripheral nerve compression, peripheral nerve injury, or periph-

eral nerve repair. In addition, Semmes et al.'s research needs did not require a technique that could measure the continuum from the lowest threshold to the high-

est because they were not doing serial measurement, but were looking for the presence or absence of a defect.

The filament as an instru-

Filament Number	Force✦ Grams	Diameter mm	Filament Marking✛	Pressure★ g/mm²
1	.0045	.0635	1.65	1.45
2	.0230	.0762	2.36	5.20
3	.0275	.1016	2.44	3.25
4	.0677	.1270	2.83	4.86
5	.1660	.1524	3.22	11.1
6	.4082	.1778	3.61	17.7
7	.6968	.2032	3.84	19.3
8	1.194	.2286	4.08	29.3
9	1.494	.2540	4.17	31.5
10	2.062	.3048	4.31	33.1
11	3.632	.3556	4.56	47.3
12	5.500	.3810	4.74	68.0
13	8.650	.4064	4.94	60.9
14	11.70	.4318	5.07	65.6
15	15.00	.4826	5.18	69.1
16	29.00	.5588	5.46	107.0
17	75.00	.7112	5.88	181.0
18	127.0	.8128	6.10	243.0
19	281.5	1.016	6.45	337.0
20	447.0	1.143	6.65	439.0

TABLE 7.3 SEMMES-WEINSTEIN NYLON MONOFILAMENTS CORRELATION OF MARKINGS WITH PRESSURE

Note:
✛ Log_{10} Force (0.1 mg)
✦ From *Somatosensory Changes After Penetrating Brain Wounds in Man,* by J. Semmes, S. Weinstein, L. Ghent, & H. L. Teuber, 1960, Cambridge, MA: Harvard University Press.
★ From "von Frey's Method of Measuring Pressure Sensibility in the Hand: An Engineering Analysis of the Weinstein-Semmes Pressure Aesthesiometer," by S. Levin, G. Pearsall, & R. S. Ruderman, 1978, *Journal of Hand Surgery, 3:*211-216, 1978.

ment has biomedical engineering flaws. As described by Levin et al. (1978), specifically the flaws are that the surface is probably not flat at the time the stimulus is given and, therefore, the actual pressure applied is probably not that theoretically calculated by dividing the force of application determined from the chemical balance by the cross-sectional area of the filament. The intervals between the filament markings are sequential, as they reflect the log value of the force, but when the pressure (stress) is calculated by division with the cross-sectional area, the resultant sequence of the filaments from lowest to highest pressure is not the same as it was for force. The test, as practiced by Semmes et al., used a brief touch, whereas use today requires the stimulus to be applied for 3 seconds. This likely causes a difference in perception from a

brief or moving touch to a constant or static touch. The effect of this duration of stimulation does affect the threshold (Mackinnon, unpublished observations, 1993).

Perhaps the biggest two misconceptions about the filaments are (a) that they give a measurement, whereas they actually give an estimate of a range (see Chapter 6, Figure 7.19 D, and Tables 6.1 & 7.5), and (b) that the value to report from the test is the numerical value on the rod handle which, as noted in the quote above, may be thought to be treated arithmetically, while in reality it is the logarithm of the force (not the pressure) in 10ths of milligrams (not milligrams or grams). This last bit of information is only available in the footnote to Tables 1 and 2 and Appendix B of Semmes et al.'s 1960 book. A further problem with the fila-

ments as stimuli for testing the touch threshold is that every filament delivers a stimulus that differs from its predecessor in force and in surface area. The difference in surface area is a critical difference because the larger the surface area of the filament, the larger will be the number of sensory receptors beneath the surface of the skin that are stimulated.

In 1993, the Weinstein Enhanced Sensory Tester, or WEST™, was introduced (see Figure 7.10). It is designed to overcome some of the criticism of the monofilaments. First, each of the five filaments that belong to the WEST™ are calibrated prior to leaving the manufacturer. This is supposed to improve the reliability of each filament. Second, each of the five filaments has the same diameter rounded ball at its tip. This permits each stimulus to be given through the

TABLE 7.4   SEMMES-WEINSTEIN NYLON MONOFILAMENTS CORRELATION OF MARKINGS WITH COLOR SCHEME

Filament Marking	Clinical Interpretation	Color Code for Report
2.36 – 2.83	normal light touch	green
3.22 – 3.61	diminished light touch	blue
3.84 – 4.31	diminished protective sensation	purple
4.56 – 6.65	loss of protective sensation	red
unresponsive	unresponsive to 6.65	red lined

Note: From "Light Touch-Deep Pressure Testing Using Semmes-Weinstein Monofilaments," by J. A. Bell, 1984, in *Rehabilitation of the Hand,* 2nd edition, J. M. Hunter, L. H. Schneider, E. J. Mackin, & A. D. Callahan, Editors. St. Louis: C. V. Mosby Company, chapter 35.

same surface area. The first information about the WEST™ device was presented at a meeting of the American Society for Peripheral Nerve in May 1994 by Michael Patel, MD and Lynn Basini, OT, CHT (Brooklyn, NY). Their data is given in Table 7.5.

The distribution of normals is very interesting in that it confirms the observations reported by Semmes et al. (1960), that a significant percentage of the normal population has a threshold greater than the 2.83 filament marking. This again demonstrates that the color scheme commonly used to indicate normal is not related to any statistical study. Unfortunately, despite the improvement in the WEST™ device,

TABLE 7.5   NORMATIVE DATA (N=125) FOR THE WEST™, CORRELATED WITH TWO-POINT DISCRIMINATION DATA

WEST™			Percentage of Normals at Each Threshold
Filament #	SWM #	Force (g)	
1	2.83	0.07	59%
2	3.61	0.20	35%
3	4.31	2.00	5%
4	4.56	4.00	1%
5	6.65	200.00	0%

DISK-CRIMINATOR™

Static two-point discrimination	(mm)	
	2	25%
	3	50%
	4	14%
	5	6%
	6	2%
	7	2%
	8	1%

Moving two-point discrimination		
	2	30%
	3	46%
	4	17%
	5	5%
	6	0%
	7	2%

Note: Unpublished data presented by Michael Patel, MD, at the May 1994 meeting of the American Society for the Peripheral Nerve in Rye, New York. Reprinted with permission of the authors.

FIGURE 7.9

(A) Normative data for the Semmes-Weinstein monofilaments obtained during evaluation of the Automated Tactile Tester™ (n = 100 subjects). The cutaneous pressure threshold data obtained in this study did not correlate with patient age, (r = .0178) in contrast to the relationship oberved with the computer-assisted stimuli, the touch trapezoid (see Figure 7.14). This implies that the two testing instruments, while each purporting to measure a cutaneous touch threshold, in fact probably measure something different from each other. (B) Normative data of the Semmes-Weinstein monofilaments obtained from 260 subjects. (A) from "An Automated Tactile Tester for Evaluation of Cutaneous Sensibility," by K. Horch, M. Hardy, S. Jimenez, M. Jabaley, 1992, Journal of Hand Surgery 17A: 829-837, Churchill Livingstone, New York. Reprinted with permission of the authors. (B) from unpublished data from Michael Patel, Brooklyn, NY, presented at the American Society for the Peripheral Nerve meeting in Rye, NY, May 1994.

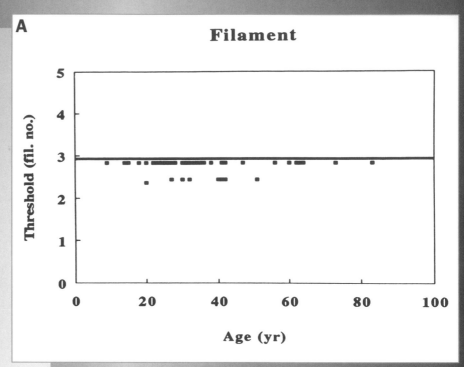

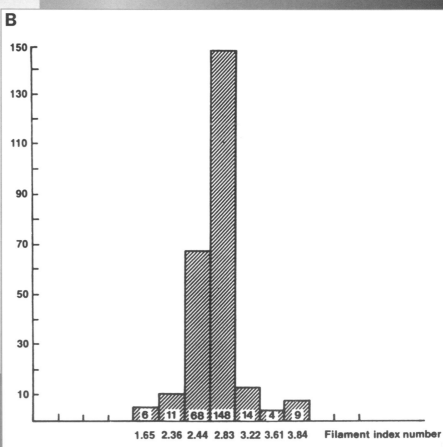

FIGURE 7.10

The Weinstein Enhanced Sensory Tester (WEST™) modification of Semmes-Weinstein nylon monofilaments. (A) This set of 5 filaments, labelled 1 through 5, is given its own color code (B) which roughly correlates with the color code in Figure 7.8 so that 1 (traditional marking 2.83) equals green, 2 (traditional marking 3.61) equals blue, 3 (traditional marking 4.31) equals purple, 4 (traditional marking 4.56) equals red, and 5 (traditional marking 6.65) equals orange. (C) The measured force (not pressure) of each of the five WEST™ filaments is given in the x–axis of the graph. The distribution of the normal population is represented here. Note that since, traditionally, the upper limit of normal is considered to be the 2.83 marked filament, with the WEST™, 40% of normals would be graded as abnormal. The distribution of (D) static and (E) moving two-point discrimination measured with the Disk-Criminator™ for this same population with the numbers on the x–axis representing distance in millimeters. Unpublished data from Michael Patel, MD, Brooklyn, NY, presented at the American Society for the Peripheral Nerve meeting in Rye, NY, May 1994. Reprinted with permission of the authors.

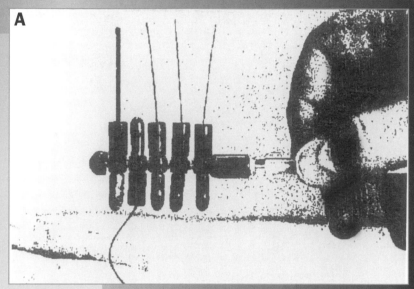

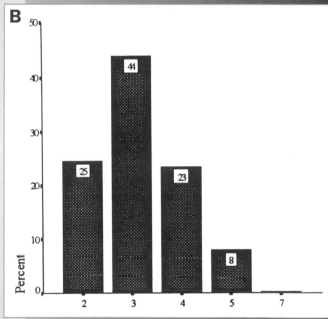

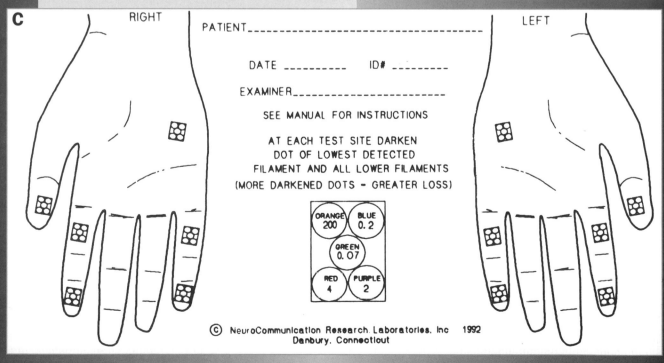

RIGHT   LEFT

PATIENT_____

DATE _____   ID# _____

EXAMINER_____

SEE MANUAL FOR INSTRUCTIONS

AT EACH TEST SITE DARKEN
DOT OF LOWEST DETECTED
FILAMENT AND ALL LOWER FILAMENTS
(MORE DARKENED DOTS – GREATER LOSS)

ORANGE 200   BLUE 0.2
GREEN 0.07
RED 4   PURPLE 2

© NeuroCommunication Research Laboratories, Inc   1992
Danbury, Connecticut

this type of filament testing still produces a range of estimates, not discrete measurements. The intervals between the filaments are spaced so distantly from one another that small changes that could indicate clinical improvement or worsening may not be detected. In the absence of any other ability to quantitate sensibility, this device may still be used, but with full awareness of its limitations as a device to make measurements (see Figure 7.19 D).

THE DISK-CRIMINATOR™

The Disk-Criminator™ was designed to provide an easy to use, inexpensive medical device for office or clinic use to measure two-point discrimination, as well as to provide a home rehabilitation device for sensory reeducation (see Chapter 11). The Disk-Criminator™ (see Figure 7.11) is a set of two plastic, octagonal-shaped discs, each side of which contains at least one metal prong. The metal prongs

have hemispherical tips, all with the same diameter. They are sufficiently long that the examiner can tilt the Disk-Criminator™ when using it to see the contact with the skin surface without the flat edge of the disc coming into contact with the skin surface. The prong interspacing ranges from 2 mm to 15 mm. If the Disk-Criminator™ is held still, static two-point discrimination can be measured; if it is moved, then moving two-point discrimina-

---

FIGURE 7.11

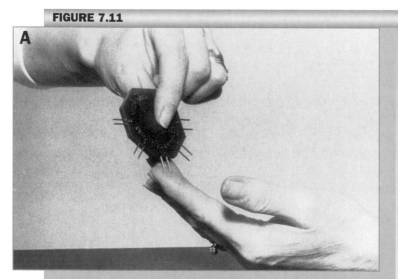

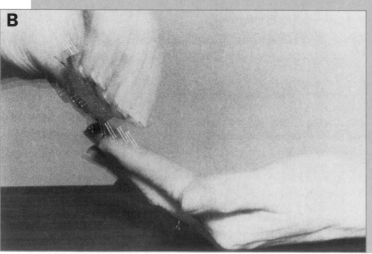

Disk-Criminator™. (A) Static two-point discrimination is tested with the two prongs transverse (right angle) to the longitudinal axis of the skin surface being tested. With a normal pattern of peripheral receptive fields, which is generally circular, doing the measurement parallel to the long axis makes no difference (±1 mm), but during nerve regeneration the field pattern varies considerably, so that a standard approach to the measurement is necessary. Note that with the Disk-Criminator™ the prongs are sufficiently long that the examiner can see them touch the surface without the transverse edge of the testing instrument touching the skin surface. (B) Moving two-point discrimination is tested by moving the two prongs, which are at a right angle with respect to the long axis of the finger (not parallel, from proximal to distal. From Surgery of the Peripheral Nerve, by S. E. Mackinnon & A. L. Dellon, 1988, New York: Thieme Publishing. Reprinted with permission of the authors.

tion can be measured. The Disk-Criminator™ is easily rotated between the examiner's fingers to change the interprong distance, and the examiner can easily rotate between one prong and two during the examination to be certain the patient is giving consistent responses.

For static two-point discrimination measurement, the prongs are held in contact with the skin surface for at least 3 seconds. The pressure of application of the two prongs should be sufficient to overcome the patient's cutaneous pressure threshold (see Chapter 6). Otherwise, the examination will not give a true picture of the skin's sensory capacity, but only a picture of its capacity to perceive two points when the pressure of application is at or below the perception threshold. The same approach is used during the moving two-point discrimination test, introduced by Dellon in 1978 to stimulate all the group A-beta fibers that were not stimulated after the first msec of application of the two prongs during the static test.

Thus, static two-point discrimination testing alone will underestimate the true number of nerve fibers innervating the skin surface being tested because after the initial contact with the skin surface the Disk-Criminator™ will only be stimulating the slowly-adapting fiber/receptor system. Information consistent with this explanation

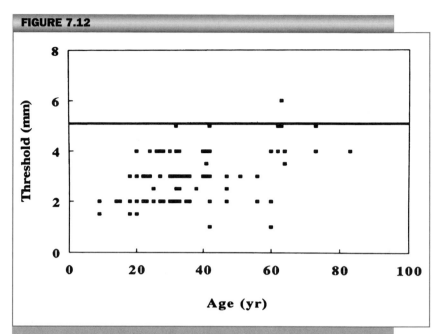

FIGURE 7.12

Normative data for the Disk-Criminator™ obtained during evaluation of the Automated Tactile Tester™ (n = 100 subjects). The threshold for distinguishing one- from two-point static-touch as measured in distance correlated with patient age, (r = 0.143), but not to the same degree that these investigators found when they used the Automated Tactile Tester™ to make this same measurement (see Figure 7.14). From "An Automated Tactile Tester for Evaluation of Cutaneous Sensibility," by K. Horch, M. Hardy, S. Jimenez, & M. Jabaley, 1992, Journal of Hand Surgery 17A:829-837, Churchill Livingstone, New York. Reprinted with permission of the authors.

was obtained by Ochoa and Torebork (1983) doing microstimulation of single unit nerve fibers through the skin in awake human subjects. During the moving two-point discrimination test, the prongs are moved parallel to each other from proximal to distal along the long axis of the finger. The patient is cautioned to say 1 or 2 only when he or she perceives two points that are moving.

Since the Disk-Criminator™ was introduced in 1986, studies have been published

demonstrating that as an instrument it is reliable and valid (Kallman & Dellon, 1983; Dellon, Mackinnon, & Crosby, 1987; Crosby & Dellon, 1989; Novak, Mackinnon, Williams, & Kelly, 1993; and Novak, Mackinnon, & Kelly, 1993). Normative data for static two-point discrimination of the fingertip, obtained with the Disk-Criminator™ by Horch et al. (1992), is given in Figure 7.12. Normative data for both static and moving two-point discrimination of the fingertip, obtained with the Disk-Criminator™ by Patel and Basini (1993), is given in Table 7.5. The Disk-Criminator™ is suggested for use with computer-assisted sensory testing systems to obtain the distance in mm, which must then be manually entered into the computer by Greenleaf's EVAL™ system, by Cedaron's Dexter™ system, and by Exos's Dextrous Hand Master™. For the Pressure-Specified Sensory Device™, the Disk-Criminator™ is a rapid method to obtain the threshold in mm for two-point discrimination prior to using the sensory device component of the computer.

For routine clinical use, 2 of 3 correct answers suffices for most situations. For a final end-assessment evaluation study of the results of nerve repair, it is reasonable to do this test, so that the correct answer must be obtained 4 of 7 times. No one has ever done an end-assessment study to determine if there is any difference in doing this test any of these different ways to determine if there is any increased certainty doing them the increased number of times. Since the test is done on a person, I get a lot of confidence about the patient's answer by changing from one to two points during the sequence in which the distance is made smaller, and by paying attention to the rapidity with which the patient gives the answer. Using these

psychological guidelines, I feel confident obtaining 2 of 3 correct responses for most routine clinical or office use of this test.

The normative values for two-point discrimination were obtained by Semmes et al., and reported in their book in 1960. This is one of the few places in which both a longitudinal and a transverse measurement were made for the same skin surface, and for that reason it is reported here. Semmes et al.'s group consisted of 33 veterans with injuries to the lower extremity nerves, but no brain injury, and with a mean age of 34.6 years. For the right palm of the hand there was a difference of 1.9 mm, and for the left palm of the hand a difference of 0.7 mm, with the longitudinal axis being the larger distance in each case. Of further interest, with respect to Chapter 6 and the definition of how much pressure should be applied in measuring two-point discrimination, Semmes et al. called two-point discrimination measurements threshold measurements, and "care was taken to apply the (blunted) compass points with firm and equal pressure; in every instance, the pressure was well above the subject's pressure 'threshold'." The mean normal value for two-point discrimination that they found for the palm was 13 mm + 2.5 mm, averaging the values for the right and left sides.

Of further interest is their

reliability testing for two-point discrimination, for which they used a separate population of 30 normal subjects, with the test/retest paradigm using a 1- to 4-day interval between tests. They found that the Pearson product-moment correlation coefficient was .64 for the right hand and .70 for the left hand, indicating excellent reliability. Semmes et al. did not find a difference in brain-injured men between abnormal pressure threshold and abnormal two-point discrimination. This suggested to them that the cortical region necessary for both of these functions was linked, perhaps by some general anatomic substrata. Their observation, viewed with respect to the unification hypothesis put forth in Chapter 6, is consistent in that threshold testing for pressure perception requires information about the ability to discriminate between both one and two pressure points required for that discrimination.

CRITICAL ANALYSIS OF THE DISK-CRIMINATOR™

The Disk-Criminator™ is the ideal tool with which to make the distance component of the threshold measurement for two-point discrimination testing. It has blunt, hemispherical, rounded tips, in contrast to compass-type instruments, or the black, rubber tipped, three-pronged device. All the prongs of the Disk-Criminator™ have the same surface area, in contrast to a bent paper clip, and the Disk-Criminator's™ prongs are set at fixed distances so that a sliding rule or a ruler need not be manipulated to arrive at the threshold distance. In 9 years of use the Disk-Criminator™ has developed no known problems. The only theoretical criticism of it is that it cannot specify the pressure at which the two points were distinguished. This was the criticism of all previous two-point discrimination measurements prior to the development of the Pressure-Specified Sensory Device™, which is a computer-assisted sensory testing device. The Disk-Criminator™ represents the best, most cost-effective device available for rapid determination of the distance at which two points can be distinguished from one.

THE AUTOMATED TACTILE TESTER™

This computer-assisted sensory testing device was invented by Ken Horch, who has a PhD in neurophysiology. Horch had done extensive research in the area of single-unit nerve fiber recordings, primarily evaluating the touch-dome in the foot pad of the cat. His interest in the neurophysiological basis of cutaneous sensibility led him to develop the Automated Tactile Tester™. The

only report on this device was in the *Journal of Hand Surgery* (Horch, Hardy, Jimenez, & Jabaley, 1992), and it was based on testing the radial side of the index finger and the ulnar side of the little finger in 62 normal volunteers. A companion report in the same issue of the *Journal of Hand Surgery* reported the use of the Automated Tactile Tester™ in 61 patients referred for the evaluation of pain or numbness in their hands (Hardy, Jimenez, Jabaley, & Horch, 1992).

The Automated Tactile Tester™ requires an IBM-compatible computer, software to run the tester, an electronic control unit, and two stimulator modules. One stimulator module includes a force-controlled probe for testing sensitivity to pinprick, a thermal stimulator, and a displacement-controlled probe for testing touch sensibility. The second stimulator module tests two-point discrimination (see Figure 7.13). During testing the patient holds the stimulator module in the hand, while the hand and the module rest on a table. The operator, or the person doing the testing, chooses the test to be done from the computer screen menu. When the patient perceives the stimulus, a button is pushed with the opposite hand, sending a message to the computer.

The operator instructs the patient on the basic procedure to be followed and

initiates the test. The operator can present one or more sample stimuli which allow him or her to adjust the stimulus parameters, and to ensure that the patient understands the instructions. Preliminary work done during development of the system showed that thresholds are not significantly affected by changes in contact pressure between the stimulator and the skin, as long as the pressure is in the range normally considered light or gentle. During testing, observation of the patient ensures that contact is maintained and that the patient is not exerting excessive pressure on the test site. Thresholds are determined by a staircase method.

The sequence starts by presentation of a stimulus with an amplitude slightly above the expected threshold. If the stimulus is detected by the patient, the next stimulus is decreased by a fixed ratio. This process is repeated until the patient fails to detect the stimulus. Subsequent stimuli are then incrementally increased in magnitude until they are again detected by the patient. At this point the stimuli are then decreased in amplitude, and so on, until a fixed number of reversals between detection and failure to detect a stimulus have occurred. This procedure produces a sawtooth-shaped record of stimulus amplitude versus time. Threshold is de-

FIGURE 7.13

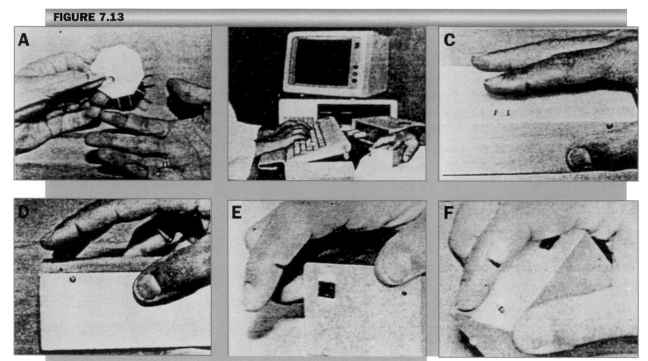

Automated Tactile Tester™. The device consists of a controlling microcomputer, an electronic control unit, and two stimulator modules (B). One stimulator module is used for testing two-point discrimination (C), and the other for testing touch and vibration (D), temperature (warming) (E), and pinprick (F). From "An Automated Tactile Tester for Evaluation of Cutaneous Sensibility," by K. Horch, M. Hardy, S. Jimenez, & M. Jabaley, 1992, Journal of Hand Surgery 17A:829-837, *Churchill Livingstone, New York. Reprinted with permission of the authors.*

fined as the midpoint between the peaks and valleys of this record. Threshold was defined as the mean of five stimulus amplitudes at which the subject went from detection to nondetection of the stimulus, or vice versa.

The measurement of the threshold for warming by this device is described above under the Perception of Temperature section (see Figure 7.1).

Perception of pain is tested with a disposable 20- or 22-gauge needle that is connected to a force-controlled probe. The threshold is that amount of force at which the stimulus perception changes from dull to sharp during a 0.2 second stimulus. The interval between successive testing was 2 seconds (see Figure 7.1).

Perception of touch is tested with a blunt-tip probe. The tip, which is 1 mm in diameter, is moved with sufficient force to displace the skin 2 mm, that is, to create a small indentation. The device provides sufficient force to overcome skin compliance. The probe is programmed to provide either a maintained indentation (constant-touch), or sinusoidal variations ranging in frequency up to 250 Hz (vibration). Vibratory stimuli are given at 50 Hz and 150 Hz, with a 1 second vibration added to a maintained 100 micron indentation of the skin. The amplitude of the vibration is varied by the computer to determine threshold. The interval between successive stimuli was 2 seconds (see Figure 7.14)

One-point static-touch is evaluated with the Automated Tactile Tester™ by what they term a *touch trapezoid*. This is an indentation of the skin at 10 mm/s, with the in-

FIGURE 7.14

Automated Tactile Tester™. Normative data for vibration at 50 Hz (A) and 150 Hz (B). Normative data for touch trapezoid and two-point discrimination, with the 99% confidence limit being shown as a line whose equation is given at the top of the graph. Note that the threshold values for both the touch trapezoid and two-point discrimination are given as microns of displacement. The correlation coefficient with age is .455 for 50 Hz and .494 for 150 Hz. From "An Automated Tactile Tester for Evaluation of Cutaneous Sensibility," by K. Horch, M. Hardy, S. Jimenez, & M. Jabaley, 1992, Journal of Hand Surgery 17A:829-837, Churchill Livingstone, New York. Reprinted with permission of the authors.

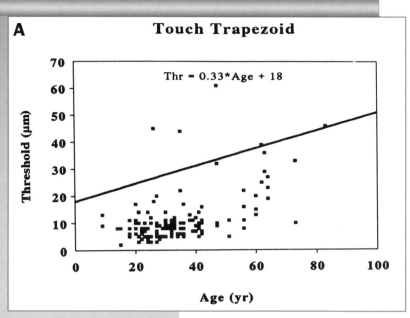

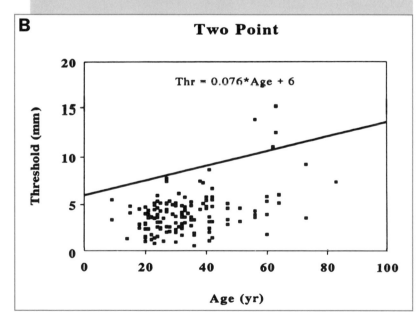

The subjects report verbally whether they feel one or two points of indentation. The amplitude of indentation is set well above threshold for the subject (typically 1 mm, but preliminary tests showed that the amplitude of indentation was not critical as long as the stimuli could be clearly felt). The separation of the points was varied to determine threshold. The interval between successive stimuli was 2 seconds. When this is done for one point, the threshold is called the touch trapezoid because of the pattern of the stimulus ramp. Normative data is given for these measurements in Figure 7.15.

In a clinical study, the Automated Tactile Tester™ was used to test 61 patients who had a variety of clinical problems. The percentage of patients detected as abnor-

dentation held for 0.5 seconds. The stimulus is then retracted at 10 mm/s. The depth of the indentation is varied between trials by the computer. Two-point discrimination is tested with a pair of 1 mm blunt-tip probes, the distance between them varying from 0 to 30 mm. The probes indent the skin simultaneously at a rate of 10 mm/s. The indentation is maintained for 1 second.

FIGURE 7.15

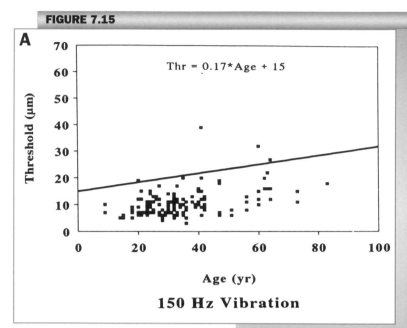

A

Thr = 0.17*Age + 15

Threshold (μm) vs *Age (yr)*

150 Hz Vibration

Automated Tactile Tester™. Normative data for touch trapezoid and two-point discrimination, with the 99% confidence limit being shown as a line whose equation is given at the top of the graph. Note that the threshold values for both the touch trapezoid and two-point discrimination are given as microns of displacement. The correlation coefficient with age is .510 for touch trapezoid and .452 for two-point discrimination. From "An Automated Tactile Tester for Evaluation of Cutaneous Sensibility," by K. Horch, M. Hardy, S. Jimenez, & M. Jabaley, 1992, Journal of Hand Surgery 17A:829-837, Churchill Livingstone, New York. Reprinted with permission of the authors.

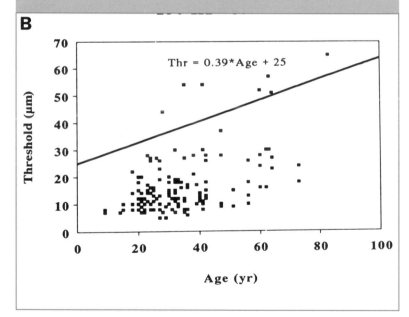

B

Thr = 0.39*Age + 25

Threshold (μm) vs *Age (yr)*

mal with computer-assisted sensory testing was compared to the percentage detected as abnormal by Semmes-Weinstein and Disk-Criminator™ testing (manual), and those considered abnormal by electrodiagnostic testing (nerve conduction studies). The comparisons are given in Table 7.6 and in Figure 7.16. Testing with the 50 Hz vibratory probe was reported as the test that gave the highest incidence of abnormalities; however, this was an incidence of 70% and is not significantly different from the incidence of abnormal touch-trapezoid (that is, one-point, static-touch) perception, which was 65%. Combined, the low-frequency vibration and touch-trapezoid abnormalities identified 78% of the patients with abnormal nerve conduction studies as having sensory abnormalities.

This means that in symptomatic patients the Automated Tactile Tester™ has a 22% false-negative rate, or that it failed to detect an abnormality in 22% of the patients that were found to be abnormal by electrodiagnostic testing. Traditional Semmes-Weinstein testing identified just 37% of this group as abnormal, and traditional two-point static-touch discrimination (in mm) identified just 39% of

FIGURE 7.16

Automated Tactile Tester™. Results of testing 61 patients who complained of pain or numbness in their hand. (A) The top set of bars is a comparison of the percentage of abnormal results obtained with each of the parameters that can be tested with the Automated Tactile Tester™ compared to the percentage of abnormal findings with monofilaments and two-point discrimination in those patients with abnormal nerve conduction studies. (B) The bottom set of bars is the same data presentation for those patients with normal nerve conduction studies. From "Evaluation of Nerve Compression With the Automated Tactile Tester™," by M. Hardy, S. Jimenez, M. Jabaley, & K. Horch, 1992, Journal of Hand Surgery 17A:838-842, Churchill Livingstone, New York. Reprinted with permission of the authors.

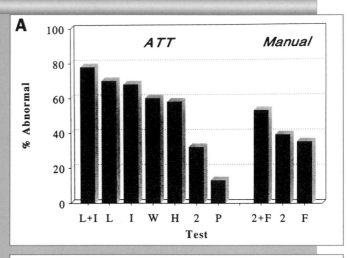

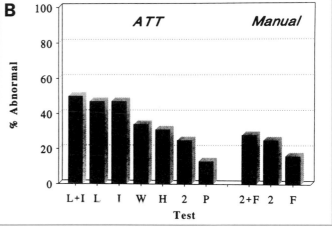

this group as abnormal. The number of patients identified by the Automated Tactile Tester™ was significantly higher (p < .05) than the number identified by traditional testing. As noted in Chapters 6 and 12, in chronic nerve compression, two-point discrimination, when measured only by the distance at which one can be distinguished from two, is present only in severe degrees of compression and, therefore, is not recommended as a screening test. However, when the threshold for distinguishing one from two points is measured as the pressure required for discrimination, then two-point discrimination testing, as done with the Pressure-Specified Sensory Device™, is suitable for screening, and correlates well with electrodiagnostic studies. (See below).

When Horch, Hardy, Jimenez, and Jabaley (1992) looked at the data the same way for index fingers in symptomatic patients whose nerve conduction studies

TABLE 7.6 AUTOMATED TACTILE TESTER™

	Incidence of Abnormality
Automated Tactile Tester™	71%
Manual Sensory Tests	44%
"Nerve Conduction"	42%

	Nerve Conduction	
	Normal	Abnormal
Automated Tactile Tester™	53%	82%
Manual	28%	51%

were normal, they found the same trend. That is, they found that the Automated Tactile Tester™ identified 53% of the patients as having sensory abnormalities, whereas traditional testing identified just 24% of the patients as having sensory abnormalities (p < .05). This portion of their study demonstrated that if patient symptoms, instead of electrodiagnostic studies, are considered as the gold standard, then computer-assisted sensory testing with the Automated Tactile Tester™ is more sensitive than the electrodiagnostic studies, since 53% of patients with normal nerve conduction values who had symptoms had abnormal computer-assisted sensory testing values. The authors did not report their sensitivity and specificity data from this study, but it can be calculated from their tables.

CRITICAL ANALYSIS OF THE AUTOMATED TACTILE TESTER™

The Automated Tactile Tester™ is unique in that it contains within just two hand-held modules the computer-assisted ability to measure the cutaneous thresholds for one-point static-touch, vibration at more than one frequency, temperature (warming), perception of sharp versus dull, and the distance at which two-point touch can be distinguished from one-point touch. Since

the instrument is held by the patient against his or her own body surface to be tested, that is, the hand, the stimulus parameters are controlled by the computer, rather than by the examiner. This very feature, however, limits the application of the Automated Tactile Tester™ to the palmar surface of the hand. While it is possible to conceive of a design that would allow application to the feet, such a design is not available and, therefore, this instrument cannot be used to evaluate the lower extremity, the face, or the breast.

While this instrument's touch trapezoid, the one-point static-touch threshold, is roughly analogous to what therapists have traditionally measured with the Semmes-Weinstein monofilaments, the analogy goes only so far. To its credit, the Automated Tactile Tester™ can measure continuously throughout the stimulus range, in contrast to the monofilaments which rather than make a measurement, give an estimate of a range for the pressure perception threshold (see Chapter 6, Table 6.1, and "Semmes-Weinstein Nylon Monofilaments" in this chapter). In their report of normative data for the Automated Tactile Tester™, the authors noted that there was no age-related change in Semmes-Weinstein monofilament values (see Figure 7.9), whereas there was a significant effect of age on the

touch trapezoid (one-point static-touch) threshold (see Figure 7.15). This further illustrates that what this instrument is measuring and what the Semmes-Weinstein monofilaments estimate are probably not physiologically the same.

The touch-trapezoid threshold is reported in microns of skin displacement, a parameter with which virtually all readers will be unfamiliar for measurement of the cutaneous pressure threshold. Microns of displacement can be converted to g/mm², that is, pressure units, if one knows the skin compliance measurement. The manufacturers would do the end-user, the therapist/clinician, a favor if they would permit the computer printout to be in units of pressure, which is what we all think we are measuring—that is, the cutaneous pressure threshold. Theoretically, it may be the precise amount of skin displacement that is related to the mechanoreceptor's threshold for stimulation, but for the device's report to be intuitive, it would be more desirable for it to read out in units of pressure.

While the Automated Tactile Tester™ can apparently be set to deliver vibratory stimuli from 8 to 250 Hz, the one clinical study with this device chose to use 50 and 150 Hz stimuli. It is clear from the discussion on vibratory perception in Chapter 1 that the quickly-adapting fiber/receptor systems are subgrouped into those responsive to low frequencies, that is, about 30 Hz (the Meissner afferents), and those responsive to high frequency, that is, about 250 Hz (the Pacinian afferents). It is not clear, therefore, why testing with 50 Hz should be any different from testing with 150 Hz, but in the study of symptomatic patients, the authors called the 150 Hz stimulation "high frequency," as discussed in Chapter 1. One-hundred-fifty Hz would not be considered characteristic of the Pacinian afferents; a frequency of 256 Hz or higher would be.

The conclusions of the study of 61 patients with symptoms of numbness was that the highest incidence of abnormalities was detected with low-frequency vibratory stimulation. However, whether you consider the patients with abnormal electrodiagnostic studies (44% of the study population), or whether you consider the patients with normal electrodiagnostic studies, it is clear from the data that although the percentage of patients with abnormal vibratory thresholds is higher for 50 Hz versus 150 Hz stimulation, that is, 70% versus 58%, or 44% versus 30%, respectively, these differences are not statistically significantly different by chi square analysis, that is, p = .369 and p = .314, respectively. Therefore, this study did not demonstrate that low-frequency vibratory stimuli are the best for detecting chronic nerve compression. The study did demonstrate, as discussed above, that either one of these frequencies may identify abnormalities in the symptomatic patient whose electrodiagnostic testing is normal.

While the study suggests that with the Automated Tactile Tester™ the best screening test would be vibration, analysis of the data again demonstrates that there is no significant difference in the percentage of patients with abnormal thresholds identified by 50 Hz vibratory stimuli and the touch trapezoid (70% versus 65% for those with abnormal electrodiagnostic testing, or 44% versus 43% with normal electrodiagnostic testing). The study did demonstrate, as discussed above, that either 50 Hz or the touch trapezoid, that is, one-point static-touch, may identify abnormalities in the symptomatic patient whose electrodiagnostic testing is normal.

Finally, the ability of the Automated Tactile Tester™ to measure the threshold for small nerve fibers offers an important option to the therapist or clinician interested in doing special evaluations. For example, the ability to test pain and temperature has applications to clinical situations (see Table 7.1) ranging from assessment of the early phase of neural regeneration, to detection and following of peripheral neuropathy, to evaluation of painful conditions, to the diagnosis of syringomyelia (a spinal cord cyst that injures the anterolateral spinothalamic tract, causing loss of pain and temperature perception, while touch perception, through the dorsal spinal tracts, is preserved). In this regard the Automated Tactile Tester™ may be compared to the Neurometer™, which also gives information on the small diameter nerve fiber population (see below). However, for complete evaluation of thermal perception, an instrument that measures both hot and cold thresholds would be required.

THE CASE IV SYSTEM

The CASE IV System is the Computer Assisted Sensory Examination, Model IV, discussed above in the section Perception of Temperature. Figure 7.17 demonstrates the overall aspects of this system. The patient is seated on a hydraulic chair that raises him or her to have the foot tested, and lowers him or her to have the hand tested. The specific device for touch-pressure is illustrated, as is the device for vibration and temperature detection thresholds. Aspects of this system have been discussed above related to the detection of the temperature threshold (see Figure 7.5), and the vibratory

FIGURE 7.17

The CASE IV System. The subject's height may be adjusted in this chair to test either the foot (A) or the hand (B). Touch (C), vibration (D), and temperature (E) perception thresholds are measured using a computer-generated forced-choice paradigm (F). From "Detection Thresholds in Cutaneous Sensation in Humans," by P. J. Dyck, J. L. Karnes, P. C. O'Brien, & I. Zimmerman, 1993, Peripheral Neuropathy, 3rd Edition, P. J. Dyck, P. K. Thomas, J. W. Griffin, P. A. Low, & J. F. Poduslo, Editors, Chapter 37, Philadelphia: W. B. Saunders Company. Reprinted with permission of the authors.

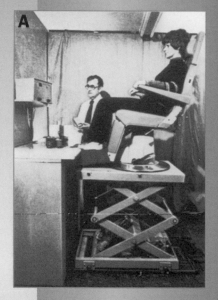

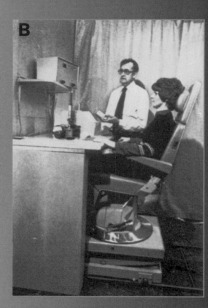

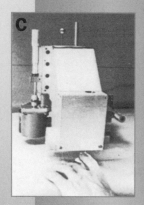

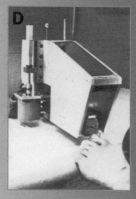

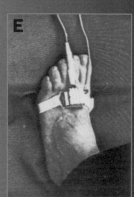

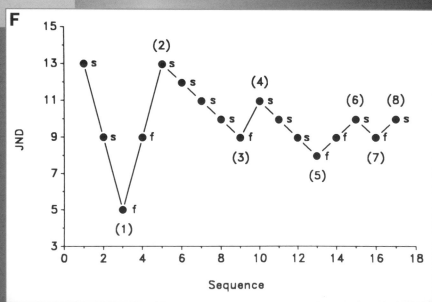

threshold (see Figure 7.18).

The detection of *touch-pressure* for the normal population is given in Figure 7.18 for the index finger, with age-related data. The normative values for the lip are given in Figure 15.11 and for the big toe in Figure 13.9. In contrast to the threshold for the lip, the touch-pressure threshold for the fingertip increases with age. However, the difference between the 99% confidence limit of the upper limit of normal for a person 10 years of age is 5.5 mg, whereas for a person 80 years of age it is about 6.5 mg. Therefore, the age-related change in the touch-pressure threshold does not appear to be of great magnitude. The 99% upper confidence limit for the lip is 6.0 mg throughout the age range, whereas the threshold for the big toe is 6.7 mg for 10 years of age, and 7.7 mg for 80 years of age (with the threshold for men being slightly higher than for women, 8.0 mg versus 7.4 mg).

It is important to note that Dyck et al. (1993) discuss the reporting of the touch-pressure threshold in terms of milligrams, a measurement of force. They developed a conversion of this into displacement of skin, a micron measurement. However, they noted that this method was only accurate for higher levels of force. When they compared the regression lines for touch-pres-

FIGURE 7.18

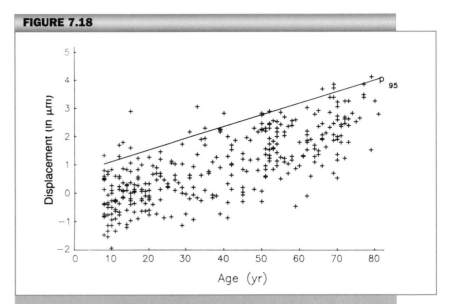

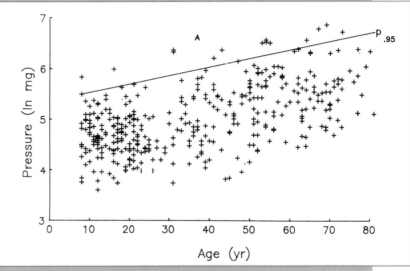

The CASE IV System examples of detection thresholds in normal subjects (151 males, 177 females) related to age for vibrations (A) and touch (B). From "Detection Thresholds of Cutaneous Sensation in Humans," by P. J. Dyck, J. L. Karnes, P. C. O'Brien, & I. Zimmerman, 1993, Peripheral Neuropathy, 3rd Edition, P. J. Dyck, P. K. Thomas, J. W. Griffin, P. A. Low, & J. F. Poduslo, Editors, Chapter 37, Philadelphia: W. B. Saunders Company. Reprinted with permission of the authors.

sure reported in force compared to those reported in displacement, they found that the *ranking* changed. This means that whereas for

force the lip had the lowest threshold at 80 years of age, when reported in displacement the finger had the lowest threshold, and the lip threshold was about the same as that for the big toe in men. Their conclusion was that displacement varied because of the different nature of the skin; that is, the facial skin was more compliant than the fingertip skin. (This observation has further significance with respect to the Automated Tactile Tester™, which reports touch-trapezoid thresholds in terms of skin displacement. While the Automated Tactile Tester™ is only used for evaluation of the hand, if its technology were to be transferred to other body surface areas, the errors identified by Dyck et al. would apply.)

Dyck, Karnes, O'Brien, and Zimmerman (1993) give case examples of the results of the CASE IV in evaluating touch-pressure detection thresholds in a variety of neuropathies, with this instrument being able to demonstrate abnormalities compared to their normative data. They conclude that this instrument, despite its cost, will permit neurology clinics to examine these types of patients more efficiently and more cost effectively because the automated nature of the computer-assisted testing will permit technicians to do the testing instead of physicians.

CRITICAL ANALYSIS OF THE CASE IV SYSTEM

The CASE IV System has been extensively documented and is reliable and valid within the concepts of its design. However, this instrument is not traceable to NIST. I can find no information on how often it needs to be calibrated. There does not appear to be a recommendation as to when vibratory perception thresholds should be tested versus when touch-pressure thresholds should be tested, since they both test the group A-beta fibers. I can find no reported information as to the diameter of the probe for the touch-pressure stimulus, so that their results, reported in terms of force, can be converted into pressure, permitting comparison of the CASE IV thresholds with those reported for the Pressure-Specified Sensory Device™.

The CASE IV System is limited by its design features to testing the top of the foot. This design feature would appear to limit its application to problems related to the plantar aspect of the foot. The hand can be supinated to test the fingertips, but this would be difficult to do for someone with arthritis and an associated peripheral nerve problem, or with certain posttraumatic deformities. In general, the instrument seems ideal for a neurologist to use when the results of electrodiagnostic testing are inconclusive, or when frequent follow-up evaluations are required and electrodiagnostic testing is believed to be either too expensive or too painful. It is also clear that this device cannot be used to test all body surfaces.

THE PRESSURE-SPECIFIED SENSORY DEVICE™

The Pressure-Specified Sensory Device™ was developed beginning in 1989 to fill the need for a device that would measure the pressure at which two points could be distinguished from one point touching the skin. The instrument that finally was developed contained, at the base of each of two prongs, a force transducer that developed an electrical signal that was processed through a signal conditioning unit and relayed into an IBM-compatible computer (see Figure 7.19). This created an instrument that was capable not only of measuring the pressure at which two-point discrimination was possible, but also of measuring the one-point static touch threshold, which is the threshold that had been estimated by the Semmes-Weinstein nylon monofilaments. Of course, the instrument can be used with or without movement across the surface of the skin.

The first report of normative values with the Pressure-Specified Sensory Device™ (E. S. Dellon, Mourey, & A. L. Dellon, 1992) reported, therefore, six different cutaneous pressure thresholds for each finger tested: one-point static-touch (1PS), one-point moving-touch (1PM), two-point static-touch (2PS), and two-point moving-touch (2PM), with each of these being reported in units of pressure, that is, grams/mm². The thresholds for 2PS and 2PM were, of course, also reported as the distance between the two prongs, that is, millimeters (see Figure 7.20).

The electromechanical concept of the Pressure-Specified Sensory Device™ must be contrasted with the traditional mechanical concept of the nylon monofilaments. This contrast will be discussed in detail below, and has been discussed in Chapter 6 from various aspects of threshold versus innervation density. Within the context of instrument design, it must be emphasized again that the finite number of filaments in a set can only define a range of sensation.

This means that the results obtained with the filaments cannot possibly be any more than qualitative or an approximation or an estimate of a range (see Figure 7.19). Furthermore, the Pressure-Specified Sensory Device™, according to the manufacturer's specifications, can measure with the hand-held device a resolution of ± 2 mg, with a threshold that is 100 mg ± 15 mg. If the Pressure-Specified Sensory Device™ is mounted on a computer-driven fixture that will lower the prongs onto the

skin surface, eliminating the examiner's hand variance, the threshold becomes 25 mg ± 7 mg. For even finer degrees of basic science investigation, there is available a six-degree of freedom remote computer-controlled stimulator.

There will always be some degree of oscillation that is intrinsic to humans, such as the cardiovascular dynamics, and some that are external, such as seismic or gravity, electrical interference, or patients' hand movements. Therefore, for this hand-held device, a damping mechanism on the surface of the Pressure-Specified Sensory Device™ is capable of reducing oscillations of the examiner's hand by 90% without reducing the resolution or accuracy of the pressure perception measurements.

To give this computer-assisted sensory measurement system the highest degree of reliability from an engineering point of view, it is recognized that the most likely source of error within the system will be electrical. To alert the user to any electrical problem within the system, the actual NK Biotechnical devices output their electrical signal into a signal conditioning "box" called the DAQ2001. This is small enough to fit into a shirt pocket and is capable of connecting many different devices into the computer, so that just one DAQ2001 is needed even if the system

contains grip and pinch and skin compliance, in addition to the Pressure-Specified Sensory Device™. The DAQ2001 contains solid-state switches and microprocessing ability and converts the electrical signal into digital form. The microprocessor is used to run the TEC2001 software that comes with the system, and acts as the internal diagnostic software that alerts the user by means of a prompt on the computer screen anytime there is any electrical malfunction, preventing the acquisition of faulty clinical data.

The initial study with the Pressure-Specified Sensory Device™ revealed several exciting aspects of this computer-assisted sensory device. First, it became clear that by just using one prong this device had the potential to correct all the criticisms that had been raised about the Semmes-Weinstein nylon monofilaments. This new device could make an actual measurement of the cutaneous pressure threshold, not just give an estimate of its range. It could do so because it could measure continuously from 0.1 to 100 gm/mm² of pressure, thus avoiding the problem of having to use several different filaments and having to accept just one as the threshold, when in fact that one represented just one end of an interval. Second, the Pressure-Specified Sensory Device™ is traceable to NIST,

FIGURE 7.19

The Pressure-Specified Sensory Device™. This is a computer-assisted sensory testing device that is used for quantitative sensory testing. (A) The Pressure-Specified Sensory Device™ is demonstrated here during testing of a patient in a therapist's clinic setting. (B) It is modular in that it is one of several devices manufactured by the NK Biotechnical Corporation that can be independently attached to a signal conditioning unit (large boxes in rear) and then to an IBM-compati-

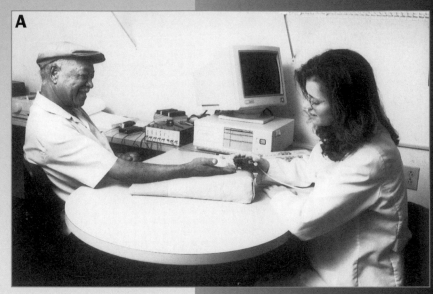

ble computer. The computer can be PC-size or a laptop. The instruments, from left to right, are the skin compliance device, the NK grip strength device, the NK pinch device, the Pressure-Specified Sensory Device™, and on the far right, above the Disk-Criminator™, are two types of goniometers.

(C) The patient's hand and the therapist's hand should be supported. In this close-up view, note that just one of the two prongs is in contact with the fingertip, so that the threshold for one-point static touch can be measured. Used in this mode, the Pressure-Specified Sensory Device™ gives improved measurements over the traditional nylon monofilament. The device is sensitive to gravity, and may be used to test any body surface, only requiring a computer key to be pressed to "zero" the device for the gravitational field in that position. For examples of this device being used to test sensibility of the upper ex-

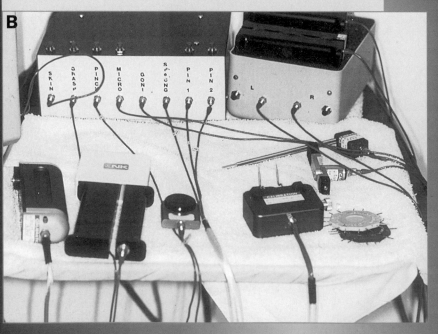

tremity after nerve repair and with carpal and cubital tunnel syndrome, and after fractures, see Chapter 12. Examples of this device being used to test sensibility of the lower extremity for nerve compression are in Chapter 13; for lead poisoning and diabetes, in Chapter 14; and for the lip, in Chapter 15.

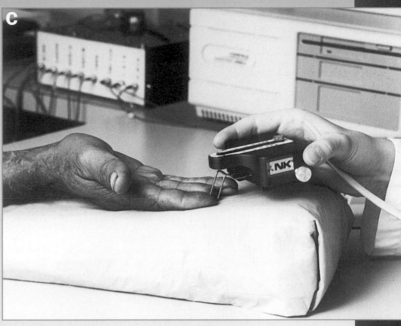

(D) The continuous measurement range of this device is exemplified by the "Tennis Ladder." If a new member joins a tennis club, he or she must play other members whose tennis ability has already been measured with respect to each other, and must be ranked from 1 to 10 on the ladder. This ladder represents the best measurement that can be made for that club (ladder on the left). If 7 of the club members who make up the ladder are not available at the time of measurement, the new member's true ability can only be estimated by comparison with those few (the ladder on the right). Note the position of the new member's face on each of the two ladders. On the left, the little angry face represents the club member with the most ability whom the new member beat. The location of the new member's face on the ladder on the right side can only provide an estimate of the range in which the new member plays tennis with respect to all other club members, and is not a true measurement. Figures (A)–(C) copyright A. Lee Dellon. Reprinted with permission.

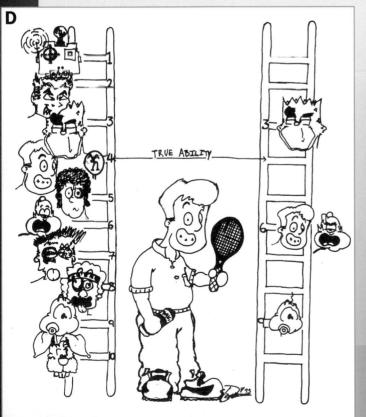

FIGURE 7.20

A

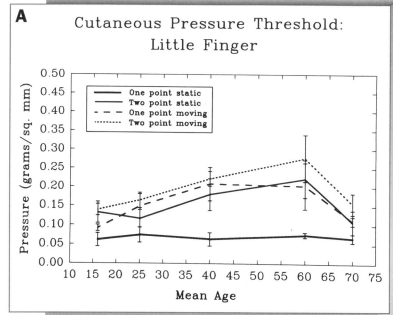

Cutaneous Pressure Threshold: Little Finger

The Pressure-Specified Device™. (A) Normative, age-related data for the little finger, and (B) comparing the index and the little finger. Note that the pressure threshold is reported directly in units of pressure, that is, g/mm^2, and that for any given surface area four different measurements of the pressure can be made, that is, one- or two-point static or moving touch, which is the unique feature of the Pressure-Specified Sensory Device™. Since the distance between the two prongs in mms is also reported, it is possible to display certain data for analysis as three-dimensional plots such as (C) a group of patients in whom the relationship between skin compliance and moving two-point discrimination is being evaluated using data from the little finger, or (D) a group of patients in whom the relationship between hand function (object recognition index) and mov-

B

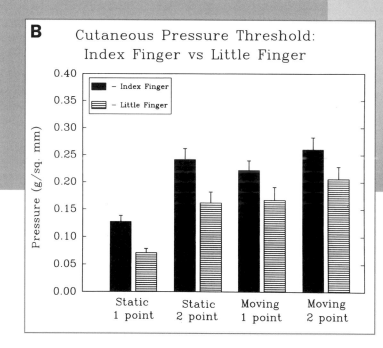

Cutaneous Pressure Threshold: Index Finger vs Little Finger

chophysical stimulus is constant. Fourth, the Pressure-Specified Sensory Device™ reads out on the computer directly in units of pressure, or g/mm^2, instead of as the filaments do in a log value of the force in 10ths of milligrams.

Another study (E. S. Dellon, Crone, Mourey, & A. L. Dellon, 1993) found a very poor correlation ($r = .211$) between the cutaneous pressure threshold measured with the Pressure-Specified

so that the value recorded as the pressure actually is what the pressure is, rather than whatever the nylon filament might be recording that day, after previously being bent many times or having never been calibrated at all. Third, the prong on the Pressure-Specified Sensory Device™ is uniform in size and does not vary from one measurement to the next, as do the different size monofilaments, with their differing cross-sectional areas, so that the psy-

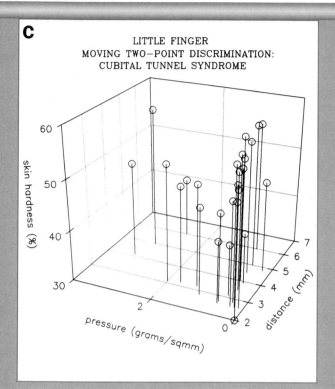

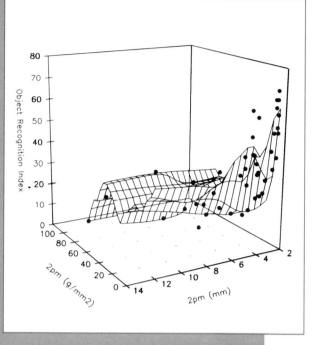

ing two-point discrimination is being evaluated uing data from the index finger. (A) and (B) from "Human Pressure Perception Values for Constant and Moving One- and Two-point Discrimination," by E. S. Dellon, R. Mourey, & A. L. Dellon, 1992, Plastic and Reconstructive Surgery 90:112-117. (C) and (D) from unpublished observations of E. S. Dellon & A. L. Dellon (1992). Reprinted with permission of the authors.

Sensory Device™ and the Semmes-Weinstein nylon monofilaments. This poor correlation is likely due, again, to the change in the filament's surface area each time it is applied to the skin. This, in turn, alters the number of receptors being tested and adds to the problem of the filaments estimating intervals. For example, the upper limit of normal is usually listed in the filament color scheme charts as the filament with the 2.83 marking,

corresponding to a pressure threshold of 4.86 g/mm².

The weight of some common objects is instructive in this regard. For example, a plastic paper clip weighs 0.1 gm, a metal paper clip weighs 0.5 g, and a penny weighs 2.47 g. When you divide their weight by their surface area to get the force per unit area or the pressure they would apply, you get a result that is clearly well below the theoretical value given by the Semmes-Weinstein filament.

In contrast, the Pressure-Specified Sensory Device™ can make a measurement down to 0.1 g/mm².

In a study (E. S. Dellon, Keller, Moratz, & A. L. Dellon, 1995) of the cutaneous pressure threshold for one-point static-touch in the normal index and little finger tip, the lowest threshold value identified for 1PS touch was 0.1 g/mm², with the mean threshold for 1PS touch being 0.5 g/mm², less than even the finest Semmes-Weinstein 1.65 nylon monofilament (which calculates out to 1.47 g/mm²). The 99% confidence limit for the upper limit of normal with the Pressure-Specified Sensory Device™ for the index or little fingertip in peo-

TABLE 7.7 PRESSURE-SPECIFIED SENSORY DEVICE™ NORMATIVE DATA FOR THE INDEX FINGER						
	Pressure Perception Threshold					
	(g/mm²)		**(mm)**	**(g/mm²)**		**(mm)**
	1PS	**2PS**	**2PS**	**1PM**	**2PM**	**2PM**
≤ 45 years of age						
mean	0.5⁺	0.7✦	2.6	0.4	0.6★	2.6
s.d.	0.2	0.2	0.1	0.2	0.2	0.1
95%	0.57	0.78	2.7	0.50	0.64	2.7
99%	0.60	0.81	2.8	0.52	0.67	2.8
min	0.1	0.3	2.5	0.1	0.2	2.5
max	0.9	1.2	3.1	0.7	1.0	3.1
> 45 years of age						
mean	0.7⁺	1.5✦	2.9	0.5	1.0★	2.7
s.d.	0.3	1.2	0.4	0.3	0.7	0.4
95%	0.87	2.1	3.1	0.64	1.3	3.0
99%	0.93	2.2	3.3	0.69	1.4	3.2
min	0.2	0.1	2.5	0.1	0.1	2.5
max	1.5	5.0	4.0	1.3	3.5	4.0

Note:

⁺ $p < .01$

✦ $p < .001$

★ $p < .008$

From "Pressure Threshold Measurements in Carpal and Cubital Tunnel Syndrome with the Pressure-Specified Sensory Device™," by A. L. Dellon & K. Keller, *Annals of Plastic Surgery, 38:* 493-502. 1997. Reprinted with permission of the authors.

ple under 45 years of age is 1.0 g/mm².

In contrast, the data in Table 7.5 suggest that 41% of the normal population have a threshold higher than the 2.83 filament (4.86 g/mm²) when the new WEST™ device is used to make the measurement. This means that the Pressure-Specified Sensory Device™ is a more sensitive measurement device than the monofilaments, which are limited by the nature of their design. The Pressure-Specified Sensory Device™ is, therefore, capable of evaluating the earliest changes in touch sensibility. Furthermore, the E. S. Dellon et al. study (1995) demonstrated an excellent interest reliability (r = .930 for 2PM and r = .970 for 1PS), for the Pressure-Specified Sensory Device™, with a 99% confidence limit for the greatest difference between the left and right index or little finger being 0.5 g/mm² .

The next exciting area opened for investigation with the Pressure-Specified Sensory Device™ is the ability to measure the threshold for two-point discrimination as both the distance at which the two points can be distinguished from one and the minimum pressure at which discrimination occurred. As reviewed in Chapter 6, Moberg's concern had always been that two different people measuring two-point discrimination might arrive

TABLE 7.8   PRESSURE-SPECIFIED SENSORY DEVICE™ NORMATIVE DATE FOR THE LITTLE FINGER

| | Pressure Perception Threshold | | | | | |
| | (g/mm²) | | (mm) | (g/mm²) | | (mm) |
	1PS	2PS	2PS	1PM	2PM	2PM
≤ 45 years of age						
mean	0.4	0.6✢	2.7	0.3	0.5✦	2.7
s.d.	0.2	0.3	0.2	0.2	0.2	0.2
95%	0.48	0.68	2.8	0.35	0.60	2.7
99%	0.50	0.70	2.9	0.37	0.63	2.8
min	0.1	0.1	2.5	0.1	0.1	2.5
max	0.8	1.0	3.5	0.8	0.9	3.1
> 45 years of age						
mean	0.4	1.3✢	3.2	0.3	0.8✦	3.1
s.d.	0.1	1.0	0.6	0.2	0.5	0.6
95%	0.50	1.7	3.4	0.37	1.1	3.4
99%	0.53	1.9	3.5	0.40	1.2	3.5
min	0.2	0.1	2.5	0.1	0.2	2.5
max	0.7	4.0	4.6	0.6	1.9	4.6

Note:
✢ $p < .01$
✦ $p < .001$
From "Pressure Threshold Measurements in Carpal and Cubital Tunnel Syndrome with the Pressure-Specified Sensory Device™," by A. L. Dellon & K. Keller, *Annals of Plastic Surgery, 38:* 493-502. 1997. Reprinted with permission of the authors.

at two different distances for the same patient because the two examiners each pressed the instrument into the skin at different pressures. This concern is eliminated if the pressure at which the two points can be distinguished is also measured by the instrument.

The ideal specification of two-point discrimination requires a measurement of both distance and pressure. It remains to be determined whether any additional in-formation about disease or nerve regeneration would result from this new ability, but the Pressure-Specified Sensory Device™ can make this ideal measurement. In a study that correlated a measure of hand function, specifically object recognition, with these two threshold measurements for two-point discrimination (E. S. Dellon et al., 1995), the data was plotted in a three-dimensional format (see Figure 7.20

While this plot is interesting, it does not give added insight into this particular data set. However, this type of analysis may prove valuable for future neurophysiological or psychophysical studies. Normative data from another study (Dellon & Keller, 1995) is given in Table 7.7 for the index finger, and in Table 7.8 for the little finger, demonstrating the relationship between the thresholds for distance and pressure in two-point discrimination

FIGURE 7.21

A

LOCATION	1 PT STATIC GM/SQmm	2 PT STATIC GM/SQmm	MM	1 PT MOVING GM/SQmm	2 PT MOVING GM/SQmm	MM
LEFT						
INDEX	2.5	0.6	2.0	1.1	0.6	2.0
LITTLE	1.2	1.3	4.5	1.1	0.9	4.5
DORSALRADIAL	15.3	1.3	4.0	1.1	0.3	4.0
PALM	17.3	4.7	6.5	4.3	2.6	6.5
RIGHT						
INDEX	12.7	3.2	4.0	2.4	6.7	4.0
LITTLE	3.7	2.3	4.0	2.5	2.3	4.0
DORSALRADIAL	12.2	?...		4.6	23.4	13.2
PALM	31.5	22.6	9.0	4.4	7.4	9.0

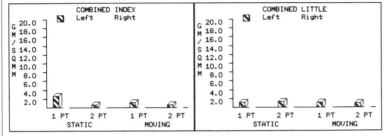

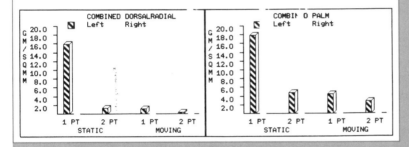

B

PRESSURE SENSORY ONE / TWO POINT DEVICE

LOCATION	1 PT STATIC GM/SQmm	2 PT STATIC GM/SQmm	MM	1 PT MOVING GM/SQmm	2 PT MOVING GM/SQmm	MM
RIGHT						
INDEX	1.7	0.6	8.0	0.4	0.4	8.0
RADIAL DIP	0.6	0.7	2.1	0.8	0.3	2.1
ULNAR DIP	1.1	1.3	2.6	0.5	1.4	2.6

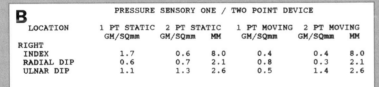

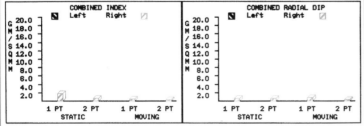

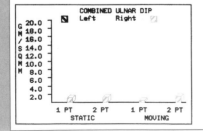

The Pressure-Specified Sensory Device™. Example of report in a patient with a proximal median nerve entrapment in the left forearm. While the numerical values for both hands are given, just the graphs for the left are shown. This patient previously had two left carpal tunnel releases and is an assembly line worker. Note that the sensory threshold is now almost normal for the left index fingertip, (A) yet the threshold is high for the palm, (B) demonstrating that the palmar cutaneous branch of the median nerve is involved. This helps to localize the site of compression, proximal to the wrist. Electrodiagnostic testing demonstrated only persistent distal latency abnormalities and decreased sensory amplitude, consistent with residual carpal tunnel syndrome. (C) This patient has abnormal radial sensory and ulnar nerve measurements as well on the left. None of the measurements on the right are normal. This patient is a good example of someone with cumulative trauma disorder (see Chapter 18).

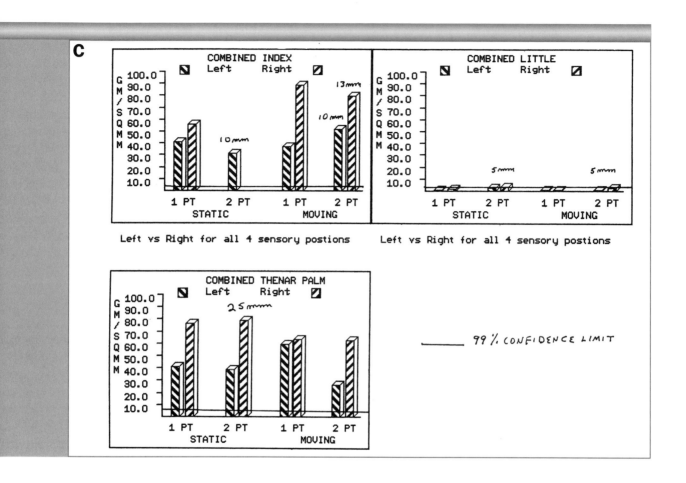

testing.

Another area of investigation was whether all the parameters that can be measured with the Pressure-Specified Sensory Device™ need to be measured, and whether they give additional information for a given disease process. This question was studied (Dellon & Keller, 1995) with the data that will be given in greater detail in Chapter 12, under "Upper Extremity Nerve Compressions." However, for purposes of this chapter it may be stated that for chronic nerve compression, such as the carpal and cubital tunnel syndrome, the information provided by the moving one-point touch and the moving two-point discrimination thresholds do not give additional information of predictive diagnostic significance (see Figure 7.21). Therefore, in the initial evaluation or screening of chronic nerve compression, just the static touch thresholds need to be measured. (See Chapter 18 on cumulative trauma for further discussion of the results of this study on establishing screening values for industry.)

Furthermore, for many patients with carpal tunnel syndrome, the one-point static threshold was normal at a time when the pressure threshold for the discrimination of one- from two-points at 3 mm was already abnormal. Thus, it was concluded that the first cutaneous pressure threshold to become abnormal in a patient with carpal tunnel syndrome or cubital tunnel syndrome is the pressure at which two points can be distinguished from one. The one-point static pressure threshold is not the first type of touch threshold to become abnormal. In a recent study of lower extremity nerve compression, these same observations were found in patients with tarsal tunnel syndrome (see Chapter 13), compression of the posterior tibial nerve at the ankle (Tassler & Dellon, 1995).

With respect to the ability to measure neural regeneration after nerve injury or nerve repair, it should be recalled from Chapter 4 that the first touch submodality to recover is that of movement, followed by constant touch, and for simple touch to recover before two-point discrimination. The Pressure-Specified Sensory Device™ has been used effectively to monitor neural regeneration (see Figure 7.21 and Chapter 12 for additional specific examples). For this specific indication of quantitative sensory testing, it is critical to have an instrument with the capacity to measure both moving- and static-touch thresholds for both one-point and two-point detection.

The Pressure-Specified Sensory Device™ has been demonstrated to be reliable and valid. The interrater correlation is excellent (r = .61 and p = .78 by ANOVA), which means that there is no significant difference between the observations made by the two different examiners (E. S. Dellon et al., 1993). The intertest correlation for the same examiner is excellent (r = .930 for 2PM and r = .970 for 1PS). Measurements obtained with this device have an excellent correlation with hand function, as measured with the

Mayo Dexterity Test and a test of timed object recognition (E. S. Dellon et al., 1995). In particular, both the pressure and the distance thresholds for two-point discrimination had a correlation coefficient of (r = .790 for pressure and r = .802 for distance, p < .0001). Whereas no previous study had demonstrated a correlation between the one-point static threshold as determined traditionally with the Semmes-Weinstein monofilaments, this study, using the measurement technology available with the Pressure-Specified Sensory Device™, did demonstrate a correlation between 1PS threshold and object identification of (r = .691, p < .001).

Finally, in terms of validity, the diagnosis obtained by traditional electrodiagnostic testing was correlated with that obtained with the Pressure-Specified Sensory Device™ for patients with clinically significant upper and lower extremity nerve compressions; that is, subsequent to testing they each had surgical decompression (Tassler & Dellon, 1995). Table 7.9 demonstrates the excellent correlation found in this study. In brief, all patients with abnormal electrodiagnostic testing had abnormal quantitative sensory testing with the Pressure-Specified Sensory Device™. Those patients with clinically significant peripheral nerve compression who had normal

electrodiagnostic testing had abnormal quantitative sensory testing with the Pressure-Specified Sensory Device™.

CRITICAL ANALYSIS OF THE PRESSURE-SPECIFIED SENSORY DEVICE™

The Pressure-Specified Sensory Device™ meets all the criteria of the consensus reports of the American Diabetes Association and the American Peripheral Neuropathy Association (Arezzo et al., 1993) for quantitative sensory testing. Although this computer-assisted sensory testing device has not yet benefitted from published, widespread, independent confirmation of its clinical utility, its utility has been proven in over 4 years of continuous use for patient evaluation at the Children's Hospital in Baltimore. Reports of normative data for the upper and lower extremity are now available, as are studies of the diagnosis of chronic nerve compression in the upper and lower extremities. The device is sufficiently sensitive to permit investigation of clinical questions of sensibility (Watts, Tassler, & Dellon, 1994), many of which are outlined in Chapter 20.

This device appears to be able to resolve the controversy as to whether it is better to do threshold or innervation density testing in patients with peripheral nerve problems. That is because

TABLE 7.9   PRESSURE-SPECIFIED SENSORY DEVICE™ CORRELATION WITH ELECTRODIAGNOSTIC TESTING* USING CLINICAL DIAGNOSIS AS THE GOLD STANDARD

Carpal Tunnel Syndrome

	CLIN+	CLIN–	SPEC	SENS
PSSD +	23	0	*	100%
PSSD–	0	0		
EDT +	20	0	*	87%
EDT–	3	0		

Cubital Tunnel Syndrome

	CLIN+	CLIN–	SPEC	SENS
PSSD +	19	0	*	83%
PSSD–	4	0		
EDT +	9	0	*	39%
EDT–	14	0		

Tarsal Tunnel Syndrome

	CLIN+	CLIN–	SPEC	SENS
PSSD +	16	0	*	100%
PSSD–	0	0		
EDT +	13	0		*81%
EDT–	3	0		

Common Peroneal Nerve Entrapment

	CLIN+	CLIN–	SPEC	SENS
PSSD +	9	0	*	90%
PSSD–	1	0		
EDT +	7	0		*70%
EDT–	3	0		

Note:

(+) Disease present

(-) Disease absent

(*) Statistically undefined

From "Correlation of Measurements of Pressure Perception Using the Pressure-Specified Sensory Device with Electrodiagnostic Testing," by P. L. Tassler & A. L. Dellon, 1995, *Journal of Occupational Medicine 37*:862-866. Reprinted with permission of the authors.

FIGURE 7.22

The Greenleaf Eval™ System. This system provides menu-driven Macintosh software that generates very detailed anatomic (A and B) and graphic (C) reports related to impairment ratings. Its own proprietary measurement device provides range-of-motion information for joints through the Data-Glove™, but otherwise the strength measurements are generated through Jamar-type devices that are linked directly to the computer, and the sensory measurements are generated through traditional noncomputer devices, the Semmes-Weinstein filaments, and the Disk-Criminator™, and then entered by hand onto the computer screen. From brochure accompanying the Greenleaf Eval™ System, published by Greenleaf Medical Systems, Palo Alto, CA. Reprinted with permission of the company.

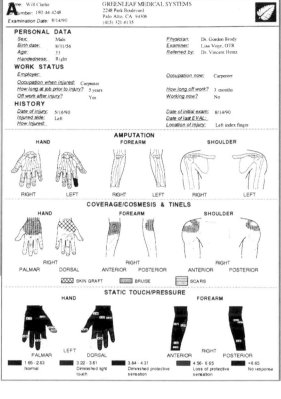

the device is the most ideal instrument to make the classic measurement of one-point static touch and to make the threshold measurements for two-point discrimination, which now can include the threshold for the pressure at which the two points can be distinguished. The relationship between the upper limits of normal for the pressure thresholds in the hands and the development of symptoms for chronic nerve compression suggest that the Pressure-Specified Sensory Device™ will be ideal for screening and surveillance in industry (see Chapter 18).

Toward that end, this device can be combined with computer-assisted motor testing in a portable case with notebook-size computer and printer. The software to operate it is extremely user-friendly. Classes for instruc-tion or certification in quantitative sensory testing with this equipment are available at the manufacturer's facility in Minneapolis.

Thus, the only disadvantage of the Pressure-Specified Sensory Device™ is its cost (Chapter 7 Appendix), which can be minimized by obtaining it in a modular, or step-wise fashion, rather than having to purchase it as part of an entire "system" of measurement, display, and reporting services. Future acceptance of this device and its unique measurement ability will depend on independent confirmation of its value by other therapists and clinicians. It is anticipated that there will be a large future demand for quantitative sensory testing that will create the need for therapists with the ability to provide this ser-vice. It is likely that this demand will originate not only from the traditional source of surgeons caring for patients with peripheral nerve problems, but also from podiatrists attempting to document progression of neuropathy to satisfy medicare requirements for documentation prior to obtaining special shoes, from oncologists attempting to monitor the development of sensory neuropathy related to vincristine, cisplatin, and taxol treatment, and from primary care physicians who will want to obtain cost-effective, valid, nonpainful measurements of their patients prior to authorizing more expensive neurologic evaluations.

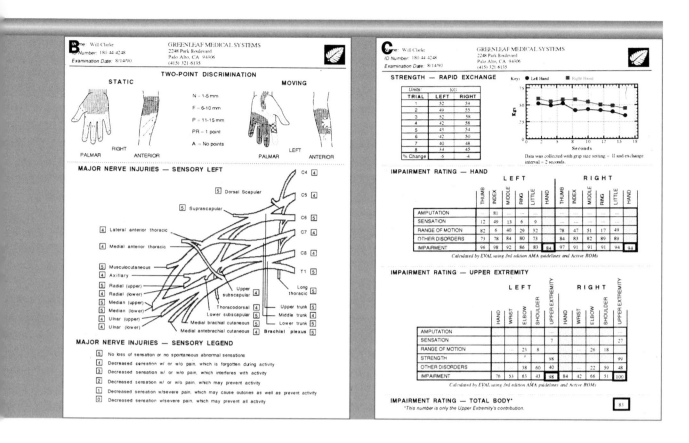

OTHERS

Four very similar systems are available that make the same general statements about their abilities and which provide about the same variety of services to the therapist/clinician. They are the Greenleaf Eval™ system, the Cedaron Dexter™ system, the Exos Clinical Hand Master system, and the newest one, the Henley system. Each of these provides a basic computer system to which they add one or more of their own proprietary products, usually ones that measure range of motion of the joints of the hand and wrist. To this they add an array of software designed primarily to convert the joint range of motion measurements, and other measurements that are made with already existing instruments, such as the Semmes-Weinstein monofilaments or the Disk-Criminator™ for sensibility, and such as a variation of the Jamar dynamometer and pinch meter for strength, into an *impairment* rating.

The rating is set into a colorful and graphic display that is designed to impress referring physicians and insurance carriers. Some of the software programs provide for photograph-like imaging of the hand deformity that can be included in the report as part of the record. One of the systems can even be voice-actuated, if you want to invest in the software. None of these systems makes computer-assisted measurements of sensibility or uses devices to measure strength that can be traced to NIST. In general, these are expensive systems that provide beautifully colored graphic and photographic displays of impairment and serial recordings of patient progress. They will make your practice more efficient only if you need to add the range of motion of a large number of joints to your reports, and if you otherwise need the computer to calculate your impairment rating for you. For comparison purposes, brief examples of the information/reports from each of these systems follow. The information has been obtained from the manufacturers' literature.

The Greenleaf Eval™ system has a proprietary Data-Glove™ that is placed on the hand which generates the range of motion measurements. The Eval™ system uses Macintosh software and hardware and is not IBM-compatible, although the company says such compatibility will be available in the future. Strength measurements are input by the patient gripping a dynamometer-type device with a curved handle. Pinch measurements are recorded by pinching a similar device, in any one the three classic forms of pinch. Sensibility measurements are input as the numerical marking on the nylon monofilament handle, that is, the log value, not as the pressure in g/mm^2, by the therapist recording separately the cutaneous pressure threshold with the Semmes-Weinstein monofilaments, whose value then appears color-coded according to the Judy Bell-Krotoski scheme (see section on "Semmes-Weinstein Nylon Monofilament" above and Figure 7.8). Two-point discrimination is measured separately by the therapist, using a Disk-Criminator™, and input into the computer as the distance in millimeters. Image capturing allows the picture of the hand to appear in the report. Examples of the reporting format are given in Figure 7.22.

There is no normative data unique to this equipment. It has recently become available in laptop computer configuration.

The Dexter™ system, manufactured by the Cedaron Corporation and distributed through Smith Nephew Corporation, is the system that offers the voice-actuated computer through licensed software. Its newest software allows the user to just "touch screen" in order to change the screen, instead of using the mouse. Its imaging system provides accurate reproductions of X rays or images of the hand to be included in the report. It has no proprietary measurement devices and relied, in the past, on Jamar-type strength measurements which are computer-linked, and on sensory measurements done traditionally with the Semmes-Weinstein nylon monofilaments and the Disk-Criminator™, which are then entered by hand into the computer (see Figure 7.23 for a sample report from their digital image processing system.) As of mid-1995, the NK measurement devices for grip and pinch, and the Pressure-Specified Sensory Device™, have been approved for inclusion with the IBM-compatible Dexter™ system, available through Cedaron or Smith-Nephew.

The Henley Hands On™ system is the most recent addition to the group of computerized evaluations of the hand and upper extremity. It offers the same options as the competing systems described above, with no apparent differences. It offers no proprietary measurement devices. Its software may offer more degrees of color shading for the Semmes-Weinstein monofilaments, and more icons, such as a key for the choice of "key-pinch," and a curved image of the Jamar for the strength choice. Its report format offers a pie graph to depict the percent loss of strength.

PERCEPTION OF VIBRATION

The perception of vibration is the interpretation of patterns of impulses transmitted to the brain by the quickly-adapting large myelinated (group A-beta) fibers. While there is the Greek word *pallesthesia* for vibratory sense, it is now clear that there is no separate "sense" of vibration the way there is for vision, smell, and hearing. Vibration is another form of touch. Vibration perception is not bone conduction, but is transmitted through the nerve fibers in the skin and dermis. To be sure, there is a transmission of the energy of the vibratory stimulus down to the bone, and nerve fibers within the periosteum may be stimulated and transmit impulses to the brain, but the perception of vibration is primarily mediated through the nerve fibers to the skin. Instru-

FIGURE 7.23

The Dexter™ System. Its graphic imager provides beautiful photographic images, such as these, which are included in the reports. This system lacks proprietary measurement products. Its unique software features include the potential for voice-actuated commands, and the "touch screen" operating system. From brochure accompanying the Dexter™ System, published by Cedaron Medical, Incorporated, Davis, CA. Reprinted with permission of the company.

Sample Report from Digital Image Processing System

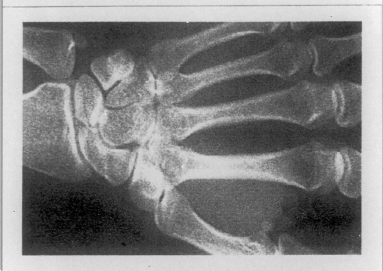

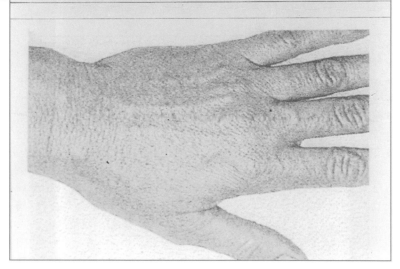

ments to test vibration may, therefore, be considered as those that can stimulate just one frequency, for example, 120 Hz, but can vary the intensity of the stimulus by increasing the amount of voltage into the vibrating probe (head or tactor), a fixed-frequency, variable-intensity vibrometer, or one that can also vary the stimulus frequency, a variable-frequency, variable-intensity vibrometer.

The quantity that is measured with the vibrometer is best understood as the distance in microns the stimulating probe must penetrate the skin to be perceived (a micron is 10^{-4} cm or 10^{-6} meters; a red blood cell is about 8 microns in diameter) . This is often called *microns of motion*. The probe tip

is calibrated in air, not against any fixed resistance, by increasing the voltage into the device and measuring the excursion of the probe tip. A calibration curve or table would accompany the instrument; therefore, reports with a given device might be reported as either voltage, amps, or microns of motion. Since different machines have varying resistance, it is difficult to compare the threshold values reported for different vibrometers unless they use microns of motion.

Another problem in reporting vibratory thresholds is that acoustical engineers speak about vibration or noise levels in terms of decibels. This is similar to the problem the psychologist found when reporting the pressure threshold, and decided to use logarithm values to construct a small, uniform interval scale from numbers that might have ranged from 10ths of milligrams to grams. Since the intensity range of vibratory stimuli can be so large, the acoustic engineers defined the decibel to be 20x the value of the logarithm to the base 10 of the ratio of the stimulus in microns to a standard reference (decibel = 20 $\log_{10}$ [observed value in microns /10^{-9} microns]). The difference between a nylon monofilament of 4.0 and 6.0 is not 2.0 but 10^2, or 100x. This difference is magnified even more for the decibel system, and in a manner such that the difference between 40 and 60 decibels is the difference between 0.1 and 1.0 microns (a difference of less than 1 micron), whereas the difference between 60 and 80 decibels (another jump of 20 decibels, an equal interval in decibels) is the difference between 10 and 100 microns (a difference of 90 microns).

It can be seen, then, that without a conversion table it is not readily clear to most people that a difference of 20 decibels, which may not appear to be a big difference, may in fact be a very large difference in microns, depending on where on the scale this change occurs (see Figure 7.24). The threshold measurement is complicated by the fact that the probe may be pressed into the skin sufficiently hard by the examiner, or the patient may press so hard against the probe, as to damp the vibrations. While initial reports with vibrometers ignored or discounted this effect, more recent studies show that the force of application of the vibrating probe against the skin surface does damp the oscillation. Thus, the reported microns of motion are larger than the actual stimulus intensity. Newer vibrometers, such as the Case IV and the Force-Defined Vibrometer, set the oscillation of the probe tip against an already applied force sufficient to overcome skin compliance.

THE OPTACON™

The Optacon™ was among the first vibrotactile testing devices to be used clinically for the evaluation of peripheral neuropathy. It was reasoned that most neuropathies are of the distal axonopathy type, meaning that the symptoms began at the tips of the toes first, then the fingers, and progressed, if they did, proximally. Therefore, a device that could test the sensory threshold at the tips of the fingers might be valuable. In 1973, engineers developed a device called the Optacon™ to translate visual (camera) cues into vibrotactile cues to permit blind people to be aware of their environment and to read without braille. Original designs used arrays of vibrating probes, or tactors, that reformatted visual cues into spatial patterns for perception by a given body surface, such as the back or the thigh.

The modified Optacon™ is a battery-powered device consisting of 144 miniature rods organized into a 24 x 6 matrix, with a 2 mm horizontal and a 1 mm vertical interrod spacing. These rods protrude through a plastic plate and contact a discrete portion of skin. They vibrate at 230 Hz. The amplitude of vibration varies with the voltage applied, and the threshold for stimulation is reported in volts. In general, testing proceeds after a period of familiarization so that the subject will know what particular pattern of stimulation is the correct stimulus. Then a series of 5 ascending and 5 descending trials is given, according to the method of limits. The high and low values are usually discarded, and the rest averaged to give the threshold. The device emits a noise, and subjects are often given a set of headphones to wear during testing (Arezzo & Schaumberg, 1980).

The device has been found useful for screening for neuropathy associated with neurotoxicity, such as acrylamide (Arezzo, Schaumberg, & Peterson, 1983). In a study of 257 workers exposed to acrylamide, a consistent age-related linear decrease in vibration sensitivity within the population was detected. Individuals with subclinical involvement of the peripheral nerves were identified with this equipment. The authors of this study felt that the Optacon™ was suited for longitudinal study of such workers. They also concluded that the

Optacon™ is most useful for rapidly surveying large populations for sensory loss, but it is clearly not as sensitive as the elaborate computer-assisted devices currently employed in some centers (e.g., the Mayo Clinic) to detect dysfunction of specific sensory systems, and due to intersubject variability is no substitute for a careful examination by a neurologist.

See also the study by Bleecker (1986) using this device in screening for carpal tunnel syndrome.

CRITICAL ANALYSIS OF THE OPTACON™

Although I have never used the Optacon™ to evaluate patients, it is clear that this device is not being used extensively clinically. On September 10, 1993 I traveled to Princeton, NJ, to visit with Roger Cholewiak, PhD, in the Cutaneous Communications Laboratory. He and his colleagues have been using the Optacon™ for more than a decade for psychophysiologic studies related to perception and learning. I had the opportunity to try the device in learning and discrimination paradigms. I felt humbled by my

inability to rapidly acquire the ability to see these patterns with my fingertip. A younger colleague of mine, however, was much more successful, clearly being far more sensitive, if not smarter, than I. Judging by the few Optacons™ in use clinically, it is clear they have been supplanted by the development of simpler-to-use vibratory testing instruments.

• PERCEPTION OF (ELECTRICAL) CURRENT •

THE NEUROMETER™

The Neurometer™ is an instrument for quantitative sensory testing that generates constant current electrical sine waves at three different frequencies, and applies them transcutaneously to directly stimulate the sensory nerve fibers. In this way, its stimulus differs from the mechanical stimuli that have been discussed above for touch and vibration, stimuli which require transduction through sensory receptors for the impulse to be stimulated. Therefore, the three different frequencies used to stimulate with the Neurometer™, 5 Hz, 250 Hz, and 2000 Hz, must not be confused with the different frequencies generated by the vibrometers, which will stimulate different subpopufibers. In this way, its stimulus differs from the mechanical stimuli that have been discussed above for touch and vibration, stimuli which require transduction through sensory receptors for the impulse to be stimulated. Therefore, the three different frequencies used to stimulate with the Neurometer™, 5 Hz, 250 Hz, and 2000 Hz, must not be confused with the different frequencies generated by the vibrometers, which will stimulate different subpopulations of the group A-beta (large myelinated) fibers.

Indeed, one of the claims for the uniqueness of the Neurometer™ is that it is neuroselective; that is, the 2000 Hz stimulation will cause the large myelinated fibers, the A-betas, to respond, whereas the 250 Hz will more likely stimulate the A-deltas, and the 5 Hz the unmyelinated C-fibers. Normative data is given in Table 7.10. This claim was substantiated in patients recovering from spinal anesthesia in whom the recovery of different new fiber populations was correlated with Neurometer™ frequencies (Liu, Kopacz, & Carpenter, 1995).

The electrical stimulation is delivered by means of electrodes that are taped to the skin (see Figure 7.25) over the dermatome or the cutaneous territory of the peripheral nerve being tested. Normative data have been accumulated

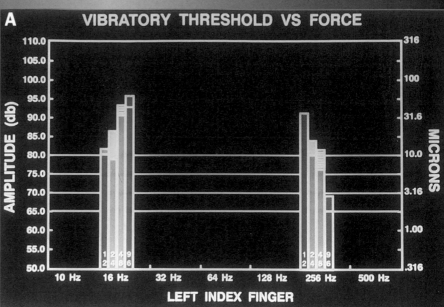

FIGURE 7.24

The Force-Defined Vibrometer. (A) A variable frequency, variable intensity vibrometer. The unique feature of this device is that prior to making the measurement of the vibratory threshold, skin compliance is tested. The skin compliance measurement is then transferred into the Force-Defined Vibrometer, which defines the force at which the oscillating probe will contact the skin surface before the vibratory stimulus is applied. Variation in cutaneous vibratory threshold for the index finger of a normal person occurs in direct relationship to the force applied to the end of the vibrating probe. Note that for the 16 Hz and the 256 Hz frequencies, the force applied has been varied from 12 to 96 g. Note the large variation in threshold with change both in applied pressure of the vibrating probe and in frequency. (B) Example of normal vibratory threshold for a given force of application, here 8 g for two different fingers. The shaded region of the top of each bar represents the range during which the stimulus is first perceived (top of bar) and last perceived (bottom of shaded region). The threshold is the average of these two values.

(C) Example of alterations in vibratory perception for different frequencies in a patient 9 months after digital nerve repair. Note that the lowest frequencies (Meissner afferents) have begun to recover, while the highest frequency (Pacinian afferents) lag behind, as expected dur-

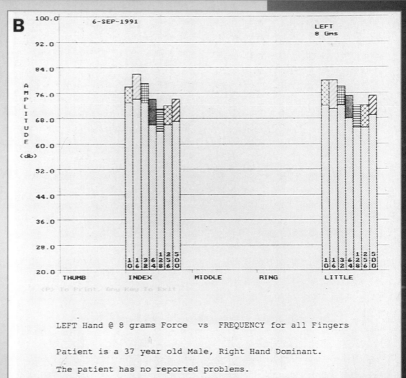

LEFT Hand @ 8 grams Force vs FREQUENCY for all Fingers

Patient is a 37 year old Male, Right Hand Dominant.

The patient has no reported problems.

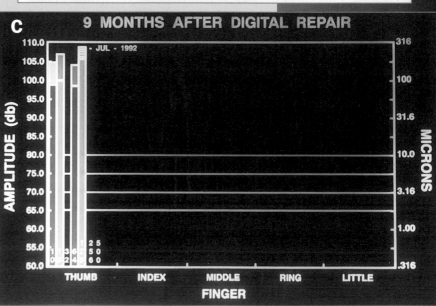

ing normal neural regeneration. *(D) Example of abnormal vibrogram for a patient with sensory loss following vincristine chemotherapy for the treatment of lymphoma. Note that the perception of the low-frequency vibration becomes abnormal first. (Similar findings for patients with neuropathy after lead poisoning are given in Chapter 14.) (E) Normative, age-related data for the index finger. (A) from "Quantitative Sensory Testing with the Force-Defined Vibrometer," by E. S. Dellon & A. L. Dellon, Journal of Reconstructive Microsurgery, submitted: 1995. Reprinted with permission of the authors. (B), (C), (D) and (E).*

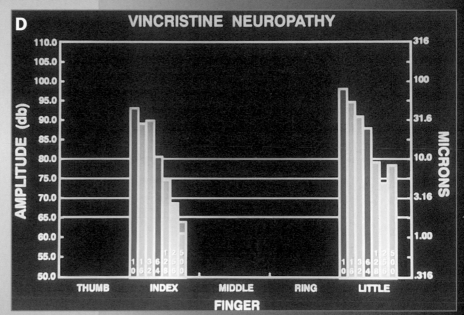

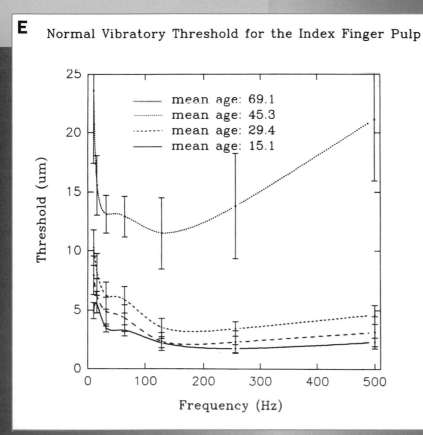

for the face (the trigeminal nerve), the hand (the median nerve), and the big toe (the peroneal nerve). The stimuli are delivered in a forced-choice paradigm generated by the computer. The test is usually set up to compare the threshold at the face to the thresholds at the hand and big toe, as well as left versus right, and for each test site itself.

The Neurometer™ was introduced in a review article by Bleecker in 1986, and then in a series of papers by Jefferson Katims, MD, a physiatrist from Baltimore who invented the device when he was a medical student at the Johns Hopkins University School of Medicine (Katims, Naviasky, Ng, Bleecker, & Rendell, 1986; Katims et al., 1991). Margit Bleecker, MD, PhD, is a neurologist working primarily with occupational medicine problems. Their studies, along with those by Masson and Boulton's group (Masson & Boulton, 1991; Masson, Veves, Fernando, & Boulton, 1989) in Manchester, England have established the Neurometer™ as an instrument capable of detecting neuropathy in diabetics, alcoholics, and uremics.

A booklet containing 45 abstracts of studies using the Neurometer™ is available from the manufacturer (see Appendix at end of this chapter). An example of the type of population study done by Katims, Naviasky,

Ng, Bleecker, & Rendell (1986) was one involving 29 patients on long-term hemodialysis. Traditional electrodiagnostic studies identified abnormalities in the median nerve distribution in 79% of the patients, while current perception threshold testing identified abnormalities in 92%, for a correlation coefficient of r = .79, p < .001. In 9 patients tested more than once over a 4-week period, the coefficient of variation for the 2000 Hz stimulus was found to be 6%.

Masson et al. (1989) studied 31 normals and 90 diabetics. They found that the current perception thresholds could distinguish between the neuropathic and nonneuropathic groups of diabetics, p < .001, and that the device was "quick [10 to 15 minutes] and easy to use." Furthermore, by studying temperature and vibratory perception in the same group of diabetic patients in whom they did current perception threshold testing, they found a strong correlation between the 2000 Hz stimulus and large diameter nerve fibers (vibratory perception, correlation, r = .42-.69, p < .001) and between the 5 Hz stimulus and small diameter nerve fibers (temperature perception, r = .34-.46, p <.005). They found the coefficient of variation at 2000 Hz to be 8-11%, and at 5 Hz 16-20%. These studies involved populations of pa-

tients, and did not serially follow individual patients.

I have used the Neurometer™ to evaluate patients with neuropathy due to lead poisoning, and have found it able to monitor the progress of the neuropathy after nerve decompressions (see Figure 14.13).

The most recent study of the use of the Neurometer™ as a potential instrument for industrial screening for carpal tunnel syndrome has not been supportive of the use of this device. Franzblau, Werner, Johnston, and Torrey (1994) evaluated 84 workers from an automotive assembly plant using a self-administered questionnaire of carpal tunnel symptoms, a limited electrodiagnostic test of median and ulnar distal sensory latency and amplitude, and the full Neurometer™ test to the index finger. The prevalence of carpal tunnel syndrome in this group of workers was 15%.

Franzblau et al. (1994) found very weak correlations (r < .20) between the current perception threshold for any frequency and any of the electrophysiologic measurements. They found that when the presence of carpal tunnel symptoms was taken as the gold standard, the Neurometer™ sensitivity was .53, the specificity was .61, the positive predictive value was .19, and the negative predictive value was .88. (The comparative values for the electrodiagnostic test ver-

TABLE 7.10 CURRENT PERCEPTION THRESHOLD TESTING: NORMATIVE DATE FOR THE NEUROMETER™				
	Minimum	**Maximum**	**Mean**	**S.D.**
Trigeminal Nerve				
5 Hz	001	038	010	008
50 Hz	004	051	021	011
2000 Hz	045	244	1390	44
Median Nerve				
5 Hz	016	100	048	020
250 Hz	022	180	084	031
2000 Hz	120	398	237	058
Peroneal Nerve				
5 Hz	018	170	078	032
250 Hz	044	190	118	037
2000 Hz	187	516	323	076

Note: Data from the manufacturer of the Neurometer™, Neurotron, Incorporated, Baltimore, MD. Reprinted with permission of the company.

sus symptoms was .44, .85, .34, and .90 respectively.) They found that when the presence of carpal tunnel syndrome was determined using electrodiagnostic testing as the gold standard, the Neurometer™ sensitivity was .60, the specificity was .63, the positive predictive value was .22, and the negative predictive value was .90. They concluded that current perception threshold testing could not be recommended as a screening procedure for identification of possible cases of carpal tunnel syndrome among active industrial workers.

Experience with the Neurometer™ in evaluating sensibility of the penis is discussed in Chapter 17. The Neurometer™ was found to be quite useful in testing this region of the body.

CRITICAL ANALYSIS OF THE NEUROMETER™

In 1988, I began to use the Neurometer™ in an attempt to quantitate the sensory changes in diabetics in whom I was doing peripheral nerve decompressions to relieve the symptoms of their neuropathy. It was clear to me then, as has actually been observed by many neurologists, that electrodiagnostic testing often did not correlate with the patient's symptomatology in diabetic neuropathy.

The Neurometer™ was used extensively during the next 2 years to evaluate diabetics with neuropathy, patients with peripheral nerve compression, patients following denervation of regions of the extremities, and patients following nerve repair or grafting. It was also used to study men with impotence, which is discussed in Chapter 17. Our experience led to some modifications in the use of the instrument, particularly in realizing that the big toe is an ambiguous region to test because it contains nerves from both the peroneal and the posterior tibial nerve. Figure 7.25 demonstrates the change in electrode placement that was suggested from our experience (Dellon & Scally, unpublished obser-

FIGURE 7.25

Current Perception Threshold testing; the Neurometer. This instrument (A) delivers a constant current sinusoidal wave of varying frequency to determine the cutaneous perception threshold. This type of stimulation differs from the mechanical stimulation of the other instruments that stimulate touch in that the electrical current theoretically directly stimulates the nerve fibers, whereas the mechanical stimuli must be trans-

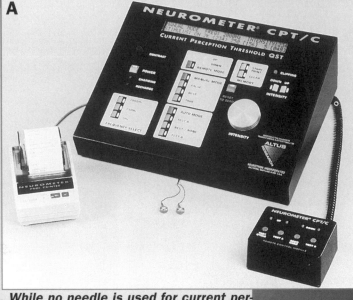

duced by the sensory receptors. While no needle is used for current perception testing, the electrical stimulation does produce sensory perceptions ranging from stinging or burning pain for the low, 5 Hz frequency, to more mechanical types of buzzing for the 2000 Hz frequency. In (B), the electrode is shown around the big toe, which was originally described as the point to stimulate the peroneal nerve. It is suggested, however, from our use of the Neurometer™ that this produces stimulation of both the peroneal and the posterior tibial nerve, with the patient's threshold being related to the more normal nerve. It is suggested further, therefore, that placement of the electrode for the peroneal nerve be as in (C), while for

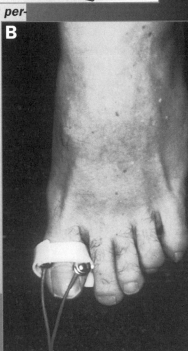

the posterior tibial nerve, as in (D). Figures (A)–(D) copyright A. Lee Dellon. Reprinted with permission.

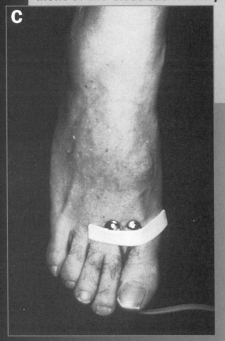

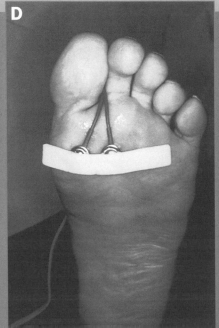

FIGURE 7.26

Current Perception Threshold testing; the Neurometer™. (A) Normative data (courtesy of Neurotron, Inc., Baltimore, MD). (B) Repeated testing with the Neurometer™ in a 19-year-old patient who had interfascicular nerve grafting of her right posterior tibial nerve over a 15 cm segment beginning proximal to the knee. The contralateral (left) foot serves as a normal control for the observations related to nerve fiber regeneration over time. Note that after a delay required for axon sprouts to reach the plantar aspect of the foot, there was first a decrease in the current perception threshold for the 5 Hz stimulus. The next stimulus perception to recover was that for the 250 Hz frequency. The last frequency stimulation to begin to recover was that for the highest frequency, 2000 Hz. This is a good correlation with the clinical observations that the first sensory perceptions to recover following nerve grafting are the perceptions of pain and temperature, all mediated by the thinly myelinated and unmyelinated fiber population. The last sensory functions to recover are those related to the larger A-beta myelinated fibers, for moving- and static-touch. The results of the above clinical observations and Neurometer™ measurements suggest that perception of the 5 Hz stimulation is related to the nerve fiber population with small diameter fibers, while perception related to 2000 Hz stimulation is related to the nerve fiber population with large diameter fibers. (A. L. Dellon, MD, unpublished observation).

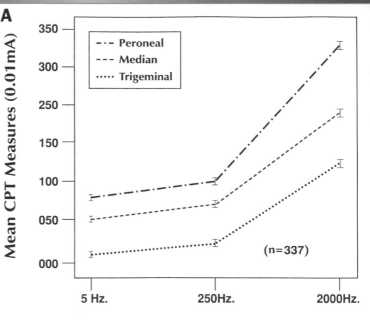

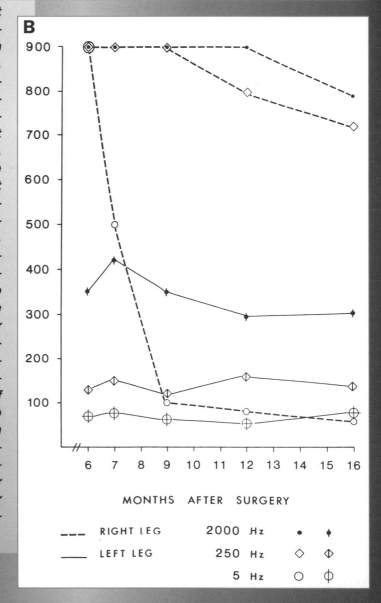

vations, 1994).

We found that the perception of stimuli in the big toe was transmitted through whichever of these two nerves was the least affected by the peripheral nerve problem. With respect to the diabetic population, we found it difficult to monitor individual patients during the postoperative period because about 50% of diabetics could not distinguish the stimuli of the different frequency electrical sine waves from the neuropathic sensations that they were experiencing from either their diabetes or from the neural regenerative phenomenon. Indeed, it was our disappointment with this particular aspect of the Neurometer™ that became part of the impetus for pursuing the development of the Pressure-Specifying Sensory Device™, the first prototype of which became available in late 1989.

However, the Neurometer™ itself was found to be reliable and easy to use. We found it valid for evaluating the recovery of neural function after nerve repair or grafting (see Figure 7.26), in that the low-frequency stimuli, reflecting the small diameter nerve fiber population, was the first to recover toward the normal threshold, followed thereafter, and in temporal sequencing, by the response to the 250 Hz and the 2000 Hz stimuli. We found that the thresholds were often below normal in patients with pain, perhaps consistent with a hypersensitivity. We also found that we could identify regions of denervation and subsequent reinnervation, consistent with the concept of collateral sprouting (see Devor, Schonfeld, Seltzer, & Wall, 1979, and Chapter 4).

THE BIO-THESIOMETER™

The Bio-Thesiometer™ may represent the first commercially available, hand-held, fixed-frequency (120 Hz), variable-intensity vibrometer (see Figure 7.27). The most recent model is the "PVD," but it differs little from the original. The scale on the vibrometer screen is calibrated to read out in volts across the top and microns of motion across the bottom, with the relationship such that 5 volts produces .25 microns of motion, 10 volts produces 1.0 microns of motion, and 25 volts produces 6.4 microns of motion. The accuracy is said by the manufacturer to be ± 1%. Normative data have been reported by Gregg (1951), and are given in Figure 7.28.

Because the Bio-Thesiometer™ can be hand held, it can be used to test the vibration perception threshold on any body surface area. The normative data for this instrument on the face can be found in Chapter 15, on the breast in Chapter 16, and on the penis in Chapter 17. The normative data for the upper extremity, from the first study in which the Bio-Thesiometer™ was introduced into the hand surgery literature (Dellon, 1983) is contained in Table 7.11.

The Bio-Thesiometer™ has been found to be an efficient device with which to test vibratory threshold. It has been useful in the research setting as well. A drawback to its use, as with most vibrometers, is that if the examiner presses the probe too hard against the skin surface to be tested, the probe's oscillations are damped, creating an error between the actual stimulus intensity delivered to the skin and that recorded on the dial, for which the probe tip calibration was done against air.

THE SENSORTEK II™

The Sensortek II™ is a fixed-frequency (120 Hz), variable-intensity vibrometer upon which the subject may place a finger or a toe for evaluation of the vibratory perception threshold (see Figure 7.29). Because it is relatively stationary, it cannot be used to test the vibratory perception threshold for other body surface areas.

The value of screening populations of patients with vibrometry has been evaluated with the Sensortek in comparison with traditional electrodiagnostic testing, and with the

Nerve Pace, a hand-held, "quick" office-type distal motor latency device (see Chapter 8). A group of 29 shipyard workers were tested with each device, and each worker was further questioned and examined by an occupational health physician with respect to the likelihood of carpal tunnel syndrome being present. A group of 10 asymptomatic hospital workers served as controls. The results of the study are abstracted in Table 7.12. This study demonstrated that there was a good correlation of the vibratory threshold in microns of motion (a sensory test) with the results of the motor testing by both the traditional electrodiagnostic study and the Nerve Pace. When used to screen the population at risk, however, the electrodiagnostic tests proved to be more sensitive, while the vibrometry was more specific. The actual value of the numbers for sensitivity and specificity changed, depending on the certainty of the clinical diagnosis.

Unfortunately, this means that if the Sensortek II™ were used to screen this population, workers with carpal tunnel syndrome would go undetected. Those workers who would be picked up by the Sensortek II™, however, would have a high probability of actually having carpal tunnel syndrome. The cost/risk benefit of using a less expensive, less painful

FIGURE 7.27

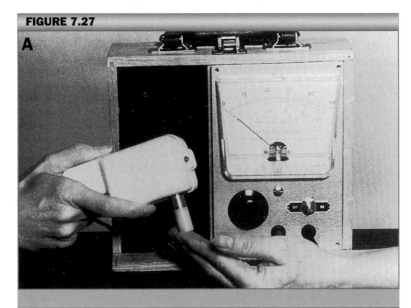

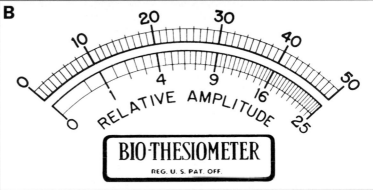

Bio-Thesiometer™. (A) A fixed-frequency (120 Hz), variable-intensity vibrometer. The hand-held probe of the instrument is applied gently to the skin surface being tested with one hand, while the examiner uses the other hand to increase the stimulus intensity. When the vibratory stimulus is perceived by the subject, the subject must indicate this verbally. (B) Several ascending trials are done, and the resulting threshold in microns of motion is averaged, after reading directly from the scale that reports both volts and microns of motion. Photo from Surgery of the Peripheral Nerve, *by S. E. Mackinnon & A. L. Dellon, 1988, New York: Thieme Publishing. Reprinted with permission of the authors.*

screening test must be weighed against the cost of not detecting true disease and the cost of having to do expensive testing anyway on those detected by screening but who, in fact, do not have the disease. This type of analysis needs to be done for each proposed screening test device.

FIGURE 7.28

A

Forehead 6.16	Trunk, anterior	Calf, distal side 2.96
Cheekbone 7.90	T2 ....2.96	First Toe Base 0.616
Jaw Bone 6.16	T4 ....2.34	First Toe Tip 0.838
Sternal notch 2.21	T6 ....3.70	Toe
Shoulder................7.40	T8 ....6.41	2 ....1.11
Upper Arm..............1.72	T11 ....9.11	3 ....1.38
Forearm 6.90	Trunk, posterior	4 ....1.12
Wrist...................0.780	T2 ....1.47	5 ....0.936
Finger Tip	T4 ....1.97	Instep 0.666
1 (thumb)............0.370	T6 ....5.42	Edge of Tibia 0.780
2 ....0.420	T8 ....14.7	Side of Knee 3.50
3 ....0.395	T11 ....6.16	Calf, proximal side 2.95
4 ....0.320	7th Vertebral Spine........6.90	Sacrum 12.3
5 ....0.370	Thigh	
	L2 ....8.88	
	L3 ....6.66	

B

Finger Tips 0.375	Upper Arm...............1.720	Trunk, anterior T8 ....6.410
First Toe Base 0.616	Trunk, posterior T4 ....1.970	Thigh L3 ....6.660
Instep 0.666	Sternal Notch 2.210	7th Vertebral Spine 6.900
Edge of Tibia 0.780	Trunk, anterior T4........2.340	Forearm 6.900
First Toe Tip 0.780	Calf, proximal side 2.950	Shoulder................7.400
Toe	Trunk, anterior T2 ....2.960	Thigh L2 ....8.880
2 ....0.946	Side of Knee 3.500	Trunk, anterior T11 ....9.110
3 ....1.110	Jaw Bone 3.700	Sacrum 12.300
4 ....1.120	Trunk, posterior T11.......5.420	Trunk, posterior T8.......14.700
5 ....1.380	Trunk, anterior T8.........6.160	
Trunk, posterior T2 ....1.470	Thigh L3................6.160	

Bio-Thesiometer™ (A & B) normative data for different body surfaces as reported by the manufacturer.

THE AUTOMATED TACTILE TESTER™

See description above under "Perception of Touch."

THE CASE IV SYSTEM

See description above under "Perception of Touch."

THE FORCE-DEFINED VIBROMETER™

The Force-Defined Vibrometer™ is a variable-frequency, variable-intensity device that began clinical trials in 1991, but which has just been described in the literature (Dellon & Dellon, 1995). This vibrometer can test the frequencies 10, 16, 32, 64, 128, 256, and 500 Hz, but differs from it in the basic principle that the vibrating probe first contacts the skin surface to be tested at a defined force. That force is defined as the force required to overcome the compliance of the skin surface being tested. Skin compliance is measured first with the NK Skin Compliance Device (see below). The force required to overcome skin compliance is set into the Force-Defined Vibrometer™, and becomes the force with which the vibrometer's probe presses against the skin. The force required to produce the vibration of the prong tip is superimposed on this initial force. Since as early as 1940, Geldard observed that vibratory threshold changed significantly with the force applied to the probe, and since this observation was verified by Gregg in 1951, Cosh in 1953, and more recently by Lowenthal and Hockaday in 1987, it was clear that a vibrometer incorporating this knowledge was needed. This unique feature of the Force-Defined Vibrometer™ permits a clear definition of the test parameters.

Figure 7.24 demonstrates

TABLE 7.11 BIO-THESIOMETER™ VIBRATORY PERCEPTION IN CHRONIC NERVE COMPRESSION

	n	Bio-Thesiometer™	Tuning Fork 30 Hz	Tuning Fork 256Hz	2PD Static ≥ 6mm	2PD Moving ≥ 4mm
Clinical Stage Carpal Tunnel Syndrome						
Early	7	0 % abnormal	28%↑	42%↑	0%	0%
Moderate	14	35% abnormal	7%↑, 42%↓	21%↑, 70%↓	0%	0%
Late	13	85% abnormal	8%↑, 84%↓	100%↓	48%	84%
Clinical Stage Cubital Tunnel Syndrome						
Early	2	50% abnormal	100%↑	100%↑	0%	0%
Moderate	3	33% abnormal	0%↑, 33%↓	0%↑, 33%↓	0%	0%
Late	5	100% abnormal	80%↓	100%↓	80%	100%

Note: Data from "The Vibrometer," by A. L. Dellon, 1983, *Plastic and Reconstructive Surgery 71:427-431.* Reprinted with permission of the author.

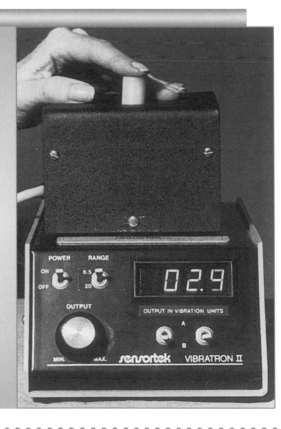

FIGURE 7.29

The Sensortek II™ vibrometer. A fixed frequency (120 Hz), variable intensity vibrometer. From **Surgery of the Peripheral Nerve, by S. E. Mackinnon & A. L. Dellon, 1988, New York: Thieme Publishing.** *Photos reprinted with permission of the authors.*

this change in vibratory threshold with change in the force of application of the stimulus. The observed pivot point is around the 64 to 128 Hz frequencies, and may be related to the known *viscoelastic* properties of skin. At low frequencies the skin behaves more like rubber, having a damping effect, such that increasing the force of stimulus application results in an increased threshold (i.e., less sensitivity). At higher frequencies, associated with a higher energy, the properties of skin behave more "ideally" elastic, such that increasing ease of transmission is manifested by lowering of the vibratory per-

TABLE 7.12 CORRELATION OF VIBROMETRY (SENSORTEK II), NERVE PACE, AND TRADITIONAL ELECTRODIAGNOSTIC TESTING OF THE INDEX FINGER

Correlation Coefficient*

Carpal tunnel symptoms (n=29)	r	
Nerve Pace	.81	p < .0001
Vibrometry	.48	p < .0003
Asymptomatic controls (n=10)		
Nerve Pace	.91	p < .0001
Vibrometry	.35	p < .18

Detection of Carpal Tunnel Syndrome

	Sensitivity	Specificity	Predictive Value
Clinical Symptoms Only			
Traditional NCS	.92	.44	.54
Nerve Pace	.86	.35	.47
Vibrometry	.29	.86	.60
Clinical Symptoms + Abnormal Physical Findings, + Abnormal NCS			
Nerve Pace	.86	.78	.86
Vibrometry	.21	.85	.80

Note:
* Correlation of distal motor latency with Nerve Pace and Vibrometry.
Data from "A Comparison of Digital Neurometry, Tactometry, and Nerve Conduction Studies in the Diagnosis of Carpal Tunnel Syndrome," by M. G. Cherniak, D. Maolli, & C. Viscolli, in press 1995, *Journal of Hand Surgery*. Reprinted with permission of the authors.

ception threshold.

The Force-Defined Vibrometer™ can vary the amplitude of stimulation from 0.1 microns to 316 microns (40 to 110 decibels). The probe tip that does the vibrating is a metal prong that is hemispherical in shape with a 1.8 m diameter (1.95 mm² hemispherical projected surface area). This prong is presented to the skin through a 3.0 mm diameter port over which the fingertip or the toe can rest. The testing paradigm is by the method of limits, using both an ascending and descending order for the stimulus. The entire sequence is repeated 3 times. The report prints out the ascending and descending limits of stimulus detection as a bar graph, and the mean of the two limits as a number. The accuracy of this vibrometer, according to the manufacturer's specifications, is ± 0.216 microns for a stimulus intensity of 40 decibels, ± 0.646 microns at 70 decibels, and ± 1.0 microns above 80 decibels.

The computer controls the stimuli, not the person doing the testing. The person doing the testing selects from the IBM-compatible software menu the force to be applied, the skin surface to be tested, and the frequency to be tested, and then pushes a button. The subject is seated so as not to be able to see the computer screen. The vibrometer is sufficiently sound-proofed so that the subject does not need to wear acoustic earphones. The subject pushes a button with the hand not being tested when the vibration is first perceived, and then when the vibration is no longer perceived.

Normative data have been obtained from the right and left index and little finger of 36 volunteers. This population was subdivided on the basis of age into 4 groups, ≤ 19 with a mean age of 15.1 (n = 9), 20-39 with a mean age of 29.4 (n = 9), 40-59 with a mean age of 45.3 (n = 8), and > 60 with a mean age of 69.1 (n = 10). The age-related normative data are given in Figure 7.24 (E) because the results of using the Force-Defined Vibrometer™, to evaluate upper extremity peripheral nerve problems are described in detail in Chapter 12.

The intertest reliability of the Force-Defined Vibrometer™ was evaluated by testing the same subject over the course of 1 year. The mean variability for all tested frequencies was 4.4 microns, with a range of 2-10 microns, with the greatest variability being at the 10 Hz end of the stimulus scale. Since the testing is done by

the computer, there is no need with this device to do interobserver reliability testing. The intratest reliability was evaluated from the three data points obtained at each test site. Repeated testing at a given frequency for a given test site had a mean variation of 3.5 microns. There is general agreement between the normative data obtained with the Force-Defined Vibrometer™ and previous work on vibratory perception in that the relationship between increasing frequency and threshold is a "U-shaped" curve, there is no difference between the right and the left hand, and there is an increase in threshold above 40 years of age.

The normative data for the Force-Defined Vibrometer™, however, is not easily comparable in the absolute number of microns to results from other vibrometers because of the uniqueness of the initial force applied to the fingertip, and because of the size of the probe's hemispherical tip. It was observed by Cosh (1953) that increasing the probe tip size from 3 to 19 to 75 mm^2 will decrease the vibratory threshold, presumably because the larger contact surface stimulates a greater number of sensory receptors. This observation has been confirmed by others, and is reviewed by Dellon and Dellon (1995). According to Mountcastle (1968), the mean peripheral nerve receptor field

size for the large myelinated nerve fibers is 3.71 mm^2 for 23 sites over the distal phalanx of the monkey. The surface area of the Force-Defined Vibrometer™ was chosen to be in about this range, or 1.95 mm^2. In contrast, the surface area of the Sensortek Vibrator II probe is 19 mm^2, while that of the Bruel & Kjaer vibrometer is 5 mm^2.

An example of the use of the Force-Defined Vibrometer™ to evaluate the results of a digital nerve repair is given in Figure 7.24 (C). From the discussion of the pattern of sensory recovery during neural regeneration (see Chapter 4), it is clear that the first vibratory perception to recover is that related to the low-frequency afferents, because it is relatively easier to reinnervate a Meissner corpuscle than a Pacinian corpuscle. From Figure 7.24 (C) it may be noted that the thresholds for the perception of the lower frequencies are still abnormally high, but they have begun to recover at a time when the highest two frequencies, 256 and 500 Hz, have not yet returned at all.

The results of using this vibrometer to evaluate patients with neuropathies, such as diabetes and lead poisoning, are described in Chapter 14 (see Figure 14.12), with one example being given in Figure 7.24 (D) for a neuropathy related to chemotherapy (vincristine). Note that the unusual "U-shaped" normal curve for threshold versus frequency (see Figure 7.24 B) is not present in this neuropathy, but rather the low-frequency thresholds are all markedly elevated with respect to normal and to the high-frequency thresholds. This pattern is similar to that seen with lead neuropathy, which is that the vibratory perception for low frequency is affected first, that is, it becomes increased. It is, therefore, possible that vibrometry may offer a method of providing a "fingerprint" for the different types of neurological problems that affect the peripheral nerve.

CRITICAL ANALYSIS OF VIBROMETRY

It is clear that evaluation of the large myelinated fiber population that subserves touch can be evaluated by the vibratory perception threshold. What remains unclear is what information can be gained from vibrometry that cannot be gained from measuring the cutaneous pressure threshold. Both the vibratory and cutaneous pressure threshold measurements are quantitative sensory testing and, as such, offer nonaversive, noninvasive, relatively inexpensive tools for evaluating the peripheral nervous system. As such, they were recommended by the consensus groups of both the American Diabetes Association and the Ameri-

can Peripheral Neuropathy Association in the spring of 1993. Neither of these techniques evaluates the small myelinated or unmyelinated classes of fibers. As will be noted in Chapter 14 on peripheral neuropathy, it is likely that there will be a different pattern of vibratory threshold abnormalities at different frequencies, related to specific neuropathies, but this is still largely anecdotal information.

The new knowledge that the force of application of the vibratory stimulus can change the threshold significantly implies that previous studies have large, systematic errors that cannot easily be rationalized. On the most simplistic level, the hand-held tuning fork, used as a qualitative screening test, remains very useful to me on a day-to-day basis in the office, and remains valuable in the emergency room setting for evaluation of compartment syndrome and peripheral nerve injury (see Chapter 12).

MEASUREMENT OF SKIN COMPLIANCE

Compliance is a measure of softness or, conversely, a measure of hardness. Infinite compliance would mean that if you pushed with a certain minimal force against a material, that material would push in for an infinite distance. For practical purposes, NIST defines compliance of a material

with respect to natural rubber. Natural rubber is by definition 100% compliant, and would therefore be 100% soft and 0% hard. For the purposes of measuring human tissues which are, in general, soft materials, and considering that for clinical purposes increasing hardness would probably be related to increasing problems or disease, it was decided, by convention, to create an instrument that would measure skin compliance but that would read out on the computer in terms of the pressure required to deform the skin. Thus, a higher pressure would relate to increased hardness, meaning less compliance, of the tissues being measured.

The NK Skin Compliance Device™ is engineered to have a pin with a fixed distance it can travel, and for the pressure required to cause that pin to travel that distance to be reported in terms that are traceable to NIST. The device is shown in Figure 7.30, and the operating parameters that correlate with the above definitions are given in Table 7.13. The force that is actually measured by the device is divided by 4.104 mm², which is the projected surface area of the hemispherical pin tip, to get the pressure value. The NK Skin Compliance Device™ is independent of the pressure applied by the examiner, and of movement of the subject. This device has a unique electromechanical circuit and hardware that will only accept "valid" measurements, and will audibly instruct the evaluator to repeat the trials until an acceptable measurement is obtained.

The first clinical study with this device evaluated the index and little finger of 25 subjects whose jobs ranged from female professionals to maintenance men (E. S. Dellon, Keller, Moratz, & A. L. Dellon, 1995). There were 13 women and 12 men from 15 to 76 years of age, with a mean age of 43. It was found that the mean hardness for the index finger was $51.0 \pm 5.1\%$, or a pressure of 12.5 ± 0.6 g/mm^2. There was no statistical difference between the hardness of the index and little finger (p = .73), between the right and the left hand (p = .6), between the dominant and nondominant hand (p = 0.9), or between men and women (p = .34). There was also no correlation between the subjects' age and skin hardness (see Figure 7.31).

The NK Skin Compliance Device™ permits investigation of many clinical problems. For example, it may be asked whether the normal variation in skin hardness has any relationship to the pressure perception threshold. This was evaluated in the Dellon et al., 1995 study, and the results are given for two of the pressure threshold measurements in Figure 7.31. In brief, there was no

significant correlation between skin hardness and pressure perception (measured with the Pressure-Specified Sensory Device™) for the population studied. The most reasonable explanation for this is that the mechanoreceptors for pressure are located directly beneath the intermediate papillary ridge and are so efficient at transducing any static-touch force that a variation in skin compliance within the normal range is not sufficient to alter the neural response to the touch stimuli. It remains to be investigated whether conditions that produce large callouses on the fingertips, the palm, or the bottom of the foot affect perception of touch stimuli. (See Chapter 20 for suggested research projects with this device.)

An additional investigation with the NK Skin Compliance Device™ looked at the claim often made by surgeons that they have less ability to feel when they double glove. The surgeons usually wear two pairs of gloves when they operate on a person known to have hepatitis or AIDS. Watts et al. (1994) demonstrated that skin hardness does increase as you go from skin to one glove to two gloves, and that the pressure perception threshold also increases from skin to one glove to two gloves, with the pressure perception being measured with the Pressure-Specified Sensory Device™.

Hand function was evaluated in this study by having the subject attempt to identify sutures, presented as pairs of different sizes, for example, 5-0 versus 6-0 nylon (see Figure 7.35), a task that simulates what the surgeon's sensory demands might be. It was found that even with two gloves, the subjects could still make the correct suture identification. The suggested interpretation of this data is that the computer-assisted measuring devices for skin compliance and pressure perception are sufficiently sensitive to detect the differences created by double gloving, and that the subject may simply increase the pressure applied by the fingertips to permit sufficient sensory stimuli for identification of the object recognition task.

CRITICAL ANALYSIS OF SKIN COMPLIANCE DEVICE™

The NK Skin Compliance Device™ is a reliable and valid computer-assisted measurement tool that may be used to evaluate changes in skin hardness. The potential clinical usefulness of this device for the rehabilitation department includes:
1. Documentation of hand edema at the beginning and end of a therapy session.
2. Documentation of changes in scar hardness during therapy.
3. Documentation of re-

FIGURE 7.30

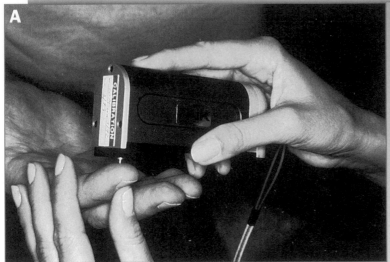

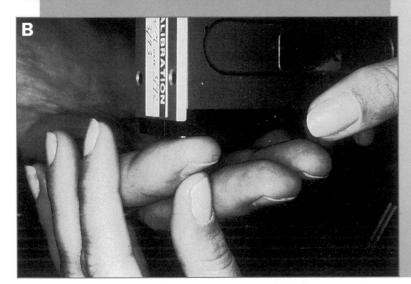

NK Skin Compliance Device. The device has a sensing pin which measures changes in pin deflection and the pressure required for deflection, both the force and the distance measurements being traceable to the National Institute of Standards and Technology natural rubber standards. (A) The device is brought into contact with the skin surface to be tested, and (B) depressed until the base of the pin touches the skin surface, at which time the skin compliance or hardness is registered on the computer. The result can be reported as the percent compliance (softness), or its inverse, hardness, or as the pressure in g/mm^2 that was required for the deflection of the pin against that skin surface. The device may be connected to a personal computer or a laptop. C) Typical printout from the computer measurement of skin compliance, stating the relationship between a measurement in terms of pressure or in terms of compliance. Copyright A. Lee Dellon. Reprinted with permission.

sponse to edema control (gloves, elevation).

The clinical disease conditions for which this device might offer measurements include:

1. Response of inflamed tissues, that is, rheumatoid arthritis, to medication.
2. Progression of dermatologic conditions, that is, scleroderma.
3. Response of dermatologic conditions to treatment.
4. Response of body to dialysis, that is, decrease tissue turgor after dialysis.
5. Response of the body to implanted material, that is, breast implants.
6. Penile rigidity (hardness), treatment of impotence.

MEASUREMENT OF GRIP AND PINCH STRENGTH

The measurement of muscle strength is, in general, a subject that is outside the scope of this book. However, peripheral nerve problems often include a motor component, and the approach that this book takes toward the science of measuring sensibility should be applicable to the science of measuring strength. Furthermore, the diagnosis of many upper extremity problems related to sensibility change may be helped by reliable and valid measurements of grip and

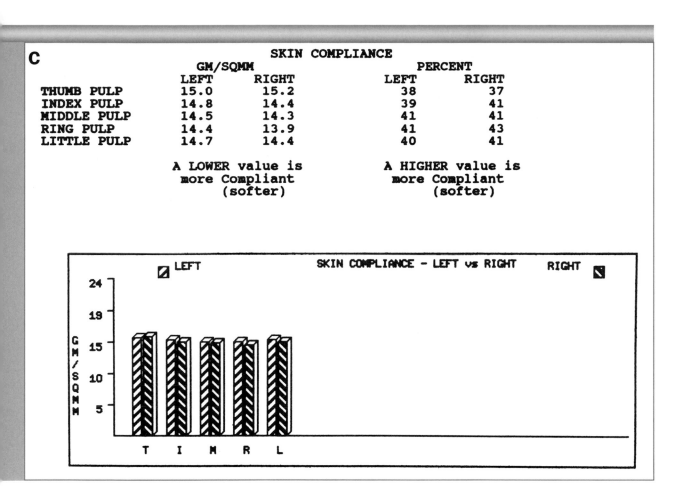

	SKIN COMPLIANCE			
	GM/SQMM		PERCENT	
	LEFT	RIGHT	LEFT	RIGHT
THUMB PULP	15.0	15.2	38	37
INDEX PULP	14.8	14.4	39	41
MIDDLE PULP	14.5	14.3	41	41
RING PULP	14.4	13.9	41	43
LITTLE PULP	14.7	14.4	40	41

A LOWER value is more Compliant (softer)

A HIGHER value is more Compliant (softer)

pinch strength.

Among the concepts for the upper extremity that are still debated and which require the use of strength testing instruments are the relationship to carpal tunnel surgery and grip strength, whether grip strength measurements can be used for screening in industry, and the relationship between abnormalities in grip strength in the patient with carpal tunnel syndrome and associated cubital tunnel syndrome. (The concept of malingering is discussed in detail in Chapter 5.) A review article in the presti-gious *New England Journal of Medicine* (Dawson, 1993) included measurement of strength as important in the diagnosis and management of patients with carpal tunnel, cubital tunnel, and thoracic outlet syndrome. Accordingly, it is essential to include a brief overview of the historical and traditional hydraulic instruments and the current state of the art of computer-assisted motor testing instruments.

There is an extensive literature on the traditional hydraulic, curved-handle, gripmeter, often called a dynamometer, and referred to specifically by the trade name "Jamar." The Jamar dynamometer, which has been in existence since the 1950s, has been manufactured and marketed by a wide variety of companies since the original company, Bechtol and Asimov Engineering, began manufacturing it. It is almost universally available in clinics and doctors' offices. In 1954, the California Medical Association wrote a report related to worker's compensation and recommended the Jamar as the "best instrument available." The number of papers in the literature that de-

TABLE 7.13 NK SKIN COMPLIANCE DEVICE™: RELATIONSHIPS BETWEEN DEFINITIONS OF COMPLIANCE

Softness (%)	Hardness (%)	Force (g)	Pressure (g/mm²)	Pin Deflection inches	Pin Deflection mm
0	100	100	24.4	0.00	0.00
10	90	90	21.9	.01	.25
20	80	80	19.5	.02	.51
30	70	70	17.1	.03	.76
40	60	60	14.6	.04	1.02
50	50	50	12.2	.05	1.27
60	40	40	9.8	.06	1.52
70	30	30	7.3	.07	1.78
80	20	20	4.9	.08	2.03
90	10	10	2.4	.09	2.28
100	0	0	0.0	.10	2.54

scribe its use, standardization of test positions, normative data, and variations on these subjects is extensive (see, for example, Mathiowetz, Rennels, & Donahoe, 1985; Smith & Benge, 1985; and Crosby & Wehbe, 1994).

The Jamar was said to be accurate to ± 5%; however, this was only for the center of the curved handle (see Figure 7.36 A). The handle had been made curved to fit into the palm of the hand, but then calibration was done by placing the instrument on a stand, which actually allowed the instrument to be slightly angled with respect to gravity, and then to be calibrated by hanging weights from its curved center. Clearly, any hand structural deformity, for example,

an amputated or arthritic finger, or a peripheral nerve problem, such as ulnar nerve compression, would redirect the force of grasp away from the center of the handle, making the recording measurement of strength inaccurate. *This is an inescapable design flaw and exists regardless of whether different examiners can obtain similar measurements with the instrument.* It was also determined, and reported by Mathiowetz (1987), that inadequate lubrication between the post and the handle could cause errors of up to 15%, and that the Jamar required frequent recalibration. Furthermore, the Jamar devices are not reported or advertised to be traceable to NIST. Jamar dynamometers are widely used because they have been the only instrument readily available, not because they are scientifically the best instrumentation.

The NK computer-assisted strength measurement devices were developed with the biomedical engineering advice of Edmund Chao, PhD, and the hand surgery clinical input of William P. Cooney, MD, from the Orthopedic Surgery Department of the Mayo Clinic. Work began in 1988, and was completed by the NK Biotechnical Corporation. The devices are illustrated in Figure 7.33 B and C. The NK Digit-Grip™ series of devices are available as a stand-alone unit, a unit joined to the computer which records the overall grip strength plus grip strength for the radial two and the ulnar two digits, and a third version that will record independently

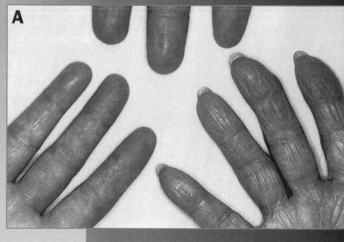

FIGURE 7.31

NK Skin Compliance Device. (A) In one study, skin compliance was measured for subjects of varying ages and varying occupations. (B) No relationship to age was noted for the index finger. C) There was only a modest correlation with one-point static touch (r = .46), and (D) with two-point moving touch (r = .40) for the index finger. From "Relationhip Between Skin Hardness and Human Touch Perception," by E. S. Dellon, K. Keller, V. Moratz, & A. L. Dellon, Journal of Hand Surgery, 20B:44-48, 1995.

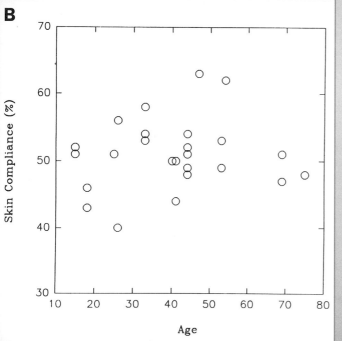

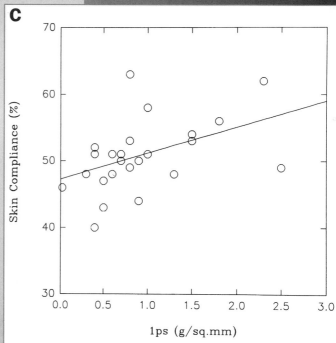

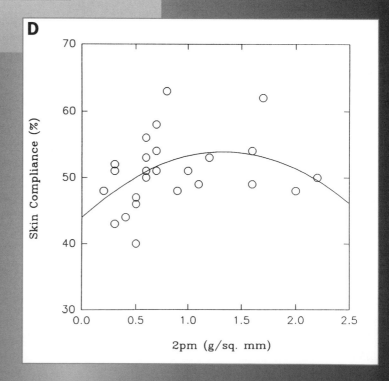

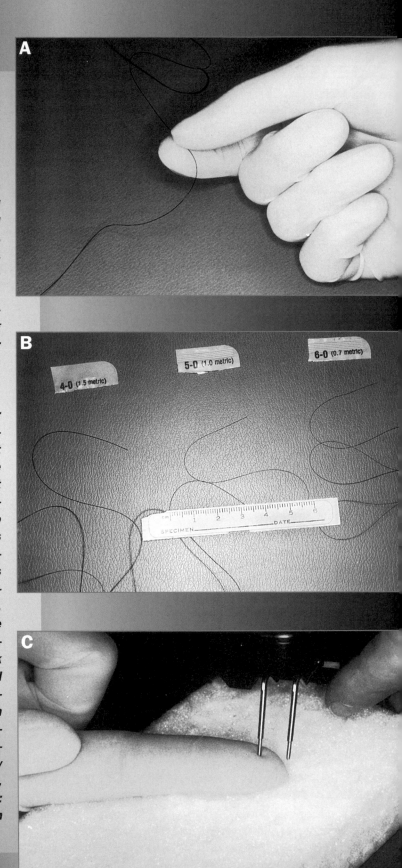

FIGURE 7.32

NK Skin Compliance Device. The device is useful for clinical investigation such as this recent example in which the question asked was the relationship between a surgeon "double gloving" for protection in surgery against hepititis or AIDS and the change in skin compliance and pressure perception related to wearing the gloves. Many surgeons report that they feel less well when they wear two pairs of gloves. (A) A test was devised in which the subject attempted to identify, by rolling the suture between the index finger and thumb, which size suture (B) was placed between the two fingers. C) Skin compliance was measured, as was the pressure threshold for one-point static touch, and the pressure at which prongs 3 mm apart could be distinguished from one prong. The study demonstrated that skin hardness increased as the subjects went from skin to one glove to two gloves. The pressure thresholds also increased during these increases in gloving. However, subjects could still correctly distinguish between suture pairs. In this study, the subjects' ability to increase the pressure applied by the fingers during the sensory discrimination task was able to overcome the measured changes in skin compliance and elevated perception thresholds. From "The Effect of Double Gloving on Cutaneous Sensibility, Skin Compliance, and Suture Identification," by D. Watt, P. L. Tassler, & A. L. Dellon, 1994, Contemporary Surgery 44: 289-292. *Reprinted with permission of the authors.*

FIGURE 7.33

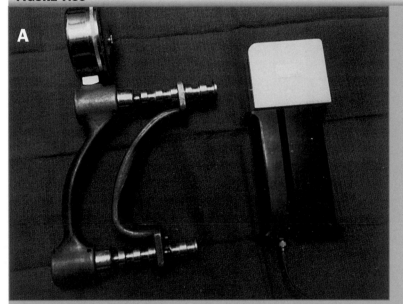

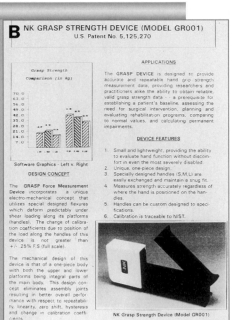

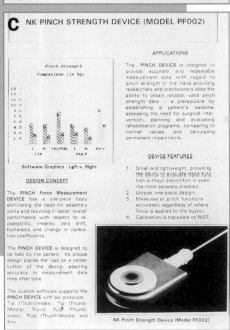

NK Biotechnical Corporation's computer-assisted strength measurement devices. (A) Engineering design differs from the historical and traditional hydraulic dynamometer devices, left, which record the force applied at the center of the curved handle. In contrast, the NK design, which is also isometric, gives accurate reading of the force applied anywhere along its handle. (B) Manufacturer's details for the grasp device and for the C) pinch device. Note that both NK devices are traceable to the National Institute for Standards and Technology and have passed the FDA 510 K evaluation and are manufactured in line with federal requirements. (A), (B), and C) from brochure accompanying the NK Grasp Strength Device, published by NK Biomedical Corporation, Lutherville, MD. Reprinted with permission of the company.

the strength for each of the five fingers. There is also a software program for rapid-exchange grip to help identify malingerers. Rapid exchange grip has been described as a means of assessing malingering (Joughlin et al., 1993). Use of the impulse made of the NK grasp device to evaluate malingering is discussed further in Chapter 5 (see Figure 5.4).

The accuracy of these computerized measurement systems is ±2%. The force is measured accurately anywhere along the surface of the handle. Different size handles are available for anthropomorphic accommodations, including a pediatric grip. The instrument makes an isometric contraction. Importantly, by means of the NK device's connection to

an IBM-compatible computer through the DAQ2001 signal conditioning device, there exists self-contained diagnostic software. This means that the device continually checks its own internal signal against NIST standards, records the checks, and reports to the screen if

FIGURE 7.34

NK Biotechnical Corporation printouts of typical reliability assessment protocol for the Digit-Grip® device. Metrology, the science of measurement, is used to make these devices traceable to the National Institute of Standards and Technology. (A) Example of electrical signal stability and accuracy related to time. (B) Printout from the computer's internal monitoring system that checks itself thoughout use to notify the end-user by means of a screen prompt if there is any electrical imbalance, in which case the comptuer will not accept an inaccurate measurement. From informaton on the NK Grasp Strength Device, published by NK Biomedical Corporation, Lutherville, MD. Reprinted with permission of the company.

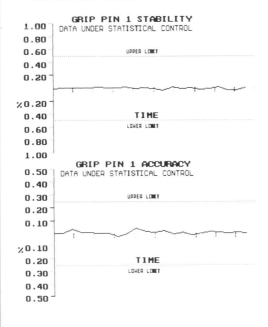

A

PART II   NK BIOTECHNICAL CORPORATION
                                   ASSESSMENT DEVICE SYSTEM REPORT

DEVICE NAME: GRIP PIN 1   DATA ACQUISITION CHANNEL: 1
DEVICE MODEL: SIGNAL CONDITIONING NAME:
DEVICE SERIAL NUMBER: 904017   SIGNAL CONDITIONING SERIAL NUMBER:
DEVICE CALIBRATION FACTOR: 0.03442   GAIN RESISTOR: OHMS +/- 1%
OUTPUT (mV/V): 0.000 mV/V at   0 KG   SHUNT RESISTOR: OHMS +/- 1%
LAST PHYSICAL CALIBRATION DATE: 07/01/93   BRIDGE OUTPUT IMPEDANCE: 0.0 OHMS (NOMINAL)
LATEST RELIABILITY REVIEW DATE: 12/28/93   BRIDGE LEAKAGE RESISTANCE: OHMS
NEXT RELIABILITY REVIEW DATE: 12/28/95   MANUFACTURING DATE:
CALIBRATION LOCATION: MANUFACTURING LOCATION:

   NOTE: The file on this device is kept at NKB METROLOGY LAB in accordance
         with "GOOD MANUFACTURING PRACTICE". The user may request specific
         information on this device at any time.

   NKB SUPPORT LINES: VOICE: 1-800-462-3751   FAX: 1-800-541-0863

        GRIP PIN 1 STABILITY
1.00 DATA UNDER STATISTICAL CONTROL   SYSTEM STABILITY
0.80
0.60   UPPER LIMIT   OFFSET MEAN   = 2054.85 COUNTS
0.40   MEAN STD. DEV. = 0.51053 COUNTS
0.20   0.01757 KG

%0.20   21 Tests
0.40   TIME   INITIAL DATE = 15-DEC-1994
0.60   LOWER LIMIT   LATEST DATE = 4-JAN-1995
0.80   24 total days
1.00

        GRIP PIN 1 ACCURACY
0.50 DATA UNDER STATISTICAL CONTROL
0.40   SYSTEM ACCURACY
0.30   UPPER LIMIT
0.20   ELECTRICAL CALIBRATION = 984.90 COUNTS
0.10   33.90 KG
                                               ELECTRICAL STD. DEV.   = 0.40493 COUNTS
%0.10   0.01394 KG
0.20   TIME
0.30   LOWER LIMIT   21 Tests
0.40
0.50

B

PART III   NK BIOTECHNICAL CORPORATION
GRIP PIN 1 ZERO AND SHUNT CALIBRATION RAW DATA
Serial No. 904017

Sample No.	Zero	Std. Dev.	Shunt	Std. Dev.	Date	Time	No. of Samples
1	2055.00	0.44721	984.10	0.30000	15-DEC-1994	3:26 PM	
2	2054.90	0.53852	985.30	0.40000	15-DEC-1994	3:26 PM	
3	2055.00	0.44721	984.90	0.30000	15-DEC-1994	3:26 PM	
4	2055.10	0.53852	984.90	0.44721	15-DEC-1994	3:26 PM	
5	2055.27	0.52083	984.83	0.48066	15-DEC-1994	3:33 PM	
6	2055.13	0.62881	984.80	0.36515	15-DEC-1994	3:35 PM	
*2070.00	0.77777	984.80	0.55555	15-DEC-1994	3:45 PM		
7	2054.97	0.41384	984.20	0.37905	16-DEC-1994	11:13 AM	
8	2055.23	0.56832	984.53	0.43018	16-DEC-1994	12:07 AM	
9	2054.83	0.37905	985.63	0.50742	16-DEC-1994	12:09 AM	
10	2055.10	0.60743	985.10	0.40684	19-DEC-1994	10:30 AM	
11	2054.87	0.43417	985.00	0.43417	20-DEC-1994	10:59 AM	
12	2054.20	0.48423	985.30	0.50855	21-DEC-1994	10:11 AM	
13	2055.27	0.52083	984.73	0.26261	22-DEC-1994	2:39 PM	
14	2054.77	0.62606	985.03	0.40684	23-DEC-1994	10:37 AM	
15	2055.00	0.45486	984.60	0.56324	27-DEC-1994	10:32 AM	
16	2054.50	0.50855	984.93	0.50401	28-DEC-1994	10:11 AM	
17	2054.70	0.46609	985.17	0.34575	29-DEC-1994	11:53 AM	
18	2055.10	0.40258	985.07	0.46113	30-DEC-1994	12:33 AM	
19	2054.13	0.62881	984.87	0.26261	2-JAN-1995	8:30 AM	
20	2053.97	0.49013	984.97	0.25371	3-JAN-1995	8:34 AM	
21	2054.97	0.61495	984.83	0.48423	4-JAN-1995	12:04 AM	
#2054.85	0.51053	984.90	0.40493	4-JAN-1995	12:04 AM	0021	

there is any error, or if the device needs to be recalibrated. Recalibration is required only every 3 years. Figure 7.34 gives examples of the self-diagnostic reporting schemes. Because of their superior engineering, rendering the devices the most reliable, it is clear that the NK strength measurement devices will become the industry standard.

• • •

APPENDIX: SUPPLIERS OF INSTRUMENTS

■ **Automated Tactile Tester**™
Ztech L.C.
P.O. Box 581215
Salt Lake City, UT 84148
Phone: 801-581-5928
Cost: $14,950

■ **Bio-Thesiometer**™
Biomedical Instrument Company
15764 Munn Road
Newbury, OH 44065
Phone: 216-543-9443
Cost: $300

■ **Breast Compliance Device**™
NeuroRegen LLC
2328 West Joppa Road
Suite 325
Lutherville, MD, 21093
Phone: 410-583-9136
Fax: 410-583-0201
Cost: $2,200⁺

NeuroRegen LLC
2328 West Joppa Road
Suite 325
Lutherville, MD 21093
Phone: 410-583-9136
Fax: 410-583-0201
Cost: $20,000

■ **Case IV System**
W.R. Medical
123 N. Second Street
Stillwater, MN 55082
Phone: 612-430-1200
Fax: 612-439-9733
Cost: $21,995

■ **Dexter**™ Cedaron Medical, Inc.
P.O. Box 2100
Davis, CA 95617

Phone: 800-424-1007
Cost: $22,000

■ **Digit-Grip**™
NeuroRegen LLC
2328 West Joppa Road
Suite 325
Lutherville, MD 21093
Phone: 410-583-9136
Fax: 410-583-0201
Cost: Stand-alone model $1,600
Computer-linked $3,600⁺
Pinch device $2,000⁺

■ **Disk-Criminator**™
NeuroRegen, LLC
2328 West Joppa Road
Suite 325
Lutherville, MD 21093
Phone: 410-583-0200
Fax: 410-583-0201
Cost: $60

■ **Eval**™
Greenleaf Medical Systems
3145 Porter Drive
Building A202
Palo Alto, CA 94304
Phone: 415-321-6135
Fax: 415-321-0419
Cost: $26,950 Desktop
$36,950 Video System

■ **Force-Defined Vibrometer**™
NeuroRegen LLC
2328 West Joppa Road
Suite 325
Lutherville, MD 21093
Phone: 410-583-9136
Fax: 410-583-0201
Cost: $20,000

■ **Hendler Pain Questionnaire**

Mensana Clinic
1718 Greenspring Valley
Road
Stevenson, MD 21153
Phone: 410-653-2403
Cost: $50 licensing fee for
unlimited use

■ **Henley**
Henley, a Division of
Maxxim Medical
104 Industrial Blvd.
Sugar Land, TX 77498
Phone: 713-240-2442
800-800-8485
Fax: 713-240-2577
Cost: $13,000

■ **Jamar Dynamometer**
Alimed
297 High Street
Dedham, MA 02026
Phone: 617-329-2900
Fax: 617-329-8392

Fred Sammons, Inc.
145 Tower Drive
Burr Ridge, IL 60521
Phone: 708-325-1700
Fax: 708-325-4602

North Coast
187 Stauffer Blvd.
San Jose, CA 95125
Phone: 408-283-1900

Smith and Nephew Rolyan
P.O.Box 1005
One Quality Drive
Germantown, WI 53022
Phone: 800-558-8633
Fax: 800-545-7758
Cost: $200-$212

■ **Mayo Dexterity** Board
NeuroRegen LLC
2328 West Joppa Road

Suite 325
Lutherville, MD 21093
Phone: 410-583-9136
Fax: 410-583-0201
Cost: $ 1,800

Nerve Pace™
Neurotron, Inc.✦
Lawrenceville, NJ

■ **Neurometer**™
Neurotron, Inc.✦
1501 Sulgrave
Suite 203
Baltimore, MD 21209
Phone: 800-345-9040
410-664-0800
Fax: 410-664-0831
Cost: $8,000-$16,000

■ **Neurotube**™
NeuroRegen, LLC
2328 West Joppa Road
Suite 325
Lutherville, MD 21093
Phone: 410-583-0200
Fax: 410-583-0201
Cost: $450

■ **Optacon**™
Telesensory Systems
P.O. Box 7455
Mountain View, CA 94039
Cost: $3,695

■ **Pressure-Specified
Sensory Device**™
NeuroRegen LLC
2328 West Joppa Road
Suite 305
Lutherville, MD 21093
Phone: 410-583-9136
Fax: 410-583-0201
Cost: $4,900✦

■ **Semmes-Weinstein
Filaments**

Alimed
297 High Street
Dedham, MA 02026
Phone: 617-329-2900
Fax: 617-329-8392

Fred Sammons, Inc.
145 Tower Drive
Burr Ridge, IL 60521
Phone: 708-325-1700
Fax: 708-325-4602

North Coast
187 Stauffer Blvd.
San Jose, CA 95125
Phone: 408-283-1900

Smith and Nephew Rolyan
P.O.Box 1005
One Quality Drive
Germantown, WI 53022
Phone: 800-558-8633
Fax: 800-545-7758
Cost: $80-$175 for set of 5
$295-395 for set of 20

■ **Sensortek**™
Clifton, NJ
Phone: 201-779-5577

■ **Skin Compliance** Device
NeuroRegen LLC
2328 West Joppa Road
Suite 305
Lutherville, MD 21093
Phone: 410-583-0200
Fax: 410-583-0201
Cost: $2,000✦

■ **Thermal Sensory
Analyzer** (TSA-2001)
Compass Medical Tech, Inc.
7300 France Avenue South
Suite 405
Minneapolis, MN 55435
Phone: 612-835-2595
Fax: 612-835-2784

Cost: $16,700 for Model
TSA-2001

■ **Vibrometers**
See also **Bio-Thesiometer**™
See also **Force-Defined**

■ **Vibrometer**™
(NK Biomedical Corp.)
See also **Sensortek**™

■ **Vitapulp**™
Pelton and Crane
Charlotte, NC
Phone: 704-523-3212

■ **West**™
*Additional information
unavailable.*

✢ For the NK Biotechnical devices, one DAQ signal conditioning unit is needed. The DAQ
costs $2,400. This cost must be
added just once for all the devices you choose to buy to create
your NK System; that is, grip,
pinch, and PSSD all can be run
from one DAQ.

✦ Please note that two different
companies are each identified by
the same name, but that they
market two different products.

• **REFERENCES** •

Arezzo, J. C., Bolton, C. F., Boulton, A., & Dyck, P. J. Quantitative sensory testing: A consensus report from the Peripheral Neuropathy Association. *Neurology 43:*1050-
1052, 1993.

Arezzo, J. C., & Schaumberg, H. H. The use of the Optacon
as a screening device: A new technique for detecting sensory loss in individuals exposed to neurotoxins. *Journal of
Occupational Medicine 22:*461- 464, 1980.

Arezzo, J. C., Schaumberg, H. H., & Laudadio, C. Thermal
sensitivity tester: Device for quantitative assessment of
thermal sense in diabetic neuropathy. *Diabetes 35:*590-
592, 1986.

Arezzo, J. C., Schaumberg, H. H., & Petersen, C. A. Rapid
screening for peripheral neuropathy: A field study with
the Optacon. *Neurology 33:*626-629, 1983.

Asbury, A. K., & Porte, D., Jr. Consensus statement of the
American Diabetes Association: Standard measures in diabetic neuropathy. *Diabetes Care 16:*2:82-92, 1993.

Bell, J. A. Light touch-deep pressure testing using Semmes-
Weinstein monofilaments. In *Rehabilitation of the Hand:
Surgery and Therapy,* 2nd edition, J. M. Hunter, L. H.
Schneider, E. J. Mackin, & A. D. Callahan, Editors. St.
Louis: C. V. Mosby Company, Chapter 35, 1984.

Bell-Krotoski, J. A. Light touch-deep pressure testing using
Semmes-Weinstein monofilaments. In *Rehabilitation of the
Hand: Surgery and Therapy,* J. M. Hunter, L. H. Schneider,
E. J. Mackin, & A. D. Callahan, Editors. St. Louis: C. V.
Mosby, 1990.

Bleecker, M. Vibration perception thresholds in entrapment
and toxic neuropathies. *Journal of Occupational Medicine
28:*991-994, 1986.

Callahan, A. D. Sensibility testing: Clinical methods. In *Re-
habilitation of the Hand: Surgery and Therapy,* 2nd Edition,
J. M. Hunter, L. H. Schneider, E. J. Mackin, & A. D.
Callahan, Editors. St. Louis: C. V. Mosby Company,
Chapter 36, 1984.

Cherniak, M. G., Moalli, D., & Viscolli, C. A comparison of
digital neurometry, tactometry, and nerve conduction
studies in the diagnosis of carpal tunnel syndrome. *Journal of Hand Surgery,* in press: 1995.

Cosh, J. A. Studies on the nature of vibration sense. *Clinical
Science 12:*131-151, 1953.

Crosby, C. A., & Wehbe, M. A. Hand strength: Normative
values. *Journal of Hand Surgery 19A:*665-670, 1994.

Dawson, D. M. Entrapment neuropathies of the upper extremities. New England *Journal of Medicine 329:*2013-
2017, 1993.

Dellon, A. L. The vibrometer. *Plastic and Reconstructive Surgery 71:*427-431, 1983.

Dellon, A. L., & Keller, K. M. Cutaneous pressure threshold measurement in carpal and cubital tunnel syndrome. *Annals of Plastic Surgery, 38:*493-502, 1997.

Dellon, E. S., Crone, S., Mourey, R., & Dellon, A. L. Comparison of the Semmes-Weinstein monofilaments with the Pressure-Specifying Sensory Device. *Restorative Neurology Neuroscience 5:*323-326, 1993.

Dellon, E. S., & Dellon, A. L. Quantitative sensory testing with the force-defined vibrometer. *Journal of Reconstructive Microsurgery,* submitted: 1995.

Dellon, E. S., Keller, K. M., Moratz, V., & Dellon, A. L. Relationship between skin hardness and human touch perception. *Journal of Hand Surgery 20B:*44-48,1995.

Dellon, E. S., Keller, K. M., Moratz, V., & Dellon, A. L. Validation of cutaneous pressure threshold measurement with the Pressure-Specified Sensory Device. *Annals of Plastic Surgery, 38:*485-492, 1997.

Dellon, E. S., Mourey, R., & Dellon, A. L. Human pressure perception values for constant and moving one- and two-point discrimination. *Plastic and Reconstructive Surgery 90:*112-117, 1992.

Devor, M., Schonfeld, D., Seltzer, Z., & Wall, P. D. Two models of cutaneous reinnervation following peripheral nerve injury. *Journal of Comparative Neurology 185:*211-220, 1979.

Dyck, P. J., Curtis, D.J., Bushek, W., & Litchy, W. J. Description of "Minnesota thermal disks" and normal values of cutaneous thermal discrimination in man. *Neurology 24:*325-330, 1974.

Dyck, P. J., Karnes, J. L., O'Brien, P. C., & Zimmerman, I. R. Detection thresholds of cutaneous sensation in humans. In *Peripheral Neuropathy,* P. J. Dyck, P. K. Thomas, J. W. Griffin, P. A. Low, & J. F. Poduslo, Editors. Philadelphia: W. B. Saunders Company, 1993.

Dyck, P. J., Zimmerman, I. R., O'Brien, P. C.,

Ness, A., Caskey, P. E., Karnes, J., & Bushek, W. Introduction of automated systems to evaluate touch-pressure, vibration, and thermal cutaneous sensation in man. *Annals of Neurology 4:*502-510, 1978.

Franzblau, A., Werner, R. A., Johnston, E., & Torrey, S. Evaluation of current perception threshold testing as a screening procedure for carpal tunnel syndrome among industrial workers. *Journal of Occupational Medicine 36:*1015-1021, 1994.

Gregg, E. C., Jr. Absolute measurement of the vibratory threshold. *Archives of Neurology and Psychology 66:*403-411, 1951.

Grunert, B. K., Wertsch, J. J., Matloub, H. S., & McCallum-Burke, S. Reliability of sensory threshold measurement using a digital vibrogram. *Journal of Occupational Medicine 32:*100-102, 1990.

Guy, R. J. C., Clark, C. A., Malcolm, P. N., & Watkins, P. J. Evaluation of thermal and vibration sensation in diabetic neuropathy. *Diabetologia 38:*131-137, 1985.

Hardy, M., Jimenez, S., Jabaley, M., & Horch, K. Evaluation of nerve compression with the automated tactile tester. *Journal of Hand Surgery 17A:*838-842, 1992.

Hendler, N., & Fenton, J. A. *Coping with Chronic Pain.* New York: Clarkson N. Potter Publishers, 1979.

Hendler, N., Mollett, A., Talo, S., & Levin, S. A comparison between the Minnesota Multiphasic Personality Inventory and the Mensana Clinic Back Pain Test for validating the complaint of chronic back pain. *Journal of Occupational Medicine 30:*98-102, 1988.

Horch, K., Hardy, M., Jimenez, S., & Jabaley, M. An automated tactile tester for evaluation of cutaneous sensibility. *Journal of Hand Surgery 17A:*829-837, 1992.

Jetzer, T. C. Use of vibration testing in the early evaluation of workers with carpal tunnel syndrome. *Journal of Occupational Medicine 33:*117-120, 1991.

Joughin, K., Gulati, P., Mackinnon, S. E., McCabe, S., Murray, J. F., Griffiths, S., & Richards, R. An evaluation of rapid exchange and simultaneous grip tests. *Journal of Hand Surgery 18A:*245-252, 1993.

Katims, J. J., Naviasky, E., Ng, L. K. Y., Bleecker, M. L., & Rendell, M. New screening device for the assessment of peripheral neuropathy. *Journal of Occupational Medicine 28:*1219-1221, 1986.

Katims, J. J., Patil, A. S., Rendell, M., Rouvelas, P., Sadler, B., Weseley, S. A., & Bleecker, M. L. Current perception threshold screening for carpal tunnel syndrome. *Archives of Environmental Health 46:*207-212, 1991.

Levin, S., Pearsall, G., & Ruderman, R. J. von Frye's method of measuring pressure sensibility in the hand: An engineering analysis of the Weinstein-Semmes pressure aesthesiometer. *Journal of Hand Surgery 3:*211-216, 1978.

Liu, S., Kopacz, D. J., & Carpenter, R. L. Quanitative assessment of differential sensory nerve block after lidocaine spinal anesthesia. *Anesthesiology 82:*60-63, 1995.

Lowenthal, L. M., & Hockaday, T. D. R. Vibration sensory thresholds depend on pressure of applied stimulus. *Diabetes Care 10:*100-102, 1987.

Lundborg, G., Lie-Stenstrom, A. K., Sollerman, C., Stromberg, T., & Pyykko, L. Digital vibrogram: A new diagnostic tool for sensory testing in compression neuropathy. *Journal of Neurology, Neurosurgery and Psychiatry 11A:*693-699, 1986.

Masson, E. A., & Boulton, A. J. M. The neurometer: Validation and comparison with conventional tests for diabetic neuropathy. *Diabetes Medicine 8:*63-366, 1991.

Masson, V. E., Veves, A., Fernando, D. J. S., & Boulton, A. J. M. Current perception thresholds: A new, quick, and reproducible method for the assessment of peripheral neuropathy in diabetes mellitus. *Diabetologia 32:*724-728, 1989.

Mathiowetz, V. Grip-strength measurement: A comparison of three Jamar Dynamometers. *Occupational Therapy Journal of Research 7:*235-243, 1987.

Mathiowetz, V., Rennels, C., & Donahoe, L.

Effect of elbow position on grip and key pinch strength. *Journal of Hand Surgery 10A:*694-697, 1985.

Mackinnon, S. E., & Dellon, A. L. *Surgery of the Peripheral Nerve.* New York: Thieme Publishers, 1988.

Melzak, R. The McGill Pain Questionnaire: Major properties and scoring methods. *Pain 1:*277-299, 1975.

Meyer, R. A., & Campbell, J. N. Peripheral neural coding of pain sensation. *Johns Hopkins APL Technical Digest 2:*164-171, 1981.

Mountcastle, V. B. Medical *Physiology.* St. Louis: C. V. Mosby Company, 1968, chapters 61-63.

Novak, C. B., Mackinnon, S. E., & Kelly, L. Correlation of two-point discrimination and hand function following median nerve injury. *Annals of Plastic Surgery 31:*495-498, 1993.

Novak, C. B., Mackinnon, S. E., Williams, J. I., & Kelly, L. Establishment of reliability in the evaluation of hand sensibility. *Plastic and Reconstructive Surgery 92:*312-322, 1993.

Ochoa, J., & Torebork, E. Sensations evoked by intraneural microstimulation of single mechanoreceptor units innervating the human hand. *Journal of Physiology 342:*633-654, 1983.

Price, D. D., McGrath, P. A., Rafii, A., & Buckingham, B. The validation of visual analogue scales as ratio scales measures for chronic and experimental pain. *Pain 83:*45-56, 1974.

Raja, S. N., Meyer, R. A., & Campbell, J. N. Hyperalgesia and sensitization of primary afferent fibers. In *Pain Syndromes in Neurology,* H. L. Fields, Editor. London: Butterworths, 1990.

Revill, S. I., Robinson, J. O., Rosen, M., & Hogg, M. I. J. The reliability of a linear analogue scale for evaluating pain. *Anaesthesiology 31:*1191-1198, 1976.

Semmes, J., Weinstein, S., Ghent, L., & Teuber, H. L. *Somatosensory Changes After Penetrating Brain Wounds in Man.* Cambridge, MA: Harvard University Press, 1960.

Smith, R. O., & Benge, M. W. Pinch and grasp strength: Standardization of terminology and protocol. *American Journal of Occupational Therapy 39:*531-535, 1985.

Tassler, P. L., & Dellon, A. L. Correlation of measurements of pressure perception using the Pressure-Specified Sensory Device with electrodiagnostic testing. *Journal of Occupational Medicine 37:*862-866, 1995.

Tassler, P., & Dellon, A. L. Pressure perception in the normal lower extremity and in the tarsal tunnel syndrome. *Muscle and Nerve, 19:*285-289, 1996.

Uematsu, S., Hendler, N., Hungerford, D., Long, D., & Ono, N. Thermography and electromyography in the differential diagnosis of chronic pain syndromes and reflex sympathetic dystrophy. *Electromyography of Clinical Neurophysiology 21:*165-182, 1981.

von Frey, M. The distribution of afferent nerves in the skin. *Journal of the American Medical Association 47:*645-648, 1906.

Wall, P. D., & Melzak, R. *Textbook of Pain.* Edinburgh: Churchill Livingstone, Inc. 1984.

Watts, D., Tassler, P. L., & Dellon, A. L. The effect of double gloving on cutaneous sensibility, skin compliance, and suture identification. *Contemporary Surgery 44:*289-292, 1994.

Weber, E. Ueber den Tatsinn. Archive fur Anatomy und Physiology. *Wissenshaft Medical Muller's Archives 1:*152-159, 1835.

• ADDITIONAL READINGS •

Asbury, A. K. Pain in generalized neuropathies. In *Pain Syndromes in Neurology,* H. L. Fields, Editor. London: Butterworths, 1990, pp. 131-142.

Borg, K., & Lindblom, U. Increase of vibration threshold during wrist flexion in patients with carpal tunnel syndrome. *Pain 26:*211-219, 1986.

Cherniak, M. G., Letz, R., Gerr, F., Brammer, A., & Pace, P. Detailed clinical assessment of neurological function in symptomatic shipyard workers. *British Journal of Industrial Medicine 47:*566-572, 1990.

Crosby, C. A., & Wehbe, M. A. Hand strength: Normal values. *Journal of Hand Surgery 19A:*665-670, 1994.

Crosby, P. M., & Dellon, A. L. A comparison of two-point discrimination test devices. *Microsurgery 10:*134-137, 1989.

Daniel, C. R., Bower, J. D., Pearson, J. E., & Holbert, R. D. Vibrometry and neuropathy. *Journal of the Mississippi State Medical Association 18:*30-34, 1977.

Dellon, A. L., & Kallman, C. H. Evaluation of functional sensation in the hand. *Journal of Hand Surgery 8:*865-870, 1983.

Dellon, A. L., & Keller, K. M. Evaluation of carpal and cubital tunnel syndrome utilizing the Pressure-Specifying Sensory Device for quantitative sensory testing. *Annals of Plastic Surgery, 38:*493-502, 1997.

Dellon, A. L., Mackinnon, S. E., & Crosby, P. M. Reliability of two-point discrimination measurements. *Journal of Hand Surgery 12:*693-696, 1987.

Dellon, E. S., Keller, K. M., Moratz, V., & Dellon, A. L. Relationship between skin hardness and human touch perception. *Journal of Hand Surgery 20B:* 44-48, 1995.

Dyck, P. J., Karnes, J. L., Gillen, D. A., O'Brien, P. C., Zimmerman, I. R., & Johnson, D. M. Comparison of algorithms of testing for use in automated evaluation of sensation. *Neurology 40:*1607-1613, 1990.

Dyck, P. J., Zimmerman, I. R., Gillen, D. A., Johnson, D., Karnes, J. L., & O'Brien, P. C. Warm, and heat-pain detection thresholds: Testing methods and inferences about anatomic distribution of receptors. *Neurology 43:*1500-1508, 1993.

Gerr, F. E., Hershman, D., & Letz, R. Vibrotactile threshold measurement for detecting neurotoxicity: Reliability and determination of age- and height-standardized normative values. *Archives of Environmental Health 45:*148-154, 1990.

Gerr, F. E., & Letz, R. Reliability of a widely used test of peripheral cutaneous vibration sensitivity and a comparison of two testing protocols. *British Journal of Industrial Medicine 45:*635-639, 1988.

Johnson, M. E., Chao, E. Y. S., & Cooney, W. P. III. Computer-assisted pinch and grip strength measurements; Normative values using a non-hydraulic system. *Journal of Hand Therapy,* submitted: 1994.

Lundborg, G., Dahlin, L. B., Lundstrom, R., Necking, L. E. & Stromberg, T. Vibrotactile function of the hand in compression and vibration-induced neuropathy. Sensibility index - A new measure. *Scandinavian Journal of Plastic Reconstructive Surgery and Hand Surgery 26:*275-281, 1992.

Talbot, W. H., Darian-Smith, I., Kornhuber, H. H., & Mountcastle, V. B. The sense of flutter-vibration: Comparison of the human capacity with response patterns of mechanoreceptive afferents from the monkey hand. *Journal of Neurophysiology 31:*301-334, 1968.

Weinstein, S. Fifty years of somatosensory research: From the Semmes-Weinstein Monofilaments to the Weinstein Enhanced Sensory Test. *Journal of Hand Therapy 6:*11-22, 1993.

• • •

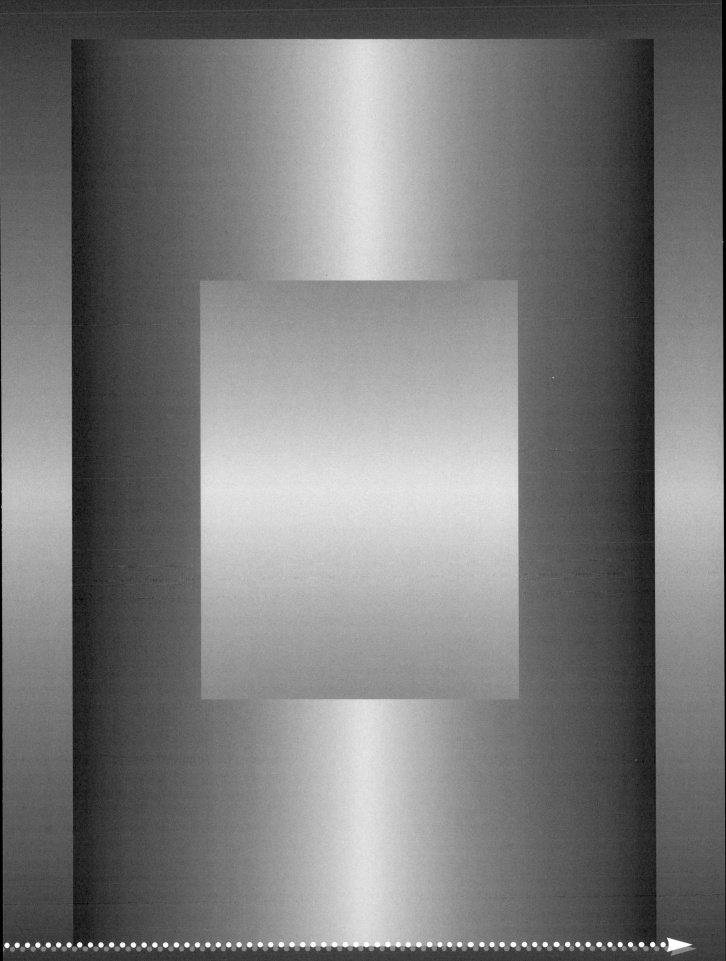

electro-
diagnostic
testing

Erlanger and Gasser, two physiologists at the Johns
Hopkins University School of Medicine, received
the Nobel Prize in Physiology for their investigations into the structure and function of the peripheral nerve. Their book, published in 1937, laid the ground-
work on which Roger W. Gilliatt, a neurologist in London,
began, in the 1960s, to describe the electrophysiologic properties of the median and ulnar nerve at the wrist (1960), diabetic neuropathy (1962), and the compression of the
brachial plexus by a cervical rib (1970). Gilliatt's basic laboratory research led to the description of, among other
things, plantar nerve compression in the guinea pig foot,
tourniquet compression effects on the peripheral nerve in
baboons, and the tourniquet test for diagnosis of carpal and
cubital tunnel syndrome in humans. When he retired from
his work in London, he accepted an appointment as Senior
Consultant to the National Institute of Neurologic Disorders
and Stroke at the National Institutes of Health (NIH) in
Bethesda, Maryland.

In April 1990, when the Plastic Surgery Research Council met in Washington, DC, I invited Dr. Gilliatt to meet
with our peripheral nerve special interest group (which the

following year became the American Society for the Peripheral Nerve). I asked him to speak about work relating to the *double crush hypothesis* (the concept that a proximal cite of nerve compression, that is, cervical disc disease, predisposes the distal nerve to chronic compression, that is, carpal tunnel syndrome).

That was an inspiring evening and led to his visiting with me in Baltimore a few months later. He agreed with a theory I put forth to him (see Chapter 14) that, from the electrodiagnostic standpoint, it would not be possible to distinguish between a distal axonopathy (such as diabetic neuropathy) and a series of chronic compression sites along the length of several peripheral nerves. He agreed that the hypothesis would be worth testing in a primate model. He declined the offer to collaborate due to clinical responsibilities at NIH. Pancreatic cancer claimed his life rather suddenly in 1991. His legacy of electrodiagnostic investigation of peripheral nerve function has become the gold standard for clinical medicine today. This chapter will briefly review some of the principles of electrodiagnosis and what its appropriate role may become in the 21st century.

Electrodiagnostic testing is critical for the diagnosis and management of many neu-

TABLE 8.1   INDICATIONS FOR ELECTRODIAGNOSTIC TESTING

Localization of Nerve Lesion
• Radiculopathy versus nerve compression, or both

Progression of Nerve Lesion
• Resolution of neurapraxia
• Reinnervation following nerve repair
• Progression of inflammatory neuropathy
• Status of brachial plexus

Evaluation of Systemic Disease
• Peripheral neuropathy
• Drug toxicity
• Neuromuscular dysfunction
• Myopathy

Verification of Suspected Nerve Problem
• Inability of patient to communicate
• Suspected malingering
• Martin-Gruber connection

romuscular and peripheral nerve problems. Table 8.1 is a list of some of the indications for electrodiagnostic testing. There are also disadvantages and inherent errors in electrodiagnostic testing, which Figure 8.1 and Table 8.2 illustrate. Another problem is that the results of electrodiagnostic testing often do not predict the success of surgery for chronic nerve entrapment. For example, electrodiagnostic test results did not provide significant data for prediction of functional recovery or reemployment after carpal tunnel release in 151 workers studied prospectively over a 5-

year period (Braun & Jackson, 1994). My view is that for many common peripheral nerve problems, such as chronic nerve compression, the high cost of the electrodiagnostic test, its invasive nature, the pain associated with it, and the frequent lack of correlation between the patient's symptoms and the test are all reasons for therapists and physicians involved with these clinical problems to go back to the basics: Take a good history, do a careful physical examination and, when needed, obtain noninvasive, low-cost, quantitative sensorimotor testing (Dellon, 1991, 1994).

• NERVE CONDUCTION STUDIES •

The speed with which an electric impulse is transmitted along the length of a sensory or motor nerve (conduction velocity), and the height of the conducted impulse, as measured on the oscilloscope screen (amplitude), can be measured by giving an electrical stimulus to the nerve through the skin and recording the impulse the stimulus generates at some distant site. If two different sites along the length of the nerve can be recorded from, and the intervening distance measured, then that distance can be divided by the time it took to transmit the impulse to obtain the conduction velocity. If only one site can be recorded from, then just the time required for the nerve to travel distally can be recorded (the *distal latency*). The magnitude of the amplitude varies between a sensory nerve, which is smaller (on the order of microvolts), and a motor nerve, where the response is measured over the muscle and is larger (on the order of millivolts). Because the small amplitudes are difficult to demonstrate due to background electrical noise, the newest computers have signal averaging, which can filter out the background noise.

There are special recording and stimulating techniques that have been developed to attempt to asses the integrity of the peripheral nerve over long distances that would include the brachial plexus and the spinal foramen. These are called the *H-reflex* and the *F-response*, and are electrical equivalents of the tendon reflex in that a graded stimulus is given, the signal travels through the spinal cord, and then back down the limb to generate a motor response. While delays in the H-reflex

FIGURE 8.1

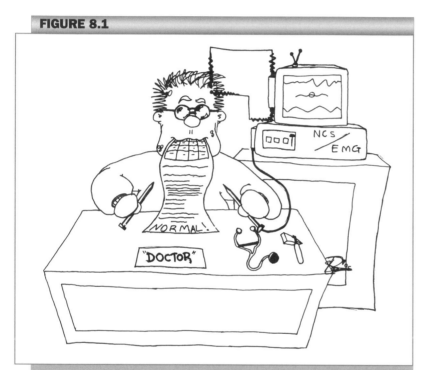

Doctor Electrophysiology. This multichannel, oscilloscope-faced tyrant conceals his objective evaluation beneath a white lab coat. Reflex hammer and stethoscope are reminders of medicine's historic past, before the days of computer-averaging, evoked potentials, and F- and H-waves. Unfortunately, many physicians call in this extremely high-priced consultant ($500-$1,500) before even carrying out their own careful history and physical examination. This consultant will often use invasive and painful stimuli, which few patients will willingly accept for a repeat follow-up examination. While Table 8.1 lists many areas in which this consultation is not only justified but is also critically necessary, this consultation is not needed for most routine peripheral nerve problems. It is for this reason that both the American Diabetes Association and the American Peripheral Neuropathy Association have recommended Quantitative Sensory Testing. Drawing by Glenn George Dellon. Reprinted with permission.

TABLE 8.2   PITFALLS IN ELECTRODIAGNOSTIC TESTING

Neurophysiology
- Large myelinated fibers preferentially recorded

Pathophysiology
- Sparing of central fascicles
- Uneven fiber loss among fascicles
- Incomplete remyelination

Anomalous Innervation
- Radial sensory nerve to thumb
- Overlap of lateral antebrachial cutaneous nerve with radial sensory nerve
- Lateral sural nerve entrapment

Technique
- Temperature
- Patient age
- Patient height
- Site along the nerve

and F-response can demonstrate a proximal conduction block, they are nonspecific delays in that any site along the long course that the impulse travels may be responsible for the delay.

The most common peripheral nerve problem being treated today in the United States is carpal tunnel syndrome. The distal median nerve is the best nerve for electrodiagnostic testing. If Kimura's (1978, 1983) inching technique is used in the palm, and if distal sensory latencies are used instead of motor latencies, and if the distal median latency is compared with the distal ulnar latency in the same hand, electro-diagnostic testing can be positive.

That is, it can identify an abnormality in up to 90% of clinically symptomatic patients. However, there are studies reported in which the false negative result is 30%, and commonly studies have 20% of symptomatic patients showing a normal result reported for their electrodiagnostic study (Spindler & Dellon, 1982; Buch-Jaeger & Foucher, 1994).

Recently, the American Academy of Electromyography carried out a literature review (meta analysis) in which all studies that met strict criteria for diagnosis for carpal tunnel syndrome were combined. Even with the strictest criteria, just 69% of symptomatic patients were found to have abnormal studies when distal motor or sensory latencies were used (see Table 8.3).

In 1993, a meta-analysis by the American Academy of Electromyography (AAEM) reported that 31% of clinically symptomatic carpal tunnel syndrome patients have normal electrodiagnostic studies (AAEM, 1993). The situation is worse for the diagnosis of ulnar nerve compression at the elbow in which, in my clinical experience, about 50% of the patients who come to me with symptoms and clinical findings compatible with ulnar nerve compression have normal electrodiagnostic studies.

Furthermore, for ulnar nerve compression at the elbow, the results of electrodiagnostic testing do not predict the results of non-operative management (Dellon et al., 1993), nor do they predict the results of submuscular transposition of the ulnar nerve at the elbow (Dellon & Coert, 1995). With the exception of being able to demonstrate denervation potentials in the flexor profundus to the index finger, or the flexor pollicis longus for the rare patient with anterior interosseous nerve syndrome, electrodiagnostic testing almost never demonstrates a proximal median nerve compression in the forearm (*pronator syndrome*). In addition, it is extremely difficult to demonstrate radial sensory nerve compression due to the overlap of the lateral antebrachial cutaneous nerve (Spindler & Dellon, 1990).

Electrodiagnostic testing for lower extremity nerve compression continues to be defined with the best results obtained when there is denervation associated with foot drop due to common per-

TABLE 8.3   COMPARISON OF ELECTRODIAGNOSIS OF MILD CARPAL TUNNEL SYNDROME

	Onset Latency ± SD	Peak Latency ± SD	Abnormal Value[+]
Median mixed nerve conduction between wrist and palm in CTS	1.54 ± 12 msec	Median sensory 2.03 ± 0.12 msec	Onset > 1.78 msec Peak > 2.27 msec
Comparison of median and ulnar mixed nervesensory conditionbetween wrist and palm in CTS	0.08 ± 0.12msec	Difference median and ulnar 0.10 ± 0.11 msec	Onset > 0.32 msec Peak > 0.31 msec
Comparison of median and ulnar sensory conduction between wrist and ring finger in CTS	0.13 ± 0.15 msec	Difference median and ulnar 0.09 ± 0.13 msec	Onset > 0.43 msec Peak > 0.35 msec
Comparison of median and radial sensory conduction between wrist and thumb in CTS	0.08 ± 0.12 msec	Difference median and radial 0.13 ± 0.12 msec	Onset > 0.32 msec Peak > 0.37 msec

Note:
[+] Criteria for abnormal value: mean +2SD.
From "Literature review of the usefulness of nerve conduction studies and electromyography for the evaluation of patients with carpal tunnel syndrome," 1993, *Muscle and Nerve 16*:1392-1414, AAEM Quality Assurance Committee. Adapted with permission.

oneal nerve entrapment at the fibular head, and compression of the posterior tibial nerve in the tarsal tunnel. However, the small distal

Specificity	Percentage Symptomatic Hands with Abnormal Studies
97%	69%
95%	66%
95%	82%
100%	69%

nerves of the foot, such as the calcaneal nerve and the deep peroneal nerve distal to its motor branch to the extensor brevis muscle, are extremely difficult to test electrodiagnostically due to their small size. Traditional electrodiagnostic testing is simply unable to document brachial plexus compression in the thoracic inlet. These discouraging comments further support the statement that was made at the beginning of this chapter that for most peripheral nerve problems, and certainly for chronic nerve entrapment, the clinician should first rely on the history and physical exam, supported by quantitative sensory testing.

In contrast, there are certain situations in which, without question, the cost and pain involved with electrodiagnostic testing is justified, and indicated. These situations are:

1. When an older patient may have a coexisting cervical disc problem with peripheral nerve entrapment
2. When a patient with multiple peripheral nerve entrapments may have a peripheral neuropathy
3. When the unusual intrinsic wasting or diffuse weakness may be due to a systemic neurologic disease
4. When there has been previous peripheral nerve surgery and it is difficult to establish a baseline
5. When there is the possible presence of anomalous innervation
6. When there is some uncertainty as to the patient's truthfulness when workmen's compensation issues, malpractice, or motor vehicle litigation is involved.

• NERVE PACE™ •

The Nerve Pace™ is an electrical stimulating device manufactured by Neurotron, Inc. of Lawrenceville, NJ (see Appendix, Chapter 7) that will give the distal motor latency for the median and ulnar nerves. The introduction of alternative electrodiagnostic tests was motivated by the recognition that nerve conduction studies have been accepted as the gold standard for diagnosis of peripheral nerve problems, that traditional electrodiagnostic testing is expensive, painful, and time consuming, and that carpal tunnel syndrome is occurring in almost epidemic proportions in industries with cumulative trauma. The Nerve Pace™ is a battery-powered, transportable device that has modest training requirements, the results of which have been reported to have a high correlation with the results of traditional electrodiagnostic testing in identifying patients with carpal tunnel syndrome (Osterman, Aversa, & Greenstein, 1995; Steinberg, Gelberman, Rydevik, & Lundborg, 1992). A surface electrode over the muscle may be used so that, theoretically, this type of testing is less painful than an electromyogram.

Among the technical differences between the use of the Nerve Pace™ and traditional testing is the longer duration reported for the distal latency with the Nerve Pace™. The Nerve Pace™ uses a variable output of 0-300 volts for a 0.5 msec duration from a square wave generator. This is not due to the distance reported between different studies, but rather to the fact that with traditional testing there is a clear takeoff point on the oscilloscope screen to define the time, whereas this is not present with the Nerve Pace™. With the Nerve Pace™, a vigorous muscle contraction must occur to discontinue the stimulus and the counter. Five consecutive readings are averaged.

The advantages of such a portable unit are obvious to an office-based therapist or physician and, therefore, the introduction of such testing may well precede epidemiologic testing necessary for establishing validity. Table 7.12 has data relative to such a determination, comparing the results of the use of the Nerve Pace™ with vibrometry and traditional electrodiagnostic testing.

UNIQUE APPLICATIONS FOR THE PERIPHERAL NERVE SURGEON

Totally apart from clinical electrodiagnosis, it is important to recognize several other valuable roles for electrodiagnosis. Dave Kline, a neurosurgeon in New Orleans, has pioneered the intraoperative use of electrical stimulation and recording for the management of the neuroma-in-continuity and brachial plexus injuries (Kline & Judice, 1983). Stuart Gaul, a hand surgeon, has pioneered the intraoperative use of electrical stimulation with an awake patient for identification of fascicles in the peripheral nerve at the time of nerve repair or reconstruction (Gaul, 1986). Julia Terzis, a plastic surgeon with a PhD in neurophysiology, has pioneered the use of electrical testing for mapping peripheral receptive fields, investigating neural regeneration, and improving intraoperative techniques for neuroma-incontinuity and brachial plexus surgery (Terzis, Dykes, & Hakstian, 1976). Most recently, Allen Van Beek, a plastic surgeon, has continued to improve clinical techniques for electrical stimulation and recording (Van Beek, 1986).

ELECTROMYOGRAPHY

The status of the innervated muscle can be evaluated by inserting a recording electrode into the muscle. The first recorded activity of a normal muscle to a needle insertion (insertional activity) is depolarization, which generates a signal of short duration, called an *M-wave*, on the oscilloscope screen. If there is no insertional activity, or if it is diminished, then the muscle may be denervated or fibrotic, or both. This activity may be increased with inflammation of the muscle. Contraction of the muscle generates a polyphasic waveform, the M-wave. If the patient attempts to activate the muscle by making it contract while the recording electrode is still in the muscle, additional motor units are progressively recruited, producing an increasing frequency of M-waves. Neuropathy, myopathy, or an uncooperative patient can each decrease the normal recruitment pattern. The normal muscle is electrically quiet. The denervated muscle spontaneously depolarizes, giving rise to what are called fibrillation potentials, which are small M-waves. A similar wave that has a sudden positive inflection on the oscilloscope screen is called the positive sharp wave, and also represents denervation.

AMYOTROPHIC LATERAL SCLEROSIS

This is an important neurologic problem for the therapist or surgeon caring for a patient with hand problems. When evaluating a patient with intrinsic muscle wasting, the first thought is usually that the problem is related to an ulnar nerve problem, either at the wrist or at the elbow. If all the intrinsics are in trouble, including the thenar muscles, the therapist or surgeon may consider that there is a problem with the median nerve and the ulnar nerve. Hopefully, however, there will be thought given to the possibility that this may represent a cervical disc problem (C8/T1), or perhaps a problem with the lower trunk or medial cord of the brachial plexus. If the problem is bilateral, consideration must be given to two other neurologic problems, *syringomyelia* (cyst of the spinal canal, associated with intrinsic muscle wasting, abnormal perception of temperature and pain, but normal perception of touch; see Chapter 19) and *amyotrophic lateral sclerosis* (ALS).

ALS was first described in 1865 by Charcot, who held the chair in pathology at the University of Paris, but its cause is still unknown. The incidence is about 1 case per 100,000 population. It presents classically with upper extremity intrinsic muscle weakness and wasting, with fasciculations of the first dorsal interosseous being the most common early sign. There is usually no associated numbness or paresthesias. It is bilateral, and progresses rapidly to involve the lower extremities, with about 20% of patients having *bulbar*

(swallowing, speech) problems. There are usually painful muscle cramps and hyperreflexia (in about 25% of cases). As lower extremity problems progress, the patient becomes confined to a wheelchair, and as the bulbar problems proceed, the patient requires ventilatory assistance. The mean survival from the time of diagnosis is about 2.5 years, with just 15% surviving 10 years.

Electromyographic examination is crucial for the diagnosis of ALS. For the diagnosis, a neurogenic pattern must be found in at least three muscles of three different limbs. This pattern consists of fasciculations, positive sharp waves, fibrillation potentials, loss of motor units during full recruitment, and increased amplitude and duration of the motor potentials. Sensory nerve conduction velocities and distal latencies are usually normal. Motor nerve conduction velocities may be slightly reduced, with slowing of distal motor latencies (Cornblath, Kuncl, & Mellits, 1992; Mondelli, Rossi, Passero, & Guazzi, 1993).

SOMATOSENSORY EVOKED POTENTIALS

Evoked potentials are similar in concept to nerve conduction studies in that they are objective, and they require an electrical stimulation of skin surface. They differ in that instead of recording the neural impulse from somewhere along the peripheral nerve, or over the muscle, they are recorded from the scalp. Thus, the recording of the evoked potential displays the cortical brain wave pattern. Special equipment is required, as is special training in interpreting the pattern. The recording consists of waveforms that go above and below the baseline, and are numbered beginning with the earliest wave, which appears as P1 (positive deflection) and N1 (negative deflection) (see Table 8.4).

Recording evoked potentials has become almost routine during certain surgical procedures, such as spinal cord surgery, since changes in the scalp recording in the unconscious patient will signal potential intraoperative complications to the surgeon.

BRACHIAL PLEXUS COMPRESSION

Brachial plexus compression in the thoracic inlet, the name I prefer for what is traditionally called the "thoracic outlet syndrome" (see Chapter 18), is difficult to diagnose. With actual division of part of the brachial plexus, or loss of function of part of the brachial plexus due to a stretch/traction injury of the plexus, such as from a motorcycle accident or birth palsy,

TABLE 8.4   EVOKED POTENTIALS: NORMATIVE DATA

Site tested	Cortical Recording Site (N1)	
	Peak Latency (msec) mean ± sd	Peak Amplitude (msec) mean ± sd
Middle finger	22.6 ± 1.3	0.5 ± 0.1
Fifth finger	24.0 ± 1.8	0.7 ± 0.3
Lateral antebrachial cutaneous	14.1 ± 0.7	0.5 ± 0.8

Note: From *Manual of Nerve Conduction Velocity and Clinical Neurophysiology*, 3rd edition, 1994, by J. A. DeLisa, H. J. Lee, E. M. Baran, K-S. Lai, & N. Spielholz, New York: Raven Press. Reprinted with permission of the authors.

traditional electrodiagnostic examination of peripheral nerve conduction velocity and selected electromyography can establish the most likely site of this proximal lesion. Traditional electrodiagnostic studies can do this because they can look at the distal target-organs, that is, muscle of selected plexus roots or trunks, and establish that the sensory conduction is normal for a dorsal root avulsion (because the dorsal root ganglion nuclei are still alive), and that there is no motor conduction velocity (because the ventral roots are avulsed from the ventral horn location of its nuclei).

With compression of portions of the brachial plexus by one or more congenital bands, or by anomalous or fibrous muscles, at one or more locations, and with all of this occurring so close to the spinal cord, it is impossible technically to demonstrate a localized region of slowing. This is made even more unre-

liable due to the impossibility of knowing the exact distance along the nerve for which the surface recording corresponds, and the effect of overlying muscle and fat on the amplitude of the action potentials. Furthermore, with the exception of the so-called "true neurogenic" thoracic outlet syndrome (< 1% of all patients with thoracic outlet syndrome), as described by Gilliatt, LeQuesne, Logue, and Sumner (1970), there is insufficient compression at any plexus site to produce muscle denervation.

Somatosensory evoked potentials offer a potential diagnostic solution to this problem because they record from the cortex with a distal stimulus, theoretically providing a testing and recording site proximal and distal to the plexus compression site. However, if just the little finger is used as the stimulus site, it cannot logically be inferred that the problem is in the lower trunk of the

brachial plexus, because the site of slowing could be at Guyon's canal or at the elbow (*cubital tunnel*).

We have tried to develop the theory, in conjunction with Michael Kaplan, MD, PhD, who does the actual evoked potential recordings, that a diagnosis of plexus compression can be made if other cutaneous nerve territories are also tested (Kaplan, Mullik, Dellon, & Hendler, 1995). For example, if the upper, inner arm is stimulated, this will give information about the medial brachial cutaneous nerve, which is a proximal branch of the medial cord, which has no intervening entrapment site between the skin and the plexus. Therefore, if both the little finger and the upper inner arm demonstrate delayed somatosensory evoked potentials, it may be inferred that the lower trunk of the brachial plexus has a site of compression (see example in Table 8.5 and Figure 8.2).

With the same reasoning, if the evoked potential is recorded after index finger stimulation and after stimulation of the volar radial surface of the forearm (lateral antebrachial cutaneous nerve, terminal branch of the lateral cord of the plexus), it may be inferred that the upper trunk of the brachial plexus is a site of compression. Note that this conclusion would not be true if the stimulus site were over the dorsal radial surface of the forearm, because a delayed evoked potential from this site might be due to entrapment of the radial sensory nerve.

TABLE 8.5   SOMATOSENSORY EVOKED POTENTIAL DIAGNOSIS: BILATERAL BRACHIAL PLEXUS COMPRESSION

| | Name of Peaks on Evoked Potential Recording | | | |
	Erbs Point	N1	P1	N2
Stimulus Location				
Fifth Finger				
Right				
Latency (msecs)	absent	absent	absent	absent
Amplitude (mvolts)				
Left				
Latency (msecs)	absent	absent	absent	absent
Amplitude (mvolts)				
Medial Brachial Cut.				
Right				
Latency (msecs)	absent	absent	absent	absent
Amplitude (μ volts)				
Left				
Latency (msecs)	absent	absent	absent	absent
Amplitude (μ volts)				
Index Finger				
Right				
Latency (msecs)	9.9	18.9	23.9	32.5
Amplitude (μ volts)		4.7	4.9	
Left				
Latency (msecs)	9.9	18.8	23.4	30.8
Amplitude (μ volts)		3.1	3.4	
Lateral Antebrach. Cut.				
Right				
Latency (msecs)	10.6	22.4	31.1	38.0
Amplitude (μ volts)		1.7	1.9	
Left				
Latency (msecs)	8.0	17.5	28.6	37.1
Amplitude (μ volts)		1.4	2.3	

FIGURE 8.2

Somatosensory Evoked Potentials. This example is from a 40-year-old women who had a motor vehicle accident in 9/92 during which she sustained significant twisting in the driver's seat with striking both palms and right elbow. She had a release of her right carpal tunnel in 11/92, her left carpal tunnel in 2/93, and a transposition of her right ulnar nerve at the elbow in 4/94. She is now 8 months after the last surgery and still has complaints of diffuse numbness in her right little and ring fingers and down the inner aspect of her arm, aching in her right neck and shoulder, and anterior chest, with worsening of her symptoms when her right arm is raised above her head. She has had 1 year of nonoperative management including muscle relaxants and shoulder girdle muscle strengthening for treatment of right brachial compression in the thoracic inlet (traditionally termed thoracic outlet syndrome). (A) Normal recording from cortex (upper tracings) and from Erb's point. The patient's recordings after stimulating right medial antebrachial (B) and right lateral antebrachial (C) cutaneous nerves. Note absent evoked potentials consistent with compression of the brachial plexus. From data provided by Michael Kaplan, MD, PhD, Baltimore, MD.

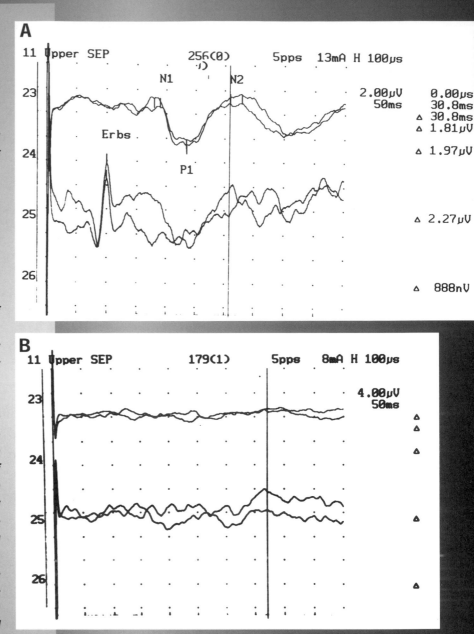

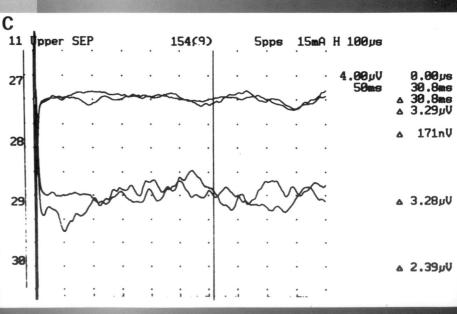

• REFERENCES •

AAEM Quality Assurance Committee, Literature review of the usefulness of nerve conduction studies and electromyography for the evaluation of patients with carpal tunnel syndrome. *Muscle and Nerve* *16*:1392-1414, 1993.

Braun, R. M., & Jackson, W. J. Electrical studies as a prognostic factor in the surgical treatment of carpal tunnel syndrome. *Journal of Hand Surgery 19A*:893-900, 1994.

Buch-Jaeger, N., & Foucher, G. Correlation of clinical signs with nerve conduction tests in the diagnosis of carpal tunnel syndrome. *Journal of Hand Surgery 19B*:720-724, 1994.

Cornblath, D. R., Kuncl, R. W., & Mellits, E. D. Nerve conduction studies in amyotrophic lateral sclerosis. *Muscle and Nerve 15*:1111-1115, 1992.

DeLisa, J. A., Lee, H. J., Baran, E. M., Lai, K-S. & Spielholz, N. *Manual of Nerve Conduction Velocity and Clinical Neurophysiology*, 3rd edition. New York: Raven Press, 1994.

Dellon, A. L. Electrodiagnosis in the management of focal neuropathies: The "WOG" Syndrome. *Muscle and Nerve 17*:1336-1342, 1994.

Dellon, A. L. Pitfalls in electrodiagnosis. In *Operative Nerve Repair and Reconstruction*, R. H. Gelberman, Editor. Philadelphia: J.B. Lippincott Company, 1991, pp. 185-196.

Dellon, A. L., & Coert, H. Results of musculofascial lengthening technique for submuscular transposition of the ulnar nerve at the elbow. *Journal of Bone and Joint Surgery*, submitted: 1997.

Erlanger, J., & Gasser, H. S. *Electrical Signs of Nervous Activity.* Philadelphia: University of Pennsylvania Press, 1937.

Gaul, J. S., Jr. Electrical fascicle identification as an adjunct to nerve repair. *Hand Clinics 2*:709-722, 1986.

Gilliatt, R. W., LeQuesne, P. M., Logue, V., & Sumner, A. J. Wasting of the hand associated with cervical rib or band. *Journal of Neurology, Neurosurgery and Psychiatry 33*:615-618, 1970.

Gilliatt, R. W., & Thomas, P. K. Changes in nerve conduction with ulnar nerve lesions at the elbow. *Journal of Neurology, Neurosurgery, and Psychiatry 23*:312-320, 1960.

Gilliatt, R. W., & Wilson, R. G. Peripheral nerve conduction in diabetic neuropathy. *Journal of Neurology, Neurosurgery, and Psychiatry 25*:11-16, 1962.

Kaplan, M., Mullik, T., Dellon, A. L., & Hendler, N. Somatosensory evoked potentials in diagnosis of brachial plexus compression in the thoracic inlet. Presented at the American Society of Peripheral Nerve, October 1995, Montreal. *Unpublished observations).

Kimura, J. A method for determining median nerve conduction velocity across the carpal tunnel. *Journal of Neurological Sciences 38*:1-10, 1978.

Kimura, J. *Electrodiagnosis in diseases of nerve and muscle.* Philadelphia: F. A. Davis Company, 1983.

Kline, D. G., & Judice, D. J. Operative management of selected brachial plexus lesions. *Journal of Neurosurgery 58*:631-649, 1983.

Mondelli, M., Rossi, A., Passero, S., & Guazzi, G. C. Involvement of peripheral sensory fibers in amyotrophic lateral sclerosis: Electrophysiological study of 64 cases. *Muscle and Nerve 16*:166-172, 1993.

Osterman, A. L., Aversa, B. A., & Greenstein, D. Use of the Nerve Pace Electroneurometer as an affective screening tool in the diagnosis of carpal tunnel syndrome. *Journal of Hand Surgery*, in press: 1995.

Spindler, H. A., & Dellon, A. L. Nerve conduction studies and sensibility testing in the carpal tunnel syndrome. *Journal of Hand Surgery 7*:260-263, 1982.

Steinberg, D. R., Gelberman, R. H., Rydevik, B., & Lundborg, G. The utility of portable nerve conduction testing for patients with carpal tunnel syndrome: A prospective clinical study. *Journal of Hand Surgery 17A*:77-81, 1992.

Terzis, J. K., Dykes, R. W., & Hahstian, R. W. Electrophysiologic recordings in peripheral nerve surgery — A review. *Journal of Hand Surgery 1*:52-66, 1976.

Van Beek, A. L. Electrodiagnostic evaluation of peripheral nerve injuries. *Hand Clinics 2*:747- 760, 1986.

• ADDITIONAL READINGS •

Black, D. L. Somatosensory evoked potential monitoring during total hip arthroplasty. *Clinical Orthopedics 262*:170-177, 1991.

Brown, W. F., & Bolton, C. F. *Clinical electromyography.* Boston: Butterworth-Heinemann, 1993.

Dellon, A. L., Hament, W., & Gittelsohn, A. Results of non-operative management of ulnar nerve compression at the elbow: A prospective study. *Neurology 43*:1673-1674, 1993.

Dykes, R. W., & Terzis, J. K. Reinnervation of glabrous skin in baboons: Properties of cutaneous mechanoreceptors subsequent to nerve crush. *Journal of Neurophysiology 42*:1461-1478, 1979.

Ebeling, P., Gilliatt, R. W., & Thomas, D. K. A clinical and electrical study of ulnar nerve lesions in the hand. *Journal of Neurology, Neurosurgery, and Psychiatry 23*:1-9, 1960.

Feierstein, M. S. The performance and usefulness of nerve conduction studies in the orthopedic office. *Orthopedic Clinics of North America 19*:859-866, 1989.

Goodman, H. V., & Gilliatt, R. W. The effect of treatment on median nerve conduction in patients with the carpal tunnel syndrome. *Annals of Physical Medicine 6:*137-155, 1961.

Kline, D. G., Hackett, E. R., & May, P. Evaluation of nerve injuries by evoked potentials and electromyography. *Journal of Neurosurgery 31*:136-138, 1969.

Pradas, J., Finison, L., Andres, P. L., Thor-nell, B., Hollander, D., & Munsant, T. L. Natural history of amyotrophic lateral sclerosis. *Neurology 43*:751-755, 1993.

Seror, P. Sensitivity of the various tests for the diagnosis of carpal tunnel syndrome. *Journal of Hand Surgery 19B*:725-728, 1994.

Spindler, H. A., & Dellon, A. L. Nerve conduction studies in the superficial radial sensory nerve entrapment syndrome. *Muscle and Nerve 13*:1-5, 1990.

Williams, H. B., & Terzis, J. K. Single fascicular recordings — An intraoperative diagnostic tool for the management of peripheral nerve lesions. *Plastic and Reconstructive Surgery 57*:562-569, 1976.

• • •

SECTION

sensory
rehabilitation

grading
peripheral
nerve function

• • •

*W*ithout assessment, we cannot
treat, we cannot communicate,
and we cannot progress.

Elaine E. Fess
1984

• • •

The modern history of clinical medicine has many instances of improved patient care as a result of a better understanding of the pathophysiology of disease. The analysis and communication of the information that forms the basis of this progress usually rely on a graded classification of the disease. Examples of diseases and other medical problems for which improved care is based on a classification are Hodgkin's disease; cancer, the treatment of which is based on a tumor's size, location, involvement of regional nodes, or distant metastases (*the* TMN *classification*); the treatment of compound fractures of the lower extremity (*the Gustillo classification*); and the treatment of congenital deformities, such as thumb duplication (*Wassel's classification*). Creating a universally acceptable numerical grading system is essential to elevating clinical care of the peripheral nerve to the scientific level it deserves. Knowledge of the pathophysiology of the peripheral nerve and of clinical assessment techniques for evaluating the peripheral nerve are now sufficiently advanced that the goal of creating a numerical grading system for the peripheral nerve is now possible to achieve.

Despite the progress made by hand therapists, neuroscientists, and surgeons in understanding and quantifying peripheral nerve function, there remains little uniformity in the reporting of end results of nerve repair, in describing the stages of chronic nerve compression, or in describing the degree of a peripheral neuropathy. Despite worldwide awareness of the existence of Highet's "British System" for classifying peripheral nerve repair results, that is, S1-4 and M1-5 (Zachary, 1954), many therapists and surgeons still employ traditional, but poorly defined descriptors, such as "poor," "fair," "good," and "excellent" to describe these results. Such descriptors fail to permit detailed statistical analysis of preoperative versus postoperative conditions, or relative improvement in motor versus sensory function. Furthermore, these traditional descriptors frustrate any attempt to do inter-center or cooperative end-result studies, now termed *meta-analysis*. Unfortunately, even when the British System is used some of its categories are too narrow, so that they have had to be qualified by adding a "+" after them, for

example, S3+. However, even that category failed to specify its meaning; for example, S3+ is defined as some two-point discrimination. But how much two-point discrimination is "some"?

It should be possible to develop a numerical grading system for peripheral nerve function. The increasing availability of therapists trained in hand evaluation techniques, the increasing emphasis on reliability and validity of testing instruments and procedures, and the recent proliferation of computer-assisted sensorimotor "systems" suggest that the time for such a grading system is now. It is the purpose of this chapter to conceptualize and formulate such a grading system.

• CRITERIA FOR A NUMERICAL GRADING SYSTEM •

A *peripheral nerve grading system* must distinguish between differing degrees of sensory and motor function. The system should be able to be applied to both upper and lower extremity nerves. It is clear, therefore, that this is not a system for evaluating hand function. Hand function may be described by a combination of the function of different nerves, of a particular hand activity, such as grip strength; and perhaps best by the function of an individual peripheral nerve, such as the ulnar nerve. But the goal is to develop a system to evaluate the function of a given peripheral nerve, such as the median or ulnar nerve.

It is desirable for a grading system to be expressed by a numerical scale so that statistical analysis will be facilitated. While a uniform scale, that is, one with the same *spacing* between points, would be ideal, it is recognized that this may not be possible either to achieve or to demonstrate. Each point on the scale must be mutually exclusive. Therefore, the statistical analysis must not assume a continuous numerical scale or a particular, that is, normal, distribution of the scale's values. Accordingly, the statistical analysis will require nonparametric statistics: That is, the descriptive statistic "average" will be the median value instead of the mean, and the test to compare the difference between two groups for significance will be the Mann-Whitney or Wilcoxon Rank Sum test instead of the Student's *t-test*. If the numerical grading system can be demonstrated to have uniform spacing, and the data obtained meet the normality test, then parametric statistics can be used. The concept of uniform spacing in the scale also implies that the scale will not be logarithmic, like that used to describe the estimates made with the Semmes-Weinstein nylon monofilaments, or the decibel scale used by many vibrometers.

Fess (1984) has emphasized the desirability of employing clinical tests that are *standardized*, that is, tests that are proven to be reliable and valid, are well described in terms of equipment specifications and methods of use, and have normative data available. Fess notes that from a practical point of view, "unfortunately only a small number of tests meet all requirements of standardization. The remaining hand assessment instruments fall at varying levels along the validity and reliability continuums....[I]nstrument selection should be predicated on satisfying as may of the standardization requisites as possible, thus ensuring an identifiable level of quality control." This statement remains important in the selection of criteria for a numerical grading system in that the instrumentation to make the measurements for the system should be standardized.

Chapter 7 provides information regarding standardization for each type of instrument that might be chosen for these measurements. It is recognized that instrumentation evolves, and that what was the industry standard a decade ago will not likely be the industry standard tomorrow. For example, the computer-assisted sensorimotor devices developed by the NK Biotechnical Corpo-

ration, the Pressure-Specified Sensory Device™, and the Digit-Grip™ will become the industry standard, but at present they are not universally available. The numerical grading scale must be constructed so that instruments are as close to being standardized as possible, while at the same time instruments that are available can be used. The scale can be such that as a more standardized instrument becomes available to a given clinic, either scientifically or economically, its measurement can be substituted into the scale.

For example, if the only equipment available to measure the cutaneous pressure threshold is a set of nylon monofilaments, then these should be used until you can upgrade your equipment to include the Pressure-Specified Sensory Device™, as this has now been demonstrated to be the more standardized instrument for this measurement. If the only equipment available to measure grip or pinch strength are the Bechtol Jamar-type dynamometers or Preston pinch meters, then these should be used until you can upgrade your equipment to include the Digit-Grip™ and NK Pinch device, as they have now been demonstrated to be the more standardized (and reliable, by virtue of being traceable to the NIST) instruments for these measurements.

With regard to measuring motor function, it must be

realized that we are trying to evaluate the function of a given muscle or muscles that are innervated by a given peripheral nerve. It is, therefore, going to require that traditional physical examination techniques be used to assess muscle function. The book by Kendall and Kendall (1949), who developed the art of physical examination of the musculoskeletal system at the Children's Hospital in Baltimore during the height of the polio epidemic, is still the bible on manual muscle testing. Where instrumentation does not exist to directly measure strength, manual muscle testing must be used. When normal muscle bulk is not present, the degree of atrophy or wasting must be estimated. It is recognized, therefore, that with the exception of grip and pinch strength, we have no instrumentation to measure motor function clinically. The numerical grading system will not incorporate electromyography, the electrodiagnostic evaluation of muscle, because it is an invasive and painful procedure and will not likely be permitted for serial evaluations.

A critical criterion for a numerical grading system is that the scale be ordered in a relationship to the known pathophysiology of the peripheral nerve. There is a certain symmetry between the progressive loss of function observed with chronic nerve compression and the recovery of sensation after nerve reconstruction. This symmetry is based on the response of nerve fibers to pressure and ischemia, and on the reinnervation of sensory and motor receptors during regeneration.

For example, the earliest change related to nerve compression is disruption of the blood–nerve barrier, causing endoneurial and subperineurial edema. This is followed by progressive demyelination of the large myelinated sensory and motor fibers, and finally by degeneration of nerve fibers. Electrophysiologic changes, such as delay in conduction, do not occur until there is thinning of the myelin, with decrease in amplitude not occurring until there is axonal loss. For the muscles, the earliest change is manifested by weakness, with wasting or atrophy not occurring until individual nerve fibers to the muscle have degenerated. For the sensory component of the nerve, the earliest changes would be symptoms of numbness or tingling (*paresthesias*), then a measurable increase in the detection threshold to a sensory stimulus and, finally, once axonal degeneration has occurred, a measurable increase in the distance required to discriminate one from two points.

During nerve regeneration following a nerve repair or graft, the same sequence

is observed. For the motor nerve, first the muscle will be noted to twitch on voluntary command, then slowly increase in strength until it can overcome gravity, and then increase in bulk and strength until it can function against resistance. For the sensory nerve, first the ability to perceive moving touch occurs, then static touch, which can be measured by their pressure detection thresholds. Then, as a sufficient number of nerve fibers regenerate into the area being tested, the ability to discriminate first one from two moving points, and then one from two static points, returns, which can be measured by the two-point discrimination pressure and distance thresholds.

It is clear from these criteria that previous attempts to grade peripheral nerve function will not prove to be acceptable for today's requirements. For example, one of the earliest attempts to grade ulnar nerve function was McGowan's (1950). This scale of ulnar nerve function only considered motor function; there was no inclusion of sensory symptoms or abnormal sensory function in the grading of ulnar nerve dysfunction. The electrophysiologic definition of an ulnar nerve grading scale by Eisen and Danen (1974) is also not suited to widespread clinical use by the hand surgeon or therapist because, in addition to the pain it caus-

es, it assumes that electrophysiological measurement correlates with patient symptoms and hand function, which it usually does not.

My own earliest attempt at grading peripheral nerve function for chronic nerve compression was too simplistic, yet heading in the right direction. I attempted to create a scale that incorporates the universally observed continuum that begins with intermittent symptoms, progresses to intermittent symptoms with clinical signs of threshold change without degeneration, then to persistent symptoms with clinical signs of threshold change without degeneration, and ends with clinical signs of nerve degeneration. At that time, 1983, I simply called these stages or degrees of nerve compression "early," "moderate," and "severe," and demonstrated progressive changes clinically by using the tuning fork, the Biothesiometer (120 Hz vibrometer), and moving and static two-point discrimination. This grading system, however, clearly did not incorporate evaluation of the motor system, nor did it permit easy statistical analysis.

A final criterion is that at each level of the grading system, the scale should have a correlation with function, which it will if the instrumentation is valid.

A final caveat is that for any classification, an exception will always be found!

● **THE BRITISH SYSTEM** ●

The British System is a prototype for a numerical grading system in that it has rank-ordered categories for sensory function and for motor function. Zachary (1954) wrote the first clear exposition I have read relating to the attempt to develop a grading scale for peripheral nerve function. He clearly delineated the principles that such a system should use (see also Seddon, 1972). Poorly defined terms such as "good" and "excellent" should not be based on the time required to reach a certain level of return. Rather, they should be based on "recording the numbers of patients who have reached particular grades of recovery when a given time has elapsed after suture, e.g. three or five years; it is preferable for recording the late and possibly final results of nerve suture."

Furthermore, Zachary stated that "an effort is made to avoid the confusion that arises from expressing recovery in terms of function of the limb, as...such expressions of recovery are not strictly related to the success of nerve suture." The belief was that "assessment of recovery must therefore be made primarily on a neurological basis, the principal guides being restoration of sensibility and the return of muscle power and control. Neurological recovery will usually improve the function of the limb, and unless disabled in some (other) way, patients with better neurological recovery will have better (limb) function."

The grading scale was first devised for the Nerve Injuries Committee of the British Medical Research Council by W. B. Highet who suggested, probably in 1942, the method of grading which we now call the British System. As I reviewed the history of nerve repair and regeneration in preparing my first book (Dellon, 1981), I noted many papers published by Highet in 1942 and 1944, and then nothing more. In Seddon's last book (1972), I discovered why. Seddon wrote:

> *W. Bremmer Highet joined us at the outbreak of the Second World War. This talented young New Zealander was awarded the Jacksonian Prize by the Royal College of Surgeons of England for an essay on nerve injuries. The closure of the Mediterranean Sea left only the Cape route for the evacuation of men injured in the fighting in the Desert War. As a result of the shortage of transport shipping, many of them piled up in South Africa. Highet was chosen to look after those who had suffered nerve injury. He was sent by sea; the ship was torpedoed and there were no survivors.*

Highet's concept of the grading system was that "motor and sensory recovery must be assessed separately and the full range from total paralysis to complete recovery should be covered by grades which represent recognizable steps in recovery." His system requires specification by two different designations, a motor designation from M1 to M5, and a sensory designation from S1 to S4, so that a given nerve would be graded, for example, M3S4. The categories are descriptive and mutually exclusive; however, they were found to be too broad in some of the sensory categories, necessitating the inclusion of the "+" to many of them (see Table 9.1).

The British System was used extensively for 30 years, and is still used for reporting end results of nerve repairs by some authors. However, since Moberg (1962) began to emphasize the relationship between two-point discrimination and hand function, most peripheral nerve reports have included a measurement of static and, since 1978, moving two-point, discrimination as the final criteria for excellence in recovery of sensory nerve function. Many authors, when using the British System for a given peripheral nerve, will have to define good or excellent nerve function as M4S3+, for example, and

TABLE 9.1   THE BRITISH SYSTEM

Sensory Recovery (Within the Autonomous Zone)

S0	Absence of sensibility
S1	Recovery of deep cutaneous pain sensibility
S1+	Recovery of superficial pain sensibility
S2	Return of some degree of superficial pain and tactile sensibility
S2+	As in S2, but with an over-response
S3	Return of superficial pain and tactile sensibility; no over-response
S3+	As in S3 but good stimulus localization and some two-point discrimination
S4	Complete recovery

Motor Recovery (of Muscles Innervated by this Nerve)

M0	No contraction of any muscle
M1	Perceptible contraction in proximal muscles
M2	Perceptible contraction in proximal and distal muscles
M3	M2 plus all muscles can act against resistance
M4	M3 plus synergistic and isolated movements are possible
M5	Complete recovery

Note: The S+ stages were added after review by the Nerve Injury Committee of the British Medical Research Council as it appears in their 1954 book. The original description of stages was proposed by W. B. Highet around 1942. In 1981, Dellon added the further definition of S3+ as 7-15 mm and S4 as ≤ 6 mm static two-point discrimination.

then report the percentage of good or excellent results they observed, again indicating the need for a better system of grading peripheral nerve function.

As reviewed by Dellon (1981), this grading system leads to disagreement regarding qualitative attempts to categorize the rank-ordered MS designations; for the ulnar nerve some have called "good" M2+ and M3S2+, and "excellent" M4S3+, whereas others have used the M3S2+ and M4S3+ for these same designations. To allow the British System categories to be related to Moberg's observations with respect to two-point discrimination, the end results of nerve repair reviewed by Dellon were correlated with the British System such that static two-point discrimination of 7-15 mm was S3+, static two-point discrimination ≤ 6 mm was S4, and static two-point discrimination > 15 was S3.

• NUMERICAL GRADING • SYSTEM

The general format of a numerical grading system is given in Table 9.2 and expanded in Table 9.3. Measurement of pain perception or temperature perception is not included in this system as they are the last functions to be lost in chronic nerve compression, and are almost always the first to recover after nerve reconstruction. Since they are of neither diagnostic nor prognostic significance, it seems unnecessary to include them in the grading system.

The grading system would begin with a value of 0 being given for normal nerve function, both sensory and motor, and 10 being given for the worst function. The worst degree of function of the motor system would be severe atrophy, and the worst degree of function of the sensory system would be anesthesia. It is theoretically impossible for a muscle to recover from severe wasting of more than 2 years duration. However, theoretically and in reality it is still possible to recover some degree of sensibility even if a finger is anesthetic. Thus, the grade of 10 is assigned logically to "severe wasting," and the grade of 9 is assigned to "anesthesia."

The first symptoms of peripheral nerve compression are intermittent numbness and tingling, or paresthesia. They are due to the early decrease in blood flow in the nerve, and usually "come and go." Therefore, the grade of 1 is assigned to these earliest symptoms, at which time the clinical exam will be normal, except for the possible "positive" provocative signs, such as wrist flexion (Phalen's sign for the carpal tunnel syndrome), elbow flexion (for cubital tunnel syndrome), hyperpronation of the forearm (radial sensory nerve compression), elevation of the arms (Roos's sign for brachial plexus compression), or pressure over the median nerve in the forearm (McMurtry's sign for median nerve compression in the forearm).

The presence of these provocative signs at this grade level is appropriate because they produce their "positive" response by increasing pressure on the nerve, thereby decreasing blood flow and, thus, producing the symptoms. In my experience, sensory complaints virtually always precede complaints of weakness; therefore, grade 1 is assigned to the sensory system. By the time a patient complains of weakness, there is usually measurable weakness, which puts this motor complaint into the category of symptoms plus signs. The one exception I can recall is that of musicians who complain of loss of coordination or control while playing, without sensory complaints,

TABLE 9.2 FORMAT FOR A NUMERICAL GRADING SYSTEM FOR THE PERIPHERAL NERVE	
Clinical Observation	**Numerical Grade**
Normal	0
Intermittent symptoms, no signs	1
Intermittent symptoms, signs of increased threshold	2,3,4
Persistent symptoms, signs of increased threshold	5
Persistent symptoms, signs of nerve degeneration	6-10

Note: Adapted from "A Numerical Grading Scale for Peripheral Nerve Function," by A. L. Dellon, 1993, *Journal of Hand Therapy 4:*152-160. Adapted with permission of the author.

Grade	Description
0	Normal
1	Intermittent sensory symptoms
2	Increased sensory threshold, mild
3	Increased motor threshold
4	Increased sensory threshold, moderate
5	Persistent sensory symptoms
6	Sensory degeneration; abnormal 2PD, mild
7	Muscle atrophy, mild
8	Sensory degeneration; abnormal 2PD, severe
9	Anesthesia
10	Muscle atrophy, severe

TABLE 9.3   NUMERICAL GRADING SYSTEM FOR ANY PERIPHERAL NERVE

Note: Adapted from "A Numerical Grading Scale for Peripheral Nerve Function," by A. L. Dellon, 1993, *Journal of Hand Therapy 4:*152-160. Adapted with permission of the author.

which may, for a violinist, for example, be related to very early ulnar nerve compression at the wrist or elbow.

A scale category that was suggested to me by the clinical observations of Curtis and Eversmann (1973) is that patients complain that their numbness is present all the time; that is, it is persistent. Dr. Curtis always indicated to me that persistent sensory change meant that there was intraneural fibrosis and that these were patients in whom he would consider doing an internal neurolysis. To me, this means that there may be a correlation between persistent sensory

symptoms and a pathophysiologic stage, with increased scarring in the nerve or sufficient external pressure being placed on the nerve to create these symptoms. This may warrant a special category within the grading system, especially if it were to prove to be an indication for a particular change in patient care, that is, if surgery were indicated instead of splinting. Dr. Curtis emphasized, and I have found it to be true in my own experience, that patients with persistent sensory complaints do not improve without surgical intervention. Accordingly, the number 5 is given

to this degree of nerve dysfunction.

Individual peripheral nerves have different relative degrees of motor versus sensory function. For example, the median nerve is generally said to be 80% sensory, while the ulnar nerve is said to be 80% motor. The numerical grading system must be able to adjust to these differences, and it is suggested that it can do so by assigning the 2, 3, and 4 categories and the 6, 7, and 8 categories to be more sensory or more motor, depending on the given nerve. This will be noted in the proposed scales given for these two nerves in

Tables 9.4 (median) and 9.5 (ulnar). It will be noted that these categories give the opportunity to "adjust" the system to individual nerves.

It should be pointed out that this concept has not been validated or approved by any other investigator or group of physicians. The proposed system will serve as a starting point for organizations such as the American Society for the Peripheral Nerve (ASPN) to create a national and, hopefully, international consensus on a peripheral nerve grading system.

• PILOT STUDIES WITH THE •
NUMERICAL GRADING SYSTEM

To know whether there was any validity to the proposed grading system, it was elected to apply it to several clinical problems to determine (a) whether it could be applied at all, (b) whether it would permit critical analysis of clinical problems, and (c) whether it gave clinically useful information. The commonest clinical problems are carpal tunnel syndrome and cubital tunnel syndrome. To determine whether the scale could be applied at all using existing clinical data gathered before the era of computer-assisted sensorimotor testing, a clinical problem or problems with a reasonably small group of patients who would have a wide degree of clinical presentation was required. These problems were recurrent carpal tunnel syndrome and recurrent cubital tunnel syndrome. To evaluate the usefulness of the system for complex statistical analysis, a prospective study of the results of the nonoperative management of cubital tunnel syndrome was chosen.

TABLE 9.4 NUMERICAL GRADING SYSTEM APPLIED TO THE MEDIAN NERVE AT THE WRIST LEVEL

| Numerical Score | | |
Sensory	Motor	Description of Impairment
0	0	None
1		Paresthesia, intermittent
2		Abnormal threshold: pressure, Semmes-Weinstein filament marking 3.22—3.61, Pressure-Specified Sensory Device™ > 1.0 g/mm²; vibration, biothesiometer 3-10 μg
	3	Weakness, thenar muscles
4		Abnormal threshold: pressure, Semmes-Weinstein filament marking 3.84-4.31, Pressure-Specified Sensory Device™ > 16.1 g/mm²; vibration, biothesiometer 11-20 μg
5		Paresthesia, persistent
6		Abnormal 2PD*—index finger: s2PD 7-10 mm; m2PD 4-6 mm
	7	Muscle wasting (1/4—2/4)
8		Abnormal 2 PD—index finger: s2PD ≥ 11 mm; m2PD ≥ 7 mm
9		Anesthesia
	10	Muscle wasting (3/4-4/4)

Note:

*2PD = two-point discrimination

Adapted from "A Numerical Grading Scale for Peripheral Nerve Function," by A. L. Dellon, 1993, *Journal of Hand Therapy 4:*152-160. Adapted with permission of the author.

Numerical Score		
Sensory	Motor	Description of Impairment
0	0	None
1		Paresthesia, intermittent
	2	Weakness—pinch/grip; female 10–14/26–39 lb; male 13–19/31–59 lb
3		Abnormal threshold: pressure, Semmes-Weinstein filament marking 3.22–3.61, Pressure-Specified Sensory Device™ > 1.0 g/mm²; vibration, biothesiometer 3–10 µg
	4	Weakness—pinch/grip; female 6–9/115–25 lb; male 6–12/315–30 lb
5		Paresthesia, persistent
6		Abnormal little finger 2PPD⁺; static 2PD 7–10 mm; moving 2PD 4–6 mm
	7	Muscle wasting (1/4–2/4)
8		Abnormal little finger 2PD⁺; static 2PD ≥ 11 mm; moving 2PD ≥ 7 mm
9		Anesthesia
	10	Muscle wasting (3/4–4/4)

TABLE 9.5 NUMERICAL GRADING SYSTEM APPLIED TO THE ULNAR NERVE AT THE ELBOW LEVEL ⁺

Note:
⁺ 2PD = two-point discrimination
⁺ Modified from "A Numerical Grading Scale for Peripheral Nerve Function," by A. L. Dellon, 1993, *Journal of Hand Therapy 4:*152-160, 1993.

RESULTS OF TREATMENT FOR RECURRENT CARPAL TUNNEL SYNDROME

The numerical grading scale in Table 9.4 for the median nerve at the wrist level was evaluated in 30 patients who had recurrent carpal tunnel syndrome. This problem was chosen because patients with it would have sufficiently severe symptoms and clinical signs and would have outcomes from surgery that might be sufficiently variable to permit application of the full range of the numerical grading scale. This study has been reported (Chang & Dellon, 1993). The patients' sensorimotor evaluations before and after neurolysis of the median nerve in the carpal tunnel were converted into the grading system in Table 9.4, and are given in Table 9.6. The mean length of postoperative follow-up was 23.5 months.

From this evaluation it was demonstrated that if a patient's worst (highest) score, whether motor or sensory, was compared to his or her worst postoperative score, whether motor or sensory, there was a statistically significant improvement resulting from the surgery (6.5 preop versus 1.8 postop, p < .001). The numerical grading scale permitted subgrouping of the entire population into those with different degrees of mo-

tor or sensory severity. This allowed for statistical analysis to be applied to determine whether the results of treatment diminished with increasing degree of preoperative severity, or whether it was relatively easier to achieve better results for sensory or for motor impairment.

It is clear from Table 9.6 that virtually any combination of preoperative conditions can be contrasted to any set of postoperative conditions. The numerical grading system proved easy to apply to this group of patients, and analysis of the results of surgery by comparing the preop with the postop numerical grading proved to be easy to do.

TABLE 9.6 NUMERICAL GRADING SYSTEM APPLIED TO RESULTS OF TREATING RECURRENT CARPAL TUNNEL SYNDROME

Patient Group Grade	Preop Grade	Postop Grade	p value
Entire Group (2-10)	6.5	1.8	< .001
Intermittent symptoms, & increased threshold (2, 3, 4)	2.0	0.0	= .014
Persistent symptoms, & degeneration, mild (5, 6, 7)	6.4	1.6	< .001
Persistent symptoms, & degeneration, severe	8.5	3.0	= .003
Motor degeneration (7, 10)	7.2	2.3	< .001
Sensory degeneration (5, 6, 8, 9)	7.3	2.0	= .003

Note: From "Surgical Management of Recurrent Carpal Tunnel Syndrome," by B. Chang & A. L. Dellon, 1993, *Journal of Hand Surgery 18B:*467-470. Reprinted with permission of the authors.

RESULTS OF TREATMENT ● FOR RECURRENT CUBITAL ● TUNNEL SYNDROME

The numerical grading scale in Table 9.5 for the ulnar nerve at the elbow level was evaluated in 40 of my patients who had recurrent cubital tunnel syndrome. The recurrent cubital tunnel syndrome was chosen because patients with this problem would have sufficiently severe symptoms and clinical signs, and would have outcomes from surgery that might be sufficiently variable to permit application of the full range of the numerical grading scale. This study has not yet been reported.

The patient's sensorimotor evaluations before and after submuscular transposition of the ulnar nerve at the elbow by the muscle slide technique (musculofascial lengthening, Dellon, 1988, 1991) were converted into the grading system in Table 9.5, and are given in Table 9.7. The mean length of postoperative follow-up was 38 months. From this evaluation it was demonstrated that if the patient's worst (highest) score, whether motor or sensory, was compared to his or her worst postoperative score, whether motor or sensory, there was a statistically significant improvement resulting from the surgery (7.1 preop versus 2.0 postop, p < .001). The numerical grading scale permitted subgrouping of the entire population into those with different degrees of motor or sensory severity, so that statistical analysis could be applied to determine whether the results of treatment diminished with increasing degree of preoperative severity, or whether it was relatively easier to achieve better results for sensory or for motor impairment.

It is clear from Table 9.7 that virtually any combination of preoperative conditions can be contrasted to any set of postoperative conditions. The numerical grading system proved easy to apply to this group of patients, and analysis of the results of surgery by comparing the preop with the postop numerical grading proved to be easy to do.

NONOPERATIVE MANAGEMENT OF CUBITAL TUNNEL SYNDROME

To determine whether this numerical grading scale would permit sufficient specificity to evaluate a patient group by the proportional hazards model, or what is usually called "life-table analysis," the scale for the ulnar nerve in Table 9.5 was applied to a cohort of cubital tunnel patients accrued from 1983 through 1987 (Dellon, Hament, & Gittelshon, 1993). This group was characterized by individuals having sufficiently early or minimal-enough symptoms and signs, or by individuals who otherwise refused surgical treatment and were treated with a standardized, nonoperative regimen to reduce pressure within the cubital tunnel.

The group was comprised of 164 individuals with cubital tunnel syndrome, with a mean length of follow up of 58.6 months. Failure of the nonoperative treatment was defined as surgical intervention. The patients were subgrouped such that the most minimally involved group would be those individuals with intermittent symptoms without signs (grade 1). The next most involved group was comprised of individuals with intermittent symptoms with signs of increased threshold (grades 2, 3, & 4). The most involved group was comprised of individuals with persistent symptoms with signs of degeneration (grades 5, 6, & 7). There was no patient in this study with a grade of 8, 9, or 10 who was treated nonoperatively.

Statistical analysis of this data is given in Figure 9.1. The data demonstrate a statistically significant increase in the percentage of patients having surgery, that is, those failing nonoperative management, in relation to the staging created by the numerical grading scale. For statistical purposes, a successful outcome of nonoperative management was defined as not having an operation; specifically, life-table analysis of the results of nonoperative management of the cubital tunnel syndrome. From the graph, 89% of patients with intermittent symptoms only (grade 1), 67% of patients with intermittent symptoms and increased sensorimotor threshold (grades 2, 3, & 4), and 38% of patients with persistent symptoms and signs of degeneration (grades 5, 6, & 7) did not have surgery. These differences were significant at the $p < .001$ level.

TABLE 9.7   NUMERICAL GRADING SYSTEM APPLIED TO RESULTS OF TREATING RECURRENT CUBITAL TUNNEL SYNDROME

Patient Group Grade	Preop Grade	Postop Grade	p value
Entire group (2-10)	7.1	2.9	< 0.001
Just motor (2, 4, 7, 10)	4.7	0.0	< 0.001
Just sensory (3, 5, 6, 8, 9)	6.4	1.6	< 0.001
Motor degeneration mild (7)	7.0	2.2	= 0.038
Sensory degeneration mild (5, 6)	5.7	0.9	< 0.001
Motor degeneration severe (10)	10.0	4.4	= 0.017
Sensory degeneration severe (8, 9)	8.2	5.2	= 0.16

Note: From "Recurrent Ulnar Nerve Compression at the Elbow Treated by the Musculofascial Lengthening Technique," by A. L. Dellon. Presented at the American Society of Surgery of the Hand meeting, Phoenix, AZ, 1992. Reprinted with permission of the author.

FIGURE 9.1

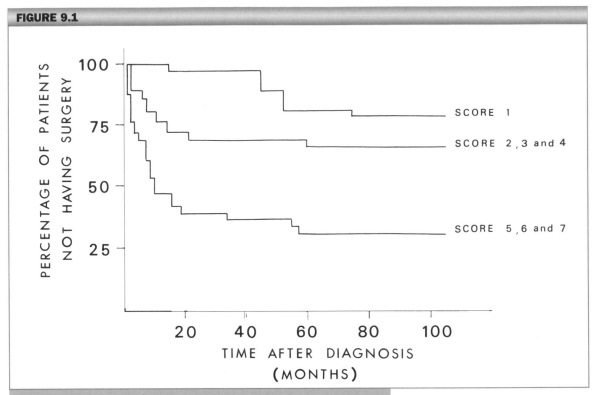

Life-table analysis of the results of nonoperative management of the cubital tunnel syndrome. For statistical purposes, a successful outcome of nonoperative management was defined as not having an operation. From the graph, 89% of patients with intermittent symptoms only (grade 1), 67% of patients with intermittent symptoms and increased sensorimotor threshold (grades 2, 3, & 4), and 38% of patients with persistent symptoms and signs of degeneration (grades 5, 6, & 7) did not have surgery. These differences were significant at the p < .001 level. From "Non-operative Management of Cubital Tunnel Syndrome: Results of an Eight-year Prospective Study," by A. L. Dellon, W. Hament, & A. Gittelsohn, Neurology 43:1673-1677, 1993. Reprinted with permission of the authors.

• TARSAL TUNNEL •
SYNDROME

Most recently, the numerical grading scale has been applied to the evaluation of the distal posterior tibial nerve, which can be entrapped at the ankle in the tarsal tunnel. This nerve would be homologous to both the median and ulnar nerve at the wrist level, but only the strength of the abductor hallucis brevis can be reliably tested manually for the medial plantar nerve and for clawing observed

for the lateral plantar nerve. The sensibility can be tested reliably at the heel and at the big toe. The numerical grading scale given in Table 9.8 has been used to evaluate the results of my approach to decompression of all the medial tunnels at the ankle for all my patients since 1987 (Mullick & Dellon, unpublished observations, 1996), and for diabetics measured with the Pressure-Specified Sensory Device™ (Azman, Kress, & Dellon, unpublished observations, 1996). This scale was developed to be analogous to that for the distal median nerve.

Grade	Description
TABLE 9.8	**NUMERICAL GRADING SYSTEM APPLIED TO THE DISTAL POSTERIOR TIBIAL NERVE**
0	Normal
1	Intermittent symptoms of numbness, tingling, paresthesia in toes, "ball" of foot, and/or heel
2	Abnormal vibratory or pressure threshold, mild (PSSD 1.0–5.0 g/mm^2)
3	Increased motor threshold (weakness) (abductor halluces brevis)
4	Abnormal vibratory or pressure threshold, moderate (PSSD >5.1–15.0 g/mm^2)
5	Persistent symptoms of numbness, tingling, paresthesia
6	Abnormal static two-point discrimination, mild; age < 45 (7–10 mm), > 45 (9–12 mm)
7	Muscle atrophy (abductor wasting)
8	Abnormal static two-point discrimination, moderate; age < 45 (11–15 mm), > 45 (13–17 mm)
9	Anesthesia (no two-point discrimination)
10	Muscle atrophy, severe (any clawing)

SURVEY OF EXPERTS ON RANK ORDERING OF THIS NUMERICAL SCALE

Thus far the conceptualization and formulation has all been the work of one individual: The rank ordering of the grading scale has come from my own personal experience. Another approach to determining the validity of this grading scale, in addition to demonstrating that it can evaluate certain clinical situations as in the three pilot projects above, would be to ask a panel of experts to rank the same categories and then compare their ranking to mine. In February 1992, a questionnaire was sent to 40 experts to do this. They were given a set of 11 cards with the category names described in Table 9.4 for the median nerve, and in Table 9.5 for the ulnar nerve. They were asked "to structure a rank/order series of events that constitute the natural history of the injured peripheral nerve." Twenty responses were received from a group that included both orthopedic and plastic surgeons who have published in the field of peripheral nerve surgery, and from hand therapists recognized for expertise in sensory rehabilitation and sensibility testing.

Figure 9.2 illustrates the responses for the median nerve and demonstrates how the responses to the questionnaire help focus on the additional information that must be ac-

quired to create a numerical grading system that has widespread acceptance. For example, it was unclear to most respondents where to place "persistent paresthesias," which is grade 5. Is this because most respondents do not ask their patients this historical question and, therefore, they have insufficient information on which to make their decision on placement of this category in the grading scale? This is the most likely explanation because most respondents simply ranked this category just after grade 1, "intermittent paresthesia." This also illustrates a methodological problem with the questionnaire in that it did not provide information as to whether the re-

FIGURE 9.2

Rank-ordering of the categories for the median nerve from Table 9.4 by 20 experts. The graph represents the distribution of the responses compared to the order to Table 9.4. (A) If all respondents agreed exactly with the author's grading scale, there would be a series of sharply defined peaks in the numerical sequence 0 through 10. This did occur, indicating excellent agreement for categories 0, 1, 9, and 10. (B) To focus on the areas of disagreement, the sensory categories are examined separately. Most respondents ranked mild increased sensory threshold before severe increased threshold (grade 2 before grade 4), and the same for sensory degeneration (grade 6 before 8). However, the relationship between the development of increased sensory threshold and sensory degeneration was uncertain (grade 6 preceded 4 for many respondents). Also note that some respondents ranked anesthesia (9) as occurring before severe sensory degeneration (8). From "Rank/ordering of the Elements of a Numerical Grading Scale for Peripheral Nerve Function: The Response of a Panel of Experts," by A. L. Dellon & A. L. Scally. Presented to the American Society for the Peripheral Nerve, 1993 meeting. Reprinted with permission of the authors.

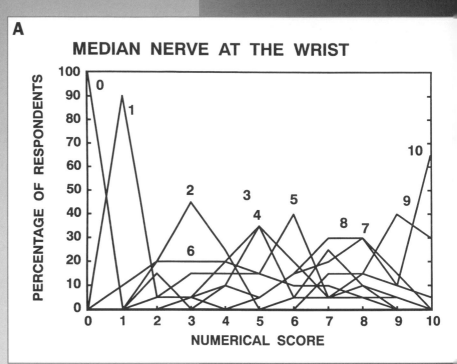

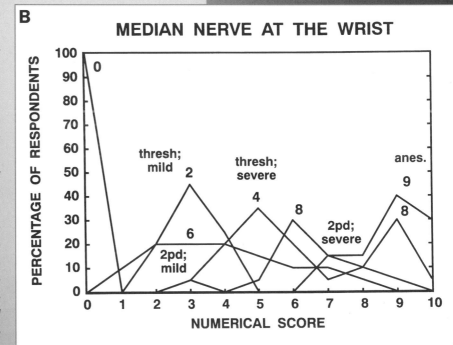

spondents truly had experience with each of the categories. This also demonstrates an area for both future investigation and educational needs.

Similarly, is the problem (Figure 9.2) with category overlap of increased sensory threshold (grade 2) and mild sensory degeneration (grade 6) due to a true difference of opinion, or does it reflect the possibility that most respondents do not measure both the cutaneous pressure threshold and the distance at whichtwo points can be distiguished? Or, the final alternative, does it reflect that these two categories do overlap and may not be mutually exclusive?

• CRITICAL ANALYSIS OF NUMERICAL GRADING SCALE FOR PERIPHERAL NERVE FUNCTION •

The numerical grading scale conceptualized and formulated in this chapter remains to be validated. By selecting two well-understood peripheral nerves, the median nerve at the wrist level and the ulnar nerve at the elbow level, it was possible to design three pilot studies to test the applicability of this grading scale. The ease with which the commonly used clinical assessment techniques can be converted into a numerical grade, the ease with which the numerical grade can be analyzed statistically, and the variety of statistical analyses possible suggest that this grading scale already may be appropriately rank ordered and may, therefore, be valid. While some of the individual clinical assessment tests, such as two-point discrimination, have been validated with respect to predicting hand function, and have been ranked, in general, in relation to threshold testing, the relationships between motor and sensory components have not been previously documented.

While the grading scale is designed to be hierarchical, it remains to be proven that it is. Recently, statistical tests have been developed to measure the degree to which a scale meets certain criteria (Mokken & Lewis, 1982; Molenaar & Sijtsma, 1988). It would be appropriate to subject this scale to such analysis. With further refinement of the scale, it may approach a series of uniform intervals, in which case the nonparametric tests applied to the pilot studies above could be changed to the more familiar Student's t-test.

The numerical grading system described here has the unique feature that it is "modular," in the sense that if the future witnesses the development of a clinical assessment technique that is clearly more reliable and more valid than an existing technique, the new device's measurement may replace the one that currently exists in the grading scale. For example, the cutaneous pressure threshold, which in the past has been estimated by the Semmes-Weinstein nylon monofilaments, should now be replaced by the Pressure-Specified Sensory Device™ (see Chapters 6 and 7). If a vibrometer were used to measure the cutaneous vibratory threshold, and it is not a vibrometer that accounts for the force of application of the applied stimulus, then the new Force-Defined (NK) Vibrometer (see Chapter 7) would be the appropriate substitution to make. If the traditional Jamar dynamometer and Preston pinch meter were used for the strength measurements, then the new NK Digit-Grip™ and NK pinch device (see Chapter 7) would be the appropriate substitution to make.

Finally, the numerical grading system has presented only the median nerve at the wrist, the ulnar nerve at the elbow, and the posterior tibial nerve at the ankle as examples. Clearly, if this concept is accepted, it would be necessary also to apply this scaling technique to each peripheral nerve for which we wish to express a diagnosis, a prognosis, and a treatment result. This will take the cooperation of an international panel of peripheral nerve experts, perhaps under the guidance of the American Society for the Peripheral Nerve.

• • •

● REFERENCES ●

Chang, B., & Dellon, A. L. Surgical management of recurrent carpal tunnel syndrome. *Journal of Hand Surgery 18B:*467-470, 1993.

Curtis, R. M., & Eversmann, W. W., Jr. Internal neurolysis as an adjunct to the treatment of the carpal tunnel syndrome. *Journal of Bone and Joint Surgery 55A*:733-740, 1973.

Dellon, A. L. A numerical grading scale for peripheral nerve function. *Journal of Hand Therapy 4*:152-160, 1993.

Dellon, A. L. *Evaluation of Sensibility and Re-education of Sensation in the Hand*. Baltimore: Williams and Wilkins, 1981.

Dellon, A. L. Operative technique for submuscular transposition of the ulnar nerve. *Contemporary Orthopedics 16*:17-24, 1988.

Dellon, A. L. Pitfalls in electrodiagnosis. In *Operative Nerve Repair and Reconstruction*, R. H. Gelberman, Editor. Philadelphia: J. B. Lipincott Company, 1991.

Dellon, A. L. Recurrent ulnar nerve compression at the elbow treated by the musculofascial lengthening technique. Presented at the American Society of Surgery of the Hand meeting, Phoenix, AZ, 1992. *Journal of Hand Surgery*, submitted: 1997.

Dellon A. L., Hament, W., & Gittelshon, A. Nonoperative management of cubital tunnel syndrome: Results of an eight-year prospective study. *Neurology 43*:1673-1677, 1993.

Dellon, A. L., & Scalley, A. L. *Rank/ordering of the Elements of a Numerical Grading Scale for Peripheral Nerve Function: The Response of a Panel of Experts*. Presented to the American Society for the Peripheral Nerve, 1993 meeting.

Eisen, A., & Danen, J. The mild cubital tunnel syndrome. *Neurology 24*:608-613, 1974.

Fess, E. E. Essential elements of an upper extremity assessment battery. In *Rehabilitation of the Hand*, J. M. Hunter, L. H. Schneider, E. J. Mackin, & A. D. Callahan, Editors. St.Louis: C. V. Mosby, 1984.

Kendall, H. O., & Kendall, F. P. *Muscles: Testing and Function*. Baltimore: Williams & Wilkins, 1949.

McGowan, A. J. Results of transposition of the ulnar nerve for traumatic ulnar neuritis. *Journal of Bone and Joint Surgery 32B*:293-301, 1950.

Moberg, E. Criticism in study of methods for examining sensibility in the hand. *Neurology 12*:8-19, 1962.

Mokken, R. J., & Lewis, C. A. Nonparametric approach to the analysis of dichotomous item responses. *Applied Psychology Measures 6*:417-430, 1982.

Molenaar, I. W., & Sijtsma, K. Mokkern's approach to reliability estimation extended to multicategory items. *Quantitative Methods 9:*115-126, 1988.

Seddon, H. J. *Surgical Disorders of the Peripheral Nerves*. Baltimore: Williams & Wilkins, 1972.

Zachary, R. B. Results of nerve suture. In *Peripheral Nerve Injuries*, H. J. Seddon, Editor. London: Her Majesty's Stationery Office, 1954.

● ADDITIONAL READINGS ●

Bechtol, C. D. Grip test: Use of a dynamometer with adjustable handle spacing. *Journal of Bone and Joint Surgery 36A*:820-823, 1954.

Dellon, A. L. The vibrometer. *Plastic and Reconstructive Surgery 71*:427-431, 1983.

Dellon, A. L., Mackinnon, S. E., & Brandt, K. E. The markings of the Semmes-Weinstein nylon monofilaments. *Journal of Hand Surgery 18A*:756-757, 1993.

Kirkpatrick, J. Evaluation of grip loss: A factor of permanent partial disability in California. *Industrial Medicine and Surgery 26*:285-289, 1957.

Mackinnon, S. E., & Dellon, A. L. Experimental study of chronic nerve compression: Clinical implications. *Clinics of Hand Surgery 2*:639-650, 1986.

Mackinnon, S. E., Dellon, A. L., Hudson, A. R., & Hunter, D. A. A primate model for chronic nerve compression. *Journal of Reconstructive Microsurgery 1*:185-194, 1985.

Mackinnon, S. E., Dellon, A. L., Hudson, A. R., & Hunter, D. A. Chronic nerve compression — An experimental model in the rat. *Annals of Plastic Surgery 13*:112-120, 1984.

Tassler, P. L., & Dellon, A.L. A draught of historical significance. *Plastic and Reconstructive Surgery 91*:400-401, 1994.

• • •

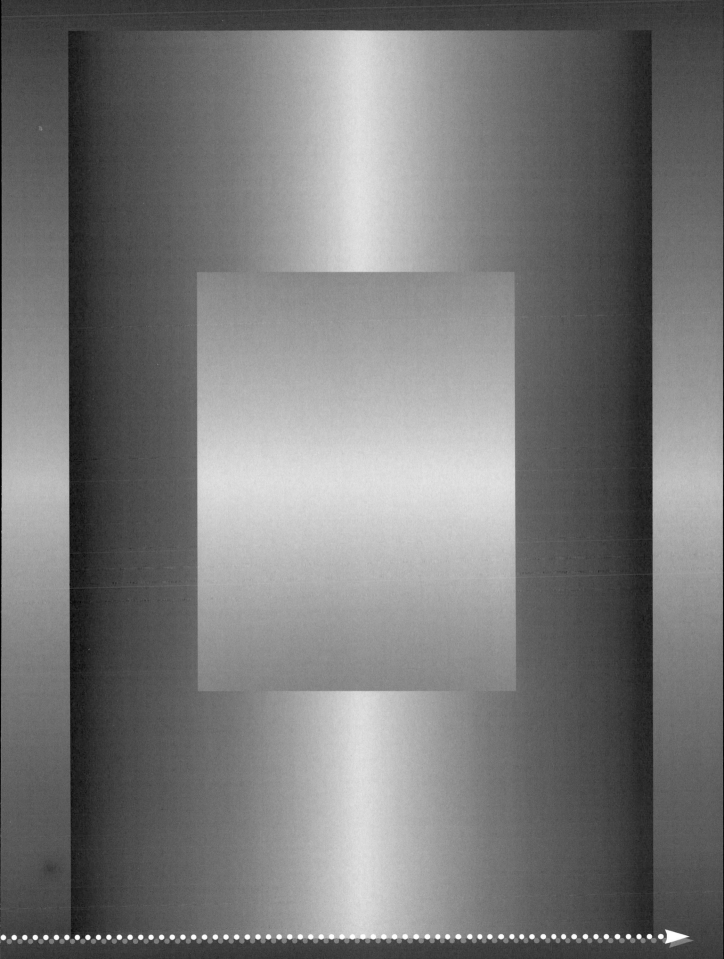

cortical plasticity

I t has always been clear that the results of sensory rehabilitation must be due to higher central nervous system
(CNS) functions. The end-result assessment of a peripheral nerve repair in the hand or wrist area traditionally
has been reported at 5 years after surgery because sensory
function has been noted to improve for that long a period of
time. And yet, we teach that the rate of axonal elongation
and, therefore, the rate at which a peripheral nerve will regenerate, is 1 mm per day, or 1 inch per month. A nerve repaired at the wrist level should have regenerated to the fingertip by 6 or 8 months after the nerve repair.

What is the explanation for the paradox, then, that when
a median nerve is repaired at the wrist level it will regenerate into the index finger pulp somewhere between 6 and 8
months later, yet the results of that nerve's function, as measured by two-point discrimination, has been observed to improve for up to 5 years after the repair? Regeneration of the
peripheral nerve cannot be the explanation for this observation of prolonged and continued improvement in function.

As another example, peripheral nerve regeneration cannot be the explanation for the observation that a patient,
several years after a peripheral nerve repair, who still lacks
the ability to discriminate objects well can, within 15 minutes of instruction in sensory reeducation, correctly identify
a nickel from a quarter when they are each placed separately
into the hand. It was these observations that initially led me,

in 1969, to begin my work on sensory reeducation (Dellon, Curtis, & Edgerton, 1974; Dellon, 1981).

Although I did not know the mechanism by which sensory reeducation worked, I knew that it did work. Over the last decade, through some ingenious research, it has become clear that changes in the CNS occur in response to peripheral nerve injury, and then will occur again in proportion to neural impulses generated by hand use. The ability of the CNS to change is called *cortical plasticity*. Cortical plasticity is the basis for sensory reeducation. This pioneering and insightful work has been done under the leadership of Michael M. Merzenich, PhD, whose doctoral studies were done with Vernon Mountcastle, MD, PhD in the Physiology Department at the Johns Hopkins University School of Medicine. Merzenich is now a professor of neuroscience and director of the Keck Center and Coleman Laboratory at the University of California, San Francisco. The work from his lab has been reviewed at intervals by Kaas (1991) and by Merzenich and Jenkins (1993).

It is the purpose of this chapter (a) briefly to explore the idea that recovery of function in the nervous system is related to development of the organism, rather than being purely a mechanism of wound healing in neural tissue (Dellon, 1990), and (b) to bring together the many experiments that have led to the current concept of cortical plasticity.

These experiments have been done in several different models, each of which has a different topographic arrangement of the brain's surface; therefore, the actual data of each experiment is difficult to compare visually. Furthermore, since the hand has its cortical representation in the contralateral side of the brain, the traditional diagrams of the results of these experiments show a hand with a reversed image of the sensory pattern than that observed on the surface of the brain, again making it difficult to conceptualize the results of the experiments. Complicating the interpretation of this research even further for the student is the presentation of the data as various points or minute diagrams on the surface of the brain, requiring the reader to do a great deal of studying of each previously published figure.

This chapter will strive, through a series of integrated illustrations, to interpret and summarize the research on cortical plasticity, presenting it in a colorful, unified manner that removes the mystery from this critical concept. It is hoped that this presentation will permit the transfer of research into rehabilitation of the patient with a sensory deficit.

• • •

*T*he earlier in life a brain lesion is sustained, the better is the overall chance of recovery.

Kennard
1936

• • •

NEURAL REGENERATION:
• **MECHANISMS OF RECOVERY OR** •
OF DEVELOPMENT?

It is natural for us to assume that the response of the nervous system to an injury is a response that exists for the system to heal itself. An alternative explanation is that the response is a *reactivation* of a sequence of events that occurred normally as part of growth and development. It is reasonable at the start of this chapter, therefore, to examine this concept, because understanding the basis for the response to injury may give insight into the most appropriate mechanisms for rehabilitation. A dramatic example is the response of an animal to removal of a large portion of its brain, such as a cortical hemisphere. A series of experiments has demonstrated that when a hemispherectomy is done in kittens, there is a much better functional outcome than when the brain resection is done on adult cats (Olmstead & Villablanca, 1980; Olmstead, Villablanca, Sonnier, McAllister, & Gomez, 1983).

In contrast to the conclusion that kittens have a better ability to reorganize their cortex following injury than do cats, the researchers suggest another explanation: It is that pathways that they have demonstrated crossing from the intact to the injured side of the brain may be there normally, and that in the process of development these are withdrawn or retracted as a response to environmental stimuli. The injured adult cat would not have these pathways, whereas the injury in the kittens would sustain preexisting crossing pathways, thereby allowing bilateral control by the remaining hemisphere. In either situation, the response to injury required training (rehabilitation) for behavioral change to occur.

Almli's group at the Washington University School of Medicine's Department of Occupational Therapy is interested in the neuropsychological behavior patterns of children and how they are affected by brain damage. Almli (1984) reviewed the research that evaluated the behavioral changes of rats with injury to their brain at the lateral hypothalamus/median forebrain bundle, a level that causes altered function relating to eating patterns and the sensorimotor system. The review demonstrated that when the brain injury occurred in the neonatal (1 to 5 days) or perinatal period (6 to 10 days) the rat demonstrated no residual behavioral changes, whereas if the brain injury occurred to the adult rat there were persistent deficiencies in eating, posture, and gait, and in the sensory systems, including vision, hearing, smell, and touch perception. Almli concluded that the behavior systems evaluated are normal developmental growth processes, and that the capacity for establishment of neuronal circuits following brain damage may very well be related to the developmental status of the neural system at the time brain damage is sustained.

In a subsequent review, Finger and Almli (1985) argued that there is little evidence to support the concept that reorganization of the brain after injury is due to a "healing" process but, rather, is an active neuronal process that recapitulates development. This active process includes (a) *reactive synaptogenesis* (intact axons sprout to occupy the sites vacated by the degenerated neuron), (b) *rerouting of axons* (regenerating axons may occupy different synaptic sites than originally), and (c) *axon retraction* (axons that do not make appropriate target organ connections are withdrawn). At the appropriate time during development, each of these processes would achieve appropriate growth. For example, at an inappropriate time after an injury, the process may cause a maladaption such as spinal reflex spasticity. These concepts are more difficult to comprehend within the CNS, and examples from the peripheral nervous system are helpful.

An example of reactive synaptogenesis is collateral sprouting (see Chapter 4), in which an intact peripheral nerve adjacent to the territory of a resected nerve (resected for the treatment of painful neuroma) sprouts to cause partial recovery of sensation (see Figures 4.12 A & B). An example of rerouting of axons would be the regeneration of a group A-beta fiber that previously innervated a Merkel cell neurite complex, into a Meissner corpuscle, causing the mechanical transduction of a touch stimulus but now with possibly dysesthetic consequences or misinterpretation of the neural input. An example of axon retraction would be the pruning back of most of the axon sprouts from a single nerve fiber once one of the regenerating sprouts has

FIGURE 10.1

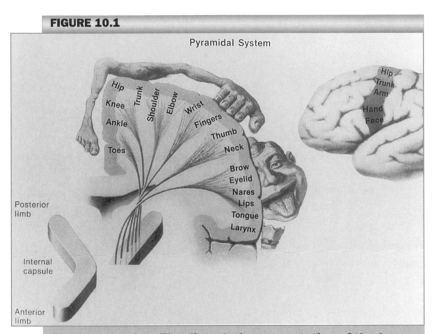

Pyramidal System

The homunculus. The distorted representation of the human form stretched out along the post-central gyrus of the human cortex was described by Penfield in the 1930s and illustrated by Nettor. In this particular view, the post-central gyrus is outlined as a band with the body regions labeled on the parietal lobe, while the homunculus is shown on a coronal section of the brain, demonstrating the continued organization of this topographic representation down through the brain by way of the pyramidal system. From The CIBA Collection of Medical Illustrations, *Volume I, by F. H. Nettor, New Jersey: Donnelly & Sons, 1983. Reprinted with permission of the author.*

made a synaptic contact with a target end-organ. Persistence of these sprouts in and about the site of nerve repair would result in a painful incontinuity neuroma.

A consequence of the hypothesis that reorganization of the brain in response to injury is a setting into motion again of the normal processes of growth and development is that measurement of the normal neonatal growth processes should provide insight for rehabilitation strategies. Almli

and Mohr (1993) have stated this nicely for the motor system, based on observations on cyclic (spontaneously active or autogenic) movement patterns of intrauterine and neonatal human infants (Almli, 1993). Almli hypothesized that autogenic movements contribute to the formation of sensorimotor neural circuits for reflexive and voluntary movements. Then, both autogenic and reflexive movements provide function for the structural development of forebrain-spinal cord/brain stem circuits that mediate voluntary movement control. Thus, movement patterns develop from autogenic to reflexive to voluntary in a developmental cascade of structure-function interactions. For example, ultrasound studies of the fetus demonstrate a certain degree of movement, which is significantly less in premature babies outside the water-supported placental environment. Decrease in movement will decrease directly sensory input to the CNS that is required for normal development. Appropriate rehabilitation for the neonatal nursery might incorporate, therefore, sensory enrichment and environmental modulation of activity.

• CORTICAL CARTOGRAPHY •

Well known is the *homunculus*—the man with the distorted body proportions draped across the surface of the human brain (see Figure 10.1). In the 1930s, Wilder Penfield, MD, a neurosurgeon at Magill University in Montreal, began to study the localization of electrical stimuli given directly to the surface of the brain (1937). A patient who was under general anesthesia for surgery on the brain was awakened once the bone flap was elevated and the cortex exposed. The stimulus was given and the patient was asked in which part of the body the evoked sensation was perceived. In this manner information was obtained that permitted the first surface mappings. These observations demonstrated that the human body's surface was not represented linearly, but rather in proportion to what could be interpreted as the relative importance or function of those body surfaces. Adrian (1941) further studied this region of the postcentral gyrus of the parietal lobe, which has become known as the Primary Somatosensory Cortex, or SI, which corresponded with the histological description of Brodman (1909) as areas 1, 2, and 3 (see Figure 10.2). Work done at Phillip Bard's Department of Physiology at the Johns Hopkins University's School of Medicine identified a second region of the brain that contained a sensory map, this region being called SII (Marshall, Woolsey, & Bard, 1941). Continuing the work on electrical stimulation of the brain through cortical penetrations, Mountcastle's group identified the unique columnar organization of cortical neurons that corresponded with quickly- and slowly-adapting properties at precise sites of the fingertips in the hand region of the homunculus (Mountcastle, 1957; Powell & Mountcastle, 1959). Merzenich's work subsequently identified two different maps of the hand within this area (Merzenich & Harrington, 1969; Merzenich, Kaas, Sur, & Lin, 1978).

Examples of the detailed anatomic localization within the brain for different species that can be related to discrete areas of the body are given in Figure 10.3. For the cat, as an example, five different representations of the sensory surface of the body have now been characterized, with the fifth area being called SV (Mori et al., 1991).

FIGURE 10.2

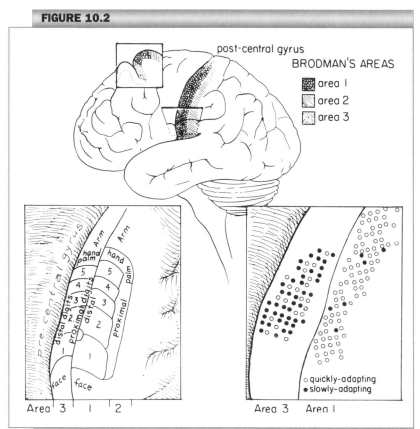

The cortical map of the primate (A) correlating the histologic description of the cellular architecture by Brodman with (C) the electrical-stimulation identification of specific sites of the hand along the post-central sulcus, the primary somatosensory area (SI). In (B), the dual representation of the hand is depicted, with an area composed of both slowly- and quickly-adapting neurons being located within the sulcus (area 3b of Brodman) and an area of primarily quickly-adapting neurons being located on the surface of the sulcus (area 1 of Brodman). From "Representaion of Slowly and Rapidly Adapting Cutaneous Mechanoreceptors of the Hand in the Brodman's Area 3 and 1 of Macaca mulatta," by R. L. Paul, M. Merzenich and H. Goodman 1972, Brain Research 36:229-249.

While the rest of this chapter will focus on understanding the SI area, it is important to know that the future will define the specific interactions of these different areas, and that this may further support our efforts at rehabilitation. For example, at least in the cat, Mori's group has suggested that areas SII, SIII, and SIV contain even smaller receptive fields for the fingertips, and fewer bilateral representations, consistent with increasing use of the forepaw during evolution, and that the newly described area SV, by virtue of receiving inputs from each of these other areas, may be the region of "higher-level sensory integration."

The typical map of the hand on the surface of the brain that will be used in this chapter comes from the observations made on New

FIGURE 10.3

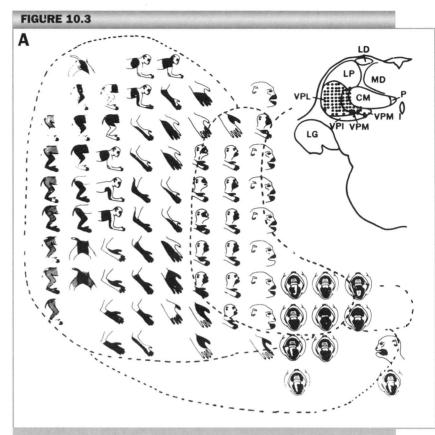

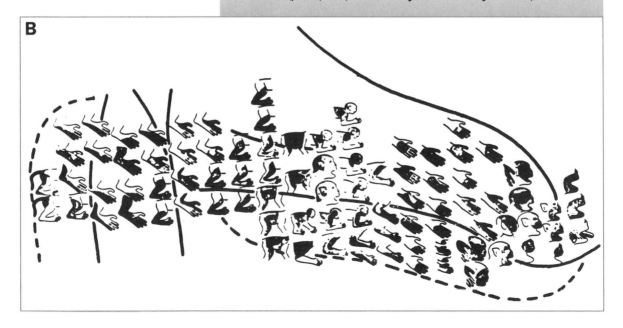

Examples of detailed cortical mapping, relating skin surfaces to brain surfaces in the monkey at the level of the thalamus (A) and cortex (B). From "The Representation of Tactile Sensibility in the Thalamus of the Monkey," by V. B. Mountcastle and E. Henneman, 1952. Journal of Comparative Neurology 97:409-440. Reprinted with permission of Wiley-Liss, Inc., a subsidiary of John Wiley & Sons, Inc.

FIGURE 10.4

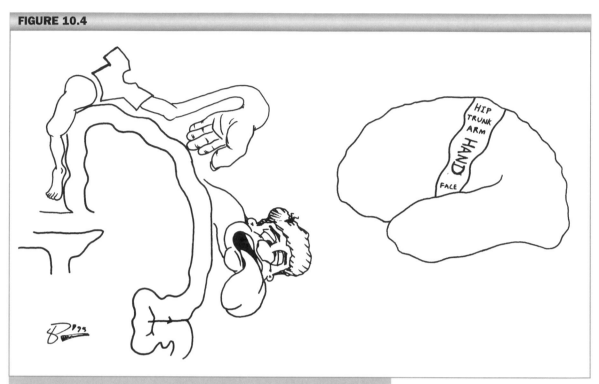

The "new" homunculus has the hand represented in the orientation in which it is now known to exist in the primary somatosensory cortex. This orientation has been demonstrated by direct cortical penetration recordings by microelectrodes of hand surface stimulation. Note that the fingertips point anteriorly, and that the thumb side of the hand is next to the neck region of the head. Drawn by Glenn George Dellon. Reprinted with permission.

World monkeys, the owl monkey, and the squirrel monkey. These species do not have the hand area of the primary somatosensory cortex interrupted by the central sulcus of the parietal lobe of the brain. From a practical point of view, this means that the entire hand region is on the flat surface of the brain, and may be reliably mapped by direct cortical penetrations of microelectrodes. When the surface of the finger is touched with a small nylon filament, an impulse is generated that can be detected by the cortical electrodes. A map will be generated from about 300 such correlations between skin surface stimulations and microelectrode penetrations. The hand region of the 3b cortical area is between 8 mm and 14 mm^2. Within this area, there is a single, simple representation of the hand, such that the fingertips are toward the precentral gyrus, or motor cortex, and the thumb or radial side of the hand is toward the neck portion of the head region of 3b (Merzenich et al., 1978; Merzenich, Nelson, & Kaas, 1987). Figure 10.4 converts the traditional view of the homunculus into this more topographically correct orientation.

The normal map of the sensory input from the hand on the surface of the brain that represents the primary somatosensory cortex (adapted as discussed above from the studies on New World monkeys) is depicted in Figure 10.5. Several conventions with regard to these drawings are created for the ease of teaching the concept of cortical plasticity. The hand will always be shown in the same anatomic orienta-

FIGURE 10.5

The normal map of the hand in 3b, the primary somatosensory cortical region. Throughout the series of cortical maps in this chapter, the following conventions will be followed: The hand is shown in a position similar to the cortical map, disregarding that the left hemisphere is related to the right hand. The thumb is digit 1, and the other fingers are numbered sequentially to digit 5, the little finger. The palmar surface of the hand is a box, with the thenar and hypothenar regions existing below the horizontal line, and distinguished from each other by color. The skin territories innervated by the cutaneous nerves are those usually found in man. The discontinuity between digits is given by a dark line. The number of each digit is presented on its distal end. The median and ulnar nerves are schematically represented at the wrist level, and demonstrate the condition of the nerve with respect to the hand for the cortical map. In this map, these two nerves are represented as being normal, with a normal number of sensory branches. Blue always represents the territory of the median nerve, green the territory of the radial nerve, orange the territory of the ulnar nerve at the wrist level, and purple, the dorsal cutaneous branch of the ulnar nerve. Note that the dorsal skin of each finger is represented by a patch that appears in the discontinuity between the palmar territory of two fingers. From "Reorganization of Cortical Representations of the Hand Following Alterations of Skin Inputs Induced by Nerve Injury, Skin Island Transfers, and Experience," by M. M. Merzenich, & W. M. Jenkins, 1993, Journal of Hand Therapy *6:89-104. Adapted with permission of the authors. Illustration drawn by Glenn George Dellon.*

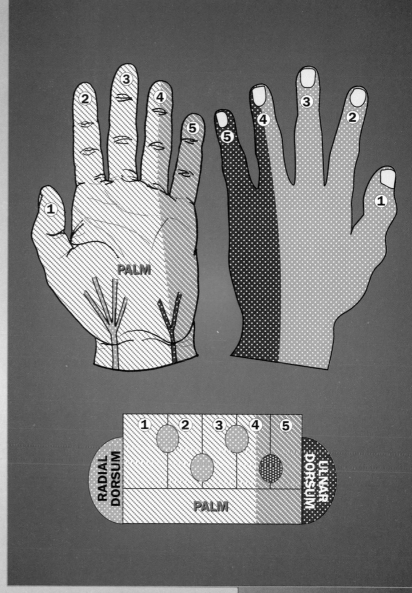

tion as the brain, even through it is the right hand that is represented in the left cortex. The pattern of innervation of the median and ulnar nerve that is most common in humans is the one illustrated, that is, the median nerve innervates the palmar surfaces of the radial digits 1 through 3 and half of the 4th, whereas the ulnar nerve innervates the entire 5th finger and the ulnar half of the 4th digit. Dorsally, the radial nerve innervates the radial three-and-one-half digits, while the ulnar nerve innervates the 5th, and the ulnar half of the 4th digit. (This is not always the situation in other species.)

Also, digits are designated numbers 1 through 5, and these numbers are always at the distal end of the digit. The palmar (volar, nonhairy, glabrous) side of the hand is represented as a box, with the palm separated from the digits by a horizontal line. The palm is split into a thenar and hypothenar region, innervated by the median and the ulnar nerve, respectively. The dorsum of the normal hand is not fully or contiguously represented on the surface of the brain, and is arranged such that the dorsoradial surface is adjacent to palmar digit 1 (the thumb), and the dorsoulnar surface is adjacent to the palmar digit 5 (the little finger). The dorsum of each digit is represented by a patch at the discontinuities that represent the borders between digits. This normal pattern is presented in different colors to facilitate the changes that occur in the cortical pattern when injury or stimulation occurs to the periphery, that is, cortical plasticity.

• REORGANIZING MAPS •

The best approach to learning about cortical plasticity involves doing something to alter the signals from the skin being received by the brain. These signals may be interrupted temporarily or permanently, partially or completely. The skin surface from which the signals are to be altered can be a small region or a large region. This type of research requires that the brain surface be mapped, the alteration to the neural input from the skin surface created and, then, at some time in the future, the brain surface must be mapped again. To illustrate the changes in the brain map, that is, cortical plasticity, after loss of a sensory neural input, which is called *deafferentation*, the clearest picture will result from models of complete loss from well-defined anatomic areas.

Amputation of a digit will create a permanent loss of neural input from a well-defined, relatively small, anatomic region. The cortical reorganization that follows amputation of a middle finger is illustrated in Figure 10.6. Loss of inputs creates an immediate effect on the cortical map, which by about 3 weeks has become reorganized. Cortical surfaces adjacent to the region now deprived of input topographically expand. The effect is that an area on an adjacent finger is now represented by a larger region of the cortex, giving it more effective representation, or what is called *finer spatial grain* (Merzenich et al., 1984). The amputation stump can be the source of a disturbing sensory phenomenon, the phantom limb syndrome.

In Figure 10.6, the skin of the stump and the skin to the radial side of digit 4 are still innervated by the median nerve fibers that had a relationship to the amputated digit, and stimulation of these skin surfaces may still evoke sensations localized to digit 3. The cortical map reorganization has the effect of "telescoping" down all the missing skin surface into a now smaller region. Touching the stump may, therefore, give a "ghost" sensation that the missing part of the extremity is still there. Two clinical observations that may be related to this are that (a) a heavy schedule of stimulation to a region of skin renders it insensate (Craig, 1993), possibly because some cortical processing mechanism chooses to ignore these "meaningless" signals, resulting in the temporary "amputation" of that region, and (b) phantom limb sensations referred to an amputated arm have been reported by stimulation of the face (Ramachandran, Rogers-Ramachandran, & Stewart, 1992), possibly because, in reference to Figure 10.4, the neck/face area would expand during cortical reorganization after amputation of the hand/arm.

A permanent loss of neural input from a well-defined, relatively large, anatomic region can be created by removing a section of the median nerve at the wrist level. The cortical reorganization that follows this type of deafferentation, *nerve division*, is illustrated in Figure 10.7. Almost immediately after the nerve resection, the cortical map begins to reorganize, and by 1 week the map has stabilized. Whereas the hairy region of the hand innervated by the radial nerve is normally represented sparsely (see Figure 10.5), it now is completely represented. Similarly, the nonhairy territory normally represented completely is now expanded two to three times its usual representational area (Merzenich et al., 1983). Note that the hand area previously innervated by the median nerve still remains, (it has not been amputated), but this skin has no cortical representation. When this skin is touched, there is no cortical recording. If, in

time, (weeks to months), sprouts from the radial or ulnar nerve were to regenerate into the skin of the hand that was previously innervated by the median nerve, then touching these newly reinnervated areas of skin would produce a cortical response, that is, sensation. This would be the phenomenon of *collateral sprouting* (see Chapter 4). Collateral sprouting has not been studied experimentally by cortical mapping.

Nerve crush is a model that permits evaluation of the effect of essentially complete neural regeneration on cortical reorganization. Crushing the median nerve, for example, will completely stop neural input from the skin territory innervated by the median nerve, but will not interrupt the fascicular arrangement, nor will it create scarring within the fascicles themselves. Therefore, neural regeneration will occur and should produce an essentially normal pattern or reinnervation. This is illustrated in Figure 10.8 (Wall, Fellerman, & Kaas, 1983).

Nerve repair is a model that permits evaluation of the effect of incomplete, and usually poor, neural regeneration on cortical reorganization. Completely transecting the median nerve at the wrist level and then repairing the nerve by suturing the two ends together will completely stop neural input from the median nerve,

completely disrupt the fascicular arrangement, and create some degree of intraneural scarring. The neural regeneration results theoretically in abnormal reinnervation because (a) there is misdirection of nerve fibers into distal sensory targets that are different in location, that is, a nerve fiber that previously innervated the thumb now reinnervates the index finger; (b) there is misdirection of nerve fibers into sensory end-organ that are different, that is, a nerve fiber that previously innervated a Meissner corpuscle now reinnervates a Merkel cell neurite complex; and (c) there is a loss of nerve fibers due to failure of some percentage of the axons ever reinnervating into the hand, that is, axons become trapped in scar at the nerve repair site.

Figure 10.9 illustrates this type of neural regeneration at 6 months after nerve repair. The hand is represented with white still throughout the area of the median nerve, indicating the persisting loss of nerve fibers. Therefore, there will be areas that are touched and yet no cortical response occurs. Because nerve fibers will regenerate into different skin territories than before, a single cortical surface area may now represent more than one skin surface area. Because nerve fibers will regenerate into different sensory end-organs, a cortical sur-

FIGURE 10.6

Cortical map after permanent deafferentation due to amputation of a finger. The hand is represented with a missing middle finger, which is completely within the territory of the median nerve. The response of the cortex to loss of neural input from digit 3 is to have the region that previously received input from digit 3 now receive input from digits 2 and 4, the immediately adjacent surface areas. Therefore, the cortical surface receiving input from digits 2 and 4 is expanded with reference to the normal map given in Figure 10.5. Note the median and ulnar nerves are normal. From "Reorganization of Cortical Representations of the Hand Following Alterations of Skin Inputs Induced by Nerve Injury, Skin Island Transfers, and Experience," by M. M. Merzenich, & W. M. Jenkins, 1993, Journal of Hand Therapy 6:89-104. Adapted with permission of the authors. Illustration drawn by Glenn George Dellon.

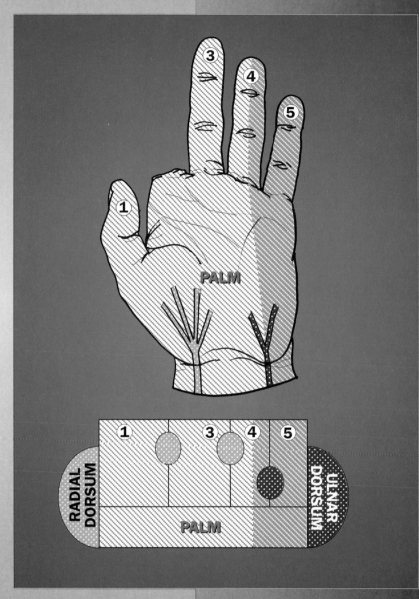

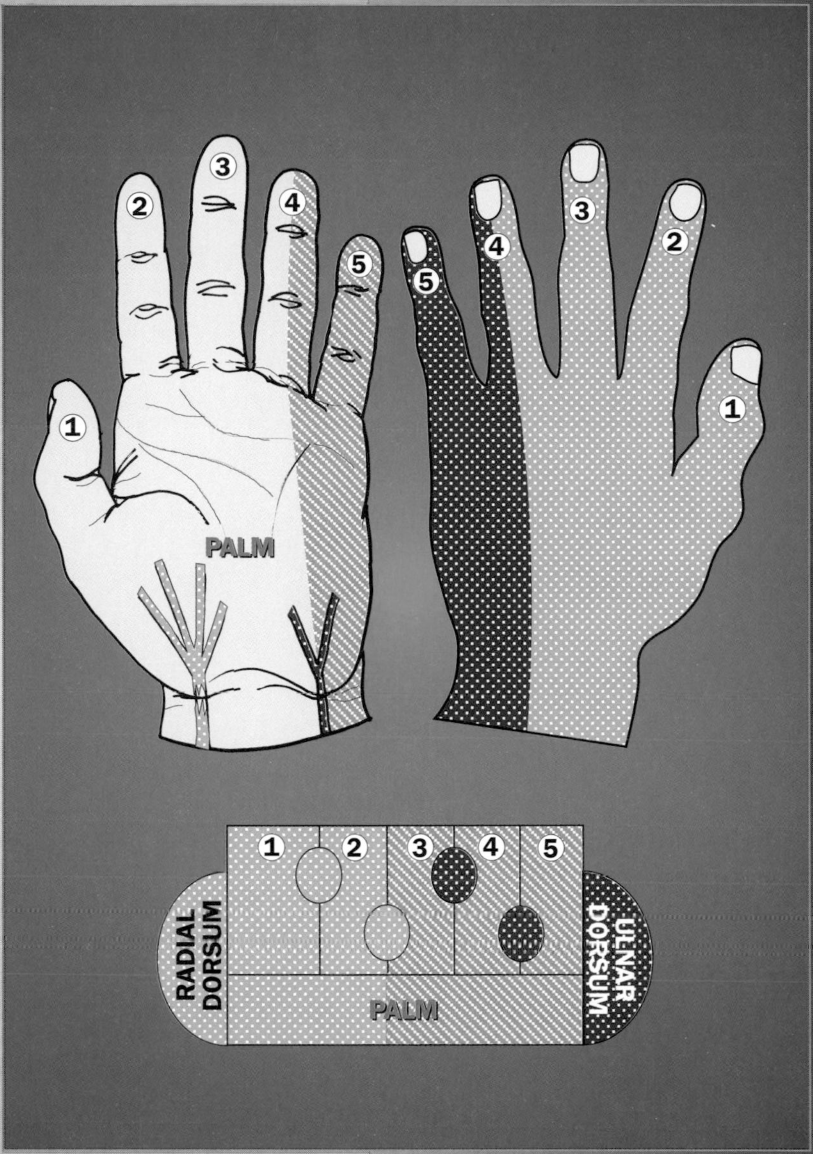

FIGURE 10.7

Cortical map after permanent deafferentation due to loss of median nerve. The hand is represented with a segment of the median nerve permanently removed at the wrist level. The hand is without color and is, therefore, white in the region previously innervated by the median nerve. The response of the cortex to loss of neural input from the median nerve is to have the region of the cortex that previously received input from the median nerve now receive inputs from the radial and ulnar nerves, the immediately adjacent surface areas. Therefore, the cortical area of the radial nerve is expanded onto the surface of cortex usually reserved for palmar neural inputs, the areas previously devoted to digits 1 and 2, while the ulnar nerve is expanded onto the surface of cortex usually reserved for digit 3 and the radial half of digit 4. From "Reorganization of Cortical Representations of the Hand Following Alterations of Skin Inputs Induced by Nerve Injury, Skin Island Transfers, and Experience," by M. M. Merzenich, & W. M. Jenkins, 1993, Journal of Hand Therapy 6:89-104. Adapted with permission of the authors. Illustration drawn by Glenn George Dellon.

FIGURE 10.8

Cortical map after temporary deafferentation, followed by excellent neural regeneration. This model may be created by a median nerve crush. The hand is represented with a segment of median nerve at the wrist level crushed, but left in continuity. This strategy causes a complete loss of neural input followed, within 3 weeks, by neural regeneration. The neural regeneration results, theoretically, in completely normal reinnervation because there is little intra-fascicular scarring to block neural regeneration, and because the perineurium remains intact permitting axons to re-generate into the exact same skin surfaces. While the cortical map should change in the immediate postcrush time period to have the same appearance as Figure 10.7, by 3 weeks after the crush, the cortex has the appearance of an essentially normal map, as in Figure 10.5. From "Reorganization of Cortical Representations of the Hand Following Alterations of Skin Inputs Induced by Nerve Injury, Skin Island Transfers, and Experience," by M. M. Merzenich, & W. M. Jenkins, 1993, Journal of Hand Therapy 6:89-104. Adapted with permission of the authors. Illustration drawn by Glenn George Dellon.

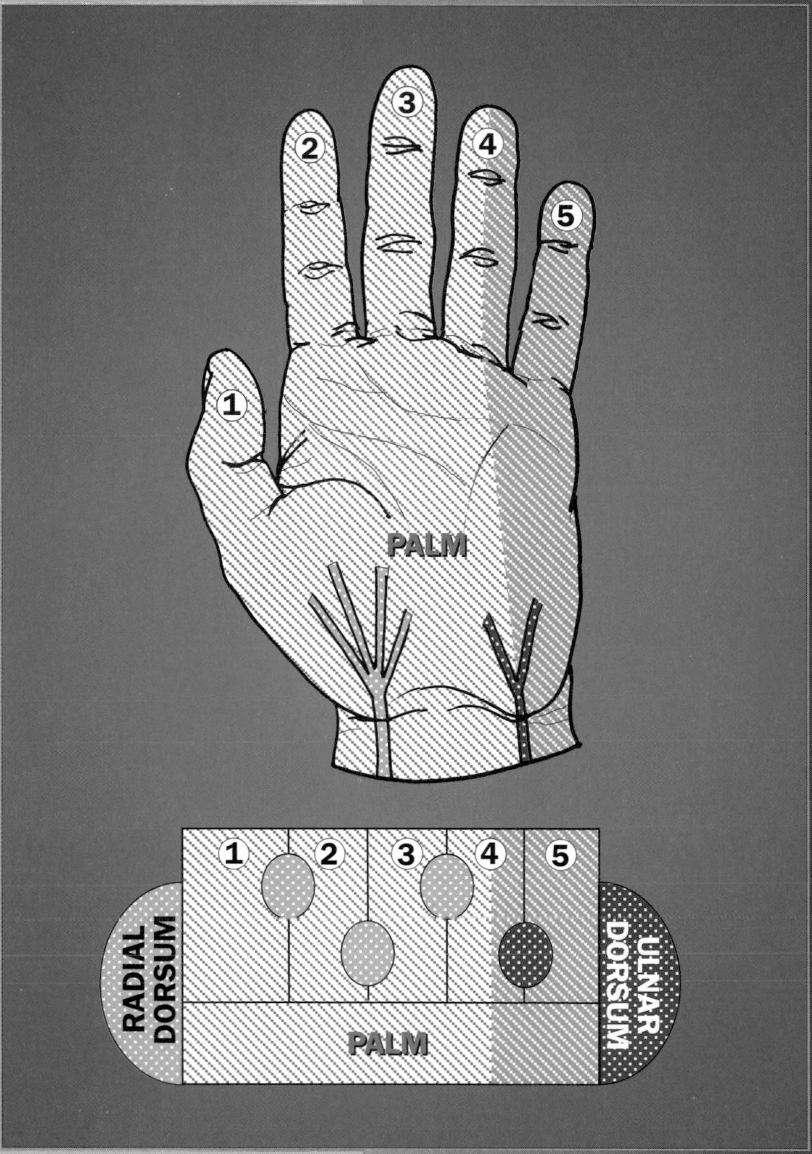

FIGURE 10.9

Cortical map after temporary deafferentation, followed by poor neural regeneration. This model may be created by a median nerve division and repair. The hand is represented with a complete transection of the median nerve at the wrist level, which has been repaired immediately. This strategy causes a complete loss of neural input followed, over the next 6 months, by neural regeneration. The neural regeneration results, theoretically, in abnormal reinnervation because (a) there is misdirection of nerve fibers into distal sensory targets that are different in location; that is, a nerve fiber that previously innervated the thumb now reinnervates the index finger, and (b) there is misdirection of nerve fibers into the sensory end-organ that are different; that is, a nerve fiber that previously innervated a Meissner corpuscle now reinnervates a Merkel cell neurite complex, and (c) there is a loss of nerve fibers due to failure of some

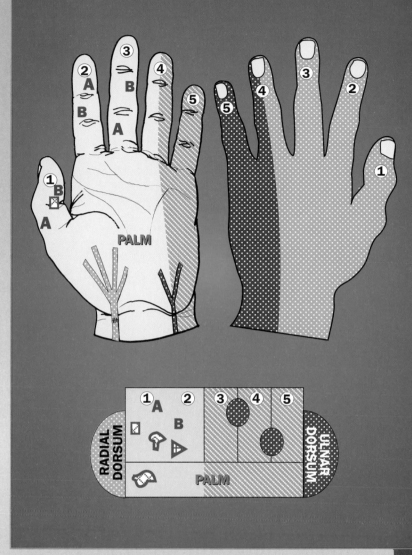

percentage of the axons ever reinnervating into the hand; that is, axons become trapped in scar at the nerve repair site. At 6 months after the nerve repair, the hand is represented with white still throughout the area of the median nerve, indicating the persisting loss of nerve fibers. There are areas of each finger that have been reinnervated, and these are represented by the letters A and B located on digits 1, 2, and 3, and by the small square on digit 1.

While the cortical map should change in the immediate postcrush time period to have the same appearance as Figure 10.7, by 6 months after the median nerve repair the cortex reflects partial reinnervation. Thus, the ulnar nerve territory is still increased compared to normal (see Figure 10.5) in that digit 3 remains in the ulnar nerve region, whereas the radial nerve territory is back to normal. Misdirection of regenerated nerve fibers is represented by (a) the letters A and B, which suggest that a single cortical region is receiving neural input now from more than one skin surface, and by (b) the several different geometric shapes in the cortical region of former digits 1 and 2 and the thenar eminence, which suggest that more than one cortical region may be receiving input from more than one skin surface. These last representations of misdirection also signify the confusion that results from a quickly-adapting fiber reinnervating a slowly-adapting receptor. From "Reorganization of Cortical Representations of the Hand Following Alterations of Skin Inputs Induced by Nerve Injury, Skin Island Transfers, and Experience," by M. M. Merzenich, & W. M. Jenkins, 1993, Journal of Hand Therapy 6:89-104. Adapted with permission of the authors. Illustration drawn by Glenn George Dellon.

face that once represented a single quickly-adapting fiber/receptor in the fingertip may now represent more than one receptor, with these receptor characteristics being different from the original ones. All of this leads to significant problems in terms of interpreting the profile of impulses generated when the hand is stimulated after a nerve repair, and is the context within which sensory reeducation developed (see Chapter 11.) I had initially attempted to portray this type of confusion that must accompany neural regeneration after any nerve repair by the photographic manipulation of Figure 10.10. This type of interpretation problem can be corrected by sensory reeducation, which I initially attempted to portray as a type of "renaming," or learning to interpret the altered profile of sensory impulses generated by stimulation of the fingertips after nerve repair (see Figure 10.10).

Behavioral training results in reorganization of cortical maps. This is perhaps a better phrase in the following circumstances than sensory reeducation because sensory reeducation suggests that some nerve injury has occurred, and that retraining the regenerated nerve is required. In contrast, if there has been no nerve injury, it is possible that intensive sensory training could result in an alteration of sensory function. This was demonstrated by Brown, Mackinnon, Dellon, and Bain (1989), who used sensory reeducation techniques to train areas of normal skin that might be used in innervated free-tissue transfers, such as the web space between the first and second toes. They found that normal subjects could improve their ability to discriminate one from two points after 3 weeks of training.

Recanzone, Merzenich, Jenkins, Grajski, and Dinse (1992) used various sensory stimulation strategies with monkeys that had normal hands. The results of two of these studies are illustrated in Figure 10.11. Their previous studies had demonstrated that to cause cortical reorganization the sensory stimuli had to (a) have attention directed to the stimulus, and (b) be meaningful, that is, provide a positive food reinforcement. Given these two prerequisites, stimuli that varied in temporal-spatial delivery could be used and the cortex mapped. In one experiment a stimulus was applied repetitively to a single site on the skin surface by applying a vibrating probe, while in the other a moving stimulus was applied to a limited skin region.

Both sets of stimuli caused a topographic expansion of the stimulated skin surface on the cortex. The stimulus that moved back and forth over the limited skin region created an expansion centered about the stimulation site, whereas the stimulus that was provided by the vibrating probe created other sites on the brain surface that also responded to the skin surface stimulation. My interpretation of the latter result is that the vibrating stimulus results in a wave that travels through the digit and, therefore, provides a less localized stimulus. The inference for rehabilitation strategies of these test results is provided in Chapter 11.

Neurotization implies that neural inputs are being provided to an area from a novel source. It is a term perhaps best applied to the motor system in which a denervated muscle, whose usual motor nerve has been injured beyond reconstruction, is reinnervated by a completely different nerve (Brunelli, 1987; Meals, Rob, & Nelissen, 1995). For example, if the lateral cord of the brachial plexus is destroyed and the musculocutaneous nerve has been avulsed from the biceps muscle, a new source of motor nerves to cause elbow flexion could be obtained by implanting the thoracodorsal nerve (the motor nerve to the latissimus dorsi muscle, originating from the posterior cord) directly into the biceps muscle, or neurotizing the biceps with the thoracodorsal nerve. Reorganization of the cortical map in response to sensory neuroti-

FIGURE 10.10

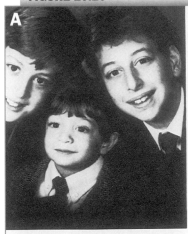
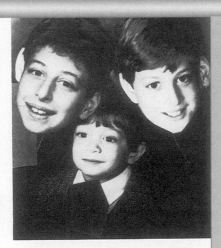
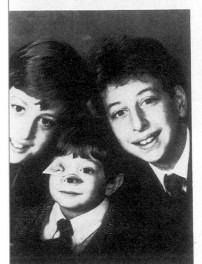
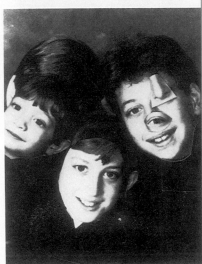

Neural regeneration after nerve repair is necessarily incomplete, generating an abnormal profile of sensory impulses after stimulation of the fingertip skin. (A) The normal perception of these faces, as in the upper left quadrant, can be altered into any one of those in the other three quadrants due to regeneration of fibers into the wrong skin territory or into the wrong sensory receptor. In (B), the normal receipt of sensory impulses has created a pattern that is named, and thereafter identified as, "Ernie." After nerve repair, in (C) the pattern of stimulated impulses is never normal, and may lead to the pattern not "matching" with a pattern in the "association cortex," thereby preventing useful or functional sensation despite neural regeneration. Sensory reeducation (D) provides the ability to "rename" this altered profile of impulses

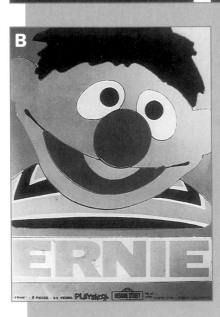
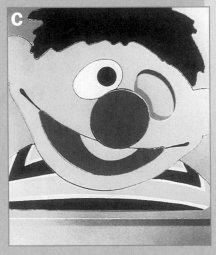
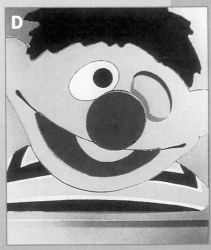

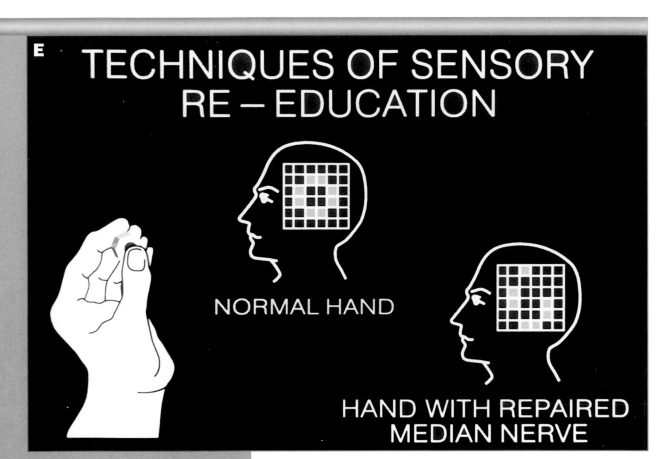

TECHNIQUES OF SENSORY RE – EDUCATION

E

NORMAL HAND

HAND WITH REPAIRED MEDIAN NERVE

providing, perhaps, an old name to a new pattern. (E) Two decades ago, the "mechanism" of sensory reeducation was illustrated by Pegge Carter, COTR, of Phoenix, Arizona, in a way that suggested cortical map reorganization. (A) From **Evaluation of Sensibility and Re-Education of Sensation in the Hand,** *by A. L. Dellon, 1981, Baltimore: Williams & Wilkins. (B), (C), (D), (E) Courtesy of A. L. Dellon, MD. Reprinted with permission of the author.*

zation was investigated through the model of relocating an innervated island skin from one finger to another, and through creating syndactyly by suturing one finger to an adjacent finger. There was always a reorganization of the cortical map in response to these manipulations of innervated skin (Clark, Allard, Jenkins, & Merzenich, 1988; Allard, Clark, Jenkins, & Merzenich, 1991; Merzenich & Jenkins, 1993).

In hand surgery, the usual situation is a correction rather than a creation of syndactyly; however, the reconstruction of a finger with a neurovascular island flap or with a nerve transfer is now in practice. A problem that remains when the nerve's origin is maintained is that, for example, if the ring finger innervation has been transferred to the thumb, when the thumb is stimulated the patient perceives it still as stimulation of the ring finger.

In Figure 10.12, an experiment is illustrated in which an ulnar innervated island of skin is transferred from the ulnar side of the ring finger and translocated into the ulnar side of the thumb, a skin territory innervated normally by the median nerve. At 3 months after the surgery, the cortical map demonstrates that stimulation of the still ulnarly-innervated island flap in the thumb gives cortical responses that are all received on the thumb cortical map. In contrast to the clinical situation, this thumb in the experiment still maintained some of its normal innervation, and perhaps this is the basis for the correct localization of the stimulus to the translocated island. In the clinical situation, the thumb reconstructed with the island flap would usually have no remaining sensibility. These observations will have direct clinical implications in terms of rehabilitation strategies.

A recent study by Rosen, Lundborg, Dohlin, Holmberg, and Karlson (1994) suggests that the capacity for sensory reeducation may be related to measurable cognitive factors. They evaluated 19 patients who were between 2 and 5 years after a peripheral nerve repair at the wrist level. They found that the patients' scores on tests of verbal learning and on visual-spatial logic were the tests of CNS function that best correlated with recovered hand function.

The results of the study imply that while cortical reorganization may be a specific biologic function of the CNS, in primates, at least, there may exist different capacities of this system in individual members of the species.

• • •

FIGURE 10.11A

Cortical map after "sensory reeducation" may be illustrated based on experiments in which a hand without a nerve injury is stimulated in a novel manner. The experiment first begins with the monkey learning to discriminate between different tactile stimuli and, perhaps, having this behavior reinforced positively with a food treat; that is, the sensory stimulus must be attended to and be meaningful. (A) A moving stimulus is applied just to the tip of the middle finger. This stimulus creates an intense pattern of neural impulses in a constant skin location that is reflected by cortical reorganization such that a larger surface of cortex becomes related to this small skin surface. Thus, behavioral training results in representing the skin surface in a finer spatial grain, that is, is better represented. Illustration drawn by Glenn George Dellon.

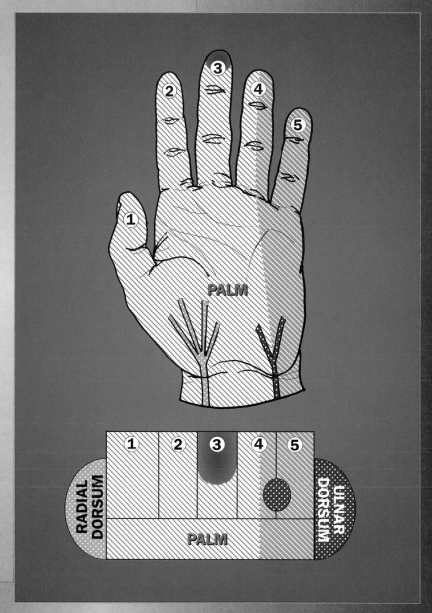

10.11 B

(B) A different behavioral training strategy is represented by stimulating with a vibrating probe at just a single "spot" of skin. While this may be thought of as a "static" stimulus, it is an oscillating stimulus at a single "spot" rather than a constant-touch stimulus at a single "spot." The cortical reorganization that results from this stimulation does increase the cortical surface related to this skin spot, but also produces a representation of this skin spot in other cortical surfaces along the same digit, perhaps reflecting the traveling wave phenomenon of the vibration. From "Reorganization of Cortical Representations of the Hand Following Alterations of Skin Inputs Induced by Nerve Injury, Skin Island Transfers, and Experience," by M. M. Merzenich, & W. M. Jenkins, 1993, Journal of Hand Therapy 6:89-104. *Adapted with permission of the authors. Illustration drawn by Glenn George Dellon.*

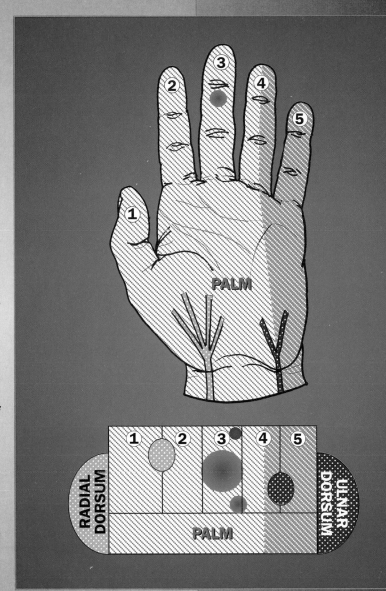

FIGURE 10.12

Cortical map after sensory neurotization. An island of skin innervated by the ul- nar nerve to the ring finger is translocated as a neuro- vascular island flap to the median-innervated thumb. At 3 months after the trans- fer, the cortical map demon- strates that stimulation of the thumb over the island flap results in cortical neu- ron discharges in the digit 1 region of the cortical map but not in the digit 4 region. The presence of me- dian nerve-innervated tis- sue adjacent to the transfer has permitted the cortical reorganization to reflect the new location of the flap. This does not occur if the ulnarly-innervated is- land flap is translocated into a still-ulnar-innervated region of the hand. From "Reorganization of Cortical Representations of the Hand Following Alterations of Skin Inputs Induced by Nerve In- jury, Skin Island Transfers, and Experience," by M. M. Merzenich, & W. M. Jenk- ins, 1993, Journal of Hand Therapy *6:89-104. Adapted with permission of the authors. Il- lustration drawn by Glenn George Dellon.*

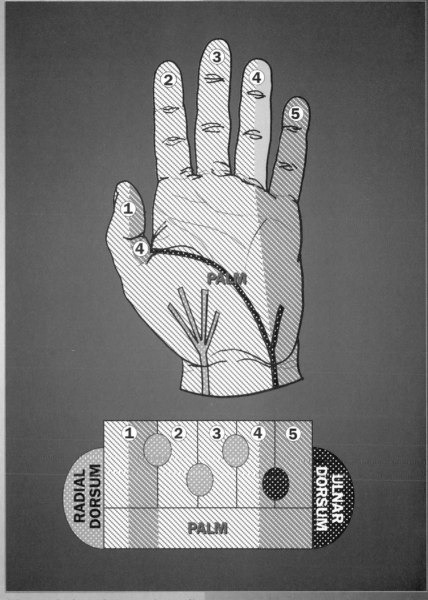

• REFERENCES •

Adrian, E. D. Afferent discharges to the cerebral cortex from peripheral sense organs. *Journal of Physiology 100*:159-191, 1941.

Allard, T. A., Clark, S. A., Jenkins, W. M., & Merzenich, M. M. Reorganization of somatosensory area 3b representations in adult owl monkeys after digital syndactyly. *Journal of Neurophysiology 66*:1048-1058, 1991.

Almli, C. R. Early brain damage and time course of behavioral dysfunction: Parallels with neural maturation. In *Early Brain Damage: Volume 2, Neurobiology and Behavior,* S. Finger & C. R. Almli, Editors. New York: Academic Press, Inc. 1984.

Almli, C. R. Influence of perinatal risk factors (preterm birth, low birth weight, and oxygen deficiency) on movement patterns: An animal model and premature human infants. In *At-risk Infants: Interventions, Families and Research,* N J. Anastasiow & S. Harel, Editors. Baltimore: Paul H. Brookes Publishing Company, 1993.

Almli, C. R., & Mohr, N. M. Born too soon: Intervention theory and research with premature infants in the NICU. In *Foundations for Practice in the Neonatal Intensive Care Unit and Early Intervention: A Self-Guided Practice Manual,* E. Vergara, Editor. Rockville: American Occupational Therapy Association, Inc., 1993.

Brodman, K. *Vergleichende Lokalisationlehre der Grosshimrinde in ihren Prinzipien dargestellt auf Grund des Zellenbaues.* Liepzig: J. A. Barth, 1909.

Brown, C. J., Mackinnon, S. E., Dellon, A. L., & Bain, J.R. The sensory potential of free flap donor sites. *Annals of Plastic Surgery 23*:135-140, 1989.

Brunelli, G. Neurotization of avulsed roots of the brachial plexus by means of anterior nerves of the cervical plexus. In *Microreconstruction of Nerve Injuries.* Philadelphia: W. B. Saunders Company, 1987.

Clark, S. A., Allard, T., Jenkins, W. M., & Merzenich, M. M. Syndactyly results in the emergence of double digit receptive fields in somatosensory cortex in adult owl monkeys. *Nature 332*:444-445, 1988.

Craig, J. Anomalous responses following prolonged tactile simulation. *Neuropsychology 31*:277-291, 1993.

Dellon, A. L. *Evaluation of Sensibility and Re-Education of Sensation in the Hand.* Baltimore: Williams & Wilkins, 1981.

Dellon, A. L. Wound healing in nerve. *Clinics in Plastic Surgery 17*:545-570, 1990.

Dellon, A. L., Curtis, R. M., & Edgerton, M. T. Re-education of sensation in the hand following nerve injury. *Plastic and Reconstructive Surgery 53*:297-305, 1974.

Finger, S., & Almli, C. R. Brain damage and neuroplasticity: Mechanisms of recovery or development? *Brain Research Review 10*:177-186, 1985.

Kaas, J. H. Plasticity of sensory and motor maps in adult mammals. *Annual Review of Neuroscience 14*:137-161, 1991.

Marshall, W. H., Woolsey, C. N., & Bard, P. Observations on cortical somatic sensory mechanisms of cat and monkey. *Journal of Neurophysiology 4*:1-24, 1941.

Meals, R. A., Rob, C. A., & Nelissen, G. H. H. The origin and meaning of "neurotization." *Journal of Hand Surgery 20A*:144-146, 1995.

Merzenich, M. M., & Harrington, T. The sense of flutter-vibration evoked by stimulation of the hairy skin of primates: Comparison of human sensory capacity with the responses of mechanoreceptive afferents innervating the hairy skin of monkeys. *Experimental Brain Research 9*:236-260, 1969.

Merzenich, M. M., & Jenkins, W. M. Reorganization of cortical representations of the hand following alterations of skin inputs induced by nerve injury, skin island transfers, and experience. *Journal of Hand Therapy 6*:89-104, 1993.

Merzenich, M. M., Kaas, J. H., Sur, M., & Lin, C. S. Double representation of the body surface within cytoarchitectonic areas 3b and 1 in "S1" in the owl monkey

(*Aortus trivirgatus*). *Journal of Comparative Neurology 181*:41-74, 1978.

Merzenich, M. M., Kaas, J. H., Wall, J. T., Sur, M., Nelson, R. J., & Fellerman, D. J. Progression of change following median nerve section in the cortical representation of the hand in areas 3b and 1 in adult owl and squirrel monkeys. *Neuroscience 10*:639-665, 1983.

Merzenich, M. M., Nelson, R. J., & Kaas, J. H. Variability in hand surface representations in areas 3b and 1 in adult owl and squirrel monkeys. *Journal of Comparative Neurology 258*:281-297, 1987.

Merzenich, M. M., Nelson, R. J., Stryker, M. P., Cyndaer, M. S., Schoppmann, A., & Zook, J. M. Somatosensory cortical map changes following digit amputation in adult monkeys. *Journal of Comparative Neurology 224*:591-605, 1984.

Mori, A., Hanashima, N., Tsuboi, Y., Hiraba, H., Goto, R., Sumino, R. Fifth somatosensory cortex (SV) representation of the whole body surface in the medial bank of the anterior suprasylvian sulcus of the cat. *Neuroscience Research 11*:198-208, 1991.

Mountcastle, V. B. Modality and topographic properties of single neurons of cat's somatic sensory cortex. *Journal of Neurophysiology 20*:408-434, 1957.

Nettor, F. H. *The CIBA Collection of Medical Illustrations, Volume 1*. New Jersey: Donnelly & Sons, 1983.

Olmstead, C. E., & Villablanca, J. R. Effects of caudate or frontal cortex ablation in cats and kittens: Passible avoidance. *Experimental Neurology 68*:335-345, 1980.

Olmstead, C. E., Villablanca, J. R., Sonnier, B. J., McAllister, J. P., & Gomez, F. Reorganization of cerebellorubral terminal fields following hemispherectomy in adult cats. *Brain Research 274*:336-340, 1983.

Powell, T. P. S., & Mountcastle, V. B. The cytoarchitecture of the post-central gyrus of the monkey Macaca mulatta. *Bulletin of Johns Hopkins Hospital 105*:108-131, 1959.

Ramachandran, V. S., Rogers-Ramachandran, D., & Stewart, M. Perceptual correlates of massive cortical reorganization. *Science 258*:1159-1160, 1992.

Recanzone, G. H., Merzenich, M. M., Jenkins, W. M., Grajski, K. A., & Dinse, H. A. Topographic reorganization of the hand representational zone in cortical area 3b paralleling improvements in frequency discrimination performance. *Journal of Neurophysiology 67*:1031-1056, 1992.

Rosen, B., Lundborg, G., Dahlin, L. B., Holmberg, J., & Karlson, B. Nerve repair: Correlation of restitution of functional sensibility with specific cognitive capacities. *Journal of Hand Surgery 19B*:452-458, 1994.

Wall, J. T., Fellerman, D. J., & Kaas, J. H. Recovery of normal topography in the somatosensory cortex of monkeys after nerve crush and regeneration. *Science 221*:771-773, 1983.

• ADDITIONAL READINGS •

Brandenberg, A., & Mann, D. Sensory nerve crush and regeneration and the receptive fields and response properties of neurons in the primary somatosensory cerebral cortex of cats. *Experimental Neurology 103*:256-266, 1989.

Jenkins, W. M., Merzenich, M. M., Ochs, M., Allard, T. T., & Guic-Robles, E. Functional reorganization of primary somatosensory cortex in adult owl monkeys after behaviorally controlled tactile stimulation. *Journal of Neurophysiology 63*:82-104, 1990.

Kennard, M. A. Age and other factors in motor recovery from precentral lesions in the monkey. *American Journal of Physiology 115*:138-146, 1936.

Nelson, R. J., Sur, M., Fellerman, D. J., & Kaas, J. H. Representation of the body surface in postcentral parietal cortex of Macaca fascicularis. *Journal of Comparative Neurology 192*:611-643, 1981.

Penfield, W., & Boldrey, E. Somatic motor and sensory representation in the cerebral cortex of man as studied by electrical stimulation. *Brain 60*:389-443, 1937.

Penfield, W., & Rasmussen, A. T. *The Cerebral Cortex of Man: A Clinical Study of Localization of Function*. New York: Macmillan Publishing Company, 1950.

Rasmussen, D. D. Reorganization of raccoon somatosensory cortex following removal of the fifth digit. *Journal of Comparative Neurology 205*:313-326, 1982.

Recanzone, G. H., Jenkins, W. M., Hradek, G. M., & Merzenich, M. M. Progressive improvement in discriminative abilities in adult owl monkeys performing a tactile frequency discrimination task. *Journal of Neurophysiology 67*:1015-1030, 1992.

Recanzone, G. H., Merzenich, M. M., & Schreiner, C. S. Changes in the distributed temporal response properties of SI cortical neurons reflect improvements in performance on a temporally-based tactile discrimination task. *Journal of Neurophysiology 67*:1071-1091, 1992.

Wall, J. T., Cusik, C. G., Migani-Wall, S. A., & Wiley, R. G. Cortical organization after treatment of a peripheral nerve with ricin: An evaluation of the relationship between sensory neuron death and cortical adjustments after nerve injury. *Journal of Comparative Neurology 277*:578-592, 1988.

Wall, J. T., Kaas, J. H., Sur, M., Nelson, R. J., Fellerman, D. J., & Merzenich, M. M. Functional reorganization in somatosensory cortical areas 3b and 1 of adult monkeys after median nerve repair: Possible relationships to sensory recovery in humans. *Journal of Neuroscience 6*:218-233, 1986.

● ● ●

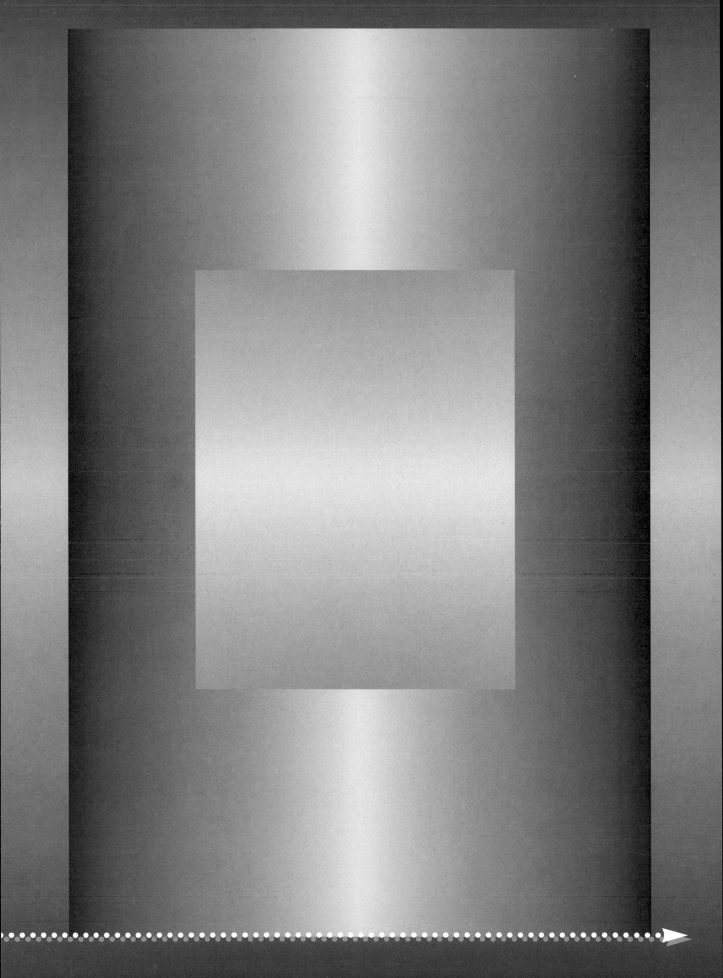

sensory reeducation

I ndividual chapters on somatosensory testing in this book describe particular aspects of sensory rehabilitation as they apply to unique anatomic regions and clinical situations. It is the purpose of this chapter to provide historical insight into sensory reeducation, to provide example protocols developed from different centers as they apply to the upper extremity, and to tabulate results of publications on recovery of sensory function in the extremities, both with and without the benefit of sensory reeducation.

Throughout the international community of health care providers, there is now virtually a universal acceptance of the concept that sensory recovery can be improved by specific sensory exercises that are carried out by the patient. It has been demonstrated that this recovery can occur even long after the initial nerve injury and reconstruction. Furthermore, it has been demonstrated that the time to recovery can be greatly reduced if the appropriate sensory exercises are instituted at the earliest point in the recovery process.

While it is true that following a nerve injury attention was devoted only to splinting to prevent joint deformities, to recover range of motion, and to provide muscle stimulation, and to exercises to increase strength, it is now recognized that sensory rehabilitation is necessary as well (see Figure 11.1). In almost every rehabilitation center there are protocols for sensory reeducation.

Although the motivated patient never needed these protocols to provide sufficient sensory input to maximize the potential given to the region by the nerve reconstruction or repair, it is human nature that without guidance and supervision, neural regeneration is as likely to be painful, underutilized, and perhaps even counterproductive as it is likely to produce a good result. Indeed, it is reasonable to say that the optimal result following nerve repair or reconstruction will not occur without an intense effort made to stimulate neural input to the brain from the earliest possible time in the recovery process.

The approach to sensory reeducation that will be detailed in this chapter has its roots in my medical school research at the Johns Hopkins University from 1969 through 1970. The concept still seems just too simple. I had noticed that during the process of testing two-point discrimination, a patient would seemingly be able to improve his or her sensory perception just through the process of being taught how to do the test. While this is perhaps just part of the "learning curve" for any new experience, it suggested that

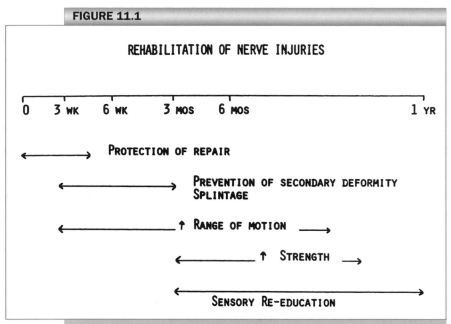

FIGURE 11.1

REHABILITATION OF NERVE INJURIES

Sensory reeducation must be a standard feature of care for the patient with a nerve injury. A suggested timetable is illustrated for the patient with a median nerve repair at the wrist. It will take about 3 months for the recovery of touch perception in the palm, but if this should occur earlier, then early phase sensory reeducation can begin even earlier.

the process of two-point discrimination was not an "all or none" phenomenon, but was an ability that could be improved through practice. This observation suggested an underutilized and underestimated capacity for sensory function.

Furthermore, I had noticed that a patient who seemingly did not have sufficient sensation to identify an object when it was first placed into his or her hand could in fact identify that object, for example, a nickel or a quarter, if (a) he or she had already recovered the ability to perceive touch and vibration, and (b) he or she re-

ceived a short training period designed to help him or her understand the meaning of the altered profile of sensory impulses received from the once-familiar stimuli. It was clear that the number and type of nerve fiber/receptor connections that occurred after nerve repair or reconstruction was likely to be quite different from what it originally had been, and that once-familiar stimuli would now generate an altered profile of sensory impulses that might at the least be confusing, and at the other extreme might be painful or uninterpretable. In a small series of patients, an

FIGURE 11.2

INJURY–ADULTS	HISTORIC CONTROLS			DELLON'S RESULTS		
	NUMBER IN GROUP	PERCENT OF RECOVERY (%)		NUMBER IN GROUP	PERCENT OF RECOVERY (%)	
		S3+	S4		S3+	S4
Median	465	33	0.5	13	39	54
Ulnar	466	34	0.7	5	20	80
Digital	381	48	11.0	17	12	82

The first group of patients to receive sensory reeducation recovered to a level that was better than was expected compared to historic controls, and the time to recovery was 2 years instead of the 5 years usually expected to reach maximum improvement. From "Re-Education of Sensation in the Hand Following Nerve Injury," by A. L. Dellon, R. M. Curtis, & M. T. Edgerton, 1974, in Plastic and Reconstructive Surgery *53:297-305) Adapted with permission of the authors.*

intense effort at sensory retraining demonstrated that a rapid improvement in recovered sensibility could be achieved (see Figures 11.2 & 11.3).

The concept of *sensory reeducation* was first presented to the American Society for Surgery of the Hand in 1971, at which time I was an intern in surgery at Columbia-Presbyterian Medical Center in New York City. The paper was presented in San Francisco. The discussor of my paper was Sevante Edsage, MD, from the faculty of Professor Erik Moberg, MD, in Gotteborg, Sweden. I was extremely nervous preparing for that presentation, which was my first at a national meeting. The opening line of my presentation was, "Without sensation the hand is blind." This is a statement that I had heard Dr. Moberg say, and which I read subsequently in Sterling Bunnell, MD's 1927 paper on nerve grafting for digital nerve defects.

After I made my presentation Dr. Edshage said from the podium that he had only one problem with my paper, and it was that "I hadn't thought of this approach myself." I was so relieved! The abstract of that paper appeared in the *Journal of Bone and Joint Surgery* in 1971. The details of these early experiences with sensory reeducation are re-

counted in my book, *Evaluation of Sensibility and Re-education of Sensation in the Hand* (1981).

Dr. Raymond M. Curtis, my mentor in hand surgery, pointed out to me that Christopher (Kit) Wynn Parry, a physiatrist and the first nonsurgeon to serve as president of the British Society of Hand Surgery, had discussed the concept of sensory rehabilitation in the first edition of his book in 1966, and actually used the words "sensory re-education." His approach was to measure the time required for a patient to identify an object placed in the hand. At a treatment session, the patient would work at identifying objects of different shapes and sizes. Improvement was noted by the decreased time required for the object to be identified. My observations in medical school were that patients could be taught to use the newly regenerated and usually incomplete sensa-

FIGURE 11.3

Early phase reeducation: *(A) A patient 8 months after a median nerve repair at the wrist has recovered perception of pain, 30 Hz, 256 Hz at the tips of the index and middle fingers, and moving- (the horizontal bar) and constant-touch (the xx) perception as well on the tip of the thumb. Since it has been demonstrated that the perception of the 256 Hz stimulus is the last to recover, the lagging behind of the touch perceptions in the index and middle finger suggest that early phase reeducation would be of value. (B) After just 1 week of early phase reeducation, the perception of moving- and constant-touch was recognized at the fingertips.* Late phase sensory reeducation: *Example of the use of two-point discrimination both to train the patient following nerve repair and to monitor recovery of function. Note that for both the median nerve (C) and the ulnar nerve (D) repair, moving two-point discrimination recovers earlier than static two-point discrimination, and recovers, ultimately, to a better degree. This is because It is not only easier to reinnervate the Meissner corpuscle* (movement detection) than the Merkel cell neurite complex (pressure detection), but also because there are more quickly-adapting fibers (Meissner and Pacinian corpuscles) than there are slowly-adapting corpuscles (Merkel cell neurite complex).

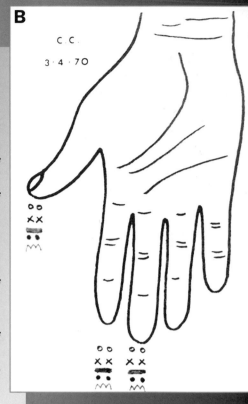

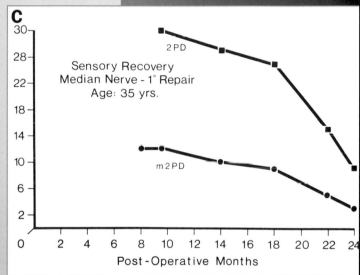

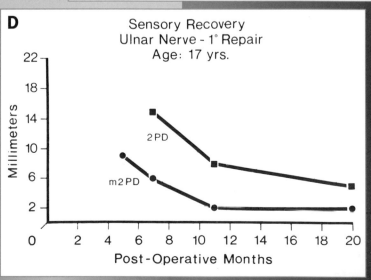

FIGURE 11.4

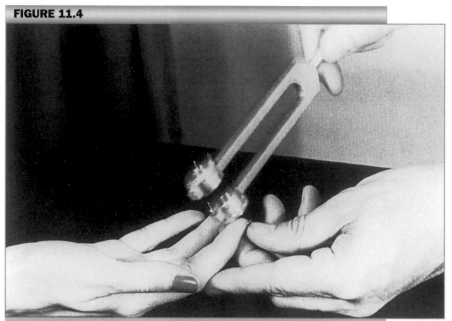

Late phase sensory reeducation can begin whenever the perception of the 256 Hz stimulus occurs in the region to be reeducated. Perception of the 256 Hz stimulus is a good screening test for late phase sensory reeducation because, according to the scheme for the recovery of sensation after nerve repair, it is the last of the touch submodalities to recover. This is because it is easier to reinnervate the Meissner corpuscle (30 Hz stimulus) than the Pacinian corpuscle (256 Hz stimulus) (see Chapter 4). Conversely, the 30 Hz tuning fork is the best screening test to determine when the first large myelinated fibers have recovered in a given region, but is not a good guide for when to begin late phase or object recognition sensory training. From Surgery of the Peripheral Nerve, by S. E. Mackinnon & A. L. Dellon, 1988, New York: Thieme Publishing. Reprinted with permission of the authors.

guide to know when to institute specific sensory exercises at the appropriate time in the recovery process. (The recovery scheme is that first the perceptions related to unmyelinated and thinly myelinated fibers recover, that is, perception of pain and temperature, and then those related to the large myelinated fibers recover in the following sequence: first 30 Hz, then moving touch, then constant touch, and finally the perception of the 256 Hz stimulus.)

The approach to sensory reeducation that evolved from an understanding of neural regeneration permitted an *early phase* of rehabilitation devoted to achieving touch submodality perception and to correct mislocalization, the problem that occurs when, for example, a nerve fiber that formerly innervated the tip of the thumb regenerates into the base of the index finger. Once the perception of the 256 Hz tuning fork had recovered to the tip of a finger (see Figure 11.4), it was found that it was possible to begin sensory rehabilitation directed toward object recognition, monitoring this process with two-point discrimination (see Figure

tions following nerve reconstruction to identify objects, but that the sensibility recovered in a predictable order, based on neural regeneration into the sensory receptors. Object identification could not logically occur until somewhat late in the recovery process, whereas the perception of touch submodalities, such as pres-

sure or touch, would occur earlier.

I also observed that this process could be monitored by measuring static two-point discrimination, once moving and static touch had been recovered in the fingertip. The sequence of recovery of the touch submodalities related to the A-beta fibers could be used as a

11.5), which, in and of itself, is a form of *late phase* sensory rehabilitation.

The scheme of sensory recovery was published in the *Johns Hopkins Medical Journal* in 1972; the first formal paper on the subject of sensory reeducation did not appear in the *Journal of Plastic and Reconstructive Surgery* until 1974. At that time, Dr. Milton Edgerton was Chief of Plastic Surgery at the Johns Hopkins Hospital and Dr. Curtis was the hand surgeon for the Johns Hopkins Hospital and the Union Memorial Hospital. Janice Maynard, the occupational therapist with whom I worked as a medical student, authored a chapter on this subject in the now classic first edition of the textbook, *Rehabilitation of the Hand* (1978). A chapter on sensory reeducation, authored by Anne Callahan, OTR, CHT, appears in the 1984, 1990, and 1995 editions. The 1995 edition has been translated into Japanese under the guidance of Dr. Tatsuya Tajima, director of the world's first Foundation for Surgery of the Hand, located in Nigata, Japan. The Hunter/Mackin yearly Philadelphia symposium on hand surgery has regularly held sessions on sensibility evaluation and sensory reeducation.

My first chapter on senso-ry reeducation appeared in George Omer's and Morton Spinner's book, *Management of Peripheral Nerve Injuries* (Curtis & Dellon, 1980). That same year, Guy Foucher, MD, an excellent microsurgeon from Strasbourg, France, published the results of his finger reconstructions with transferred toes, in which he did sensory reedu-cation. This was followed in 1984 by a similar report of excellent sensory recovery in sensory rehabilitated toe-to-hand transfers by Minami, Masamichi, Hiroyuki, and Seiichi in Saporo, Japan. In 1981 my first book, *Evaluation of Sensibility and Re-education of Sensation in the Hand*, was published. That year, Mayumi Aoki, OTR

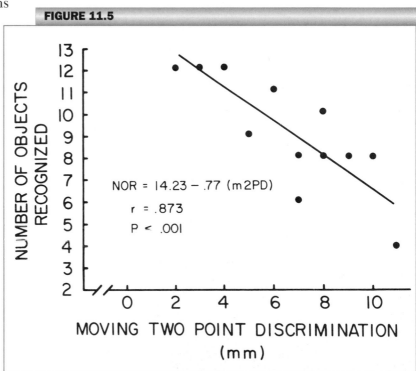

FIGURE 11.5

$$NOR = 14.23 - .77 \ (m2PD)$$
$$r = .873$$
$$P < .001$$

NUMBER OF OBJECTS RECOGNIZED

MOVING TWO POINT DISCRIMINATION (mm)

Two-point discrimination testing is a method for documenting both the level of sensory recovery and late phase sensory reeducation. While the goal of sensory reeducation is not to create "two-point discriminators" of our patients, the use of this test for home practice causes the patient to focus intently on the new patterns of neural impulses the cortex is receiving during the training, and the result, improved ability to distinguish one from two points, has been demonstrated to correlate significantly with object recognition, critical for good hand function. From "Evaluation of Functional Sensation in the Hand," by A. L. Dellon & C. H. Kallman, 1983, in Journal of Hand Surgery 8:865-870. Reprinted with permission of the authors.

(now Mayumi Nakada), from the Tokyo Metropolitan Hospital, visited me in Baltimore and brought my scheme for testing sensibility and reeducating sensation back to Japan. Her first report with these techniques, published in 1986, was about patients with leprosy (see Chapter 14, Figures 14.14, 14.15, & 14.16).

I had the honor to speak at the 1985 meeting of the Japanese Society of Surgery of the Hand and to introduce these concepts formally into Japan at that time. Thereafter, Dr. Tatsuya Tajima, who at that time was Chief of Orthopedic Surgery in Nigata, and who was the pioneer of hand surgery in Japan, instituted these concepts into his hand surgery program and yearly teaching seminars. He published his group's efforts with sensory rehabilitation techniques, confirming their usefulness (Imai, Tajima, & Natsuma, 1989, 1991).

Surgery of the Peripheral Nerve, authored by Susan Mackinnon and myself, contains an exhaustive review of the subject of sensory reeducation through 1988 (see Chapter 18). That book was translated into both Chinese and Japanese in 1993. When Dr. Mackinnon returned to Toronto, Canada to practice peripheral nerve surgery, following her hand surgery fellowship in Baltimore (1981-1982), she worked with two therapists, Chris-

tine Novak, PT, MSc, and Louise Kelly, OTR. They initiated sensory reeducation in all of her patients, and reviewed the results of her median nerve repairs and median nerve grafts (1993a, 1993b). These results demonstrated the excellent recovery that can be achieved when sensory rehabilitation is initiated as soon as possible after excellent microsurgical nerve repair and reconstruction.

Pegge Carter-Wilson, OTR, CHT, from Phoenix, Arizona, and past president of the American Society for Hand Therapy, wrote a chapter on sensory reeducation in *Operative Nerve Repair and Reconstruction* (1991). The extensive experience with toe-to-hand transfer that has developed at the Chang Gung Memorial Hospital in Taipei, Taiwan, under the leadership of Fu-Chan Wei, MD, advanced to a new level of excellence. Already his toe reconstructions demonstrated excellent survival, mastery of technical contouring, and tendon function. Now his results had recovered excellent sensation in the transplanted toes. This was made possible by the introduction in about 1991 of sensory reeducation by Helena Ma, OTR, CHT, the director of Dr. Wei's rehabilitation unit. The results of her successful techniques will appear in print soon (Ma, El-Gammal, & Wei, 1996; Wei & Ma, 1996).

In 1993, the microsurgery group from Russia's First Leningrad Medical Institute reported a series of replanted fingers. They expressed the need for rehabilitation in their patients and did extensive sensibility testing. Eighty-four percent of their reported replanted digits had good or excellent functional sensibility (Lebedev et al., 1993).

The most recent book on hand rehabilitation, *Hand Rehabilitation: A Practical Guide* (1993), contains a chapter on sensory reeducation by Mallory Anthony, OTR.

As if in confirmation of the worldwide acceptance of this concept, the Japanese Society for Sensory Rehabilitation was begun in 1990, under the direction of Mayumi Nakada, OTR, of the Ibaraki Prefectural University of Health Sciences, and Teruko Iwasaki, OTR, from the Tokyo National Rehabilitation Hospital. They have translated *Evaluation of Sensibility and Re-education of Sensation* into Japanese, under the direction of Professor Uchinishi, of Keio University, and it serves as the textbook for their schools of occupational therapy. In May 1995, I had the honor to speak on this subject before this new society, a meeting attended by 255 therapists. These therapists have extended the concepts of sensory rehabilitation beyond the acute and chronic peripheral nerve injury patients with whom I worked to patients with stoke and leprosy. A session on sensory reeducation was given by Tina Jerosch-Herrald, an occupational therapist from Great Britain, at the International Federation of Hand Therapists meeting in Helsinki, Finland in July 1995.

Erik Moberg published his first paper discussing the relationship of classic two-point discrimination in 1958. One of his last papers (1990) was also on this subject. Over that 32-year span, he had the satisfaction of knowing that clinicians interested in the function of the hand were attempting to make measurements, and were using two-point discrimination testing (even though Moberg still wished for a better instrument to make those measurements). Today, as I look back on 26 years of teaching the concepts of sensory reeducation, it appears that sensory reha-

bilitation has become incorporated into the mainstream of hand therapy.

As is clear from Chapter 10, there is no single correct way to do sensory reeducation. Success can be achieved as long as the main goal of stimulating patterns of impulses from the given skin area is realized and the patient is given cause to focus on the functional implications of those stimuli. I look forward to the future, not to see especially new or innovative techniques in sensory rehabilitation, although I am confident these will occur (for example, the virtual reality glove or touch box?), but rather to see further applications of sensory reeducation to other areas of somatosensory problems related to denervation and reinnervation, perhaps along the plans outlined in other chapters of this textbook.

REEDUCATION OF PAIN: DESENSITIZATION

Therapists have traditionally received referrals to desensitize a painful body part. The most common region of the body seen for such referrals is the hand, where the source of the pain is most commonly a neuroma. Frequently, the part to be desensitized has a painful scar. It is of interest that despite the extensive energy devoted by therapists to the actual treatment of pain, there is very little scientific study of this problem. With the exception of a few early reports by Wilson (1981), Hardy, Moran, and Merritt (1982), and Barber (1984), there has been nothing specifically written about desensitization. Certainly there has been no controlled study done to demonstrate the efficacy of a given regimen of desensitization, or to demonstrate that simply being seen by a concerned therapist or psychologist may be

as effective as any interventional treatment. Indeed, there is no proof that desensitization versus just "tincture of time" is effective. And yet, the common belief is that doing something for these patients with pain is essential for a caring clinician. Treatments directed at desensitization universally fit into the category of things that will not worsen the patient's condition, so it seems appropriate to institute such desensitization techniques.

The very name we call this treatment, desensitization, implies that the region being treated is hypersensitive, or has a lower than normal sensory threshold. Even this concept has eluded definitive documentation (Campbell, Meyer, LaMotte, 1979; Campbell, Raja, Meyer, & Mackinnon, 1988; and Raja, Meyer, & Campbell, 1990). The threshold for normal sensibility is usually so low that it exists just at the measurement levels of our instrumentation, and this may account for the problem in detecting a truly lower than normal threshold for stimulation. If we knew that the thresholds were lower than normal, than our therapeutic approach would be designed to raise them.

In contrast, the painful area is usually one in which a cutaneous nerve has been cut or entrapped in scar, and this would suggest that the thresholds are in fact higher than normal. If we knew that the thresholds were higher than normal, then our therapeutic approach would be designed to lower them. It is not even clear which of the subpopulations of nerve fibers contribute to the painful state. In that regard, the Neurometer™, which is a modified tens unit capable of stimulating at three different frequencies (see Chapter 7), may help delineate a specific treatment approach to these patients. This is because a Neurometer™ is designed, theoretically, to be able to give measurements that are above or below the threshold for C-fibers (5 Hz stimuli), A-delta fibers (250 Hz stimuli), and A-beta fibers (2000 Hz stimuli). Pain patients, however, are often reluctant to permit this electrical stimulation of their painful site.

We come then to the conclusion that pain states exist due to various causes, that an initial period of 6 months of desensitization is appropriate before any surgical intervention, and that the techniques that have been historically successful on an empirical level should be continued. It is my belief that desensitization is sensory reeducation of the C-fibers and A-delta fibers. When desensitization is effective, as judged by the patient's decrease in complaints, decreased use of analgesics, and increased use of the affected part, it must be because either (a) the massage portion of the therapy has disentangled nerve endings from the scar, and/or (b) cortical reorganization has occurred to the extent that the new pattern of impulses has been correctly localized and correctly identified, and are no longer interpreted as distractingly painful.

Understood in this context, desensitization is not directed at some hypothetical threshold realignment, but is an attempt to stimulate sufficient neural impulses under guidance so that they can become interpreted in a less painful manner. This is the concept that has always been applied to those patients who have had a nerve repair or graft and whose traditional sensory reeducation has had to be temporarily discontinued because they enter a period of dysesthesias or pain, for which they are desensitized. Understood as reeducation of sensation, desensitization (a) can be explained to the patient as helping the brain to learn the true meaning of these new impulse patterns, even as attempts are made to actually decrease the impulses from the pain fibers;

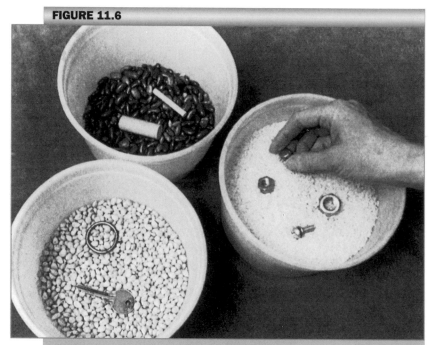

FIGURE 11.6

Desensitization. The region of the hand to be desensitized is placed into a bowl of objects, which can be changed as the hand improves. The bowl may contain items such as coffee beans or marbles. From "Desensitization," by M. S. Anthony, 1993, in Hand Rehabilitation: A Practical Guide, *G. L. Clark, E. F. S. Wilgis, B. Aiello, D. Eckhaus, & L. V. Eddington, Editors, New York: Churchill Livingstone. Reprinted with permission of the authors.*

(b) must be done on a continuing basis several times throughout the day, with the patient being aware of what is being done; and (c) must have as its goal not just relief of pain, but restoration of function to the affected part.

Anthony's review of desensitization (1993) provides an excellent treatment of the techniques that have proven clinically valuable over the years. Almost standard now are insertion of the painful hand into media of various densities, such as coffee beans or sand (see Figure 11.6), leading up to the more vigorous air blowing through different media (fluidotherapy) (see Figure 11.7). Also standard now is the rubbing of the painful part with materials of different textures, beginning first with wisps of cotton, and possibly progressing through rough material like burlap or even a fine grade of sand paper.

Hand-held instruments that apply vibratory stimulation at a fixed frequency but with variable intensity are available (see Figure 11.8). Discussion of the use of the transcutaneous nerve stimulators or tens units is beyond the scope of this text, but these devices, patterned on the "gate control" concept of pain management, are also available for use (see Figure 11.9). I find that only about one-half of patients get some relief from these, whereas most patients "enjoy" the circumstances, the parapher-

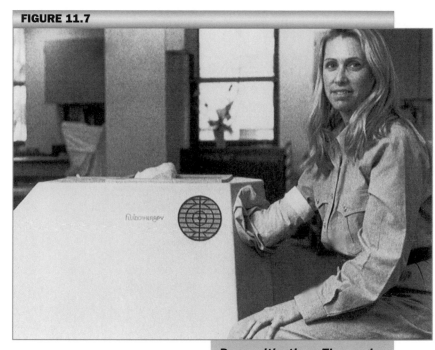

FIGURE 11.7

Desensitization. The region of the hand to be desensitized may be placed into a fluidotherapy box, in which the air-driven particles will constantly bombard the hand, creating a desensitizing stimulus. From "Desensitization," by M. S. Anthony, 1993, in Hand Rehabilitation: A Practical Guide, G. L. Clark, E. F. S. Wilgis, B. Aiello, D. Eckhaus, & L. V. Eddington, Editors, New York: Churchill Livingstone. Reprinted with permission of the authors.

nalia, and the ability to constantly attempt to manipulate their environment that comes with the unit. Many of these patients might equally well be helped by biofeedback techniques and group counseling sessions.

All patients in whom the desensitization program is directed to a region in which there is a surgical scar less than 6 months old should have twice-daily massage with a steroid-containing cream designed to reduce inflammation and separate the nerve endings from the cross-linking collagen fibers. A glove or splint with an elastomer insert that presses on the scar may be helpful. A short course of ultrasound-mediated iontophoresis of the steroid can be tried for particularly thick scars.

Recently, as I have begun to do more lower extremity peripheral nerve surgery, I see the value of water therapy. By this I mean sending patients to a pool in which they can walk. The water relieves them of about 40% of their bodyweight, making it easier for them to ambulate

FIGURE 11.8

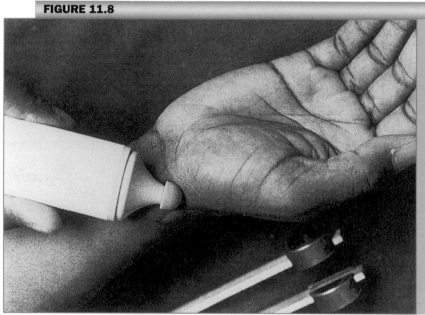

Desensitization. A battery-operated vibrating unit may be used to desensitize the painful region. This vibration unit should be stroked back and forth across the area, with the intensity of the vibration increased as tolerated by the patient. This is excellent for the patient to take home to continue the desensitization program throughout the day. From "Desensitization," by M. S. Anthony, 1993, in Hand Rehabilitation: A Practical Guide, *G. L. Clark, E. F. S. Wilgis, B. Aiello, D. Eckhaus, & L. V. Eddington, Editors, New York: Churchill Livingstone. Reprinted with permission of the authors.*

FIGURE 11.9

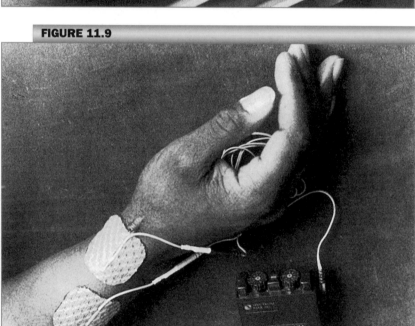

Transcutaneous nerve stimulators send an electric current, whose current intensity can be varied by the patient, through the skin in the region of pain. The electrodes may be placed by the patient to localize the stimulus to the most effective area for pain relief. This form of desensitization is effective about 50% of the time. From "Desensitization," by M. S. Anthony, 1993, in Hand Rehabilitation: A Practical Guide, *G. L. Clark, E. F. S. Wilgis, B. Aiello, D. Eckhaus, & L. V. Eddington, Editors, New York: Churchill Livingstone. Reprinted with permission of the authors.*

so they can concentrate on their gait. Also, the water brushing up against their painful skin region serves as a desensitization technique. The same concept can be achieved in a whirlpool or by a home shower-massager.

Collateral sprouting (see Chapter 4) may create a pain problem that is best treated by desensitization techniques. After deafferentation of a region of skin, either because a painful neuroma has been resected or because a nerve has been harvested as donor tissue, there may ensue in the patient a period of unpleasant sensations or pain in the denervated territory. The usual period of this discomfort may range from days to 3 months, but typically lasts about 3 weeks. Clinical examination of these initially deafferented skin territories is almost universally observed to shrink in area, a phenomenon which has been called collateral sprouting, but which has rarely been documented clinically. There is no reason to suspect that this form of neural regeneration should be any less uncomfortable than that accompanying neural regeneration after a nerve repair or nerve graft.

While the above desensitization techniques are given to the patient to help with the discomfort of collateral sprouting, documentation of the sensory changes provides visual proof for the patient that sensation is recovering and that the "bad" nerves, those removed to treat the painful neuroma, are not "coming back." Examples of the types of documentation that are now possible with quantitative sensory testing with the Pressure-Specified Sensory Device™ are given in Chapter 4 (see Figures 4.12 A & B).

Reflex sympathetic dystrophy (RSD) (see Chapter 4) is a pain state that is often referred for desensitization technique, but for which desensitization alone is usually not sufficient. These patients should not be made to wait 6 months before instituting interventional measures, such as stellate ganglion or lumbar sympathetic blocks. The blocks can now be done intravenously with phentolamine, an alpha-1 histamine blocker (Raja, Davis, & Campbell, 1992). Therapy directed at range of motion, edema control, and gentle strengthening is encouraged throughout the course of pain management, affording the therapist the opportunity to try desensitization techniques.

The therapist should be encouraged to attempt to document sensory thresholds in the part affected by RSD. An example of this for the foot is given in Figure 11.10. Such documentation may suggest subclinical nerve compression, due either to the initial trauma, or secondary to the chronic edema, suggesting that surgical intervention to decompress these nerves may diminish the pain signal that now may have become the continuing source of the dystrophy.

• REEDUCATION OF TOUCH •

The cumulative experience of the past quarter-century confirms that sensory reeducation is effective in achieving touch sensibility that is capable of better discrimination and, therefore, of better hand function. The end of this chapter contains sensory reeducation protocols that have proven effective for the institution submitting the protocol. The protocols listed for the Union Memorial Hospital in Baltimore and the Sunnybrook Hospital in Toronto clearly follow the basic design of the method that I developed in 1970 and described in detail in *Evaluation of Sensibility and Re-education of Sensation in the Hand* (1981). This technique is described again in Chapter 12 with regard to rehabilitation after nerve repair and grafting in the upper extremity.

It is the purpose of this section to develop the basic principles that may permit the design of even more effective sensory rehabilitation strategies for the future. This section draws on the collective experience of the past, and on the inferences for sensory rehabilitation that can be drawn from experimental work on cortical plasticity (Merzenich & Jenkins, 1993). Cortical plasticity is discussed in chapter 10.

• FOCUS •

Because the sensory input from the given area to be rehabilitated may be disturbing (*dysesthetic*) and distracting (*paresthetic*), the patient may deliberately block its sensations from consciousness and avoid using the part. While blocking dysesthesia may be a goal of chronic pain manage-

FIGURE 11.10

A

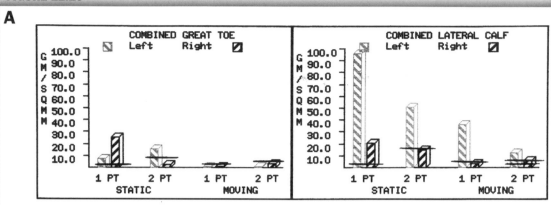

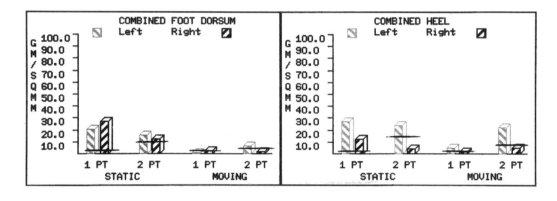

Reflex sympathetic dystrophy (RSD) can be approached through desensitization techniques alone, but this is usually not sufficient to achieve lasting pain relief. The reflex cycle must be "broken" either by interrupting the pain-generating signal, that is, by a neuroma resection and/or decompression of the peripheral nerves, or by interrupting the sympathetic supply, that is, pharmacologically or surgically. Theoretically, RSD is a hypersensitive state, implying a lowering of sensory thresholds. Quantitative sensory testing with the Pressure-Specified Sensory Device™ can document elevated cutaneous pressure thresholds in the patient with RSD that document the presence of chronic nerve compression in these patients, in whom electrodiagnostic testing is often not possible. (A) Note the elevated thresholds for the left foot at the big toe and foot dorsum consistent with tarsal tunnel syndrome and peroneal stretch traction injury, in this young woman 6 months after an ankle inversion injury with 4th and 5th metatarsal fractures. In (B), the improvement in her quantitative sensory testing is apparent by 3 months after decompression of the peroneal nerve at the knee and over the dorsum of the foot and a release of the tarsal, calcaneal, medial, and lateral plantar tunnels.

ment, it is counterproductive in sensory rehabilitation. Rather, the patient must be made to focus attention on the sensory input and learn to interpret what this altered profile of impulses means. Practicing sensory reeducation exercises for 5 to 10 minutes 2 or 3 times a day serves this purpose. Requiring the patient to observe the sensory stimulus and then to repeat it with eyes closed reinforces the true meaning of the impulses the patient's brain is receiving.

An example of this type of exercise is one that should

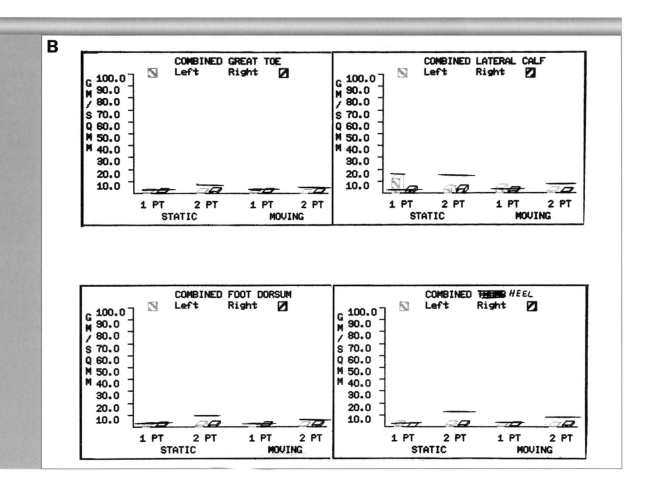

be done in the early phase of sensory reeducation after nerve repair or grafting. The problem being overcome is that fewer than normal numbers of axons will be in contact with the appropriate receptor, and many axons will be without a receptor at all, leading to the phenomenon of mislocalization and sensory input that cannot be matched with any previously stored recognition patterns. The nerve reconstruction has given the patient a certain potential for recovery, and the reeducation will enable the patient to achieve this full potential. This may be accomplished by having the patient take the eraser end of a pencil and either stroke or press the given area, while the patient first observes the stimulus (eyes open), and then concentrates on what is being perceived (eyes closed) (see Figure 11.11).

• FREQUENCY •

The more neural input the brain receives, the more it pays attention to the part sending the signals, and the greater the portion of the somatosensory cortex that is devoted to that area. Therefore, the more the part can be stimulated, the better the chance that correct interpretation of the stimuli will occur and that better function will follow.

The regimen must be one that the patient will carry out, and this brings up the subject of motivation. If the patient is sufficiently motivated, he or she may have retrained himself or herself even without the therapist's guidance. If the patient has no incentive to recover, he or she will simply disre-

FIGURE 11.11

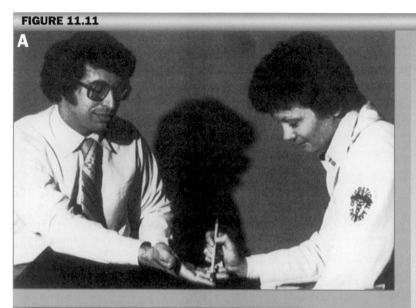

A

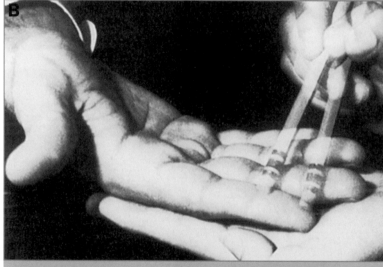

B

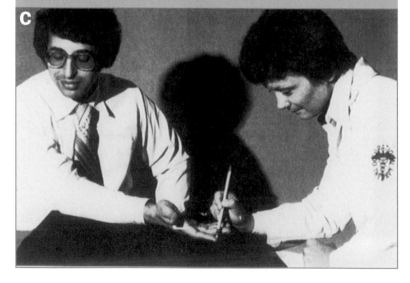

C

An example of an early phase of sensory reeducation exercise that causes the patient to focus on the recovering sensations after nerve repair or grafting. The problem being overcome is mislocalization and lack of touch-submodality recognition patterns. This may be accomplished by having the patient take the eraser end of a pencil and either stroke or press the given area, while the patient (A) first observes the stimulus (eyes open), and then (C) concentrates on what is being perceived (eyes closed). The stimulus may also be moving touch (B). From Evaluation of Sensibility and Re-Education of Sensation in the Hand, *by A. L. Dellon, 1981, Baltimore: Williams & Wilkins. Reprinted with permission of the author.*

gard the therapist's advice. The therapist must get to know the patient's home and job circumstances and design a rehabilitation home practice schedule that can be followed. The therapist must set sufficiently frequent follow-up visits that the patient's progress can be measured. The patient must be rewarded at each success, as this reinforcement adds strength to the learning session.

Giving the patient a home sensory reeducation kit or device will provide him or

FIGURE 11.12

The Disk-Criminator™ can be used for early phase sensory reeducation because it has two different surfaces. (A and B) These differ in the shape of the central depression and in the number of raised surface elements. (C) Close-up of raised numbers. The patient can actively rub the given surface area over the Disk-Criminator™, and someone else can test the patient's ability to distinguish one side from the other by passively rubbing the Disk-Criminator™ over the area.

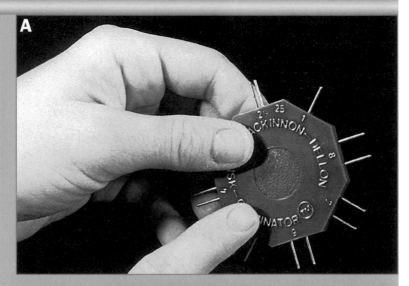

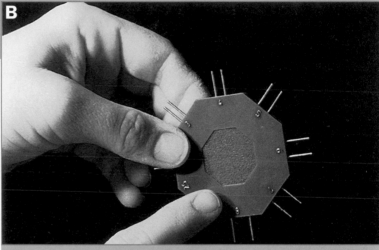

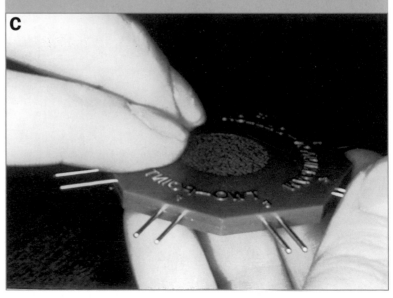

her with a reminder that there is something to do, and that he or she must do it. If the goal is to return the patient to a given type of employment, incorporating some of those work-related discrimination tasks is essential. The patient should be given a Disk-Criminator™ as a home reeducation device after being instructed in its use. In early phase sensory reeducation the finger can be moved actively over the surfaces to attempt to distinguish the raised from the smooth surfaces, and to determine one side of the device from the other (each side has a different-shaped central depression and a different amount of raised surface elements; see Figure 11.12). The Disk-Criminator™ can be billed to third-party insurance carriers either using the procedure codes related to neuromuscular testing or supply items. Alternatively, a sensory reeducation kit can be prepared from whatever materials you deem appropriate (see Figure 11.13).

• FUNCTION •

Sensory reeducation may be maximized if the rehabilitation activity is meaningful to the patient and additional stimuli can be generated from adjacent joints, muscles, and tendons. These are inferences that come from studies that have observed influences of extremity movement on sensory neuron activity in the cortex, that have observed the effect of an active versus a passive finger during sensory stimulation on cortical-evoked potentials, and that have demonstrated cortical plasticity in response to adding motivation to the training paradigms of primates (Papakostopoulos, Cooper, & Crow, 1975; Jiang, Chapman, & Lamarre, 1991; Dannenbaum & Jones, 1993; Merzenich & Jenkins, 1993; Chapman, 1994).

Although motor rehabilitation is not within the scope of this book, many of the same rehabilitation principles should apply. A potentially useful suggestion comes from the basic research that has identified the ability of stimulated cortical sensory neurons to cause facial muscle twitching in the cat (Mori, Yamaguchi, Kikuta, Furukawa, & Sumino, 1993). With regard to rehabilitation of the facial palsy patient, we have always instructed the patient to view the face in the mirror while gently touching the part from which movement is desired. Perhaps this sensory stimulation is effective by means of the mechanisms discussed in this article.

Another facet of sensory/motor interaction has been observed in stroke patients. I have little experience with stroke patients, as reflected by the paucity of information in this book about that subject. Recently, an excellent study relating sensibility testing and hand function in patients who had a left-sided middle cerebral artery occlusion (Robertson & Jones, 1994) demonstrated abnormal pressure thresholds and abnormal two-point discrimination in these patients' right hands, but noted that they still could function on the Jebsen Hand Function test. These patients could use excessive force to overcome their sensory deficit, but this increased force limited their ability to do fine manipulative tasks. These sensory/actions offer multiple channels for rehabilitation stimuli to reach cortical levels, and application of such rehabilitation can be monitored by the battery of tests Robertson and Jones describe.

Translation of these experimental studies into practical sensory rehabilitation remains a challenge for the individual therapist and patient. If a patient has enjoyed sewing or knitting, then a sensory reeducation activity might involve feeling different texture wools, yarns, string, and thread, or selecting a wide from a narrow knitting needle. If a patient has been employed as a carpenter, similar activities may be structured with grades of sandpaper and different-sized nails, and with differentiating nails from screws, or washers from bolts. Clearly, as the patient's degree of sensation recovers, these activities will progress from those of early phase reeducation to those of late phase reeducation, in which object identification is required. The objects may be placed into a bag and the patient asked to identify the object before it is removed from the bag. Such a "game" may be observed by another member of the household to add an element of motivation.

It must be remembered that implicit in the concept of sensory reeducation is that the patient will be frustrated if asked to perform a sensory function for which the appropriate number of axons have not regenerated. Frustration leads to disappointment and disenchantment with the sensory rehabilitation program. That is why the program has always been structured to increase the level of difficulty at the

FIGURE 11.13

A sensory reeducation "kit" can be prepared for the patient to take home. In this way specialized devices may be added that relate to the patient's job or leisure activities. These decrease in size and become more similar from (A) to (B) to (C). Texture differences are emphasized in (A), while shape is emphasized in (B). From Surgery of the Peripheral Nerve, by S. E. Mackinnon & A. L. Dellon, 1988, New York: Thieme Publishing. Reprinted with permission of the authors.

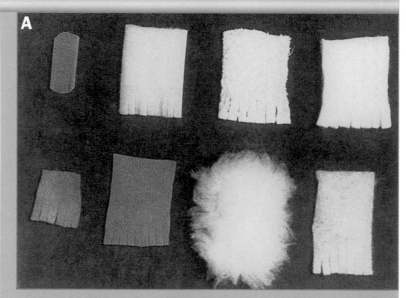

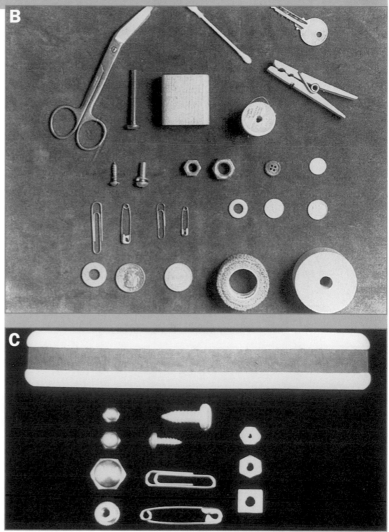

appropriate time in the recovery process. It is pointless to attempt object recognition before all sensory submodalities have regenerated to the fingertip.

The extent to which the fingertip may function as a sensory input device has been evaluated by studies in blind subjects (Nakada & Dellon, 1989; Novak, Mackinnon, Williams, & Kelly, 1993), and by studies in which skin of normal-sighted subjects is reeducated (Brown, Mackinnon, Dellon, & Bain, 1989). Taken together, these studies demonstrate that even fingertip skin has unused potential which can be improved by sensory retraining in an environment in which the subject is motivated and in which the training paradigm includes movement and functional activity of the part being retrained.

● FACILITATION ●

There may be facets to sensory reeducation exercises that can be added that will facilitate the primary rehabilitation activity. For example, when I first became involved in this area of study, Janice Maynard, OTR, the first therapist with whom I worked, noted that some patients seemed to do better at sensory reeducation exercises if they were manipulating an object with their opposite, noninjured hand, as well. Bilateral extremity activity has been found to be useful in the rehabilitation of stroke patients, perhaps related to patterning activity (Dannebaum & Dykes, 1988). This facilitation may be made more concrete by having the patient move the noninjured fingertip across material at the same time that the injured fingertip is moving across material. Of course, for a given patient, this may prove too confusing. In this context, Rosen, Lundborg, Dahlin, Holmberg, and Karlson (1994) observed that in 19 patients who were studied several years after median and ulnar nerve repairs, the functional outcome could be correlated with the patients' spatial/verbal logic capabilities.

Facilitation can be negative, too. For example, in a 1983 report on object identification with measures of sensibility (Dellon & Kallman, 1983), if two different fingers were being used for object identification during active touch, for example, the thumb and index finger, the ability to recognize objects correlated with the finger which had the best two-point discrimination. Thus, the brain chose to ignore the signals from one finger. An application of this might be the patient who had a medi-

TABLE 11.1 RESULTS OF DIGITAL NERVE REPAIRS

Reference, Date	Type of Trauma	Repair/ Timing	No. of Cases	Age (yr)	% of Children
Bunnell, 1927	Civilian	All	105		
Larson & Posch, 1958	Civilian	All	142		16
Weckesser, 1961	Civilian	Primary	12	7-55	8
Weckesser, 1961	Civilian	Secondary	12	7-48	8
Önne, 1962	Civilian	Primary	8	<14	100
Önne, 1962	Civilian	Primary	14	>14	0
Honner et al., 1970	Civilian	Primary	24	<19	100
Honner et al., 1970	Civilian	Primary	50	>19	0
Buncke, 1972	Civilian	All	18	6-51	5
Poppin et al., 1979	Civilian	Primary	62	6-67	22
Posch & delaCruz-Saddul, 1980	Civilian	Primary	71		6
Young et al., 1981	Civilian	Primary	27	3-67	
Berger et al., 1988	Civilian	Primary	129		
Goldie et al., 1992	Civilian	Primary	30	17-71	0
Kallio, 1993	Civilian	Secondary	151	1-61	28

Note: From *Surgery of the Peripheral Nerve*, by S. E. Mackinnon & A. L. Dellon, 1988, New York: Thieme Publishing. Adapted with permission of the authors.

an nerve graft in whom the middle finger lags behind the index and thumb in terms of sensory recovery (see Figure 12.13). In such a situation the therapist might need to direct individual attention to the middle finger, and discontinue use of the combined index and thumb in object identification tasks, switching to passive stimulation of each fingertip pulp.

The therapist should, therefore, be encouraged to try different strategies with the individual patient based on his or her background, education, and experience.

• RESULTS OF SENSORY REEDUCATION •

The results obtained from a program of sensory reeducation can be measured both in terms of the absolute level of sensory function achieved and in terms of the time required to achieve that end result. The results of sensory reeducation are best considered with respect to what was able to be achieved historically before the introduction of sensory reeducation.

I reviewed the available reports from the worldwide literature with this particular goal in mind, and published them in Chapter 11 of *Evaluation of Sensibility and Re-education of Sensation in the Hand* (Dellon, 1981). I reviewed the results from replanted fingers and transplanted toes in 1986 (Dellon, 1986). All of these tables were updated by Susan Mackinnon for our book, *Surgery of the Peripheral Nerve* (Mackinnon & Dellon, 1988). Where applicable, these tables have been further updated by reviewing the few papers on this subject that have appeared recently and including those results in this chapter. Another review of sensory recovery following digital replantation was reported by Glickman and Mackinnon (1990). Recently, a review of sensory recovery in innervated free tissue transfers has appeared (Graham & Dellon, 1995). Where it is clear that a formal sensory reeducation program has been used, this fact is noted in the tables.

It is unlikely that a prospective, randomized trial of peripheral nerve repair with and without sensory reeducation will ever be done because in the absence of another major military conflict, there are unlikely to be sufficient cases generated to provide the information needed for such a study. There are three methods of analysis, however, that may be used to demonstrate that sensory reeducation does make a difference in the

Follow-up (yr)	Nerve Block	Sensory Recovery (%)				
		S2	S2+	S3	S3+	S4
	No					
1-7	No	7	0	29	64	0
	No	0	0	16	42	25
	No	0	16	16	21	63
4-15	Yes	0	0	0	0	100
4-15	Yes	28	0	29	43	0
2-6	Yes	12	0	20	20	48
2-6	Yes	28	0	28	28	16
	No	0	0	22	28	50
5-15	Yes	0	10	16	55	19
2-11	No	20	0	32	48	0
2-4	No	0	0	10	57	33
2	No	0	9	0	0	91
1-4	No	13		13	44	30
2-5	No	20		38	17	25

outcome following peripheral nerve repair or reconstruction. They are (a) comparison of the results of patients receiving sensory reeducation with those results published in the past about patients who have not received sensory reeducation; (b) plotting the results of sensory recovery against the patient's age at a given time period after surgery, when that program has been instituted in the immediate postoperative period; and (c) studying the effect of instituting a course in sensory reeducation for a group of patients already assumed to have reached their maximum potential, that is, sufficiently long after nerve repair or reconstruction that no further neural regeneration is occurring peripherally, and it can be assumed that all the changes that occur over a 3-week course of sensory reeducation are due to the reeducation. The conclu-

TABLE 11.2 RESULTS OF LOW MEDIAN NERVE REPAIRS

Reference, Date	Type of Trauma	Repair Timing	No. of Cases	Age (yr)
Kirklin et al., 1949	War	All	235	Adults
Zachary, 1954	War	Secondary	290	Adults
Yahr, Beebe, Oester & Davis, 1956	War	Secondary	244	Adults
Nicholson & Seddon, 1957	Civilian	Secondary	52	
Larson & Posch, 1958	Civilian	Primary	54	
Larson & Posch, 1958	Civilian	Secondary	24	
Stromberg et al., 1961	Civilian	All	46	
McEwan, 1962	Civilian	All	27	<14
McEwan, 1962	Civilian	All	16	>14
Sakellarides, 1962	Civilian	Primary	38	3-81
Sakellarides, 1962	Civilian	Secondary	20	3-81
Flynn & Flynn, 1962	Civilian	Primary	40	
Önne, 1962	Civilian	Primary	15	<14
Önne, 1962	Civilian	Primary	17	>14
Nielsen & Torup, 1964	Civilian	All	10	5-58
Boswick et al., 1965	Civilian	All	26	
Seddon, 1972	Civilian	Secondary	110	
Omer, 1974	War	Secondary	95	Adults
Posch & delaCruz-Saddul, 1980	Civilian	Primary	14	
Tajima & Imai, 1989	Civilian	Primary	7	1-13
Kallio & Vastamaki, 1993	Civilian	Secondary	34	5-58

Note: From *Surgery of the Peripheral Nerve*, by S. E. Mackinnon & A. L. Dellon, 1988, New York: Thieme Publishing. Adapted with permission of the authors.

sion from all three types of analyses confirms the value of sensory reeducation in achieving a better, more functional level of sensory recovery, and in achieving that level in a shorter time period than has been accomplished without such a program.

To provide data to support the above conclusion, Tables 11.1 through 11.13 contain the results of nerve repair and grafting for upper and lower extremity nerves. Tables 11.14 through 11.16 contain the results of nerve repair and grafting in which sensory reeducation has been part of the rehabilitation program, and the results for replants, transplants, and other innervated soft tissue transfers. The individual, published reports from which this data were abstracted are given in the References list for this chapter.

A clinical example of the

% of Children	Follow-up (yr)	Motor Recovery (%)				Sensory Recovery (%)				
		M2	M3	M4	M5	S2	S2+	S3	S3+	S4
0	2	67				27		73		
0	5	31	14	18	0	47	15	30	9	0.2
0	4	11	23	29	31	17	28	14	18	
16	5	21	27	39	0	21	15	40	25	0
16	1-7	35	0	65	0					
16	1-7	50	0	50	0	3	0	26	71	0
?	2-24									9
100	Long	0	0	27	65	4	0	4	7	86
0	Long	13	20	27	13	17	0	17	61	0
26	2-31	13	37	11	0	15	33	13	5	0
26	2-31	25	35	25	0	20	29	32	4	0
	1-12	25	38	15	7	50	0	7	10	3
100	4-11	20	13	40	27	0	0	0	27	73
0	4-11	30	23	18	29	22	18	18	41	0
33	1-3	30		70		30		70		
35	1					0		88	8	4
?	5	5	47		44	4	5	47	44	0
0	1	61		39	0	61		39		0
6	2-11	0	43	57	0	7	7	29	57	0
100	4-7					0	0	0	0	100
10	10	30	30	30	10	29	13	18	30	10

TABLE 11.3 RESULTS OF HIGH MEDIAN NERVE REPAIRS

Reference, Date	Type of Trauma	Repair/ Timing	No. of Cases	Age (yr)	Follow-up (yr)
Kirklin et al., 1949	War	All		Adult	<2
Zachary, 1954	War	Secondary	95	Adult	5
Yahr, Beebe, Oester, & Davis, 1956	War	Secondary	124	Adult	>4
Nicholson & Seddon, 1957	Civilian	Secondary	6	Adult	5
Larson & Posch, 1958	Civilian	Primary	14		1-7
Sakellarides, 1962	Civilian	All	7	Adult	2-31
Seddon, 1972	Civilian	Secondary	100		>5
Omer, 1974	War	Secondary	48	Adult	>1
Posch & delaCruz-Saddul, 1980	Civilian	Primary	12	Adult	2-11

Note: From *Surgery of the Peripheral Nerve,* by S. E. Mackinnon & A. L. Dellon, 1988, New York: Thieme Publishing. Adapted with permission of the authors.

TABLE 11.4 RESULTS OF LOW ULNAR NERVE REPAIRS

Reference, Date	Type of Trauma	Repair Timing	No. of Cases	Age (yr)
Kirklin et al., 1949	War	All	158	Adults
Zachary, 1954	War	Secondary	384	Adults
Yahr, Beebe, Oester, & Davis, 1956	War	Secondary	441	Adults
Nicholson & Seddon, 1957	Civilian	Secondary	60	
Larson & Posch, 1958	Civilian	All	62	
Stromberg et al., 1961	Civilian	All	32	
McEwan, 1962	Civilian	All	23	<14
McEwan, 1962	Civilian	All	23	>14
Sakellarides, 1962	Civilian	Primary	39	3-81
Sakellarides, 1962	Civilian	Secondary	29	3-81
Flynn & Flynn, 1962	Civilian	Primary	40	
Önne, 1962	Civilian	Primary	10	<14
Önne, 1962	Civilian	Primary	7	>14
Nielsen & Torup, 1964	Civilian	All	16	5-58
Boswick et al., 1965	Civilian	All	19	
Seddon, 1972	Civilian	Secondary	119	
Omer, 1974	War	Secondary	95	Adults
Posch & delaCruz-Saddul, 1980	Civilian	Primary	20	
Vastamaki et al., 1993	Civilian	Secondary	34	5-58

Note: From *Surgery of the Peripheral Nerve,* by S. E. Mackinnon & A. L. Dellon, 1988, New York: Thieme Publishing. Adapted with permission of the authors.

Motor Recovery (%)				Sensory Recovery (%)				
M2	M3	M4	M5	S2	S2+	S3	S3+	S4
					37	47		
42	13	6	0	47	23	25	6	0
17	25	30	13					
33	0	50	0	50	0	34	16	0
0	14	36	0		8	50	42	0
42	14	0	0	42	0	14	0	0
6	61		30	3	6	61	30	
7	3	27	0	7	3	27	0	0
16	60	8	0	8	8	60	17	0

% of Children	Follow-up (yr)	Motor Recovery (%)				Sensory Recovery (%)				
		M2	M3	M4	M5	S2	S2+	S3	S3+	S4
0	<2					0	31	69	0	0
0	>5	72	14	5	0	54	15	28	3	0
0	>4	5	34	38	16	16	24	19	13	0
16	>5	32	32	35	0	18	14	47	21	0
16	1-7	63	0	37	0	4	0	33	63	0
	2-24									3
100	Long	4	25	67	4	0	0	5	23	72
0	Long	32	36	23	0	8	0	24	48	12
26	2-31	30	6	0	0	25	15	23	5	0
26	2-31	20	7	3	0	30	13	27	13	0
	1-12	57	15	18	0	50	0	13	7	0
100	5-10	8	30	30	32	0	0	10	30	60
0	5-10					0	0	57	43	0
33	1-3	30		70			38		62	
35	1					4		76	20	0
	>5	10	43		45	2	10	43	45	0
0	>1		61		39	0	61		39	0
6	2-11	55	30	10	0	50	0	10	30	0
10	3-20	2	14	10	74	27	13	26	20	14

TABLE 11.5 RESULTS OF HIGH ULNAR NERVE REPAIRS

Reference, Date	Type of Trauma	Repair/ Timing	No. of Cases	Age (yr)
Kirklin et al., 1949	War	All	158	Adults
Zachary, 1954	War	Secondary	384	Adults
Yahr, Beebe, Oester & Davis, 1956	War	Secondary	441	Adults
Nicholson & Seddon, 1957	Civilian	Secondary	60	
Larson & Posch, 1958	Civilian	All	62	
Stromberg et al., 1961	Civilian	All	32	
McEwan, 1962	Civilian	All	23	<14
McEwan, 1962	Civilian	All	23	>14
Sakellarides, 1962	Civilian	Primary	39	3-81
Sakellarides, 1962	Civilian	Secondary	29	3-81
Flynn & Flynn, 1962	Civilian	Primary	40	
Önne, 1962	Civilian	Primary	10	<14
Önne, 1962	Civilian	Primary	7	>14
Nielsen & Torup, 1964	Civilian	All	16	5-58
Boswick et al., 1965	Civilian	All	19	
Seddon, 1972	Civilian	Secondary	119	
Omer, 1974	War	Secondary	95	Adults
Posch & delaCruz-Saddul, 1980	Civilian	Primary	20	

Note: From *Surgery of the Peripheral Nerve,* by S. E. Mackinnon & A. L. Dellon, 1988, New York: Thieme Publishing. Reprinted with permission of the authors.

TABLE 11.6 RESULTS OF COMBINED MEDIAN AND ULNAR NERVE REPAIRS

Nerve	Type of Trauma	Sensory Recovery (%) S3+	S4	Motor Recovery (%) M4	M5
Median low	War	20	<1	40	0
	Civilian	33	<1	40	5
Median high	War	3	0	20	5
	Civilian	17	0	30	0
Ulnar low	War	15	0	40	0
	Civilian	34	<1	32	0
Ulnar high	War	0	0	23	6
	Civilian	20	0	17	0

Note: From *Surgery of the Peripheral Nerve,* by S. E. Mackinnon & A. L. Dellon, 1988, New York: Thieme Publishing. Reprinted with permission of the authors.

% of Children	Follow-up (yr)	Motor Recovery (%)				Sensory Recovery (%)				
		M2	M3	M4	M5	S2	S2+	S3	S3+	S4
0	<2					0	31	69	0	0
0	>5	72	14	5	0	54	15	28	3	0
0	>4	5	34	38	16	16	24	19	13	0
16	>5	32	32	35	0	18	14	47	21	0
16	1-7	63	0	37	0	4	0	33	63	0
	2-24									3
100	Long	4	25	67	4	0	0	5	23	72
0	Long	32	36	23	0	8	0	24	48	12
26	2-31	30	6	0	0	25	15	23	5	0
26	2-31	20	7	3	0	30	13	27	13	0
	1-12	57	15	18	0	50	0	13	7	0
100	5-10	8	30	30	32	0	0	10	30	60
0	5-10					0	0	57	43	0
33	1-3	30	70			38		62		
35	1					4		76	20	0
	>5	10	43		45	2	10	43	45	0
0	>1	61		39	0	61		39		0
6	2-11	55	30	100	50	0	10	30	0	

TABLE 11.7 RESULTS OF RADIAL NERVE REPAIRS

Reference, Date	Type of Trauma	No. of Cases	% Motor Recovery M4 and M5
Seddon, 1954	War	114	37
Woodall & Beebe, 1956	War	197	21
Sakellarides, 1962	Civilian	13	14
Brown, 1970	War	5	Some return 40%
Kallio et al., 1993	Civilian	12	33

Note: From *Surgery of the Peripheral Nerve*, by S. E. Mackinnon & A. L. Dellon, 1988, New York: Thieme Publishing. Adapted with permission of the authors.

TABLE 11.8 RESULTS OF POSTERIOR INTEROSSEOUS NERVE GRAFT

Author	Type of Trauma	Gap Grafted (cm)	No. of Cases	Age (yr)	Follow-up (yr)	M0 to M2 %	Grade M3 %	M4 to M5 %
Kallio et al., 1993	Civilian	2-10	21	7-54	5-20	24	38	38

Note: From *Surgery of the Peripheral Nerve,* by S. E. Mackinnon & A. L. Dellon, 1988, New York: Thieme Publishing. Adapted with permission of the authors.

TABLE 11.9 RESULTS OF DIGITAL NERVE GRAFTS

Reference, Date	Type of Trauma	Gap Grafted (cm)	No. of Cases	Age (yr)
Seddon, 1947	War	3-8	15	Adults
Brooks, 1955	Civilian	>2	17	
McFarlane & Moyer, 1976	Civilian	1.5-3.5	17	20-59
Young et al., 1980	Civilian	>2	27	15-57
Yamano et al., 1982	Replant	2-5	5	28-56
Wilgis & Maxwell, 1979	Civilian	1-2.5	11	17-54
Beazley et al., 1984	Civilian	1-5	12	0.5-71
Rose & Kowalski, 1985	Civilian	5-8	5	Adults
Rose et al., 1987	Civilian	4.5	13	19-55
Mackinnon, 1988	Civilian	1-5	31	18-62
Berger et al., 1988	Civilian	1-6		
Rose et al., 1989	Civilian	4-5	13	19-55
Kallio, 1993	Civilian	1-6	103	1-61

Note: From *Surgery of the Peripheral Nerve,* by S. E. Mackinnon & A. L. Dellon, 1988, New York: Thieme Publishing. Adapted with permission of the authors.

Follow-up (yr)	Nerve Block	Sensory Recovery (%)				
		S2	S2+	S3	S3+	S4
2-4	No	46	12	29	6	12
>5	No	18	0	47	0	0
0.75-2	No	0	15	39	46	0
0.5-5	Yes	0	0	60	25	15
2	No	0	0	0	100	0
0.9-2	Yes	0	0	0	33	67
2-6	No	42			58	
3-7	No	0	20	0	20	60
1	No	0	0	7	55	38
4	No	6	0	0	40	54
3-7	No			85		
1	No	0	0	7	55	38
2-5	No	49		19	19	13

TABLE 11.10   RESULTS OF MEDIAN NERVE GRAFTS

Reference, Date	Type of Trauma	Gap Grafted (cm)	No. of Cases	Age (yr)	% Children
Bunnell & Boyes, 1939	Civilian	3-15	32		
Seddon, 1947	War	5-15	11	Adult	
Brooks, 1955	Civilian	>7	33		
Millesi et al., 1972, 1976	Civilian	2-20	38	8-62	3
Walton & Finseth, 1977	Civilian	5-10	8	17-38	0
Tallas et al., 1978	Civilian	4-15	6		
Young et al., 1980	Civilian	>2	8	15-57	0
Beazley et al., 1984	Civilian	4-6	5	0.5-71	2-6
Novak et al., 1992	Civilian	1-12	14	41	0
Kallio & Vastamaka, 1993	Civilian	2-10	98	5-58	15

Note: From *Surgery of the Peripheral Nerve,* by S. E. Mackinnon & A. L. Dellon, 1988, New York: Thieme Publishing. Adapted with permission of the authors.

TABLE 11.11   RESULTS OF ULNAR NERVE GRAFTS

Reference, Date	Type of Trauma	Gap Grafted (cm)	No. of Cases	Age (yr)	% Children
Bunnell & Boyes, 1939	Civilian	3-15	32		
Millesi et al., 1972, 1976	Civilian	2-20	39	11-69	23
Walton & Finseth, 1977	Civilian	2-6	2	16-50	
Tallas et al., 1978	Civilian	3-7	10		
Young et al., 1980	Civilian	>2	5	15-57	
Hoase et al., 1980	Civilian	1.5-7	26	9-73	
Yamano, 1982	Civilian	5-9	2	6.5	100
Beazley et al., 1984	Civilian	2-7	6	0.5-71	
Vastamaki et al., 1993	Civilian	2-10	76	5-58	10

Note: From *Surgery of the Peripheral Nerve,* by S. E. Mackinnon, & A. L. Dellon 1988, New York: Thieme Publishing. Adapted with permission of the authors.

Follow-up (yr)	Motor Recovery (%)								
	M2	M3	M4	M5	S2	S2+	S3	S3+	S4
1-15									3
2-3	0	36	18	0	10	18	45	18	0
>5	0	69	0	0	21	0	69	0	0
5-11	7	21	14	46	3	0	60	34	3
1.5-2.5	12	0	50	0	13	0	12	63	12
1.5-2.5		33	16	33				33	
1-5		0	0	0	0	37	38	25	0
average M2+	0				average S2				0
4					0	0	22	28	50
10		32	48	20	38	15	25	14	9

Follow-up (yr)	Motor Recovery (%)				Sensory Recovery (%)				
	M2	M3	M4	M5	S2	S2+	S3	S3+	S4
1-15									0
5-11	8	31	18	31	0	15	65	15	5
1.5-2.5	0	50	0	0	50	0	50	0	0
1.5-3.5	20	50	30	0	20	20	40	24	0
1-5				20		0	0	60	0
2.5-5	7	45	48	0	30	5	15		50
2.5-5	0	0	100	0			?		
2-6	average M2			0		average S1			0
3-20	36	10	26	26	32	20	22	11	15

TABLE 11.12   RESULTS OF PERONEAL NERVE REPAIR/GRAFT

Author	No. of Cases Repair/ Graft	Surgery Timing Related to Injury							
		<6 Months Result				>6 Months Result			
		M4 & M5	M3	M2	M0 & M1	M4 & M5	M3	M2	M1 & M0
Millesi, 1986*	4/29	3	0	2	2	13	5	1	7
Wilkinson & Birch, 1995	3/24	8	1	0	4	3	2	1	8

Note:
*The last 9 patients in the series had a posterior tibialis transfer to the anterior tibialis at the time of nerve grafting.
From "Secondary Repair of Sciatic Nerve Lesions," by H. Millesi, 1986, *Peripheral Nerve Regeneration and Repair 4:*39-43; and "Repair of Common Peroneal Nerve," by M. C. P. Wilkinson & R. Birch, 1995, *Journal of Bone and Joint Surgery 77B:*501-503. Adapted with permission of the authors.

TABLE 11.13   RESULTS OF SCIATIC NERVE RECONSTRUCTION

Level	Results	All Cases
3	Good	28
3(T+P)	Tibial and peroneal nerves	6
3(T)	Tibial Nerve only	22
2	Satisfactory	6
1	Poor	5
0	Nil	—
Total		39

Note:
*NL = neurolysis; NG = nerve graft
From *Surgery of the Peripheral Nerve,* by S. E. Mackinnon & A. L. Dellon, 1988, New York: Thieme Publishing. Reprinted with permission of the authors.

	Sensory Reeducation	
	With	**Without**
Replanted Thumb	Schlenker, Kleinert, & Tsai, 1980 mean of 6 mm s2PD	Tamai, 1982 70 % > S3+
Big Toe-to-Thumb Transfers	Lister, Kalisman, & Tsai, 1983 75% < 10 mm s2PD	Poppen, Norris, & Buncke, 1983 mean 14.8 mm s2PD
Second Toe-to-Thumb Transfers	Minami et al., 1984 mean 6.7 mm s2PD	Poppen, Norris, & Buncke, 1983 mean 13.5 ms2PD Morrison, O'Brien, & MacLeod, 1984 mean 17 mm s2PD
Second and Third Toe Transfers	Tsai et al., 1981 mean 10.5 mm s2PD	O'Brien, Brenner, & MacLeod, 1978 > 20 mm s2PD

Note: From "Sensory Recovery in Replanted Digits and Transplanted Toes: A Review," by A. L. Dellon, 1986, *Journal of Reconstructive Microsurgery 2:*123-129. Reprinted with permission of the author.

According to Site of Lesion and Type of Operation

Foramen Infrapiriforme NL+NG*	Gluteal Area NL (Injection Lesion)	NG	Thigh NG+NL	NL
9	5	7	2	5
2	1	2	1	—
7	4	5	1	5
1	1	3	1	—
—	—	4	—	1
—	—	—	—	—
10	6	14	3	6

TABLE 11.15   SENSORY RECOVERY IN INNERVATED FREE-TISSUE TRANSFERS FOOT TO THE HAND

Author/Year	Area Reconstruction	Flap Utilized	Donor Nerve	Recipient Nerve
Morrison et al., 1977	thumb	big toe hemipulp	plantar	digital
Strauch & Tsur, 1978	palm thumb web	1st web 1st web	deep peroneal common plantar	common volar digital
Morrison et al., 1980	thumb	big toe wrap around	deep peroneal	radial sensory
Leung et al., 1980	thumb finger	2nd toe 2nd toe	plantar plantar	digital digital
Foucher, 1980	thumb finger	big toe hemipulp big toe hemipulp	plantar plantar	digital digital
Morrison et al., 1982	thumb thumb	big toe 2nd toe	plantar plantar	digital digital
Lister et al., 1983	thumb fingers	big toe 2nd/3rd toe	plantar plantar	digital digital
Gordon et al., 1985	thumb fingers	big toe 2nd toe	plantar plantar	digital digital
Kato et al., 1989	thumb thumb	big toe hemipulp 2nd toe	plantar plantar	digital digital

Note:

*Sensory reeducation given post-operatively
From "Sensory Recovery in Innervated Free-tissue Transfers", by B. Graham & A. L. Dellon, 1995, *Journal of Reconstructive Surgery 11:*157-166. Reprinted with permission of the authors.

Result
3/7 > 20 mm s2PD
4/7 x 14 mm s2PD
3-7 mm m2PD
6-8 mm m2PD
7-20 mm s2PD
3-15 mm s2PD*
3-15 mm s2PD*
4-7 mm s2PD*
10 mm s2PD
3-7 mm s2PD*
6-14 mm s2PD
17 mm s2PD
15 mm s2PD
6/16 <10 mm s2PD*
9/12 <10 mm s2PD*
6 to >15 mm s2PD
5 to >15 mm s2PD
10.7 mm s2PD*
8.1 mm m2PD*
13.3 mm s2PD*
9.8 mm m2PD*

TABLE 11.16   SENSORY RECOVERY IN REPLANTED FINGERS

| Digit | Number | Mean Static Two-Point Related to Injury | | S3+ and S4 |
		Clean Cut	Crush/Avulsion	
Thumb	87	9.3 mm	12.1 mm	61%
Finger	367	8.1 mm	15.4 mm	54%

Note: From "Sensory Recovery Following Digit Replantation," by L. Glickman & S. E. Mackinnon, 1990, *Microsurgery 11:*236-242. Reprinted with permission of the authors.

FIGURE 11.14

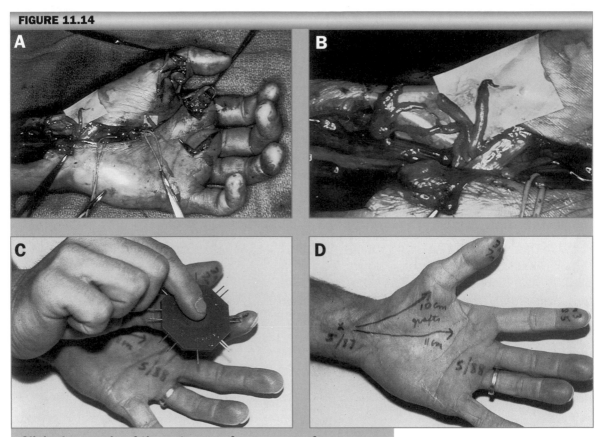

*Clinical example of the outcome of a program of sensory re-
education begun as soon as possible in the postoperative period.
(A) This 35-year-old man sustained a crush/avulsion injury to
his palm. (B) The intact median nerve did not recover any
sensation by 3 months after the injury, and it was elected to
reconstruct the median nerve with interfascicular sural nerve
grafts from the wrist to the metacarpophalangeal level with
nerve grafts. Two 10 cm grafts were placed into the thumb
and two 11 cm grafts were placed into the index finger. (C)
The Disk-Criminator™ was used for late phase sensory reeducation. (D) By 1 year after the nerve reconstruction, moving
and static two-point discrimination had been recovered in the
thumb and index fingertips.*

results of nerve grafting in the hand is given in Figure 11.14. Figure 11.15 plots a small series of digital, median, and ulnar nerve repairs against the patient's age, and includes *Önne's line* to make clear the level of sensory recovery that might have been expected if sensory reeducation had not been included. Önne's line plots were suggested by Moberg because Lars Önne, in reviewing the results of Moberg's best nerve repair cases, arrived at the conclusion that the results recovered as measured by (static) two-point discrimination, at 5 years following the repair, would be equal to the patient's age (Önne, 1962). Thus, any data point that lies below the diagonal line suggests that the therapeutic intervention, in addition to the nerve repair itself, achieved an improved result.

In Figure 11.15, all plotted data points are for 2 years, not 5 years, supporting the statement that sensory reeducation not only improved the final level of recovery, but permitted it to be reached in a shorter period of time.

FIGURE 11.15

Results of sensory reeducation demonstrated by plotting each patient's end result, as measured by static two- point discrimination testing, against the patient's age. (A) Each patient has the potential to achieve a certain level of recovery based on the mechanism of injury, the nerve reconstruction itself, and the patient's age. Most patients will achieve less than this potential. Sensory reeducation provides the basis for the patient to achieve the full level of potential. "Önne's line" represents the best results achieved in ideal cases of nerve repair at 5 years after the repair (Önne, 1962). A rehabilitation strategy, or surgical technique, that improves the results compared with traditional results will appear on the plot below Önne's line. The results of my first small series of patients plotted in this manner; (B) digital nerve repair; and (C) ulnar nerve repair. The dots that are filled-in circles represent median and ulnar nerve repairs that were in the forearm; all others are at wrist level. From Evaluation of Sensibility and Re-Education in the Hand, *by A. L. Dellon, 1981, Baltimore: Williams & Wilkins.*

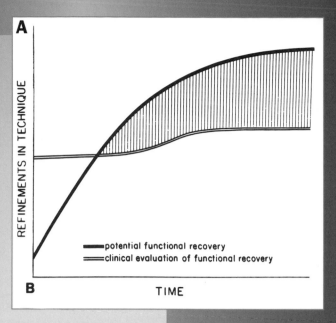

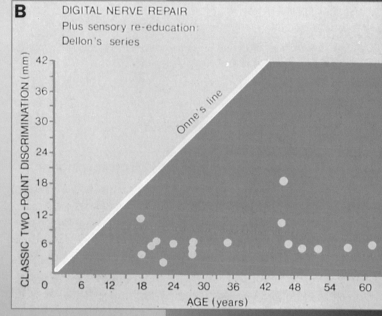

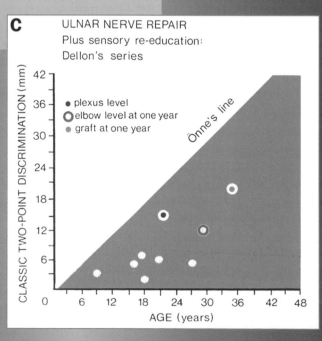

PROTOCOLS FOR SENSORY REEDUCATION

F ollowing are protocols for sensory reeducation that have worked for 5 institutions.

• • •

Raymond M. Curtis Hand Center
Union Memorial Hospital
Baltimore, Maryland

TECHNIQUES OF SENSORY REEDUCATION

S ensory reeducation is a method or combination of techniques that help the patient with sensory impairment learn to reinterpret the altered profile of neural impulses reaching his or her conscious level after the injured hand has been stimulated. In the normal state, stimulation of the hand by contact with the external environment stimulates the sensory receptors and a profile of neural impulses is elicited. These impact on the sensory cortex, associate with previous memory or experiences, and ultimately become a recognized perception. After a nerve division and nerve repair, the same contact with the external world, or the same stimulus, now elicits a different or altered profile of neural impulses. When these reach the sensory cortex, they may find no match in the association cortex. Thus, the sensation is new, cannot be named, and may even pass unnoticed.

This is the basic philosophy for sensory reeducation treatment after nerve laceration or compression. Unless these neural impulses are trained, sensation will be nonfunctional.

EARLY-PHASE SENSORY REEDUCATION

W hen 30 cps and moving touch have returned to an area, the palm, for example, early phase reeducation may begin. It is most critical to begin by the time recovery has reached the proximal phalanges.

Goals at this Stage
The goals of this stage are:
1. To reeducate specific perceptions, movements versus constant touch, and pressure, and
2. To reeducate misdirection or incorrect localization. The exercise is for the patient to use a soft in-

strument, like a pencil eraser, or someone else may use their fingertip, to stroke up and down the length of the area being reeducated. The patient observes what is happening, shuts his eyes, and concentrates on what he or she is perceiving, then opens his or her eyes to confirm again what is really happening. The patient should verbalize to himself or herself what he is perceiving as specifically as possible (e.g., "I feel something moving up (down) my index finger near the palm" [may draw numbers]).

When the patient can perceive constant touch, the same type of early phase reeducation is done for this touch submodality (e.g., the eraser is pressed down into one spot on the palm or finger within the area of recovered constant-touch perception and the patient first directly observes what is occurring, then shuts his or her eyes and repeats the stimulus, verbalizes to himself or herself what he or she is perceiving, opens his or her eyes, and reaffirms the stimulus and perception). Again, the patient should be saying, "I feel something pressing (hard or soft) on my index finger near my palm."

How hard should the stimulus be pressed into the finger? The newly reunited fiber or receptor system is "immature;" therefore, its threshold is high, and early in the recovery of sensation greater stimulus intensity must be used for perception to occur. Press the moving or stationary eraser as hard as necessary for the patient to perceive constant touch or movement. (Stimulus intensity should never evoke perception of pain. We are not reeducating the pain perception.)

Who Performs Early Phase Sensory Reeducation?

The surgeon, when examining the patient, will do these exercises to ascertain the degree of recovery. This may be about once a month and should reinforce the whole motivational and emotional system and the need for reeducation.

The therapist should be seeing the patient in a quiet, distraction-free room, 2 or 3 times a week, if possible, for approximately 10 to 15 minutes, to reinforce the goals, check the progress, and provide reassurance.

The patient should be encouraged to practice early phase sensory reeducation 3 to 4 times a day, even if just for 5 minutes a day, in a quiet, distraction-free room.

Any interested person (spouse, mother, sister, boyfriend) can be shown the sensory reeducation techniques and be pressed into service.

Early phase sensory reeducation should be introduced to the fingertip 4 to 6 months after a median or ulnar nerve repair at wrist level.

LATE-PHASE SENSORY REEDUCATION

Late phase sensory reeducation should begin as soon as moving touch and constant touch can be perceived at the fingertip with good localization. This can be as early as 6 to 8 months after median or ulnar nerve repair at the wrist. It is important at the beginning of this phase that the patient be told that he or she will continue slow improvement in his or her ability to recognize objects. The patient will not be able to differentiate the smallest objects until 10 to 12 months after nerve repair at the wrist.

Goal at this Stage

The goal at this stage is to guide the patient to recovery of tactilegnosis (object identification).

Sensory reeducation cannot induce axonal regeneration; it can only help the patient achieve the fullest potential provided by the nerve repair.

Since the goal of late phase sensory reeducation is recovery of functional sensation, the specific exercises should involve object identification.

Tactile discrimination recovers progressively over time as measured by both static and moving two-point discrimination. At any given time in the recovery process that moving two-point discrimination has recovered to a greater degree than static two-point discrimination, the object recognition tasks should incorporate movement.

The exercises should be graded, beginning with the discrimination of larger objects, with great differences among them in size, shape, and texture, if possible, and progressing to more subtle differences.

Late phase sensory reeducation is begun with a set of familiar household objects, differing widely in shape, size, and texture. Again, the sequence of object grabs with eyes open and shut with concentration of perception, eyes open for reinforcement, is utilized. After the patient has practice with the object, the therapist may test him or her and record either the number of objects identified correctly or the time required (in seconds with a stop watch) for object identification. A record such as this provides evidence to the patient, therapist, and referring physician that progress is occurring. Also, it assists patient motivation by giving the patient a goal "to beat" next time.

Late phase sensory reeducation is continued by progressing to objects differing primarily in texture, and then to objects that are smaller, differing in size and shape, but not in texture and requiring subtle discrimination. At this stage, the patient will be clinically recovering; static two-point discrimination will be less than 7 mm.

As moving two-point discrimination drops below 5 mm, patients will be able to identify the smallest objects correctly, although they may fall from the patient's grasp because the slowly-adapting fiber and receptor system has not regenerated and matured sufficiently. A Disk-Criminator™ can be given to the patient for continuation of late phase reeducation at home.

Late phase sensory reeducation also provides motor education. Activities that duplicate or incorporate work motions or activities should be included in the patient's therapy.

It is ideal to have the patient attend the workshop, working on a work simulator, to practice specific sensory grips before the patient is ready to try the actual tool at his job.

Who Performs Late Phase Sensory Reeducation?

The surgeon, whenever he or she examines the patient, should test moving and static two-point discrimination and object recognition. In so doing, praise, reinforcement, reassurance, and motivation are provided to sustain the patient and

back up what the therapist has been doing. At this point, the surgeon should be seeing the patient every 3 months.

The therapist should be seeing the patient weekly, progressing to biweekly and perhaps monthly, between the start of late phase reeducation (6 to 9 months after repair) and the patient's return to work. The therapist should be working through the exercises, testing and recording the results of object recognition, encouraging and reinforcing the patient. At each session, both static and two-point discrimination should be recorded.

The patient should be practicing at home 3 to 4 times a day, 5 to 10 minutes each time. Frequent short sessions are more productive than longer, less frequent sessions. Late phase exercises can be modified, depending on the nerve involved.

Median Nerve

All of the exercises described are applicable and essentially involve three-jaw chuck pinch or gripping of objects between thumb, index, and middle fingers and manipulating the object. A glove may be cut and modified to cover the ulnar digits leaving the thumb, index, and long fingers exposed. This will facilitate mobility of the hand but decrease sensory input from the ulnar nerve.

Ulnar Nerve or Digital Nerve Injuries

A second person's presence during exercise is helpful. That person can place objects for recognition onto the surface of the fingertip being reeducated. Less precise but still helpful is for the patient to manipulate an object between the thumb and the fingertip being reeducated. Here, the patient must try to concentrate on the perceptions being transmitted via the injured finger instead of those coming from the thumb.

OTHER TECHNIQUES OF REEDUCATION

Also useful are bilateral exercises in which the patient differentiates between various textures of material and grades of sandpaper first with vision, and then without vision.

Sand, rice, or bean media can be used for sensory reeducation. Without visual clues, patients must identify objects within a pile of sand, rice, or beans.

Once the patient has recovered functional sensationsensory reeducation should be continued.

The program should be followed for a long time. If the patient returns to work, or resumes housekeeping, or is a child, the reeducation is continued at this level and no formal program is required.

If the patient discontinues sensory reeducation exercises and active daily use of the hand, the effect of the reeducation program is lost by the time the patient is next tested. If reeducation exercises are resumed, function is quickly recovered. After recovery has proceeded for some time, the patient becomes increasingly able to maintain his or her reeducated status.

This reeducation program must be designed and modified on an individual basis.

• • •

SUNNYBROOK MEDICAL CENTER HAND SERVICE UNIVERSITY OF TORONTO TORONTO, ONTARIO, CANADA

GUIDELINES FOR PERSONS WITH DECREASED SENSATION

1. Avoid exposing your hand to sharp, hot, or very cold objects.
2. To keep skin soft and smooth, follow a daily routine of skin care, including soaking in warm water and massaging with NIVEA cream or Vitamin E cream.
3. If blisters, cuts, or other wounds occur, treat them with the utmost care to avoid further injury and possible infection. If you are uncertain about an injury, please call the office.
4. When gripping an object, do not apply more force than is necessary.
5. Avoid work that requires use of one tool for a long period of time. (Especially if the hand is unable to change its manner of grip.)
6. Change tools or objects you use frequently to rest tissue and skin.
7. Watch the skin for signs of stress: redness, swelling, warmth. Rest hand if these signs occur.
8. Begin sensory reeducation program as soon as the doctor or therapist advises you.

SENSORY REEDUCATION HOME PROGRAM

"In the normal state, stimulation of the hand by contact with the external environment stimulates the sensory receptors, a profile of neural impulses is elicited, these impact upon the sensory cortex, associate with previous memory or experiences, and ultimately become consciousness, a perception. After a nerve division and nerve repair, the same contact with the external world, the same stimulus now elicits a different or an altered profile of neural impulses. When these reach the sensory cortex, they may find no match in the association cortex. Thus, the sensation is new, cannot by named, and may even pass unnoticed."

(Dellon, A. L. *Evaluation of Sensibility and Re-education of Sensation in the Hand*. Baltimore: Williams & Wilkins, 1981, p. 210.)

- *Purpose:* To *concentrate* on sensations until your brain learns the correct responses.
- *Procedure:* Choose a quiet area with few distractions. Complete the exercises 3 times each day.
- *Sequence:* Follow an eyes open, eyes closed, eyes open sequence for each exercise.

EARLY PHASE

Localization exercises:
1. *Moving touch/pressure*
   (a) Use a pencil eraser. Stroke up and down the area indicated with eyes open and think about how it feels. Notice where you placed it.
   (b) Close eyes and repeat. Try to describe where the eraser was felt.
   (c) Open eyes and check on what is happening.
   (d) Repeat entire se-

quence 5 times. Move to another area.

Keeping to the sequence outlined, progress to doing this with lighter pressure, working up to a light touch with cotton wool or from a helper's fingertips.

2. *Constant touch/pressure*
   (a) Press the pencil eraser into one spot in the area indicated. Hold it for one second with eyes open and think about how it feels.
   (b) Close eyes and repeat. Concentrate on where you feel it and how it feels.
   (c) Open eyes and check on what is happening.
   (d) Repeat entire sequence 5 times. Move to another area.

Keeping to the sequence outlined, progress to doing this with lighter pressure, working up to light touch with cotton wool or from a helper's fingertip.

Discrimination:
1. *Texture discrimination*
   (a) Use the dowels provided (with different texture at each end, for example, moleskin and velcro).
   (b) Rub the two ends of each dowel in the area indicated. Watch as you do it and ask yourself: Are the textures the same or different? How are they different? Describe to yourself the texture

felt at each end.
   (c) Close eyes and repeat.
   (d) Open eyes and check your accuracy.
   (e) Repeat the sequence 5 times with each dowel. Move to another area.

LATE PHASE

When you can successfully identify and localize moving and constant light touch at the fingertip, late phase reeducation is introduced. The object now is to recognize common objects by touch alone—*stereognosis*.

1. *Two-point discrimination*
   (a) Use Disk-Criminator™ provided. Move the pins lengthwise in the area indicated. Try different spacings, watch as you do it and think about how it feels. Compare one moving point with two. Can you tell the difference at 8 mm, 6 mm, 3 mm, etc.?
   (b) Repeat the sequence (eyes open, eyes closed, eyes open) 5 times asking the question each time. Move to another area.
   (c) Have someone test you from time to time, and compare with your noninjured hand to see how accurate you are.
   (d) Repeat the whole procedure applying pressure in the area indi

cated, but not moving the device.

2. *Large Object Identification*
   (a) Collect everyday objects of different size, shape, and texture, or use kit provided. Pick out one object at a time and manipulate it with eyes open. Describe its shape, texture, and weight.
   (b) Close eyes and repeat for all objects.
   (c) Have someone test you from time to time to see how many you get right and how quickly you do it in seconds.
   (d) Change the objects frequently.

3. *Small Object Identification*
   (a) Collect small everyday objects, or use kit provided. Follow the sequence given above for large objects. Keep a few small objects in a pocket and try identifying them by feel.

4. *Shape/Letter/Number Recognition:*
   (a) Cut shapes, letters, or numbers out of sandpaper and stick into pieces of wood or cardboard. Feel with fingertips and eyes open.
   (b) Place face down on table, turn over with eyes closed and feel again. Try to identify

by touch.

(c) Open eyes and see if you were correct.

● ● ●

LUBBOCK ORTHOPEDIC SURGERY CLINIC AND HAND SURGERY SERVICE, DEPARTMENT OF ORTHOPEDIC SURGERY, TEXAS TECH UNIVERSITY SCHOOL OF MEDICINE
LUBBOCK, TEXAS

SENSORY REEDUCATION PROGRAM

GUIDELINES FOR PERSONS WITH DECREASED SENSATION

1. Avoid exposing your hand to sharp, hot, or very cold objects.
2. To keep skin soft and smooth, follow a daily routine of skin care, including soaking in warm water and massaging with NIVEA creme.
3. If blisters, cuts, or other wounds occur, treat them with the utmost care to avoid further injury and possible infection. If you are uncertain about an injury, please call the office.
4. When gripping an object, do not apply more force than is necessary.
5. Avoid work that requires use of one tool for a long period of time. (Especially if the hand is unable to change its manner of grip.)
6. Change tools or objects you use frequently to rest tissue and skin.
7. Watch the skin for signs of stress: redness, swelling, warmth. Rest the hand if these signs occur.
8. Begin sensory reeducation program as soon as the doctor or therapist advises you to do so.

SENSORY REEDUCATION HOME PROGRAM

For the early phase see the protocol for the Sunnybrook Medical Center Hand Service (see Figure 11.16).

LATE PHASE

Stereognosis: The ability to recognize common objects by touch alone.

1. Good motor function
   (a) Place objects provided in a bowl in front of you. Pick out one object at a time and manipulate it with eyes open. Describe its shape.
   (b) Close your eyes and manipulate the object. Describe the object.
   (c) Open your eyes and repeat. Do this sequence with each object.
   (d) Replace all objects in bowl.
   (e) With eyes closed, pick out one object at a time and try to identify it.
   (f) Open your eyes and see if you were correct.
   (g) Repeat this with each object until all are removed from the bowl.

2. Poor motor function
   (a) Using your hand (or with assistance), place one object at a time into your affected hand and move it around. Describe its shape.
   (b) Close your eyes and move the object around in your palm. Describe its shape.
   (c) Open your eyes and repeat. Do this sequence with each object.
   (d) Follow the same directions for d, e, f, and g above.

Note: When you are able to identify correctly all the objects provided with eyes open and closed, gather your own set of ten household items and repeat the exercises. Try to find objects that are similar in shape.

● ● ●

NORTH PALM BEACH HAND REHABILITATION NORTH PALM BEACH FLORIDA

DEWEY DISC SENSORY REEDUCATION SYSTEM

As hand therapists, we instruct patients in various methods and techniques to reeducate their damaged cutaneous sensory nerves. There are a few home programs, such as the Dellon program utilized at the Curtis Hand Center, that are simple to use and cost-effective for the patient to perform on a repetitive basis at home.

The Dewey Disc program has 3 cm plastic discs with a ¹⁄₁₆ and ¹⁄₃₂ inch raised number (1.5 cm width) from 0 to 9. Once the ¹⁄₁₆ numbers can be correctly identified by the affected digit with vision occluded, the patient progresses to the ¹⁄₃₂ inch raised numbers at 1.5 cm width and then possibly to smaller numbers as sensation improves. The discs are small and can easily be carried during the day for frequent manipulation. They can be held flat on a table for single digit manipulation, or held against the thumb for manipulation.

We suggest this program for patients with more advanced cutaneous sensibility because we have found that static two-point discrimination must be present at the

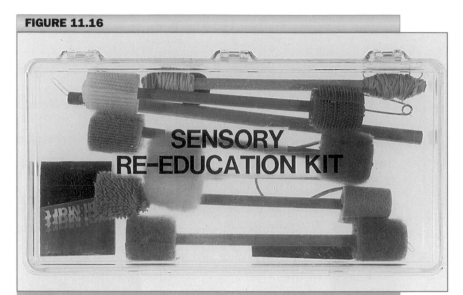

FIGURE 11.16

Royce Lewis's deceased Sensory Reeducation Kit. This is given to patients at his Lubbock, Texas clinic to take home with them. Note objects differing in size and texture. Photo taken by Lee Dellon, with permission.

digit pulp for success with identification of the ¹⁄₃₂ inch raised numbers. We anticipate that identification of geometric shapes with ¹⁄₁₆ inch rise will be easier to identify.

We issue the patient with nerve-injured digits three to four discs to begin a sensory reeducation program. We request that he or she begin by manipulating the discs with their involved digits by looking and feeling first, and then by feeling without looking. We ask that the patient carry the discs in their pocket and manipulate them constantly throughout the day, or that they work on this reeducation program for 15 to 20 minutes at least 4 times

a day. We initially give patients unlike numbers such as 1, 3, and 7, and when they have mastered identification of unlike numbers, we exchange their discs for like numbers, such as 3, 8, and 9. We record progress on a weekly or bimonthly basis by asking the patient to identify the discs at the clinic with vision occluded. We give the patient trials and record the number of correct responses.

The discs are packaged as a complete sensory reeducation kit, including three geometric shapes and numbers 1 through 8. The number 6 can also be correctly identified as a 9, and the number 0 can be used as the circle in the geometric shapes.

● ● ●

CHANG GUNG MEMORIAL HOSPITAL MICROSURGERY REHABILITATION DEPARTMENT TAIPEI, TAIWAN

Toe-to-Hand Transfer

EARLY-PHASE SENSORY REEDUCATION

Designed to promote recognition of touch submodalities, such as constant touch and moving touch (see Figure 11.17). Blunt object is either pressed or moved along the surface of the transplanted toe. This is begun in the 6th week after transplantation, by which time the perception of a 30 Hz tuning fork has usually occurred. These specific sensory exercises are utilized while the patient is both looking at the tips of the transplanted toe(s) and verbalizing, "I feel something moving on my finger," or "I feel something pressing on my finger." This exercise is then repeated with the patient's eyes closed. The patient is seen weekly in the rehabilitation unit, if possible, depending upon their geographic location. They are instructed to practice this at home four times, for five minutes, every day. This is done in addition to their motor exercises.

LATE-PHASE SENSORY REEDUCATION

When moving and constant touch can be distinguished from each other, the goal then becomes identification of objects with the tips of the transplanted toe (toes), either between themselves, or between the transplanted toe and a remaining finger (see Figure 11.18). The object is picked up between the digits, accomplishing a motor task, and the object is manipulated between the digits while the patient directly observes the sensory stimulus. Then the patient closes the eyes and concentrates on the perception of that stimulus.

If the motor ability is not sufficient for picking up the objects, then the therapist will place them between the digits. If the object is to be grasped between a toe and a finger, the patient is instructed to try to pay attention or focus upon the stimulus received from the transplant. A small finger "cot" or cut off glove piece may be placed upon the normal finger to minimize sensory input from this finger during reeducation. The patient is instructed to do this four times a day, for five minutes each time. The patient is observed in the rehabilitation unit weekly, if geography permits.

Progress is charted both by changes in moving and static two-point discrimination, by the types of objects recognized, and sometimes by the time required to recognize the object when it is placed between the digits (Ma, El-Gammal, & Wei, 1996; Wei & Ma, 1996).

● ● ●

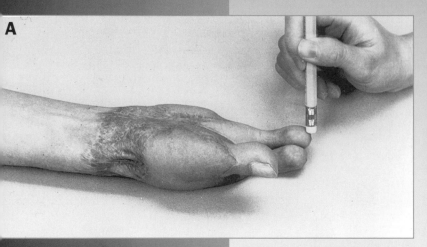

A

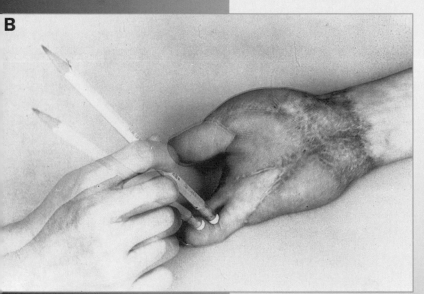

B

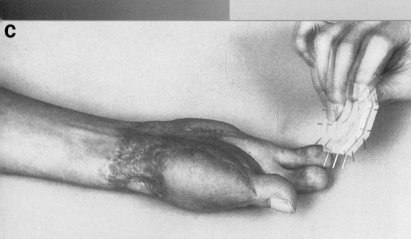

C

FIGURE 11.17

Sensory Reeducation, Early Phase, for Toe-to-Hand Transfer. This patient has had the big toe transferred to the thumb position from one foot and a composite 2nd/3rd toe transferred to the ulnar border of the hand from the second foot. In (A), the perception of constant touch and pressure is being reeducated. In (B), the pencil is being used to train the perception of moving touch. In (C), the Disk-Criminator™ is illustrated for the use of reeducation of moving touch. Note that if just one prong is used, this is considered early phase. In this illustration, two prongs are being used, which is appropriate for late phase, as in Figure 11.14C. Photos courtesy of Helena S. Ma, OTR, Chief of Rehabilitation and F. C. Wei, MD., Chang Gung Memorial Hospital, Taipai, Taiwan.

FIGURE 11.18

Sensory Reeducation, Late Phase, for Toe-to-Hand Transfer. Three different patients are used to illustrate (A) the placement of an object between the digits prior to accomplishing the motor ability to do this, as in (B). In (A) and (B), note the range of small objects used for late phase sensory reeducation, differing in size, shape, and texture. In (C), perhaps the ultimate in sensorimotor requirements, holding an object between chopsticks, without visual cues for feedback. Photos courtesy of Helena S. Ma, OTR Chief of Rehabilitation and F.-C. Wei, MD., Chang Gung Memorial Hospital, Taipai, Taiwan.

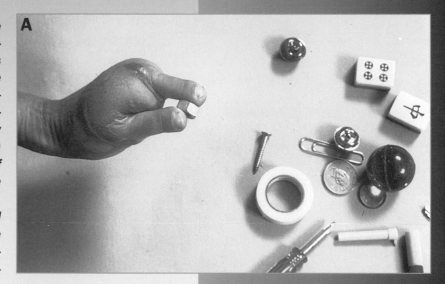

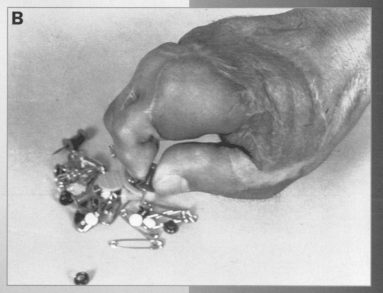

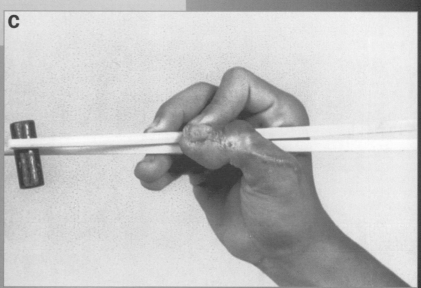

• REFERENCES •

Anthony, M. S. Sensory Re-education. In *Hand Rehabilitation: A Practical Guide*, G. L. Clark, E. F. S. Wilgis, B. Aiello, D. Eckhaus, & L. V. Eddington, Editors. New York: Churchill Livingstone, 1993.

Anthony, M. S. Desensitization. In *Hand Rehabilitation: A Practical Guide*, G. L. Clark, E. F. S. Wilgis, B. Aiello, D. Eckhaus, & L. V. Eddington, Editors. New York: Churchill Livingstone, 1993.

Azman, O., Muse, V., & Dellon, A. L. Evidence in support of collateral sprouting in the human. *Annals of Plastic Surgery*, in press: 1996.

Barber, L. M. Desensitization of the traumatized hand. In *Rehabilitation of the Hand: Surgery and Therapy*, J. M. Hunter, L. H. Schneider, E. J. Mackin, & A. D. Callahan, Editors. St. Louis: C. V. Mosby Company, 1984.

Brown, C. J., Mackinnon, S. E., Dellon, A. L., & Bain, J. R. The sensory potential of free flap donor sites. *Annals of Plastic Surgery 23*:135-140, 1989.

Callahan, A. D. Methods of compensation and reeducation of sensory dysfunction. In *Rehabilitation of the Hand: Surgery and Therapy*, J. M. Hunter, L. H. Schneider, E. J. Mackin, & A. D. Callahan, Editors. St. Louis: C. V. Mosby Company, 1984, Chapter 37.

Campbell, J. N., Meyer, R. A., & La Motte, R. H. Sensitization of myelinated nociceptive afferents that innervate the monkey's hand. *Journal of Neurophysiology 42*:1669-1679, 1979.

Campbell, J. N., Raja, S. N., Meyer, R. A., & Mackinnon, S. E. Myelinated fibers in peripheral nerves signal hyperalgesia that follows nerve injury. *Pain 32*:89-94, 1988.

Carter-Wilson, M. Sensory Re-Education. In *Operative Nerve Repair and Reconstruction*, R. H. Gelberman, Editor. Philadelphia: J. B. Lippincott Company, 1991.

Chapman, C. E. Active versus passive touch: Factors influencing the transmission of somatosensory signals to primary somatosensory cortex. *Canadian Journal of Physiologic Pharmacology 72*:558-570, 1994.

Curtis, R. T., & Dellon, A. L. Sensory re-education after peripheral nerve injury. In *Management of Peripheral Nerve Injuries,* M. Spinner & G. Omer, Editors. Philadelphia: W. B. Saunders Company, 1980.

Dannenbaum, R.M., & Dykes, R.W. Sensory loss in the hand after sensory stroke: Therapeutic rationale. *Archives of Physical Medicine and Rehabilitation 69*:833-839, 1988.

Dannenbaum, R. M., & Jones, L. A. The assessment and treatment of patients who have sensory loss following cortical lesions. *Journal of Hand Therapy 6*:130-138, 1993.

Dellon, A. L. *Evaluation of Sensibility and Re-Education of Sensation in the Hand*. Baltimore: Williams & Wilkins, 1981.

Dellon, A. L., Curtis, R. M., & Edgerton, M. T. Reeducation of sensation in the hand following hand injury. *Journal of Bone and Joint Surgery 53A*:813, 1971.

Dellon, A. L. Sensory recovery in replanted digits and transplanted toes; A review. *Journal of Reconstructive Microsurgery 2*:123-129, 1986.

Dellon, A. L., Curtis, R. M., & Edgerton, M. T. Re-education of sensation in the hand following nerve injury. *Plastic and Reconstructive Surgery 53*:297-305, 1974.

Dellon, A. L., & Kallman, C. H. Evaluation of functional sensation in the hand. *Journal of Hand Surgery 8*:865-870, 1983.

Glickman, L. T., & Mackinnon, S. E. Sensory recovery following digital replantation. *Microsurgery 11*:236-240, 1990.

Graham, B., & Dellon, A. L. Sensory recovery in innervated free-tissue transfers. Journal of *Reconstructive Microsurgery 11*:157-166, 1995.

Hardy, M. A., Moran, C. A., & Merritt, W. H. Desensitization of the traumatized hand. *Virginia Medicine 109*:134-140, 1982.

Imai, H., Tajima, T., & Natsuma, Y. Interpretation of cutaneous pressure threshold

(Semmes-Weinstein monofilament measurement) following median nerve repair and sensory re-education. *Microsurgery* *10*:142-145, 1989.

Imai, H., Tajima, T., & Natsuma, Y. Successful re-education of functional sensibility after median nerve repair at the wrist. *Journal of Hand Surgery 16A:*60-65, 1991.

Jiang, W., Chapman, C. E., & Lamarre, Y. Modulation of the cutaneous responsiveness of neurones in the primary somatosensory cortex during conditioned arm movements in the monkey. *Experimental Brain Research 84*:342-354, 1991.

Lebedev, L. V., Bogomolov, M. S., Vavylov, V. N., Slomin, V. V., Tokavetich, K. K., Yustaev, E. A., Garbunov, G. N., & Dadalov, M. I. Long-term results of hand function after digital replantation. Annals of Plastic Surgery 31:322-326, 1993.

Ma, H. S., El-Gammal, T. A., & Wei, F. C. Current concepts of toe-to-hand transfer: Surgery and Rehabilitation. Journal of Hand Therapy, in press: 1997.

Mackinnon, S. E., & Dellon, A. L. Surgery of the Peripheral Nerve. New York: Thieme, 1988.

Merzenich, M. M., & Jenkins, W. M. Reorganization of cortical representations of the hand following alterations of skin inputs induced by nerve injury, skin island transfers, and experience. Journal of Hand Therapy 6:89-104, 1993.

Minami, A., Masamichi, V., Hiroyuki, K., & Seiichi, J. Thumb reconstruction by free sensory flaps from the foot using microsurgical techniques. Journal of Hand Surgery (British) 9:239-244, 1984.

Moberg, E. Objective methods of determining functional value of sensibility in the hand. Journal of Bone and Joint Surgery (British) 40:454-466, 1958.

Moberg, E. Two-point discrimination test. Scandinavian Journal of Rehabilitation Medicine 22:127-134, 1990.

Mori, A., Yamaguchi, Y., Kikuta, R., Furukawa, T., & Sumino, R. Low threshold motor effects produced by stimulation of the facial area of the fifth somatosensory cortex in the cat. Brain Research 602:143-147, 1993.

Nakada, M., & Dellon, A. L. Relationship between sensibility and ability to read braille in diabetics. *Microsurgery 10*:138-141, 1989.

Novak, C. B., Mackinnon, S. E., & Kelly, L. Correlation of two-point discrimination and hand function following median nerve injury. *Annals of Plastic Surgery 31:*495-498, 1993.

Novak, C. B., Mackinnon, S. E., Williams, J. I., & Kelly, L. Development of a new measure of fine sensory function. *Plastic and Reconstructive Surgery 92*:301-311, 1993.

Önne, L. Recovery of sensibility and submotor activity in the hand after nerve suture. *Acta Chirugia (Scandinavia) (Supplement) 300*:1-70, 1962.

Papakostopoulos, D., Cooper, R., & Crow, H. J. Inhibition of cortical evoked potentials and sensation by self-initiated movement in man. *Nature 258*:321-324, 1975.

Raja, S. N., Davis, K., & Campbell, J. N. Alpha-adranertic pharmacology in sympathetically-maintained pain. *Journal of Reconstructive Microsurgery 8*:63-69, 1992.

Raja, S. N., Meyer, R. A., & Campbell, J. N. Hyperalgesia and sensitization of primary afferent fibers. In *Pain Syndromes in Neurology*, H. L. Fields, Editor. London: Butterworths, 1990.

Robertson, S. L., & Jones, L. A. Tactile sensory impairments and prehensile function in subjects with left-hemisphere cerebral lesions. *Archives of Physical Medicine and Rehabilitation 75*:1108-1117, 1994.

Rosen, B., Lundborg, G., Dahlin, L. B., Holmberg, J., & Karlson, B. Nerve repair: Correlation of restitution of functional sensibility with specific cognitive capacities. *Journal of Hand Surgery 19B*:452-458, 1994.

Wei, F., & Ma, H. S. Delayed sensory reeducation after toe- to-hand transfer. *Journal of Reconstructive Microsurgery,* in press: 1997.

Wilson, R. L. Management of pain following peripheral nerve injuries. *Orthopedic Clinics of North America* 12:343-353, 1981.

• ADDITIONAL READINGS •

Anthony, M. S. Sensory re-education helps patients regain function of hands. *Advances in Physical Therapy* 21:19-21, March 1994.

Callahan, A. D. Methods of compensation and reeducation for sensory dysfunction. In *Rehabilitation of the Hand: Surgery and Therapy*, J. M. Hunter, L. H. Schneider, E. J. Mackin, & A. D. Callahan, Editors. St. Louis: C. V. Mosby Company, 1984.

Chassard, M., Pham, E., & Comtet, J. J. Two-point discrimination tests versus functional sensory recovery in both median and ulnar nerve complete transections. *Journal of Hand Surgery* 18B:790- 796, 1993.

Dellon, A. L., Curtis, R. M., & Edgerton, M. T. Re-education of sensation in the hand following nerve injury (abstract). *Journal of Bone and Joint Surgery* 53A:813, 1971.

Dellon, A. L., Curtis, R. M., & Edgerton, M. T. Evaluating recovery of sensation in the hand following nerve injury. *Johns Hopkins Medical Journal* 130:235-243, 1972.

Dijkstra, R., & Box, K. E. Functional results of thumb reconstruction. *Hand* 14:120-128, 1982.

Foucher, G., Merle, M., Maneaud, M., & Michon, J. Microsurgical free partial toe transfer in hand construction: A report of 12 cases. *Plastic and Reconstructive Surgery* 65:616-626, 1980.

Frykman, G. K., O'Brien, B. McC., Morrison, W. A., & MacLeod, A. M. Functional evaluation of the hand and foot after one-stage toe-to-hand transfer. *Journal of Hand Surgery* 11A:9-17, 1986.

Goldie, B. S., Coates, C. J., & Birch, R. The long-term results of digital nerve repair in no-man's land. *Journal of Hand Surgery* 17B:75-77, 1992.

Hunter, J. M., Schneider, L. H., Mackin, E. J., & Callahan, A. D. *Rehabilitation of the Hand: Surgery and Therapy*. St. Louis: C. V. Mosby Company, 1978.

Kallio, P. K. The results of secondary repair of 254 digital nerves. *Journal of Hand Surgery* 18B:327-330, 1993.

Kallio, P. K., & Vastamaki, M. An analysis of the results of late reconstruction of 132 median nerves. *Journal of Hand Surgery* 18B:97-105, 1993.

Maynard, J. Sensory re-education after peripheral nerve injury. In *Rehabilitation of the Hand: Surgery and Therapy*, J. M. Hunter, E. J. Mackin, L. H. Schneider, & A. D. Callahan, Editors. Baltimore: Williams & Wilkins, 1977.

Nakada, M. Localization of a constant-touch and moving-touch stimulus in the hand: A preliminary study. *Journal of Hand Therapy* 6:23-28, 1993.

Narita, M., & Aoki, M. Clinical study on sensory disturbance of the hand in leprosy. *Japanese Journal of Leprosy* 55:1-12, 1986.

Novak, C. B., Kelly, L., & Mackinnon, S. E. Sensory recovery after median nerve grafting. *Journal of Hand Surgery* 17A:59-66, 1992.

Rose, E. H., Kowalski, T. A., & Norris, M. S. The reversed venous arterialized nerve graft in digital nerve reconstruction across scarred beds. *Plastic and Reconstructive Surgery* 83:593-602, 1989.

Sinclair, R. J., & Burton, H. Neuronal activity in the second somatosensory cortex of monkeys (Macaca mulatta) during active touch of gratings. *Journal of Neurophysiology* 70:331-350, 1993.

Vastamaki, M., Kallio, P. K., & Solonen, K. A. The results of secondary microsurgical repair of ulnar nerve injury. *Journal of Hand Surgery* 18B:323-326, 1993.

Wei, F-C., Chien, Y. Y., Ma, H. S., & Dellon, A. L. The myelinated nerve fiber population of digital nerves in the fingers and toes. *Plastic and Reconstructive Surgery*, submitted: 1997.

Wynn Parry, C. *Rehabilitation of the Hand*.

London: Butterworths, 1966.

Yoshimura, M., Nomura, S., Yamauchi, S., Umeda, S., Uneo, T. & Iwai, Y. Toe-to-hand transfer: Experience with thirty-eight digits. *Australian and New Zealand Journal of Surgery 50*:248-254, 1980.

● ● ●

specific applications & normative data

12

upper extremity

T he hand serves as the model for sensibility testing and rehabilitation. The information presented in this chapter has wide application for many other areas of the body, and for many systemic diseases which traditionally might not have been considered the appropriate realm for interventional treatment, that is, the neuropathies (see Chapter 14). This chapter will explore the most common upper extremity problems that the therapist will encounter. Much other information related to the upper extremity is available in this book. For example, normative sensibility data is given in Chapter 7 as it relates to the different types of sensory testing equipment used to obtain that data. Problems related to hemiplegia are covered in Chapter 19. The results of upper extremity nerve repair and grafting, along with upper extremity rehabilitation in general and as related to pain management, are covered in Chapter 11. Some specific rehabilitation techniques will be discussed here related to clinical syndromes, and the involvement of the upper extremity in cumulative trauma is covered in Chapter 18.

This chapter will highlight the ability of computer-assisted sensorimotor testing to (a) measure upper extremity impairment; (b) document changes consistent with symptomatology, even in the presence of normal electrodiagnostic findings; (c) demonstrate sequential changes in a patient's neurologic status; and (d) increase the physician's efficiency in managing the patient's problems. The involvement of the therapist in

FIGURE 12.1

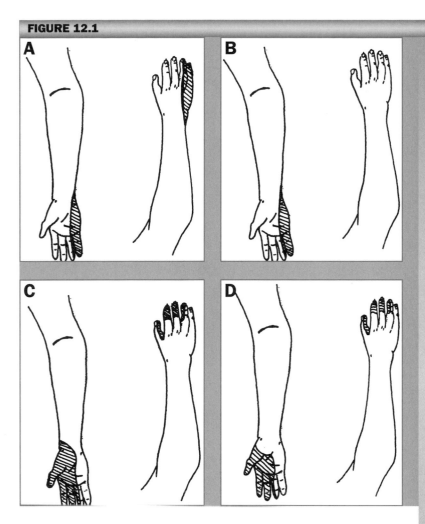

Representation of sensory territories of upper extremity nerves. (A) Proximal median nerve entrapment in the mid-forearm, beneath the deep head of the pronator teres and the sublimis muscle, causes the palmar cutaneous branch of the median nerve, and the thumb, index, middle, and half of the ring finger to have abnormal sensibility. This is in contrast to the more common entrapment of the median nerve at the wrist level (B), in which case there is normal sensibility over the thenar eminence, with just these fingers having abnormal sensibility. (C) Proximal ulnar nerve entrapment at the elbow causes the dorsal cutaneous branch of the ulnar nerve and the little finger and half of the ring finger to have abnormal sensibility. This is in contrast to the less common entrapment of the ulnar nerve at the wrist level in Guyon's canal (D), in which case there is normal sensibility over the ulnar dorsal half of the hand, with just these fingers having abnormal sensibility. Drawing by Glenn George Dellon. Reprinted with permission.

accomplishing these goals is crucial. In that regard, this chapter ends with the proto- col used to do sensory testing with the Pressure-Specified Sensory Device™.

• RELEVANT NEUROANATOMY •

Knowledge of the skin territories innervated by the different peripheral nerves (see Figure 12.1) and by the spinal cord sensory (posterior) roots (see Figure 12.2) is critical to doing the appropriate sensory test in the appropriate area of skin. The most common clinical problem to be associated with these skin territories is given in Table 12.1, along with the skin area to be tested that has the least anatomic variation associated with it.

The median nerve is formed by the joining of the terminal branch of the lateral cord of the brachial plexus with the terminal branch of the medial cord of the brachial plexus

FIGURE 12.2

Representation of the sensory territories supplied by the spinal roots to the upper extremity. (A) The C6 dermatome includes the palmar and dorsal surfaces of the hand on the radial side, in contrast to the radial sensory nerve (B) which innervates just the dorsoradial aspect of the hand and whose territory extends laterally toward the ring finger. (C) The C7 dermatome, and (D) the C8 dermatome. Drawing by Glenn George Dellon. Reprinted with permission.

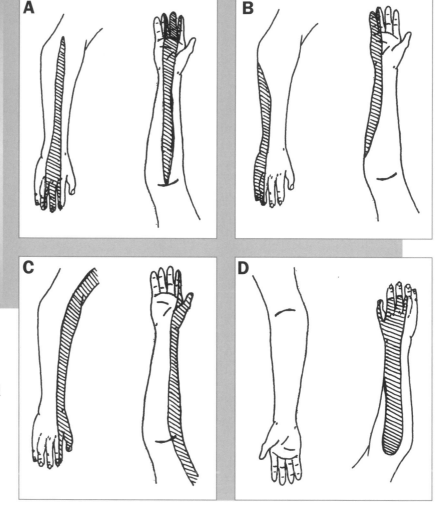

(see Figure 12.3). The lateral cord is located lateral to the axillary artery and contains the anterior division of the upper trunk. This contribution to the median nerve, therefore, contains C6 and C7 sensory fibers, thereby being responsible for the sensation of the thumb, index, middle, and half of the ring finger, including the dorsal skin to the tips of these fingers (through the dorsal branch of the volar digital nerves). The medial cord contains the posterior division of the lower trunk and, therefore, contributes C8 and T1 motor roots to the median nerve, with these innervating the abductor pollices brevis in 98% of specimens, the opponens pollices in 95% of people,

and the flexor halluces brevis, which is innervated by the median nerve, in 40% of patients. Less than 1% of hands have median nerve innervation to the little finger (Rowntree, 1949).

A division of the median nerve at the wrist level would give the sensory deficit just described plus loss of the median innervated intrinsic muscles, and is the deficit associated with severe carpal tunnel syndrome. The palmar cutaneous branch of the

median nerve originates 5 cm proximal to the wrist. Division of the median nerve proximal to the wrist, or compression of the median nerve in the forearm, such as the pronator syndrome (see Figure 12.4), will cause the additional sensory deficit of decreased sensation over the thenar eminence.

The palmar cutaneous branch of the median nerve travels in its own small tunnel adjacent to the flexor carpi radialis and may have

TABLE 12.1 CLINICO-ANATOMIC CORRELATES FOR SENSORY TESTING

Clinical Problem	Anatomic Site	Skin Test Area
Neck (C4/5 disc) pain	C5 root	lateral shoulder
Neck (C5/6 disc) pain	C6 root	dorsoradial hand/forearm
Neck (C6/7 disc) pain	C7 root	middle Finger
Neck (C7/T1 disc) pain	C8 root	little Finger/ulnar forearm
Brachial plexus injury	upper trunk	combination C5 & C6 roots
Brachial plexus injury	lateral cord	combination C5,6 & 7 roots
Brachial plexus injury	middle trunk	C7 Root
Brachial plexus injury	lower trunk/medial cord	C8 Root & upper inner arm
Brachial plexus injury	musculocutaneous nerve	proximal dorsoradial forearm
Carpal tunnel syndrome	median nerve; wrist level	index finger pulp
Pronator syndrome	median nerve; forearm	index & thenar eminence
Radial sensory entrapment	radial nerve in forearm	dorsoradial hand
Guyon's canal entrapment	ulnar nerve; wrist level	little finger pulp
Cubital tunnel syndrome	ulnar nerve; elbow	little finger & dorsoulnar hand
Quadrangular space syndrome	axillary nerve	C5 root

its own entrapment or pain syndrome (Naff, Dellon, & Mackinnon, 1993). The anterior interosseous nerve arises from either the posterior or the radial side of the median nerve in the proximal third of the forearm. If this branch is in the radial location and is associated with a fibrous origin of either the deep head of the pronator teres or the sublimis muscle bellies from the interosseous membrane, compression of the anterior interosseous nerve can occur, giving varying degrees of motor loss to the flexor pollices longus, the profundus to the index and middle finger. The anterior interosseous nerve also supplies sensation to the anterior wrist capsule after it innervates the pronator quadratus muscle (Mackinnon & Dellon, 1984). Problems at this level can cause anterior interosseous nerve syndrome which, in classical description and in distinction from the pronator syndrome is a motor nerve entrapment, and is not associated with any sensory deficit.

The ulnar nerve is one of the terminal divisions of the medial cord (the other division going to form the median nerve) of the brachial plexus (see Figure 12.3). The medial cord is located medial to the axillary artery and is the direct continuation of the anterior division of the lower trunk of the brachial plexus. Therefore, the ulnar nerve is composed of fibers from the C8 and T1 nerve roots. The ulnar nerve supplies sensation to the little finger, the ulnar half of the ring finger, and the ulnar half of the dorsum of the hand. The dorsoulnar half of the hand is innervated by the dorsal cutaneous branch of the ulnar nerve that originates about 9 cm proximal to the wrist, and crosses over the ulnar styloid to reach this dorsal skin territory.

Although it is described, there is most often not a true palmar cutaneous branch of the ulnar nerve. Therefore, the ulnar side of the palm receives its innervation directly from the sensory branches of the digital nerves as they go through Guyon's canal. The ulnar nerve innervates all the intrinsic muscles of the hand, but is generally not considered to innervate the abductor pollices brevis, the opponens pollices, or the flexor brevis pollices, with the exception of the innervation anomalies noted at the end of the preceding paragraph. Less than 1% of hands have ulnar nerve innervation to the thumb. The ulnar nerve, just proximal to the elbow, gives off the motor branch to the flexor carpi ulnaris. Therefore, this wrist flexor is usually not weak with ulnar nerve compression at the elbow level. Compression of

the ulnar nerve in the post-condylar groove, cubital tunnel syndrome, does include weakness of the grip strength due to compression of the motor branch to the profundus muscles, and weakness of pinch, due to the motor branch to the adductor pollices and the first dorsal interosseous nerve.

The radial nerve is the terminal branch of the posterior cord of the brachial plexus (see Figure 12.3). The posterior cord is located posterior to the axillary artery. The posterior cord contains the posterior divisions of all three trunks of the brachial plexus, but just those from C6 and C7 travel in the radial nerve to innervate the dorsoradial aspect of the hand from the middle finger toward the thumb. Though rare, it is well documented that the radial sensory nerve may innervate the thumb pulp to varying degrees (Dellon & Mackinnon, 1986). The radial nerve innervates no intrinsic muscles in the hand, but it does innervate all the wrist and finger extensor muscles.

A division of the radial nerve at the elbow level creates the sensory deficit associated with the radial sensory nerve and leaves the patient with a complete wrist drop and loss of all finger extension except interphalangeal extension, which is caused by the ulnar innervated intrinsic muscles. A division of the radial nerve

just distal to the elbow, at the level of the posterior interosseous nerve, may spare the sensory branch of the radial nerve and the innervation to the extensor carpi radialis longus, which arises just proximal to the supinator. This leaves the patient with only the ability to extend the wrist in a radial deviation, with all fingers being flexed at the metacarpophalangeal joint, and the thumb adducted. This is the motor deficit associated with the complete palsy of the posterior interosseous nerve syndrome. A division of the radial nerve in the distal third of the radius will cause a loss of the brachioradialis muscle, in addition to all of the above sensorimotor deficits, and a division in the proximal third will also cause a loss of triceps function.

An interesting variation in hand muscle innervation is the Martin-Gruber *anastomosis*. This is said to exist in about 25% of people, but the percentage is probably lower. I have only had one patient in whom the presence of this connection required special attention. When this arrangement is present, some of the ulnar nerve motor fibers to the intrinsic muscles travel through the anterior interosseous nerve at the elbow level, to enter the ulnar nerve in the distal forearm. Thus a complete transection of the ulnar nerve at the el-

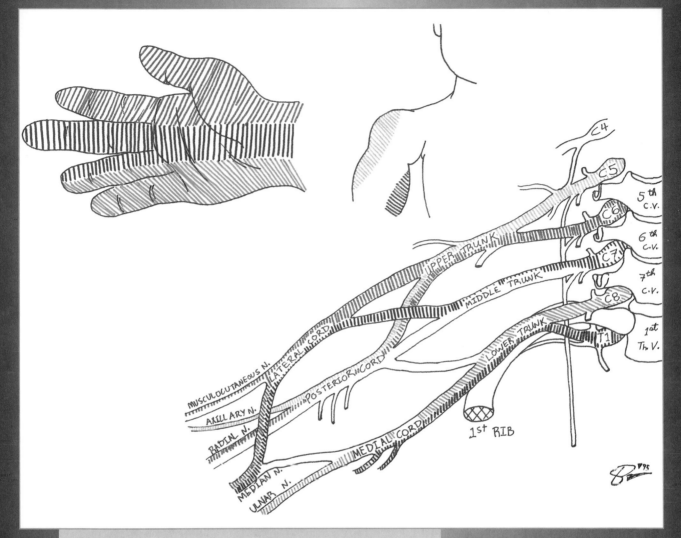

FIGURE 12.3

Representation of the brachial plexus demonstrating spinal cord roots that comprise the upper trunks, division of trunks to form cords that are named in relationship to the axillary artery, and the final formation of the major peripheral nerves in the upper extremity from the cords. The colors link the sensory roots with their unique innervated skin territories. Drawing by Glenn George Dellon. Reprinted with permission.

bow level does not result in intrinsic muscle loss. The presence of this variation can be determined by stimulating the median nerve at the elbow level and recording from the normally ulnar-innervated intrinsic muscles in the hand, that is, the first dorsal interosseous or the abductor digiti minimi.

The cutaneous nerves in the arm will be a source of pain for which referral to the therapist is appropriate. For example, the innervation to the thenar eminence by the palmar cutaneous branch of the median nerve becomes a source of pain when the terminal branches of this small nerve become embedded in the scar of a carpal tunnel release. The diagnosis of this source of pain may be made by doing a nerve block proximal to the wrist, just ulnar to the flexor carpi radialis tendon. If desensitization does not work for this pain problem (see Chapter 11), the appropriate treatment is to resect this nerve proximal to the wrist, without having to re-open the carpal tunnel. The distal end of the nerve may be implanted into the pronator quadratus muscle (Evans & Dellon, 1994), with good relief of pain.

The lateral antebrachial cutaneous nerve is generally depicted as innervating the radial volar forearm, but it has been demonstrated to overlap the radial sensory nerve either partially or

completely in 75% of cadavers (Mackinnon & Dellon, 1985). This means that in the patient complaining of pain over the dorsoradial aspect of the hand, the possibility must be considered that two nerves are involved in the pain mechanism. This is often found as a complication after excision of a dorsal wrist ganglion or after release of the first dorsal extensor compartment for DeQuervain's extensor tenosynovitisly (Saplys, Mackinnon, & Dellon, 1987). The therapist preparing a splint for the treatment of pain after this type of surgery should be aware of the possibility of neuroma formation, and should consider suggesting desensitization in addition to splinting. When conservative measures are not successful in relieving the pain, resection of one or both of these nerves (as determined by nerve block), and implantation of the nerves into the brachioradialis muscle can be highly effective in achieving pain relief (Mackinnon & Dellon, 1987).

Another common pain syndrome is that related to entrapment or injury of the medial antebrachial cutaneous nerve after ulnar nerve transposition (Dellon & Mackinnon, 1985). Cutaneous nerves can be a source of concern following their harvesting for nerve graft donor material. The first one to be described for this

purpose was the lateral antebrachial cutaneous nerve, by McFarlane and Moyer (1976). This nerve leaves a sensory territory that is denervated in the distal radial-volar forearm, but this region is seldom of concern to the patient because of overlap with the radial sensory nerve and the medial antebrachial cutaneous nerve. A donor nerve that leaves no region denervated is the terminal branch of the posterior interosseous nerve (Dellon, 1985), which can be harvested through a small incision in the distal dorsal wrist, proximal to the wrist joint. The medial antebrachial cutaneous nerve has become a source of nerve graft material with increasing frequency (Mackinnon & Dellon, 1988), but care should be taken to harvest the anterior branch. Harvesting the posterior branch can cause sufficient numbness over the elbow to cause ulceration. This nerve can be taken with a length that extends from distal to the elbow to the axilla, where it originates from the medial cord of the brachial plexus.

There are some sensory problems associated with the brachial plexus itself. The axillary nerve can be compressed in a space in the axilla that is called the quadrangular space. This space is bordered by the long head of the triceps, the humerus, and the teres major and minor. The axillary nerve, accompanied by the posterior circumflex humeral artery, goes through this space before innervating the deltoid and terminating in a sensory branch to the lateral shoulder, overlying the deltoid muscle. Numbness in this skin territory, which derives from C5, is present in the quadrangular space syndrome, in addition to weakness or paralysis of the deltoid muscle (Francel, Dellon, & Campbell, 1991). This syndrome can exist itself, usually after a stretch injury or posterior shoulder dislocation, or it can be a distal site or double lesion that accompanies a stretch/traction injury to the upper trunk of the brachial plexus. The suprascapular nerve, associated with weakness or wasting of the supra- and infraspinatus muscles, when a stretch injury or entrapment occurs, has no cutaneous sensory component, although it does innervate the anterior shoulder (glenohumeral) joint, and can be a source of shoulder pain (Azman, Dellon, Birely, & McFarlane, 1995).

Injury to the upper trunk of the plexus (C5 and C6) results in sensory change over the lateral deltoid and extending all the way down to the tips of the thumb and index finger, volarly and dorsally. Thus, this trunk includes the territories of the lateral antebrachial cutaneous nerve, the radial sensory nerve, the palmar cuta-

neous branch of the median nerve, and fibers from the median nerve. This information is useful in the clinical testing of sensation related to diagnosis of brachial plexus compression in the thoracic inlet, the so-called *thoracic outlet syndrome* (see Chapter 18). For example, since there is no known entrapment site for the lateral antebrachial cutaneous nerve, abnormal somatosensory-evoked potentials from the index and proximal radial volar forearm (lateral antebrachial cutaneous nerve) suggest that the entrapment site is likely to be the upper trunk of the brachial plexus. By analogy, injury to the lower trunk of the brachial plexus (C8 and T1) results in sensory changes from the inner medial upper arm (the medial brachial cutaneous nerve), down the ulnar volar forearm (medial antebrachial cutaneous nerve), and out to the little finger and dorsal ulnar aspect of the hand. There is no known entrapment site for the medial brachial cutaneous nerve, so that abnormal somatosensory-evoked potentials from the little finger and from the inner upper arm suggest that the entrapment site is likely to be the upper trunk of the brachial plexus (Kaplan, Mullick, Dellon, & Hendler, 1995).

Finally, remember that the upper extremity has its neural origins in the oppo-

site cerebral cortex. The therapist must be aware that sooner or later there will be a patient encountered who, despite being referred for a "hand" problem, will, in fact, have a problem related to a brain tumor, a cervical disc, a spinal cord cyst (syrinx, see Chapter 19), a tumor at the apex of the lung, a Schwannoma of the brachial plexus, or a systemic neurologic disease such as amyotrophic lateral sclerosis. With regard to sensory testing, it is important to realize that, because of anterior growth of a spinal cord cyst, the patient with a syrinx will present with intrinsic wasting of both median and ulnar innervated muscles, but in contrast to a C8 or T1 cervical disc, there will be no shooting pains and cutaneous pressure thresholds will be normal (these are posterior column spinal cord tracts).

The syrinx is the one instance in which pain and temperature testing is clearly indicated because these nerve tracts pass anteriorly (anterior spinothalamic tracts) in the spinal cord, so that there is a classic dissociation of preserved touch with lost pain and temperature sense. The patient with amyotrophic lateral sclerosis will have intrinsic muscle wasting of both the median and ulnar innervated muscles, but will have normal sensory testing. All the therapist can do is to be aware of these possibilities, and to call any unusual or discrepant physical examination findings or patient complaints to the attention of the referring physician.

CHRONIC NERVE COMPRESSION

SENSIBILITY TESTING

Chronic nerve compression implies that there has been a region of the peripheral nerve subjected to pressure for a period of time sufficient to cause well-defined pathophysiologic changes, each of which has clinical symptoms and signs associated with it. Chronic nerve compression differs from acute nerve compression with respect to the degree and time of application of the pressure. For example, if you sit with your legs crossed for a while, that pressure may cause your leg to "go to sleep." The same will occur to your hand if you sleep with your arm under your pillow or with your head on your forearm. This amount of pressure is sufficient to stop blood flow to the nerve, and the resultant ischemia generates the paresthesias that we call numbness and tingling, but not really pain. Release of that pressure results in more severe tingling for a brief period of time as circulation is reestablished and the nerve begins to conduct impulses normally again.

If that severe degree of pressure were maintained for a greater degree of time or over a narrow region of the nerve, for example, by a suture placed around the nerve inadvertently in the operating room, the nerve itself would die, undergoing acute degeneration. This is associated with pain and the paresthesias. Release of this degree of pressure may result in recovery of sensibility through neural regeneration at the rate of 1 mm/day, but may not occur if the injury to the nerve is associated with intraneural scarring. In contrast, the application of as little as 20 mm Hg pressure to the peripheral nerve is sufficient to decrease blood flow within the nerve, initiate intraneural edema, and begin the process of chronic nerve compression (Rydevik & Lundborg, 1977).

The experimental model for chronic nerve compression suggests that a region of compression about two or three times as long as the diameter of the nerve that does not externally narrow the nerve, such as can be created by placing a silastic tube about the nerve, will create sufficient endoneurial pressure to cause a change in the blood-nerve barrier. This permits the fluid to leak from the endoneurial microvessels to create endoneurial edema. This can occur by about 2 months of compression. By about 6 months of compression, epineural and perineurial fibrosis begins, accompanied by thinning of the myelin. This is accompanied by slowing of the nerve conduction. By about 1 year, actual Wallerian degeneration can occur. This has been demonstrated in both the rat sciatic nerve and the monkey median nerve (Mackinnon, Dellon, Hudson, & Hunter, 1984, 1985; Mackinnon & Dellon, 1986) and has been extensively related to clinical diagnosis (Lundborg, 1988; Mackinnon & Dellon, 1988).

The generally held concept is that both the mechanical result of compression and the decreased oxygen content within the nerve manifest their effects first on the larger nerve fibers. Therefore, the findings on physical examination are related to changes in the perception of touch, rather than to the perception of pain or temperature or sweating. These findings form the basis for the staging system or grading of chronic nerve compression that is discussed in Chapter 9, and provide the rationale for sensibility testing in the patient with chronic nerve compression.

In the earliest stage of nerve compression, which may be termed mild or *minimal degree* of nerve compression, the patient most commonly first will have intermittent symptoms of numbness involving the fingers innervated by the compression, with a less common presentation of the problem being loss of motor control or weakness. At this time, the only clinical findings will be the ability to duplicate or bring on the patient's complaints by increasing pressure over the nerve. For median nerve compression at the wrist, carpal tunnel syndrome, this is accomplished by flexing the wrist (Phalen, 1966). For ulnar nerve compression at the elbow, cubital tunnel syndrome, this is accomplished by elbow flexion (Fine & Wongjirad, 1985). For radial sensory nerve compression in the forearm, this is accomplished by hyperpronation of the forearm (Dellon & Mackinnon, 1986). For brachial plexus compression in the thoracic inlet, thoracic outlet syndrome, this is accomplished by elevating the hands above the shoulders (Roos, 1966).

At any given site of suspected nerve compression, additional pressure may be gently applied directly over the nerve with the expectation that sensory symptoms may be elicited. This is often useful in attempting to make the diagnosis of median nerve compression in the forearm, pronator syndrome (see Figure 12.4), which can also be provoked by resisted

middle finger sublimis flexion, resisted forearm pronation, or resisted elbow flexion (Spinner, 1978). Finally, there is present in about 75% of patients a positive Tinel sign at the site of anatomic constriction of the nerve. This sign is best understood as the presence of regenerating nerve fibers, either myelinated or unmyelinated, which exist at this site as a result of the chronic compression (Tinel, 1978; Dellon, 1984).

As the stage of nerve compression progresses to a *moderate degree*, the patients' symptoms are still intermittent, but the degree of intraneural change now is sufficient for the physical examination to demonstrate abnormalities related to the threshold for stimulation of pressure perception and vibratory perception. Qualitatively, application of a tuning fork to the skin surface in the territory of the compressed nerve will result in a perception of vibration, but this perception will be different from that in the contralateral territory. At the earliest change, this perception is sometimes one of increased sensory perception, although the mechanism for this remains unclear, followed by a decrease in the perception of the vibration, that is, "it doesn't feel as loud" (Dellon, 1980, 1983). Tuning forks are excellent for a rapid screening examination in the office, but do

not provide the type of documentation required for serial assessments of the clinical condition. Quantitatively, the change in vibratory threshold may be measured with a vibrometer of either a single frequency (Dellon, 1983) or of multiple frequencies (Lundborg, Lie-Stenstrom, Sollerman, Stromberg, & Pyykko, 1986; Lundborg, Dahlin, Lundstrom, Necking, & Stromberg, 1992; Dellon & Dellon, 1995). This can provide the measurement required to document clinical progress.

The measurement of pressure perception is best accomplished with the Pressure-Specified Sensory Device™ since, as discussed extensively in Chapters 6 and 7, the Semmes-Weinstein nylon monofilaments provide only an estimate of the range of abnormal pressure perception. The normative, age-related, database for the upper extremity pressure perception thresholds are given in Tables 12.2 through 12.6 for the Pressure-Specified Sensory Device™. In screening for nerve compression, it has been demonstrated that the first measurable parameter to change is the pressure required to distinguish one from two points held in constant contact with the fingertip. Therefore, in screening for chronic nerve compression, one-point moving touch and moving two-point discrimination do

FIGURE 12.4

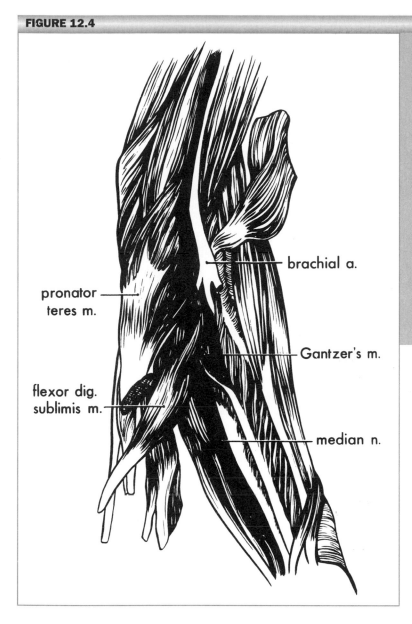

pronator
teres m.

flexor dig.
sublimis m.

brachial a.

Gantzer's m.

median n.

Illustration of the median nerve in the proximal forearm. In this location the median nerve can become compressed between the various muscle bellies of the pronator teres or the flexor digitorum sublimis. This can cause numbness in the thumb, index, and middle fingers known as the pronator syndrome. From Surgery of the Peripheral Nerve, *by S. E. Mackinnon & A. L. Dellon, 1988, New York: Thieme Publishing. Reprinted with permission of the authors.*

sults in decreased innervation density, so that in addition to the increased pressure required to distinguish one from two points, the actual distance measured for this distinction will increase, as well. This is what has been noted for a severe degree of carpal and cubital tunnel syndrome (Dellon, 1983), and is the reason why screening for the presence of chronic nerve compression by two-point discrimination testing alone does not identify patients with a minimal or moderate degree of compression.

For routine or quick office evaluation, two-point discrimination can be measured best with the Disk-Criminator™ (see Chapter 7). However, for precise documentation, the pressure required for the two points to be distinguished must be

not need to be tested (Dellon & Kress, 1995). With a moderate degree of nerve compression, muscle weakness will be present. At least for the ulnar nerve, measurement of muscle strength is possible. As discussed in Chapter 7, the hydraulic types of devices are not as reliable or valid as the electromechanical, comput-

er-assisted Digit-Grip™ and pinch device.

As the stage of nerve compression progresses to a *severe degree*, the patient's symptoms become persistent, meaning they are always present, and the degree of intraneural fibrosis is now sufficiently severe that there is Wallerian degeneration with a loss of axons. This re-

TABLE 12.2 NORMAL INDEX FINGER PULP PRESSURE PERCEPTION THRESHOLD						
	(g/mm²)		(mm)	(g/mm²)		(mm)
	1PS	2PS	2PS	1PM	2PM	2PM
≤ 45 years of age						
mean	0.5	0.7	2.6	0.4	0.6	2.6
s.d.	0.2	0.2	0.1	0.2	0.2	0.1
95%	0.57	0.78	2.7	0.50	0.64	2.7
99%	0.60	0.81	2.8	0.52	0.67	2.8
min	0.1	0.3	2.5	0.1	0.2	2.5
max	0.9	1.2	3.1	0.7	1.0	3.1
> 45 years of age						
mean	0.7	1.5	2.9	0.5	1.0	2.7
s.d.	0.3	1.2	0.4	0.3	0.7	0.4
95%	0.87	2.1	3.1	0.64	1.3	3.0
99%	0.93	2.2	3.3	0.69	1.4	3.2
min	0.2	0.1	2.5	0.1	0.1	2.5
max	1.5	5.0	4.0	1.3	3.5	4.0

Note:
⁺ p < .01
✦ p < .001
★ p < .008

From: "Computer-Assisted Quantitative Sensorimotor Testing: Patients with Carpal and Cubital Tunnel Syndrome Compared to an Age-Matched Control Population," by A. L. Dellon & K. Keller, *Annals of Plastic Surgery, 38:* 493-502. 1997. Reprinted with permission.

measured as well, and this requires measuring with the Pressure-Specified Sensory Device™. Similarly, at this stage, muscle will become denervated, with the clinical consequence that not only will there be measurable weakness, but there will also be muscle wasting or atrophy.

CARPAL TUNNEL SYNDROME

Compression of the median nerve within the carpal tunnel will give symptoms of numbness and tingling in the thumb, index, middle, and sometimes the ring finger. It will not give symptoms in the little finger. It will not cause pain. It will cause nighttime awakening because the wrist drops into a flexed position during sleep due to the greater strength of the flexor over the extensor muscles. There is usually an associated flexor tenosynovitis. In the mild degree of compression stage, the appropriate treatment is splinting with the wrist in

TABLE 12.3 NORMAL LITTLE FINGER PULP

	Pressure Perception Threshold					
	(g/mm²)		(mm)	(g/mm²)		(mm)
	1PS	2PS	2PS	1PM	2PM	2PM
≤ 45 years of age						
mean	0.4	0.6[+]	2.7	0.3	0.5[*]	2.7
s.d.	0.2	0.3	0.2	0.2	0.2	0.2
95%	0.48	0.68	2.8	0.35	0.60	2.7
99%	0.50	0.70	2.9	0.37	0.63	2.8
min	0.1	0.1	2.5	0.1	0.1	2.5
max	0.8	1.0	3.5	0.8	0.9	3.1
> 45 years of age						
mean	0.4	1.3[+]	3.2	0.3	0.8[*]	3.1
s.d.	0.1	1.0	0.6	0.2	0.5	0.6
95%	0.50	1.7	3.4	0.37	1.1	3.4
99%	0.53	1.9	3.5	0.40	1.2	3.5
min	0.2	0.1	2.5	0.1	0.2	2.5
max	0.7	4.0	4.6	0.6	1.9	4.6

Note:
[+] $p < .001$
[*] $p < .001$

From: "Computer-Assisted Quantitative Sensorimotor Testing: Patients with Carpal and Cubital Tunnel Syndrome Compared to an Age-Matched Control Population," by A. L. Dellon & K. Keller, *Annals of Plastic Surgery, 38:* 493-502. 1997. Reprinted with permission.

the neutral position. The "over-the-counter" splints, unfortunately, have the wrist in 20° of dorsiflexion. Therefore, the therapist should prepare a comfortable, supporting splint. Antiinflammatory medication and perhaps a trial of 100 mg of vitamin B6 a day are indicated, since there is no bloodtest available to determine the B6 level, and an animal model has demonstrated that B6 deficiency causes a neuropathy that is reversible with dietary supplementation (Dellon, A. L., Dellon, E. S., Tassler, Ellefson, Hendrickson, Francel, 1995). The patient should improve under this regimen.

Attention to altering activities of daily living and the work environment are indicated if there is no response to this regimen. When the

TABLE 12.4 PRESSURE-SPECIFIED SENSORY DEVICE™ NORMATIVE DATA: LEFT VERSUS RIGHT

	Mean Difference in Pressure Perception Threshold					
	(g/mm²)		(mm)	(g/mm²)		(mm)
	1PS	2PS	2PS	1PM	2PM	2PM
Index Finger						
mean	.12	.23	.10	.13	.16	.05
s.d.	.12	.16	.18	.13	.12	.12
99%	.22	.37	.24	.24	.26	.15
Little Finger						
mean	.13	.27	.21	.14	.27	.14
s.d.	.10	.31	.28	.12	.25	.19
99%	.21	.50	.43	.23	.46	.29

Note: From: "Computer-Assisted Quantitative Sensorimotor Testing: Patients with Carpal and Cubital Tunnel Syndrome Compared to an Age-Matched Control Population," by A. L. Dellon & K. Keller, *Annals of Plastic Surgery, 38:* 493-502. 1997. Reprinted with permission.

TABLE 12.5 PRESSURE-SPECIFIED SENSORY DEVICE™: NORMATIVE DATA. HAND: THENAR EMINENCE

	Pressure Perception Threshold					
	(g/mm²)		(mm)	(g/mm²)		(mm)
	1PS	2PS	2PS	1PM	2PM	2PM
< 45 years of age[+]						
mean	1.2	1.5	6.9	0.7	0.8	6.6
s.d.	1.1	1.4	1.8	0.6	0.7	1.9
> 45 years of age[*]						
mean	0.9	3.1	10.4	1.0	3.3	11.7
s.d.	0.8	4.0	1.7	1.2	4.9	1.5

Note:
[+] n = 11, mean age 33.4 years, range 10 to 43 years, data for the right hand.
[*] n = 8, mean age 48.8 years, range 46 to 55 years, data for the right hand.

From: A. L. Dellon & K. Keller, *Annals of Plastic Surgery, 38:* 493-502. 1997. Reprinted with permission.

FIGURE 12.5

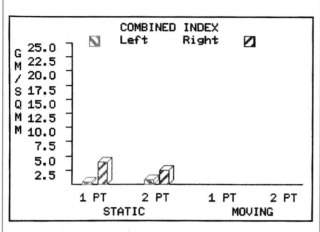

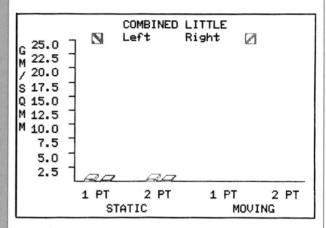

Carpal Tunnel Syndrome; Quantitative Sensory Testing. This 30-year-old typist has had symptoms of numbness and tingling in her right hand for 6 months, associated with nighttime awakening. There has been no previous treatment. Two-point discrimination is normal at 3 mm. Note that the pressure threshold for both one-point static and static two-point discrimination are above the 99% confidence level, which would be < 1.0 g/mm², and that the values for the little finger are normal. Electrodiagnostic testing is normal. Measurements made with the Pressure-Specified Sensory Device™. From: A. L. Dellon, unpublished observations, 1997.

TABLE 12.6 PRESSURE-SPECIFIED SENSORY DEVICE™: NORMATIVE DATA. HAND: DORSUM

	Pressure Perception Threshold (g/mm²)	
	1PS	1PM
mean	0.5	0.2
s.d.	0.2	0.1
95%	0.5	0.3
99%	0.6	0.4
min	0.1	0.1
max	0.7	0.6

Note: From: "Computer-Assisted Quantitative Sensorimotor Testing: Patients with Carpal and Cubital Tunnel Syndrome Compared to an Age-Matched Control Population," by A. L. Dellon & K. Keller, *Annals of Plastic Surgery, 38:* 493-502. 1997. Reprinted with permission.

patient's symptoms continue, quantitative sensory testing will demonstrate an elevated threshold for static two-point discrimination as the measurable abnormal finding (Dellon & Kress, 1995). As the compression persists, the threshold for one-point static touch will also elevate. About 20% to 30% of patients will have normal electrodiagnostic testing at this point. An example of the results of quantitative sensory testing with the Pressure-Specified Sensory Device™ is given in Figure 12.5. Another example is given in Figure 12.6 for a patient who did not improve with nonoperative measures and had a carpal tunnel release with complete resolution of symptoms. Serial quantitative sensory testing documents the improvement in pressure thresholds. An example of both median and ulnar nerve compression at the wrist level in a patient who had a motor vehicle accident and who had normal electrodiagnostic testing is given in Figure 12.7.

Tables 12.7 and 12.8 give detailed results of quantitative sensory testing with the Pressure-Specified Sensory Device™ in 125 patients with carpal tunnel syndrome. This data gives the spectrum of values obtained when this device is used. This is the data that has been used to determine that the pressure required to distinguish one from two points is the first

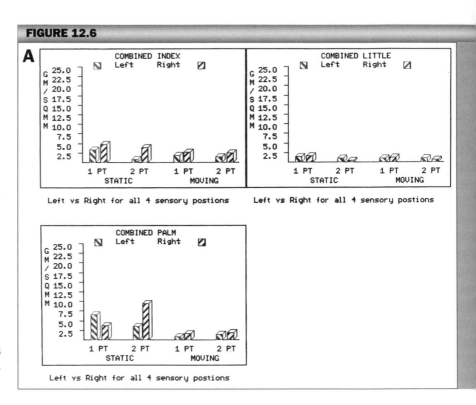

FIGURE 12.6

parameter that can be demonstrated to become abnormal, that is, greater than the 99% confidence limit, in patients with carpal tunnel syndrome. This value becomes abnormal before one-point static touch, and before either one-point moving touch or the moving two-point discrimination thresholds. Thus, this data, in conjunction with the normative data for the index finger given in Table 12.2, can be used to arrive at screening/surveillance values of industry, which are given in Table 12.9.

To do this, the minimal values for a patient 44 years of age with clinical evidence of carpal tunnel syndrome are examined, and are noted to have a pressure threshold

for static two-point discrimination at 1.1 g/mm² at a time when all other values are within normal limits, including the distance for distinguishing one from two, which was 2.5 mm. The 99% confidence limit for normal for a person less than 45 years of age is < 1.0 g/mm². Therefore, the screening parameters for a person less than 45 years of age for carpal tunnel would be a distance of 3 mm, and a pressure threshold for this distance of 1.0 g/mm². The use of computer-assisted sensory testing for industrial surveillance is typified by the reports that can be generated comparing sequential evaluations. For example, the report in Figure 12.6 C would typify a worker who was im-

Carpal Tunnel Syndrome. Preop versus Postop Quantitative Sensory Testing. For 2 years, this 36-year-old machinist has had numbness and tingling in both hands, but worse in the right, dominant hand, associated with nighttime awakening. He has had a trial of 3 months of splinting and antiinflammatory medication, but his symptoms persist and he must continue to work at his current job. (A) Quantitative sensory testing done preoperatively demonstrates elevated thresholds for the right index finger for all measurements of the right hand, with abnormal measurements being present for the left hand as well. Two-point discrimination is normal. The little finger pressure thresholds are at the 99% confidence level, and the thresholds for the thenar eminence suggest that there may be a moderate degree of median nerve compression in the forearm, as well. (B) Quantitative sensory testing done just on the right hand at 6 weeks after surgery demonstrates that the thresholds for the index finger have returned to normal. Of interest is the improvement in the thresholds to the little finger, which may relate to the known change in the shape of Guyon's canal when the transverse carpal ligament is divided. The proximal median nerve thresholds have improved, probably as a result of the time off from work. (C) The computer-generated report of sequential improvement of the right index finger. Measurements made with the Pressure-Specified Sensory Device™.

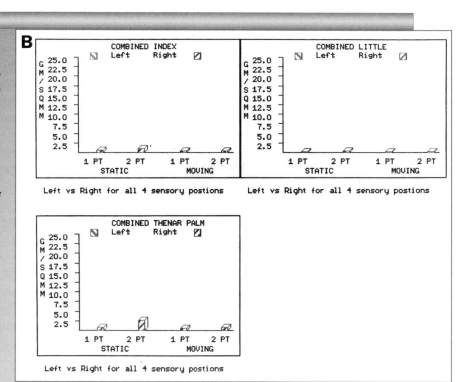

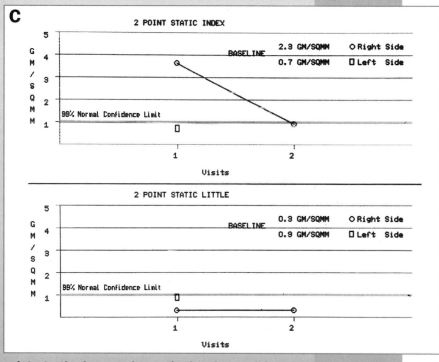

proving following appropriate treatment, while that in Figure 12.10 C would typify a worker who was becoming worse, perhaps during the initial break-in phase of a new job.

Recurrent carpal tunnel syndrome must be distinguished from other causes of index finger numbness. In Figure 12.8 the intraoperative pathology of a patient who did have recurrent carpal tunnel syndrome is illustrated. If a patient complains of numbness in the index finger and thumb, it is most commonly due to median nerve compression in the carpal tunnel. It is most appropriate to test the index and little finger of each hand. The thumb may have radial sensory nerve innervation to its tip, and the middle finger may have ulnar nerve innervation to its tip. The little finger is tested to get an appraisal of the possibility of the presence of a neuropathy (more than one nerve in more than one extremity).

FIGURE 12.7

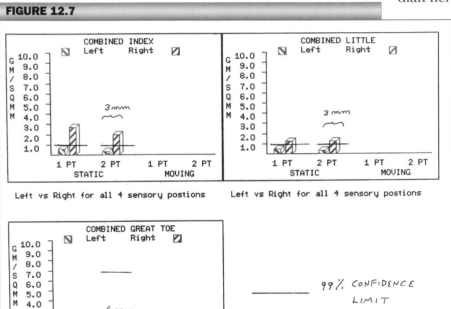

Median and Ulnar Nerve Compression at the Wrist. Quantitative Sensory Testing. Twenty-eight year old man 1 year after a motor vehicle accident in which he had his right hand on the steering wheel and his car was struck in the rear while he was stopped at a traffic light. He has had intermittent numbness in his hand for the past 6 months, including all his fingers. Note that while the two-point discrimination is normal, the thresholds for one-point static touch and static two-point discrimination are elevated above the 99% confidence limit for both the right index and right little fingers. Because of the presence of two abnormal nerves in one hand, a measurement of the posterior tibial nerve was obtained to screen for the presence of a neuropathy. The big toe measurements are normal. Electrodiagnostic testing is normal. This documentation is consistent with posttraumatic median and ulnar nerve compression at the wrist. Measurements made with the Pressure-Specified Sensory Device™.

Figure 12.7 illustrates the inclusion of sensory testing of the plantar surface of the big toe to screen for the presence of a neuropathy. Measurement of the little finger pressure threshold also serves as a comparison value for the median nerve exam. That is, with the Pressure Specified Sensory Device™ there should normally be less than a 0.5 g/mm² difference in the cutaneous pressure threshold between the index and the little fin-

FIGURE 12.8

Recurrent carpal tunnel syndrome. (A) The dotted line indicates the incision from the first operation, which did not relieve this patient's carpal tunnel symptoms. A new incision is made to avoid damaging the median nerve, which is usually adherent to the previously incised transverse carpal ligament. (B) The opened carpal canal reveals no median nerve, since it is adherent to the transverse carpal ligament. (C) The median nerve required external and internal neurolysis. From "Reoperative Peripheral Nerve Surgery," by A. L. Dellon, 1995, in Reoperative Surgery, *J. Grotting, Editor, St. Louis: Quality Medical Publishers. Reprinted with permission of the author.*

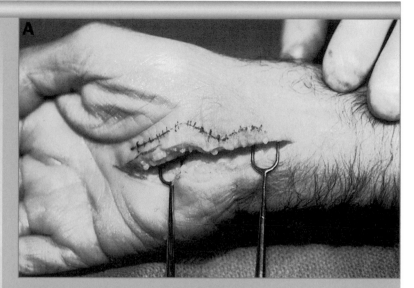

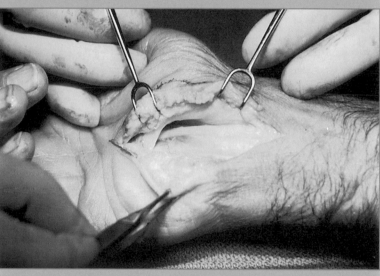

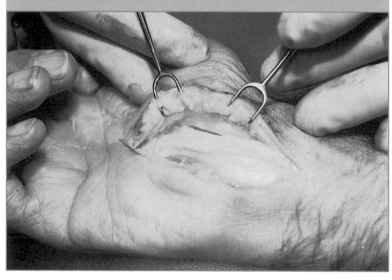

ger, and between the left and the right index or the left and the right little finger (see Table 12.4). The normative data for this sensory testing equipment for the index and little finger is given in Tables 12.2 and 12.3.

However, if a patient has numbness of the index finger and thumb, and the threshold for the fingertip or pulp is normal, it is reasonable to test the dorsoradial surface of the hand because the patient's complaints may be poorly expressed, and may represent a radial sensory nerve compression. There is no signifi-

TABLE 12.7 PATIENT POPULATION			
Carpal Tunnel Syndrome	**Unilateral**	**Bilateral**	**Total**
≤ 45 years old	11	34	79
> 45 years old	8	19	46
Total	19	53	125
Cubital Tunnel Syndrome	**Unilateral**	**Bilateral**	**Total**
≤ 45 years old	9	18	45
> 45 years old	4	11	26
Total	13	29	71
Total Compressions	**32**	**82**	**196**

Note: From "Computer-Assisted Quantitative Sensorimotor Testing: Patients with Carpal and Cubital Tunnel Syndrome" by A. L. Dellon & K. Keller, *Annals of Plastic Surgery, 38:* 493-502. 1997. Reprinted with permission of the authors.

cant difference in the cutaneous pressure thresholds between the dorsoradial and the dorsoulnar side of the hand. The normative data with the Pressure-Specified Sensory Device™ for this region is given in Figure 12.6, and an example is given in Figure 12.10. If a patient were to have a C6 disc problem, there might be abnormal sensibility threshold testing results for the index finger, the dorsoradial hand, and the lateral antebrachial cutaneous nerve. Such a patient would likely also have neck complaints, and would be a good candidate to be referred for electrodiagnostic testing.

Following are specific guidelines for sensibility testing in a patient with carpal tunnel syndrome:

Whenever possible, quantitative sensory testing of the large myelinated fibers has been shown to be the most sensitive technique for the early detection of median nerve compression, by measuring the pressure threshold required for static two-point discrimination. In the absence of this computerized sensory testing, the change in perception of a vibratory stimulus is the next best screening test. Serial measurements of the pressure threshold for one-point static touch and two-point static

touch are the best way to record progression of the chronic nerve compression or response to nonoperative management.

Once there is an increase in the distance at which one point can be distinguished from two points, the degree of compression has worsened significantly, consistent with loss of axons. At this stage, after nerve decompression, recovery depends on axonal regeneration. The best way to quantitate changes after surgery in this advanced degree of compression is to follow the improvement, that is, the decrease, in both the distance and the pressure threshold

TABLE 12.8 CARPAL TUNNEL SYNDROME

	Pressure Perception Threshold					
	(g/mm²)		(mm)	(g/mm²)		(mm)
	1PS	2PS	2PS	1PM	2PM	2PM
≤ 45 years of age						
mean	8.3	15.9⁺	3.6	4.3	6.8⁺	3.3
s.d.	18.6	19.3	1.1	13	9.4	0.9
95%	12.4	20.3	3.8	7.2	9.0	3.5
99%	13.8	21.8	3.9	8.1	9.6	3.6
min	0.1	1.1	2.5	0.1	0.3	2.5
max	97	69	6.6	97	51	5.7
> 45 years of age						
mean	5.5	14.8★	4.3	2.1	7.8★	3.9
s.d.	9.0	14.0	1.0	3.0	8.6	0.9
95%	8.2	19.0	4.6	3.0	10.3	4.2
99%	9.1	20.4	4.7	3.3	11.2	4.3
min	0.4	3.0	2.5	0.2	1.0	2.5
max	39	66	7.1	95	37	6.2

Note:
⁺ $p < .0003$
★ $p < .005$
From "Computer-Assisted Quantitative Sensorimotor Testing: Patients with Carpal and Cubital Tunnel Syndrome" by A. L. Dellon & K. Keller, *Annals of Plastic Surgery, 38:* 493-502. 1997. Reprinted with permission of the authors.

required for two-point discrimination.

However, now, because we are following neural regeneration, the earliest signs of improvement will be noted in one-point moving and moving two-point discrimination. Therefore, in the set of measurements taken in anticipation of surgery on a person with an advanced degree of compression, it is recommended to obtain the values of both static and moving one- and two-point thresholds. In the absence of computerized sensory testing equipment, progress can be recorded by qualitatively noting the changes in vibratory perception, which should trend toward normal, or even toward a hypersensitivity during neural regeneration, and by quantitatively measuring moving two-point discrimination with the Disk-Criminator™. It is not necessary to measure perception of pain or temperature in a patient with carpal tunnel syndrome.

TABLE 12.9 SUGGESTED SCREENING/SURVEILLANCE VALUES FOR NERVE COMPRESSION SYNDROMES IN INDUSTRY

	Two-Point Static Pressure Perception Threshold[+]	
	(g/mm²)	(mm)
Carpal Tunnel Syndrome		
≤ 45 years old	1.0	3.0
> 45 years old	2.2	4.0
Cubital Tunnel Syndrome		
≤ 45 years old	1.0	3.0
> 45 years old	1.9	4.0

Note:
[+] Values greater than these are considered abnormal. From "Computer-Assisted Quantitative Sensorimotor Testing: Patients with Carpal and Cubital Tunnel Syndrome" by A. L. Dellon & K. Keller, *Annals of Plastic Surgery, 38:* 493-502. 1997. Reprinted with permission of the authors.

PRONATOR SYNDROME

A more difficult situation is the patient referred with a previous carpal tunnel release who still has numbness in the index finger and thumb. This might be due to proximal median nerve compression in the forearm. Proximal median nerve compression that does not involve the motor fibers of the anterior interosseous nerve is especially difficult to diagnose because motor function is almost always normal. As discussed above, provocative testing can be useful, such as those tests described by Spinner (1978) of resisted middle or ring finger sublimis function or resisted forearm pronation. These tests are useful because they cause compression of the median nerve by the fibrous portions of the muscles that cross the nerve and support this anatomic diagnosis.

However, since the palmar cutaneous branch of the median nerve originates proximal to the carpal tunnel, quantitative sensory testing of the thenar eminence may demonstrate elevated thresholds in the patient with median nerve compression in the forearm. Such a test result is given in Figure 12.9. The degree to which these values for the thenar eminence are elevated can be appreciated by comparison with Figures 12.6 and 12.10. Quantitative sensory testing in this type of problem is especially valuable because traditional electrodiagnostic testing is almost always normal in patients with pronator syndrome. The use of quantitative sensory testing to support this diagnosis is new (Dellon, & Muse, unpublished observations, 1995) (See Table 12.5). Rarely, the palmar cutaneous branch of the median nerve can be compressed at the wrist level, in which case the Tinel will be at the wrist and provocative signs for pronator syndrome will be absent (Duncan, Yaspur, Gomez-Garcia, & Lesavay, 1995).

ULNAR NERVE COMPRESSION IN GUYON'S CANAL

Compression of the ulnar nerve in Guyon's canal is unusual as an isolated nerve entrapment. When it presents as an isolated nerve entrapment, it is usually due to the presence of a ganglion or a lipoma in this canal, and in this location there is only compression of the deep motor branch. Thus, there is normal sensation with weakness of pinch. Grip strength would be near normal. Quantitative sensory testing would demonstrate normal sensory and grip measurements, but abnormal pinch measurements.

FIGURE 12.9

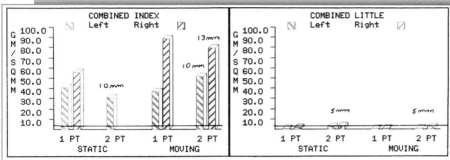

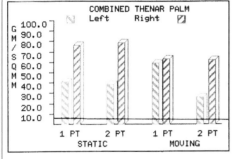

99 % CONFIDENCE LIMIT

3/30/95

Left vs Right for all 4 sensory postions

Proximal Median Nerve Compression in the Forearm; Quantitative Sensory Testing. This 48-year-old assembly-line worker had previously undergone bilateral carpal tunnel releases which only partially relieved the numbness in his thumb, index, and middle finger. He has returned to work. Electrodiagnostic studies demonstrate mild slowing of the median nerve at the wrist, bilaterally, consistent with previous carpal tunnel syndrome. There is no cervical radiculopathy. Physical examination demonstrates discomfort in the forearm with resisted middle finger sublimis flexion and resisted pronation. There is no Tinel sign over the wrist incisions, which are not painful. Moving two-point discrimination is abnormal for both index fingers, and static two-point discrimination is abnormal in the left index finger and absent in the right Index finger, so that this patient has a severe degree of median nerve compression. The pressure thresholds are markedly elevated both at the index finger and at the thenar eminence level. (For comparison of thenar eminence values, see Figure 12.6. and Table 12.5.) Note, too, the normal values for the ulnar nerve as measured in the little finger. These findings are consistent with bilateral median nerve compression in the forearm, pronator syndrome. Measurements made with the Pressure-Specified Sensory Device™.

With slightly more proximal compression, ulnar nerve compression in Guyon's canal would demonstrate abnormal sensory thresholds for the little finger, with normal grip strength measurements, and normal measurements for sensibility over the dorsoulnar aspect of the hand. This is also unusual as an isolated nerve entrapment.

An example of this occurring in conjunction with a blunt trauma to the wrist is given in Figure 12.7. Compression of the ulnar nerve in this location as part of the double crush phenomenon, described in detail in Chapter 14, related to peripheral neuropathy, is difficult to document, and reliance on a positive Tinel sign over the ulnar nerve adjacent to the pisiform is often the only way this can be determined. It should be clear, therefore, that abnormal sensibility testing for the little finger may be due to problems any-where along the course of the C8 sensory nerve root, and that the history and physical exam are critical to making the diagnosis, with the sensory documentation being supportive of it. It should also be clear that

FIGURE 12.10

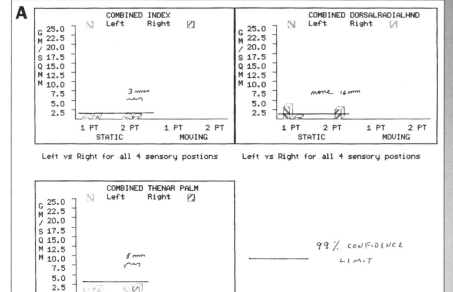

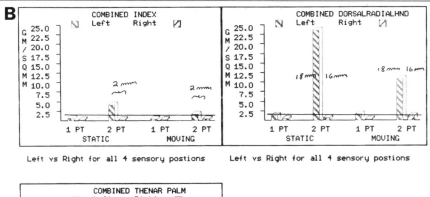

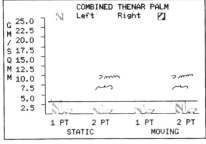

Radial Sensory Nerve Compression in the Forearm; Quantitative Sensory Testing. This 24-year-old carpenter had a wooden plank fall onto the dorsoradial aspect of his left wrist, resulting in immediate dorsoradial pain and swelling of his entire wrist. There was no laceration. (A) The first quantitative sensory testing done at 2 weeks after the injury demonstrated absent static two-point discrimination in the left radial nerve territory, but static touch perception was preserved. Thresholds for the index finger and thenar eminence were normal, consistent with the diagnosis of crush injury to the radial sensory nerve, with some residual function. It was elected to observe this injury, rather than operate, and he was retested 3 weeks later. (B) The repeat testing demonstrates recovery of static two-point discrimination. Although the pressure required to distinguish one from two points was markedly abnormal, this demonstrated that the neuropraxia was recovering and that surgical intervention would likely not be needed. Note increased threshold now for the index finger as the swelling in the wrist area appears to have caused compression of the median nerve in the carpal tunnel. (C) This computer printout is noted by the serial measurements.

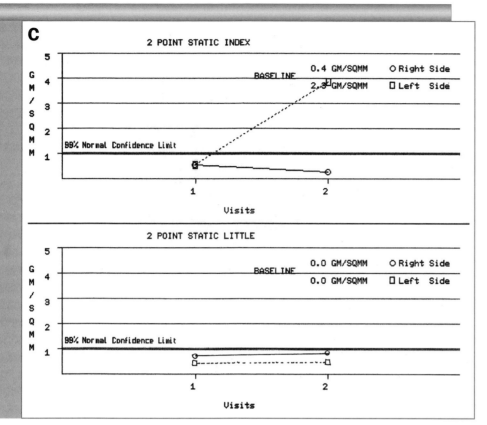

abnormal intrinsic muscle function may be due to problems anywhere along the course of the C8 and T1 motor roots, and that in addition to the history and physical examination, electrodiagnostic studies may be needed. Radiographic imaging of the cervical spine, the apex of the lung, and Guyon's canal may be required as well.

CUBITAL TUNNEL SYNDROME

Cubital tunnel syndrome is the second most common nerve compression syndrome in the upper extremity. Patients will complain of numbness in the little and ring finger, which has usually been present for awhile before they began to notice weakness of pinch and grip strength. The degree to which the motor symptoms predominate often is more related to the patient's job or hobby, such that it is frequently a problem in carrying out some activity of daily living or job-related activity that calls the motor dysfunction to their attention. Thus, for example, a violinist or pianist may complain of some inability to do a technical exercise or a portion of a piece of music, or of the inability to play as long as they used to without fatigue. These are most often ulnar nerve-related complaints, even though virtually every traditional test of nerve function will be normal. In these types of circumstances in which the patient is so keenly aware of their motor function and, therefore, of its subtle limitation, they may not yet even complain of sensory symptoms.

Table 12.10 gives detailed results of quantitative sensory testing with the Pressure-Specified Sensory Device™ in 71 patients with cubital tunnel syndrome. This data gives the spectrum of values obtained when this device is used. This is the data that has been used to determine that the pressure required to distinguish one from two points is the first parameter that can be demonstrated to become abnormal, that is, greater than the 99% confidence limit, in patients with cubital tunnel syndrome. This value becomes abnormal before one-point static touch, and before either one-point moving touch or the moving two-point discrimination thresholds.

Thus, this data, in conjunction with the normative data for the little finger, given in Table 12.3, can be used to arrive at screening/surveillance values of industry, which are given in Table

TABLE 12.10	CUBITAL TUNNEL SYNDROME									
				Pressure Perception Threshold						
	(g/mm²)		(mm)	(g/mm²)		(mm)		(g/mm²)		
	1PS	2PS	2PS	1PM	2PM	2PM dorsal		1PS	1PM	
≤ 45 years of age										
s.d.	24.8	18.9	1.6	20.6	12.4	1.5		35.0	33.0	
99%	23.6	26.4	5.3	13.5	15.8	4.8				
max	97	70	8.6	97	49	8.6				
> 45 years of age										
s.d.	14.6	16.8	1.3	2.8	10.7	1.1		9.0	1.3	
99%	16.2	28.2	5.5	3.9	16.8	5.1				
max	59	58	7.7	11.5	48	7.4				

Note:
⁺ p < .02
⁺ p < .001
From "Computer-Assisted Quantitative Sensorimotor Testing: Patients with Carpal and Cubital Tunnel Syndrome Compared to an Age-Matched Control Population," by A. L. Dellon & K. Keller, *Annals of Plastic Surgery, 38:* 493-502. 1997. Reprinted with permission.

12.9. To do this, the minimal values for a patient 44 years of age with clinical evidence of cubital tunnel syndrome are examined, and are noted to have the pressure threshold for static two-point discrimination of 1.5 g/mm² at a time when all other values are within normal limits, including the distance for distinguishing one from two, which was 2.5 mm. The 99% confidence limit for normal for a person less than 45 years of age is < 1.0 g/mm². Therefore, the screening parameters for a person less than 45 years of age for cubital tunnel would be a distance of 3 mm, and a pressure threshold for this distance of 1.0 g/mm².

For the diagnosis of cubital tunnel syndrome with quantitative sensory testing, there should be abnormal sensory thresholds for both the little finger and for the dorsoulnar aspect of the hand, and abnormal pinch and grip measurements. An example of such a patient is given in Figure 12.11. The values obtained for abnormal pinch and grip measurements using the Digit-Grip™ and the NK pinch device in patients with cubital tunnel syndrome are those for patients younger than or actually 45 years of age; the mean pinch strength is 69.6%, and the mean grasp strength is 48.8% of predicted strength (Dellon & Keller, 1995). As discussed above, weakness is not a complaint of the patient with isolated carpal tunnel syndrome. When a patient with sensory complaints compatible with carpal tunnel syndrome complains about weakness or dropping things, do not consider these complaints to be part of carpal tunnel syndrome. Rather, attempt to identify any coexisting associated ulnar nerve problem.

To demonstrate this, a group of patients with carpal tunnel syndrome had their grip and pinch strength tested with computerized sensorimotor equipment. For those carpal tunnel syndrome patients younger than or actually 45 years of age, the mean pinch strength is 118% and the mean grasp strength is 80% of predicted strength. For those patients older than 45 years of age, the mean pinch strength is 146 percent and the mean grasp strength is 90% of predicted strength. These values are essentially no different from normal (Dellon & Keller, 1995).

When compared to the mean strengths for those patients with carpal tunnel syndrome of the same age group, the cubital tunnel syndrome patients are significantly weaker in pinch ($p < .002$) and grip ($p < .04$). For those cubital tunnel syndrome patients older than 45 years of age, the mean pinch strength is 71.1% and the mean grasp is 45.6% of predicted strength. When compared to the mean strengths for those patients with carpal tunnel syndrome, the cubital tunnel syndrome patients are significantly weaker. For those patients younger than 45 years of age, the significance level for pinch is $p < .002$, and for grip $p < .004$, while for those older than 45 years of age, the pinch is $p < .003$, and grip $p < .006$. Weakness in the presence of normal sensory measurements may be related to painful conditions at the wrist, such as arthritis, carpal instability, or flexor tenosynovitis. Clearly, the history and physical examination will be important in arriving at both a correct diagnosis and an appropriate treatment plan.

Another possible source of weakness associated with normal sensibility may be related to radial tunnel syndrome, which will be discussed below. The possibility of a primary muscle disease, a myopathy, must be considered. Diagnosis of myopathy is greatly aided by electromyography. The strength/duration component of the Digit-Grip™ computerized testing equipment will become valuable in this regard, but is outside the scope of this textbook. For patients with "instantaneous" strength but no endurance, the curve will rise sharply and then fall sharply, in contrast to the usual gradual decline in strength over the 3 sec measuring period. For patients being treated medically for myopathy, that is, for myasthenia gravis, the results of the treatment may be tracked by noting an increase in the area of the curve during the 3 sec measuring period.

The therapist may become involved in the treatment of ulnar nerve entrapment at the elbow because of the value of splinting to treat the early stages of this compression. Eighty percent of patients with a minimal degree of compression can be treated successfully without surgery by a regimen that minimizes elbow flexion beyond 30°, and that changes both job activity and activities of daily living to accomplish this same purpose (Dellon, Hament, & Gittelsohn, 1993). Unfortunately, the splint is often found to be extremely confining for the patient. Some have found the splint that is fabricated so that it covers the volar aspect of the forearm to be more comfortable than one that covers the posterior aspect, but individualization of the splint is as critical here as it is in most other instances.

When nonoperative man-

FIGURE 12.11

A

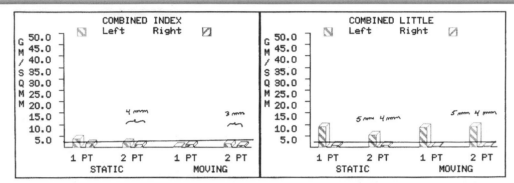

Left vs Right for all 4 sensory postions   Left vs Right for all 4 sensory postions

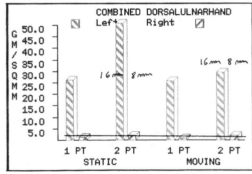

99 % CONFIDENCE
LIMIT

Left vs Right for all 4 sensory postions

Cubital Tunnel Syndrome; Quantitative Sensory Testing. This 39-year-old woman has had complaints of numbness in the left little and ring finger for about 2 years, associated with weakness and clumsiness in the use of the left hand. She has no complaints of numbness in the index finger or thumb, and her hand does not awaken her at night. She works as a telephone operator, holding the phone in her left hand, and does not use a headset. She is aware that when her left elbow is bent, her symptoms worsen. She has no systemic diseases. (A) The sensory testing demonstrates normal values for the index finger, but elevated values for both the left little finger and the dorsoulnar aspect of the left hand with respect to the right side. Not only is the pressure required to distinguish one from two points elevated, but so, too, is the distance at which the points can be distinguished. (B) The grip strength is reduced in the left hand. The variance between measurements, the relationship of the variance between the left and the right hand, and the relative strength of the radial versus the ulnar digits for each impulse measurement are consistent with a person making an honest attempt to give their best effort during the testing procedure. From "Detection of Submaximal Effort with Computer-assisted Grip Strength Measurements," by M.D. Mitterhauser, V. L. Muse, A. L. Dellon, & T. C. Jetzer, Journal of Occupational Medicine, submitted: 1996. Reprinted with permission of the authors.

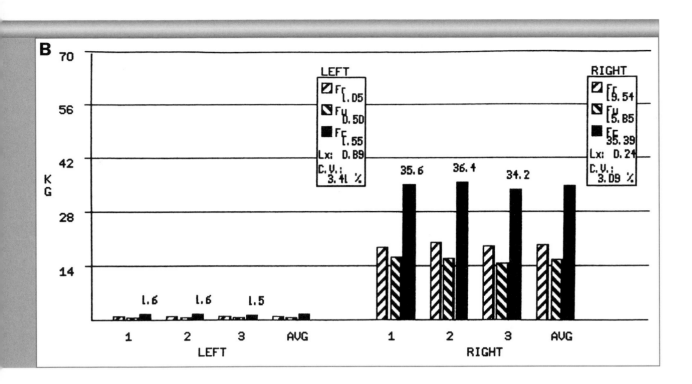

B

LEFT
☑ Fᵣ	[.05
◪ Fᵤ	0.50
■ Fₑ	[.55
Lx:	0.89
C.V.:	3.41 %

RIGHT
☑ Fᵣ	[9.54
◪ Fᵤ	[5.85
■ Fₑ	35.39
Lx:	0.24
C.V.:	3.09 %

agement is unsuccessful, or the patient tires of restricted work and vocational activities, surgical decompression is indicated. In my experience, the most predictable results are achieved by a submuscular placement of the ulnar nerve using a technique that lengthens the musculofascial origins of the flexor/pronator muscle mass (Dellon, 1988; Dellon, 1991; Dellon, Chang, Coert, & Campbell, 1994). This approach reduces pressure on the ulnar nerve in its new location, permits surgical treatment of every anatomic structure that may cross the path of the ulnar nerve, and has just an 8% recurrence rate (Dellon & Coert, 1995).

Following are specific guidelines for sensibility testing in the patient with cu-

bital tunnel syndrome:

Whenever possible, quantitative sensory testing of the large myelinated fibers has been shown to be the most sensitive technique for the early detection of ulnar nerve compression, by measuring the pressure threshold required for static two-point discrimination. In the absence of this computerized sensory testing, the change in perception of a vibratory stimulus is the next best screening test. Serial measurements of the pressure threshold for one-point static touch and two-point static touch are the best way to record progression of chronic nerve compression or the response to nonoperative management.

Once there is an increase in the distance at which one

point can be distinguished from two points, the degree of compression has worsened significantly, consistent with loss of axons. Similarly, the best technique to measure the early changes in the motor system related to ulnar nerve compression is to use the Digit-Grip™ to record grip, and the NK Sensory Device to record pinch. The individual intrinsic muscles must be inspected, principally, the first dorsal interosseous and the abductor pollices brevis, and the hypothenar muscles. Persistent abduction of the little finger should also be noted. Once there is muscle wasting, this must be recorded as degrees of muscle wasting, as subjective and imprecise as that is.

At this stage, after nerve

decompression, recovery will depend on axonal regeneration. The best way to quantitate changes after surgery in this advanced degree of compression is to follow the improvement, that is, the decrease, in both the distance and the pressure threshold required for two-point discrimination. However, now, because we are following neural regeneration, the earliest signs of improvement will be noted in one-point moving and moving two-point discrimination. Therefore, in the set of measurements taken in anticipation of surgery in the person with an advanced degree of compression, it is recommended to have obtained the values from both static and moving one- and two-point thresholds.

In the absence of computerized sensory testing equipment, progress can be recorded by qualitatively noting the changes in vibratory perception, which should trend toward normal, or even toward a hypersensitivity during neural regeneration, and by quantitatively measuring moving two-point discrimination with the Disk-Criminator™. It is not necessary to measure perception of pain or temperature in a person with carpal tunnel syndrome. Clearly, improvement in motor function will be noted by reversal of muscle wasting, and strength may improve even without complete reversal of muscle wasting.

RADIAL SENSORY NERVE ENTRAPMENT

Compression of the radial sensory nerve in the forearm has now been well documented (Dellon & Mackinnon, 1986), and should be detected by testing sensibility. There should be an abnormal threshold over the dorsoradial border of the hand in contrast to the contralateral hand, and in contrast to the index finger, unless there is an associated carpal tunnel syndrome or a bilateral radial sensory nerve entrapment. Figure 12.10 presents an example of a patient who sustained a crush injury to the dorsoradial aspect of the left hand, with associated pain. The initial quantitative sensory testing with the Pressure-Specified Sensory Device™ demonstrated normal sensibility over the index pulp and thenar eminence, but an absent static two-point discrimination over the dorsoradial aspect of the hand. One-point static touch perception was still present, but with an elevated threshold, consistent with a severe injury to the radial sensory nerve, but an injury in which the nerve was still in continuity. Accordingly, the appropriate treatment was splinting, massage, antiinflammatory medication, edema control, and repeat quantitative sensory testing. The repeat testing demonstrated recovering two-point discrimination 3 weeks later,

and surgical intervention was not done. Of interest is that over that period of time, due perhaps to the residual edema within the carpal tunnel, there was gradual onset of carpal tunnel syndrome at the same time the radial sensory nerve was recovering. Quantitative sensory testing documented this, and the patient had steroid injections into the carpal tunnel with subsequent relief of symptoms and return to work. The report generated from the computer measurements (see Figure 12.10 C) documents this change for the worse in the median nerve function. Such a serial measurement is of the type that would be generated during industrial surveillance.

Radial sensory nerve entrapment in the forearm can be associated with pain, as the stretch/traction test demonstrates. If the thumb is held adducted and the wrist taken through a forceful ulnar deviation, the radial sensory nerve is pulled against its proximal entrapment site between the brachioradialis and the extensor carpi radialis longus tendon, producing a sharp pain. This pain is similar to that seen from extensor tenosynovitis of the first dorsal extensor compartment.

On physical examination, the best way to distinguish these two diagnoses is to test for resisted thumb extension. This produces pain even without wrist or thumb movement, demonstrating the presence of tendinitis. In the presence of tendinitis, the radial styloid is often swollen and tender. There will be a Tinel sign at the site of passage of the radial sensory nerve over the brachioradialis tendon in the presence of nerve entrapment. There may be a more distal site if the compression has been caused by a tight watch band (or handcuffs!) (Dellon & Mackinnon, 1986; Mackinnon & Dellon, 1988). The therapist may be the first to detect this clinical syndrome in patients being treated for forearm fractures, and especially if the patient has had an external fixation device, whose pins often pass in close proximity to the radial sensory nerve.

Because radial sensory nerve entrapment may cause pain associated with wrist movement, there may be an associated decrease in pinch and grip strength. This would be distinguished from ulnar nerve entrapment by evaluating the sensibility of the little finger. The nonoperative management of radial sensory nerve entrapment is to splint the wrist in neutral with the thumb in an abducted and slightly extended position, combined with the use of job or daily activity modification and antiinflammatory medication. When this proves unsuccessful, neurolysis of the radial sensory nerve usually gives excellent relief.

Specific guidelines for sensibility testing in the patient with radial sensory nerve entrapment mirror those for carpal tunnel syndrome (see above).

POSTERIOR INTEROSSEOUS NERVE ENTRAPMENT

Entrapment of the radial nerve's motor branch just distal to the elbow is called posterior interosseous nerve entrapment. The only sensory component of this nerve relates to the dorsal wrist capsule, so evaluation of sensibility is normal with this syndrome, although the patient may complain of an aching wrist as part of the syndrome. There is weakness of all thumb and finger extensors, and of the extensor carpi radialis brevis. Because the motor branch to the extensor carpi radialis longus comes off proximal to the entrapment site, the patient can extend the wrist weakly toward the radial side. Because wrist extension is weak, grip strength will usually be measurably weak. Pinch strength may be weak because of inability to stabilize the thumb during forceful pinching. Because muscle weakness may quickly progress to paralysis, surgical decompression is indicated unless there has been recent blunt trauma that may suggest that within a few weeks of observation recovery is possible. During such a period of observation before surgery, or during the postoperative period, a "wrist cock-up" splint is indicated.

RADIAL TUNNEL SYNDROME

Entrapment of the radial nerve at the elbow has been called radial tunnel syndrome. There are no sensory changes distally, and perhaps the only motor weakness will be related to grip strength. The patient usually complains of pain referred to the lateral side of the elbow; thus, differentiating this syndrome from tennis elbow, or lateral humeral epicondylitis, is required. The best description of the physical findings in this problem is by Lister (Lister, Belsoe, & Kleinert, 1979; Lister, 1993).

In the radial tunnel syndrome there should (a) be no tenderness directly over the lateral humeral condyle, but rather tenderness directly over the radial nerve when palpated beneath the brachioradialis muscle mass, and (b) pain referred to the elbow with resisted middle finger extension (because the extensor carpi radialis brevis tendon crosses the radial nerve and inserts into the base of the middle finger). Treatment may be directed at reducing inflammation about the elbow by splinting and with nonsteroidal antiinflammatory medications. In many patients with tennis elbow, the counterforce brace used to protect the origin of the wrist and finger extensors from the impact of the tennis ball can, unfortunately, cause compression of the radial nerve in the proximal forearm or elbow, causing a concomitant radial tunnel syndrome. Attention by the therapist to the splints created for lateral humeral epicondylitis will be required to prevent this problem.

• NERVE RECONSTRUCTION •

NERVE REPAIR, NERVE GRAFT, NERVE ALLOGRAFT, NERVE CONDUIT

The patient referred to the therapist following a nerve reconstruction will require, in general, an initial sensorimotor assessment, attention to possible splinting requirements, motor and sensory reeducation, serial sensorimotor examinations to assess progress of neural regeneration, and then a final assessment suitable for evaluation of impairment. With the exception of the splinting and motor rehabilitation, all of these goals of therapy have in common evaluation of sensibility. Current textbooks (Clark, Wilgis, Aiello, Eckhaus, & Eddington, 1993; Hunter, Schneider, Mackin, & Callahan, 1978, 1994) deal comprehensively with splinting and motor rehabilitation, while Chapter 11 in this textbook deals with sensory reeducation. It is the purpose of this section to be specific about exactly what sensibility tests are required for a thorough yet efficient examination and report.

The first concept is that neural regeneration is the common denominator among nerve repair, autograft, allograft, or conduit reconstruction. The mechanism by which the two ends of the nerve are joined will determine, in part, the degree to which neural regeneration is successful, but that mechanism does not alter the method of assessment employed by the therapist. In a repair, after the injured ends of the nerve are trimmed, sutures are used to join the proximal and distal ends of the nerve. If the injury produced enough damage to the nerve that trimming the injured tissue requires the two ends of the nerve to be joined under tension, then something must be interposed between the two ends of the nerve to prevent scar formation as a response to that tension from interfering with neural regeneration. Either the patient's own (autograft) nerve or another person's (allograft) nerve may be placed into that nerve gap.

Following their success in subhuman primates (Bain et al., 1992), the first human nerve allograft was done successfully by Mackinnon's group, initially in Toronto (Mackinnon & Hudson, 1993), for a sciatic nerve reconstruction, and in 1994 in St. Louis, for an upper extremity nerve defect (Mackinnon, 1994). Currently, the allograft, which requires immunosuppression, is being performed only on patients who require a large length of nerve graft. The neural regeneration proceeds along the length of the allograft nerve, whose Schwann cells support the regeneration while the immunosuppression prevents their rejection. Once the host nerve has regenerated across the allograft, the immunosuppression may be stopped.

In contrast, if a nerve gap of 3 cm or less is needed, then the distance can be bridged successfully by a bioabsorbable conduit, for example, one made from polyglycolic acid (PGA), a suture material.

Following demonstration of their success in subhuman primates (Dellon & Mackinnon, 1988), the first human nerve reconstruction with these tubes, called a Neurotube™, was reported (Mackinnon & Dellon, 1990). The neural regeneration proceeds along the length of the tube, which will be absorbed by hydrolysis, losing its strength by 3 months, at which time the neural regeneration will have reached the distal segment of the injured nerve. The tables of Chapter 11 demonstrate the evaluation of sensibility reported for the traditional nerve repair and nerve graft, while Tables 12.11 and 12.12 demonstrate the evaluation of sensibility required for the end-results assessment of the first reported human nerve allograft and of the first reported results with the Neurotube™. It is clear that the therapist must be able to measure the result of neural regeneration regardless of which of these techniques is used by the surgeon for nerve reconstruction.

At the initial assessment of the patient following nerve reconstruction, the question to be answered by the evaluation of sensibility is whether neural regeneration is progressing appropriately for what will be a successful result. The sequence of recovery of sensation (Dellon, Curtis, & Edgerton, 1972; Gelberman, Urbaniak, & Bright, 1978) is that the unmyelinated and small myelinated fibers regenerate first, but their functions— sweating and the perception of pain and temperature— do not correlate with hand function, whereas the function—moving and static touch—of the large myelinated fibers that regenerate thereafter do correlate with hand function (Moberg, 1958; Dellon & Kallman, 1983; Novak, Mackinnon, & Kelly, 1993; Dellon, E. S., Kress, Moratz, & Dellon, A. L., 1995). Therefore, it is rarely indicated to test for the perception of temperature and pain. I only do this if in doubt that any regeneration is occurring at all, as might be the case if there

were no advancing Tinel sign. If the Tinel sign does advance over time, then moving-touch and, finally, static touch will be recovered at the fingertip or within the area being tested.

The sequence of recovery within the large myelinated fiber population is that the first perception to return is the perception of the 30 Hz tuning fork. This is followed shortly thereafter by the perception of moving-touch. This is related to the ease with which the Meissner corpuscle rather than the Merkel cell neurite complex is reinnervated. Constant-touch perception will then follow and, finally, the last to recover, the perception of the 256 Hz tuning fork. Therefore, the initial examination should include a tapping along the course of expected regeneration from distal to proximal to identify the most distal the Tinel sign has advanced. Then, usually at a site further distal than this Tinel sign, there will be the first site at which the 30 Hz tuning fork will be perceived. The examiner may then simply stroke the skin with his or her fingertip to determine the perception of moving-touch, and press on the skin with his or her fingertip to determine the perception of constant-touch.

In general, by the time the 256 Hz stimulus is perceived at a spot on the skin, the perception of constant-

touch has usually occurred at the spot, as well. So, testing with the 256 Hz tuning fork is an easy way to screen a large skin surface area, such as the regions of the palm or the fingertips, after median nerve reconstruction. These techniques are qualitative, but are sufficient to determine if neural regeneration is occurring appropriately. Once these touch submodalities have recovered to an area, it may be anticipated that further appropriate regeneration will result in an increasing number of these large myelinated fibers reinnervating the skin surface. This will result in the recovery of first moving and then static two-point discrimination. The Disk-Criminator™, with its smooth, rounded, uniform prongs, preset distances between the prongs, and ease of rotation is the preferred testing instrument (see Chapter 7).

Ideally, the therapist's work place will become a "center for excellence" in quantitative sensory testing, and the therapist will be able to quantitate the degree of sensory recovery. During the initial assessment, then, if there is a vibrometer present, even if it is just a single-frequency, variable-intensity vibrometer (see Chapter 7), the vibratory threshold at several sites from proximal to distal along the course of neural regeneration can be measured. If there is a variable

A

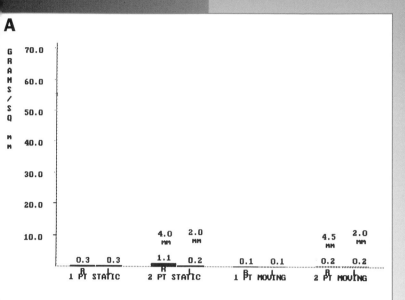

B

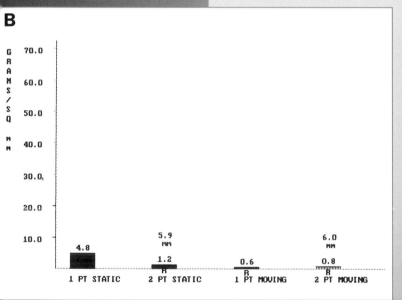

C

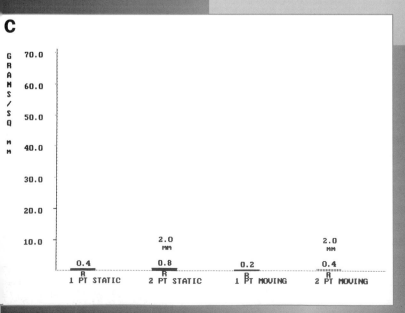

FIGURE 12.12
Neural Regeneration after Digital Nerve Repair; Quantitative Sensory Testing. The sensibility is measured in this 22-year-old woman 6 months after the right radial digital nerve to the index finger was repaired in the hand. (A) Measurements at the tip of the right and left index finger show excellent recovery already, but there is crossover innervation at the tip. The patient received sensory reeducation. Measurements have been made in the autonomous zone of the digital nerve on both the (B) radial and (C) ulnar digital nerve sides of the finger. Note that the pressure threshold for one-point moving touch has recovered to a better level than one-point static touch, over the radial, reinnervated side of the finger, and that two-point discrimination, at 6 mm, is just beginning to recover in the autonomous zone. Measurements made with the Pressure-Specified Sensory Device™.

FIGURE 12.13

Neural Regeneration after Median Nerve Graft; Quantitative Sensory Testing. The sensibility is measured at 18 months in (A) and 24 months in (B) in the left hand of a 47-year-old woman after a four strand, interposition, interfascicular sural nerve graft to the median nerve. Each sural nerve fascicle was 5 cm in length. She received intensive sensory reeducation. Note that the middle finger continues to lag behind the recovery of the thumb and index finger. This is because the common volar digital nerve to the middle/ ring web space was not reconstructed with a graft to permit as many axons as possible to regenerate from the proximal median nerve into the most critical sensory regions, the thumb and the radial sides of the index and middle finger. At 18 months the index has recovered already exceptional functional sensation. The thumb and middle finger at 18 months demonstrate the precise pattern of sensory recovery that must be observed for the therapist to assure the surgeon that neural regeneration is proceeding appropriately, that is, one-point moving-touch has recovered earlier, and to a

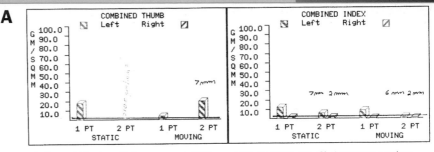

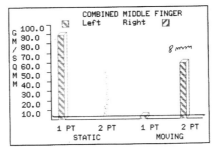

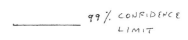

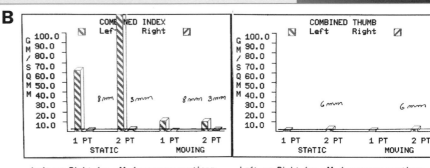

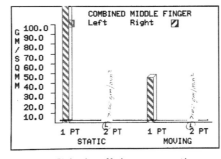

better level, than has one-point static-touch, and that moving two-point discrimination has recovered earlier and to a better level than has static two-point discrimination. These measurements, made with the Pressure-Specified Sensory Device™, permit the substitution of quantitative testing for the qualitative testing done previously with the 30 Hz tuning fork. By 24 months, the index finger has recovered static two-point discrimination and the thumb has continued to improve, while the middle finger, perhaps because the patient is using the thumb and index finger inputs to the cortex most of the time, has not demonstrated further improvement. From: A. L. Dellon, unpublished observations. 1997.

frequency vibrometer, it will be able to measure that there is recovery of the low-frequency stimulus first, then both the low and high at the same skin site, with the lower frequency having the lower threshold for stimulation. If there is a Neurotron™, it will be able to document that there is recovery of the 5 Hz stimulus first, then the 250 Hz stimulus and, finally, the 2000 Hz stimulus at the same skin site over time. (Remember that this is an electrical and not a vibratory mechanical stimulus, an example of which is given in Figure 7.27.)

I believe, however, that the best way to document sensory recovery, is with the Pressure-Specified Sensory Device™. As illustrated in Figure 12.12 for a digital nerve, and in Figure 12.13 for a median nerve, the one-point moving touch will be the first to recover, substituting for the 30 Hz and moving-touch stimulus described in the preceding paragraph, but now this is quantitated in terms of g/mm² for the one-point moving touch threshold. The next to recover will be the one-point static touch, quantitated (measured) in terms of g/mm². (This is what is estimated by the Semmes-Weinstein nylon monofilament and by the West™). Next to recover will be moving two-point discrimination, measured in terms of both the distance at which the two points can be

distinguished and the pressure required for this discrimination. Finally, static two-point discrimination will be recovered, measured in terms of both the distance at which the two points can be distinguished, and the pressure required for this discrimination.

Assessment of the progress of neural regeneration will use the identical scheme as delineated above for the initial assessment, but embodies the concept that once moving touch and static touch have recovered to an area, they each no longer need to be documented. At that point, just the continued improvement in moving and static two-point discrimination need to be measured. In Figures 12.12 and 12.13, using the Pressure-Specified Sensory Device™, it will be noted that the one point moving- and static-touch thresholds were still measured, but this was more for the interest of the tester than for the need to have these measurements to document progression. To restate this concept, and in the interest of the therapist doing the most efficient sensory evaluation possible, once two-point discrimination has begun to recover, only two-point discrimination needs to be measured to document appropriate neural regeneration related to functional sensation.

If the one-point moving and one-point static touch

thresholds improved, but two-point discrimination did not recover, or stopped recovering, then it would be clear that appropriate neural regeneration had stopped. If no two-point discrimination recovers, the therapist provides the basis by this quantitative documentation that reoperation is indicated, and that probably a resection of the first nerve repair site is required and reconstruction by a nerve graft or nerve conduit is most likely indicated. If two-point discrimination recovers, but then stops improving, and the patient desires improved sensory function, the therapist provides the basis by this quantitative documentation that reoperation is indicated, and that probably a neurolysis is indicated. This circumstance is illustrated in Figures 12.14 and 12.15.

End-results assessment of neural regeneration primarily uses the concept that functional sensation in the digit or hand is best correlated with two-point discrimination. At the time neural regeneration is considered complete and the patient will not be seen for another year, and a disability or other report is needed, both moving and static two-point discrimination should be measured. Again, ideally, the pressure required to distinguish the two points should be specified if computerized equipment is available.

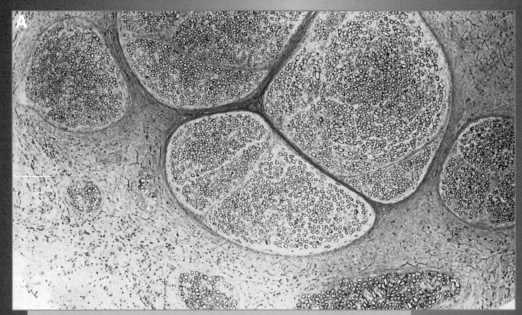

FIGURE 12.14

(A) Histologic appearance of interfascicular fibrosis that is present with chronic nerve compression and that permits intraneural microdissection within this plane, resulting in (B), the appearance of the median nerve after an internal neurolysis. This is shown to demonstrate what may not be done following a nerve reconstruction, because such a dissection would disrupt the regenerated axons. Therefore, following a nerve reconstruction, (C), if there is less than the desired recovery, an external neurolysis may still be offered (D). From Surgery of the Peripheral Nerve, *by S. E. Mackinnon & A. L. Dellon, 1988, New York: Thieme Publishing. Reprinted with permission of the authors.*

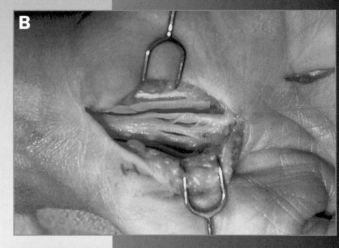

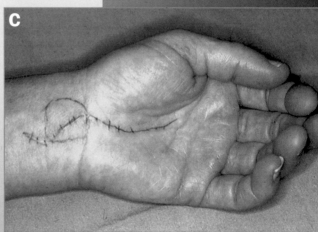

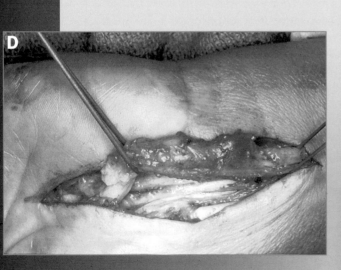

FIGURE 12.15

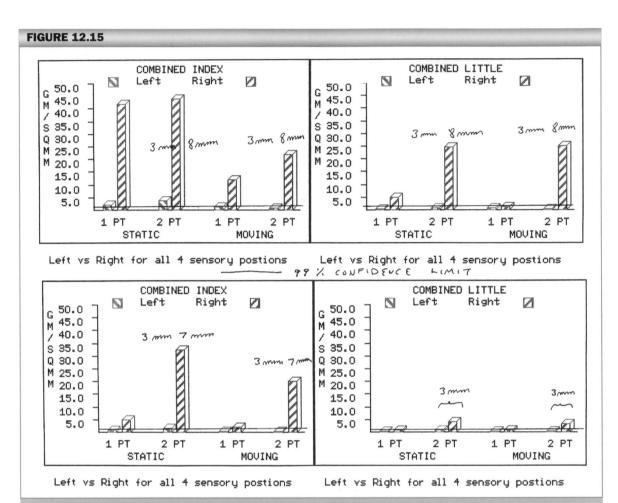

Left vs Right for all 4 sensory postions

Left vs Right for all 4 sensory postions

99 % CONFIDENCE LIMIT

Left vs Right for all 4 sensory postions

Left vs Right for all 4 sensory postions

Neural Regeneration after Neurolysis; Quantitative Sensory Testing. The top index and little finger measurements were taken 2 years after a median and an ulnar nerve repair done at the wrist level in a 26-year-old woman. Her repaired tendons have been functioning well, and she uses this right, dominant hand, at work, but wishes her sensation could be further improved. This is already a good result after nerve repair. She has already had sensory reeducation. The mass in her palm is slightly painful. Because she has recovered two-point discrimination, nerve grafting would be inappropriate because there is the chance the results of a nerve graft at this time would not give better results after 2 years of regeneration than she now has; however, a microsurgical external neurolysis of both nerves may give some improvement. The bottom measurements, six months after the neurolysis, demonstrate that the sensibility of the little finger has improved into the normal range, while the index finger has improved just a little. The measurements were made with the Pressure-Specified Sensory Device™. The computerized sensory testing equipment is sensitive enough to document these changes.

PRESSURE-SPECIFIED
SENSORY DEVICE™:
HAND TESTING PROTOCOL

The Pressure-Specified Sensory Device™ (PSSD) is an instrument designed to measure the threshold for the perception of pressure stimuli on the surface of the human body. These stimuli may consist of either static (non-moving) touch or moving touch applied to the body surface being tested, such as the fingertip pulp. Since the position of the testing instrument will vary with respect to gravity, the instrument must be zeroed to correct for this force at the start of each testing procedure for each different body surface, or for each different positioning of the part being tested with respect to the examiner's positioning of the instrument.

The instrument consists of two metal prongs, each with an identical hemispherical-shaped tip. If just one of these prongs is used as the testing stimulus, the test is called "one point," with the adjective "static" or "moving" used depending on whether the examiner positions the prong so that there is no movement with respect to the skin surface other than increasing the depth of skin indentation (static touch), or the examiner moves the prong from proximal to distal along the surface of the fingertip while increasing the depth of skin indentation (moving touch). If both prongs are used simultaneously as the testing stimulus, the test is called "two point," with the adjective "static" or "moving" depending on whether the examiner positions the prongs horizontally across the fingertip pulp so there is movement with respect to the skin surface in addition to increasing the depth of skin indentation, (moving two-point discrimination), or the examiner just increases the depth of skin indentation (static two-point discrimination). The threshold is the pressure at which the subject can first detect the stimulus. The stimuli are designated as 1PS (one-point static touch), 2PS (static two-point discrimination), 1PM (one-point moving touch), and 2PM (moving two-point discrimination).

The PSSD provides a threshold measurement throughout a continuous range of applied pressures, whose perception threshold will be reported as pressure in grams per square millimeter, or g/mm^2. The distance at which the perception of two points being pressed against the skin surface can be distinguished from just one point is called two-point discrimination. When the PSSD is used for this measurement, the distance, as is traditional, is expressed in millimeters. In contrast to tradition, the PSSD also permits the specification of the minimum pressure required for the discrimination of two points from one point. That pressure threshold is expressed in g/mm^2. While the PSSD itself may be used to determine the smallest distance for two-point discrimination, it is more practical in terms of efficiency for this distance to be approximated first with a Disk-Criminator™, using as much pressure as required to be sure that the patient is receiving a supramaximal pressure stimulus. This distance will be taken as the starting point for two-point discrimination testing with the PSSD.

A complete test of any given surface area using the PSSD will, therefore, be reported in terms of 6 different values. The value for 1PS and for 1PM will be given as a single number, the pressure threshold expressed as g/mm^2. The value of both 2PS and 2PM will be expressed as two separate numbers for each test, one in millimeters and one in gm/mm^2. Thus, a report will state that for the index fingertip 1PS is 0.5 g/mm^2, whereas 2PS is 3 mm at 0.5 g/mm^2.

GENERAL SEQUENCE
OF TESTING

The patient must be seated in a comfortable manner, with the body part to be tested placed in a supported position that minimizes movement without physically restraining the surface. The examiner must be seated in a comfortable position with the arm that will be holding the PSSD supported. The room in which the testing is done must be distraction free. The tester must have confidence that the patient is (a) intelligent enough to understand the testing procedure, (b) not mentally impaired by pain medication or alcohol, and (c) cooperative and not primarily motivated by workmen's compensation or other legal issues that preclude the patient giving an honest response to the testing. Otherwise, the testing should be discontinued or the causes for the tester's concern listed on the report so that anyone interpreting the testing results will be able to make the correct interpretation. This information will become apparent during the entering of the demographic data at the start of the session and during the familiarization period prior to obtaining data.

The patient must be familiarized with the testing procedure, and the first set of measurements obtained should not be considered definitive test results. The testing routine should be done on a body surface presumed to be normal so that the patient will know what type of touch response is caused by the one- and two-point, static and moving stimuli. During the familiarization period the subject may see the computer screen, but the view of the screen must be blocked during the testing sequence. As indicated above, the PSSD must be zeroed against gravity and for each new stimulus at each new test site, but not between every trial for each

stimulus.

For a given test site and a given stimulus, there will be 5 trials recorded. Each trial consists of the examiner bringing the prong into contact with the skin surface, the subject perceiving that a stimulus has been delivered, and the subject responding to the stimulus. In general, these 5 data points will be displayed on the screen for the examiner to review. At that time, the examiner will select the 3 data points that are most closely grouped as representing the data to be averaged and saved. These are selected by eliminating the highest and lowest values recorded. Clearly, if the examiner jams the prong onto the test area, the response measured will be falsely high. If the subject anticipates the touch sequence and presses the button too soon, the response measured will be falsely low. The examiner must be aware of these testing errors and correct for them by giving another test trial. These errors may occur without the examiner being aware of them, in which case they will become apparent when the time comes to average the responses. For example, if the 5 responses obtained for 1PS were, in g/mm^2, 2.2, 0.5, 0.7, 0.1, and 0.6, then the 3 data points chosen for averaging should be 0.5, 0.7, and 0.6, with the reported 1PS pressure threshold being 0.6 g/mm^2.

MEASURING THE ONE-POINT TOUCH PRESSURE THRESHOLD

The patient is instructed to respond to the stimulus by pressing either the hand-held response button or, if the hand is too impaired, the foot-controlled switch. The examiner selects the appropriate computer screens to arrive at the choice of which one-point touch stimulus is to be delivered to which body surface. If the one-point static touch threshold is being measured, the patient is then instructed to "make the response at the first detection of the prong touching the skin," followed by, "as soon as you know you are being touched, press the button." If the one-point moving touch threshold is being measured, the verbal instruction is to "make the response at the first detection of the prong moving along the surface of the skin," followed by "do not press the button as soon as you are touched, but only when you can tell that something is moving."

The testing sequence then begins with the examiner alerting the subject that the stimulus is coming by saying, "Shut your eyes and get ready, the test is beginning now." The examiner then slowly brings the prong of the PSSD into contact with the surface to be tested. The examiner must directly observe the prong's approach to, and contact with, the skin surface to get visual feedback of the testing procedure. The examiner uses visual cues related to the degree of skin indentation and tactile cues related to the feeling in the examiner's own hand as the PSSD is guided onto the test site. These cues permit the examiner to slowly increase the pressure of stimulus application until the subject presses the response button. The subject may open his or her eyes between each test. The examiner should check the subject's eyes and realert the subject at the start of each test by saying, "Get ready, close your eyes, the test is beginning again." After 5 satisfactory trials the 1PS test sequence is stopped and the data is averaged by the examiner, while the subject is instructed to open his or her eyes and relax. Reassure the subject that the procedures were followed appropriately, if they were, and correct the subject's understanding of the procedures if they were not followed correctly.

MEASURING THE DISTANCE THRESHOLD FOR DETECTION OF TWO POINTS

The uniqueness of the PSSD measurement is its ability to record the pressure threshold and the distance. It is easier to revolve the Disk-Criminator™ through the examiner's fingers than it is to adjust the interprong distance on the PSSD, so the Disk-Criminator™ is used to

determine the actual distance measurement. In the absence of a Disk-Criminator™, the PSSD certainly can be used to make the final determination of distance by turning the knob and observing the value in millimeters in the small window on the computer screen.

The threshold distance for the subject's ability to detect one from two prongs touching the test skin surface is estimated quickly with the Disk-Criminator™. The patient is first shown the instrument to alleviate any fears of pain and is informed that he or she is to give a particular verbal response (not press a button) when the touch stimulus that is perceived is either one or two "points." The subject is then instructed to shut his or her eyes. The examiner begins by touching one prong to the skin, pressing it moderately hard into the surface to be sure that the test is above the pressure threshold. The examiner asks, "Is that one or two?" The patient should say, "one," following which the examiner should provide positive reinforcement by saying, "That is correct, now what is this, one or two?" at which time the examiner does the next test with the Disk-Criminator™ at a distance of 6 mm. If the patient says "two," the examiner goes on to a 5 mm distance. If the subject says "one," then the subject is asked to open his or her eyes and

directly view the stimulus. The sequence is then repeated with first the 1 mm and then the 6 mm distance. If the subject still incorrectly identifies the 6 mm stimulus as two points, then the examiner must increase the distance to 8 mm and repeat the sequence entirely from the beginning.

On the way down to smaller distances, the examiner may proceed from 5 mm, to 4 mm, to 3 mm. If the subject gives quick and correct responses, then the examiner has confidence that, in fact, the stimulus is being correctly perceived, and he or she may continue down to smaller distances without requiring "7 out of 10" correct responses. As the two-point limen, or threshold, is approached, the patient's responses will become slower and more thoughtful. At this time, the one-prong stimulus should be alternated with the two-prong stimulus to be sure that the patient can still detect one from two correctly. At the distance selected for the "end-point," the subject must get 2 out of 3 trials correct with the answer of "two." If the subject incorrectly identifies the two prongs as one, or as a single broad one, the distance selected for the PSSD test should be the next millimeter higher or wider spacing; that is, if the 2 mm distance is not identified as two, set the PSSD at 3 mm for testing. If the 5 mm distance is not identified as two, set the PSSD at 6 mm for testing.

For routine testing in the clinical setting or for screening/surveillance in industry, it is sufficient to set the PSSD interprong spacing to the nearest whole number, that is, 5 mm rather than 5.5 mm. If the computer electronically records the distance as 5.1 mm or 4.9 mm, that is acceptable and not statistically or clinically significantly different from 5.0 mm, and the examiner should not be concerned about that difference in distance. For routine clinical testing or screening/ surveillance examinations, the final distance threshold may be accepted as 2 of 3 correct responses, whereas for an outcome study, a research protocol, or a repeat of an abnormal screening examination, more strict criteria, such as 3 out of 5 or 7 out of 10, may be required.

MEASURING THE TWO-POINT DISCRIMINATION PRESSURE THRESHOLD

Once the distance has been entered into the computer by setting the interprong distance with the knob at the undersurface of the PSSD, and the desired distance is checked by the examiner by observing the distance displayed on the computer screen's viewing window, the subject must be instructed again. If 2PS is being tested, the examiner

says, "You are to press the button when you first detect that two points are touching you. Do not push the button as soon as you feel something touch you. Be sure that you can distinguish two separate points. I may sometimes touch you with just one point to be sure that you are responding to the correct stimulus." If 2PM is being tested, the examiner says, "You are to press the button when you first detect that two points are moving along the surface of your skin. Do not push the button as soon as you feel something touch you. Do not push the button as soon as you feel two different points touch you but be sure that you feel two points moving. I may sometimes touch you with just one point or not move the two points just to be sure that you are responding to the correct stimulus."

The testing sequence then begins with the examiner alerting the subject that the stimulus is coming by saying, "Shut your eyes and get ready, the test is beginning now." The examiner then slowly brings the prongs of the PSSD into contact with the surface to be tested, striving to touch the skin surface with both prongs simultaneously. The examiner must directly observe the prong's approach to, and the prong's contact with, the skin surface to get visual feedback of the testing procedure. The examiner uses visual cues relat-

ed to the degree of skin indentation, and tactile cues related to the feeling in the examiner's own hand as the PSSD is guided onto the test site. These cues permit the examiner to slowly increase the pressure of stimulus application until the subject presses the response button.

In contrast to testing 1PS or 1PM, the examiner should also view the computer screen once the prongs have contacted the skin surface, as the test must deliver as close to the same pressure with each of the two prongs. This goal is monitored visually on the computer screen, where each prong's applied pressure is displayed as the height of the bar. The examiner's goal is to keep the two bars at the same height as the PSSD is slowly applied to the test skin site with increasing pressure. The subject may open his or her eyes between each test. The examiner should check the subject's eyes and realert the subject at the start of each test by saying, "Get ready, close your eyes, the test is beginning again." After 5 satisfactory trials, the 2PS or 2PM test sequence is stopped and the data is averaged by the examiner while the subject is instructed to open his or her eyes and relax. Reassure the subject that the procedures were followed appropriately, if they were, and correct the subject's understanding of the procedures if they were not followed correctly.

• **REFERENCES** •

Azman, O., Dellon, A. L., Birely, B., McFarlane, E. Clinical implications of innervation of the human shoulder joint. *Clinical Orthopedics and Related Research*, submitted: 1995.

Bain, J. R., Mackinnon, S. E., Hudson, A. R., Wade, J., Evans, P., Mackin, A., & Hunter, D. Peripheral nerve allograft in primate immunosupressed with Cyclosporin A: I. Histologic and electrophysiologic assessment. *Plastic and Reconstructive Surgery* 90:1036-1046, 1992.

Clark, G. L., Wilgis, E. F. S., Aiello, B., Eckhaus, D., & Eddington, L. V. *Rehabilitation of the Hand: A Practical Guide*. New York: Churchill Livingstone, Inc., 1993.

Dellon, A. L. Clinical use of vibratory stimuli to evaluate peripheral nerve injury and compression neuropathy. *Plastic and Reconstructive Surgery* 65: 466-476, 1980.

Dellon, A. L. Operative technique for submuscular transposition of the ulnar nerve. *Contemporary Orthopedics* 16:17-24, 1988.

Dellon, A. L. Partial dorsal wrist denervation; Resection of distal posterior interosseous nerve. *Journal of Hand Surgery* 10A:527-533, 1985.

Dellon, A. L. Reoperative peripheral nerve surgery. In *Reoperative Surgery*, J. Grotting, Editor. St. Louis: Quarterly Medical Publishers, 1995, pp.1561-1602.

Dellon, A. L. Techniques for successful management of ulnar nerve entrapment at the elbow. *Neurosurgical Clinics-North America* 2:227-234, 1991.

Dellon, A. L. The vibrometer. *Plastic and Reconstructive Surgery* 71:427-431, 1983.

Dellon, A. L. Tinel or not Tinel? *Journal of Hand Surgery (British)* 9:216, 1984.

Dellon, A. L., Chang, E., Coert, H. J., & Campbell, K. R. Intraneural ulnar pressure changes related to operative techniques for cubital tunnel decompression. *Journal of Hand Surgery* 19A:923-930, 1994.

Dellon, A. L., & Coert, H. Results of the treatment of ulnar nerve compression at the elbow by the musculofascial lengthening technique. *Journal of Bone and Joint Surgery*, submitted: 1997.

Dellon, A. L., Curtis, R. M., & Edgerton, M. T. Evaluating recovery of sensation in the hand following nerve injury. *Johns Hopkins Journal of Medicine* 130:235-243, 1972.

Dellon, A. L., Dellon, E. S., Tassler, P. L., Ellefson, R. E., Hendrickson, M., & Francel, T. G. Experimental model of pyridoxine (B6) deficiency-induced neuropathy. *Annals of Plastic Surgery*, submitted: 1997.

Dellon, A. L., Hament, W., Gittelsohn, A. Non-operative management of cubital tunnel syndrome; Results of eight-year prospective study. *Neurology* 43:1673-1677, 1993.

Dellon, A. L., & Kallman, C. H. Evaluation of functional sensation in the hand. *Journal of Hand Surgery* 8:865-870, 1983.

Dellon, A. L., & Keller, K. Computer-assisted quantitative sensorimotor testing in patients with carpal and cubital tunnel syndrome. *Annals of Plastic Surgery*, 38: 493-502. 1997.

Dellon, E. S., Keller, K., Moratz, V., & Dellon, A. L. Validation of cutaneous pressure threshold measurements for the evaluation of hand function. *Annals of Plastic Surgery* 38: 493-502. 1997.

Dellon, A. L., & Mackinnon, S. E. An alternative to the classical nerve graft for the management of the short nerve gap. *Plastic and Reconstructive Surgery* 82:849-856, 1988.

Dellon, A. L., & Mackinnon, S. E. Injury to the medial antebrachial cutaneous nerve during cubital tunnel surgery. *Journal of Hand Surgery* 10B:33-36, 1985.

Dellon, A. L., & Mackinnon, S. E. Radial sensory nerve entrapment. *Archives of Neurology* 43:833-837, 1986.

Dellon, E. S., & Dellon, A. L. Quantitative sensory testing with the force-defined vibrometer. *Journal of Reconstructive Microsurgery*: submitted 1997.

Duncan, G. J., Yospur, G., Gomez-Garcia, A., & Lesavay, M. A. Entrapment of the palmar cutaneous branch of the median nerve by a normal palmaris longus tendon. *Annals of Plastic Surgery 35*:534-536, 1995.

Evans, G. R. D., & Dellon, A. L. Implantation of the palmar cutaneous branch of the median nerve into the pronator quadratus for treatment of painful neuroma. *Journal of Hand Surgery 19A*:203-206, 1994.

Fine, E. J., & Wongjirad, C. The ulnar flexion maneuver. *Muscle and Nerve 8*:612, 1985.

Francel, T. J., Dellon, A. L., & Campbell, J. N. Quadrilateral space syndrome. *Plastic and Reconstructive Surgery 87*:911-916, 1991.

Gelberman, R. H., Urbaniak, J. R., & Bright, D. S. Digital sensibility following replantation. *Journal of Hand Surgery 3*:313-319, 1978.

Hunter, J. M., Schneider, L. H., Mackin, E. J., & Callahan, A. *Rehabilitation of the Hand*, 1st Edition. Philadelphia: C. V. Mosby, 1978.

Hunter, J. M., Schneider, L. H., Mackin, E. J., & Callahan, A. *Rehabilitation of the Hand*, 4th Edition, 1994.

Kaplan, M., Mullick, T., Dellon, A. L., & Hendler, N. Value of somatosensory evoked potentials in the diagnosis of brachial plexus compression in the thoracic inlet (thoracic outlet syndrome), unpublished observations, 1997.

Lister, G. *The Hand: Diagnosis and Indications*. 3rd edition. Edinburgh: Churchill Livingstone, Inc., 1993.

Lister, G. D., Belsoe, R. B., & Kleinert, H. E. The radial tunnel syndrome. *Journal of Hand Surgery 4*:52-59, 1979.

Lundborg, G. *Nerve Injury and Repair*. Edinburgh: Churchill Livingstone, 1988.

Lundborg, G., Lie-Stenstrom, A. K., Sollerman, C., Stromberg, T., Pyykko, L. Digital vibrogram: A new diagnostic tool for sensory testing in compression neuropathy. *Journal of Neurology, Neurosurgery, and Psychiatry 11A*:693-699, 1986.

Lundborg, G., Dahlin, L. B., Lundstrom, R., Necking, L. E., & Stromberg, T. Vibrotactile function of the hand in compression and vibration-induced neuropathy. Sensibility index—A new measure. *Scandinavian Journal of Plastic and Reconstructive Hand Surgery 26*:275-281, 1992.

Mackinnon, S. E. Invited discussion on nerve allografting. *Annals of Plastic Surgery 33*:516-517, 1994.

Mackinnon, S. E., & Dellon, A. L. Clinical nerve reconstruction with a bioabsorbable polyglycolic tube. *Plastic and Reconstructive Surgery 85*:419-424, 1990.

Mackinnon, S. E., & Dellon, A. L. Experimental study of chronic nerve compression: Clinical implications. *Clinics of Hand Surgery 2*:639-650, 1986.

Mackinnon, S. E., & Dellon, A. L. Overlap of lateral antebrachial cutaneous nerve and superficial sensory radial nerve. *Journal of Hand Surgery 10A*:522-526, 1985.

Mackinnon, S. E., & Dellon, A. L. Results of treatment of recurrent dorsoradial wrist neuromas. *Annals of Plastic Surgery 19*:54-61, 1987.

Mackinnon, S. E., & Dellon, A. L. *Surgery of the Peripheral Nerve*. New York: Thieme, 1988.

Mackinnon, S. E., & Dellon, A. L. Terminal branch of anterior interosseous nerve as source of wrist pain. *Journal of Hand Surgery 9B*:316-322, 1984.

Mackinnon, S. E., Dellon, A. L., Hudson, A. R., & Hunter, D. A primate model for chronic nerve compression. *Journal of Reconstructive Microsurgery 1*:185-194, 1985.

Mackinnon, S. E., Dellon, A. L., Hudson, A. R., & Hunter, D. Chronic nerve compression: An experimental model in the rat. *Annals of Plastic Surgery 13*:112-120, 1984.

Mackinnon, S. E., & Hudson, A. R. Clinical application of peripheral nerve transplantation. *Plastic and Reconstructive Surgery 90*:695-699, 1993.

McFarlane, R. M., & Moyer, J. R. Digital nerve grafts with the lateral antebrachial cutaneous nerve. *Journal of Hand Surgery*

1:169-173, 1976.

Mitterhauser, M. D., Muse, V. L., Dellon, A. L., Jetzer, T. C. Detection of submaximal effort with computer-assisted grip strength measurements. *Journal of Occupational Medicine,* submitted: 1995.

Moberg, E. Objective methods of determining functional value of sensibility in the hand. *Journal of Bone and Joint Surgery (British) 40B*:454-466, 1958.

Naff, N., Dellon, A. L., & Mackinnon, S. E. The anatomic source of the palmar cutaneous branch of the median nerve, including a description of its own unique tunnel. *Journal of Hand Surgery 18B*:316-317, 1993.

Novak, C. B., Mackinnon, S. E., & Kelly, L. Correlation of two-point discrimination and hand function following median nerve injury. *Annals of Plastic Surgery 31*:495-498, 1993.

Phalen, G. S. The carpal tunnel syndrome: Seventeen years experience in diagnosis and treatment of 654 hands. *Journal of Bone and Joint Surgery 48A*:211-228, 1966.

Roos, D. B., & Owens, J. C. Thoracic outlet syndrome. *Archives of Surgery 93*:71-74, 1966.

Rowntree, T. Anomalous innervation of hand muscles. *Journal of Bone and Joint Surgery 31B*:505-510, 1949.

Rydevik, B., & Lundborg, G. Permeability of intraneural microvessels in perineum following acute graded experimental nerve compression. *Scandinavian Journal of Plastic and Reconstructive Surgery 11*:179-183, 1977.

Saplys, R., Mackinnon, S. E., & Dellon, A. L. The relationship between nerve entrapment versus neuroma complications and the misdiagnosis of DeQuervain's Disease. *Contemporary Orthopedics 15*:51-57, 1987.

Spinner, M. *Injuries to the Major Branches of the Peripheral Nerves of the Forearm,* 2nd edition. Philadelphia: W. B. Saunders Company, 1978.

Tinel, J. The tingling sign in peripheral nerve lesions. Translation by Emmanuel B. Kaplan. In *Injuries to the Major Branches of Peripheral Nerves of the Forearm*, M. Spinner, Editor. Philadelphia: W. B. Saunders Company, 1978.

• ADDITIONAL READINGS •

Arezzo, J. S., Schaumberg, H. H., & Laudadio, C. Thermal sensitivity tester: Device for quantitative assessment of thermal sense in diabetic neuropathy. *Diabetes 35*:590-592, 1986.

Gelberman, R. H. *Operative Nerve Repair and Reconstruction*. Philadelphia: J. B. Lippincott Company, 1991.

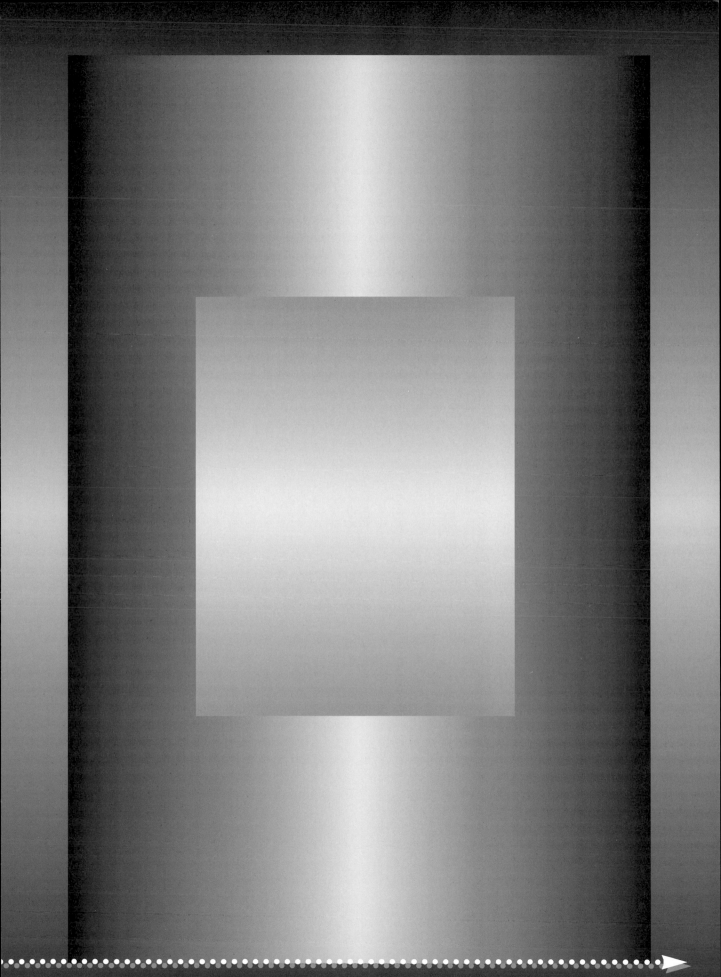

CHAPTER 1

lower extremity

I t is my belief that therapists will become increasingly in-volved in the care of lower extremity peripheral nerve problems. As we have become more expert in under-standing the mechanisms involved with upper extremity peripheral nerve problems, and more experienced with the nonoperative and operative management of these problems, it has become clear that there are direct applications of this knowledge to the lower extremity. To be sure, there are med-ical specialists who are devoted to the care of the foot, such as the orthopedic surgeons who are members of the Foot and Ankle Society, and the members of the American Soci-ety for Podiatric Medicine and Surgery. But, for the most part, physicians and therapists have not put in the same ef-fort with respect to the diagnosis, treatment, and rehabilita-tion of the foot as they have with respect to the hand.

I clearly recall the day in my office, when, accompanied by a resident, I evaluated the improved sensation that had been recovered in the hands of a patient with diabetes after pe-ripheral nerve decompression. The patient asked, "You've helped my hands so much, can you do the same for my feet?" My initial response was, "We don't do feet." But, being in a teaching mode, my next response was, "Why not try?" Over the past 10 years I have found that the concepts that have been developed for the treatment of upper extremity nerve problems can be successfully applied to the lower extremity. As the results of this work are published and confirmed by other investigators and surgeons, it may be anticipated that there will be increased numbers of patients with lower extremity nerve problems referred to therapists for quantitative sensory testing and rehabilitation.

Perhaps the most common role the therapist will have in the care of lower extremity nerve problems will be documenting the degree of sensibility in the skin territories supplied by the peripheral nerves. This documentation, which requires measurement, is necessary for diagnosis, for evaluating progress after treatment, and for determining treatment results.

• RELEVANT NEUROANATOMY •

Figure 13.1 illustrates the most typical areas of skin innervation by the sensory nerves that are the most common causes of clinical problems in the lower extremities. Figure 13.2 illustrates the most common distribution of the sensory dermatomes of the spinal nerves that might be a cause of lower extremity symptoms that may be similar to those from the peripheral nerves.

• THE POSTERIOR TIBIAL NERVE •

The relationships of the posterior tibial nerve and its branches to the surrounding structures are crucial to understanding the symptoms related to compression of this nerve and to its surgical decompression. The posterior tibial nerve begins as a branch from the sciatic nerve in the popliteal fossa. In this location it will give off the medial sural branch (see below), which is most commonly used as a source for nerve graft donor material. In the popliteal fossa it will also give off the motor branches to the gastrocnemius muscles. Then the posterior tibial nerve will travel toward the medial malleolus, giving off the branches to the long toe flexors. As it approaches the ankle, it will enter the tarsal tunnel. The tarsal tunnel is that space covered by the flexor retinaculum (previously termed the lancinate ligament), bounded anteriorly by the medial malleolus and posteriorly by the calcaneus, and having at its floor the tendon sheaths of the posterior tibialis, flexor digitorum communis, and the flexor hallucis longus.

It is important to note that there is normally no synovium within the tarsal tunnel as there is surrounding the flexor tendons in the carpal tunnel. The tarsal tunnel, in addition to the posterior tibial nerve, contains the posterior tibial artery and its accompanying veins. The roof of the tarsal tunnel, the flexor retinaculum, is the thickened extension of the deep fascia of the leg. The posterior tibial nerve divides into the medial and lateral plantar nerve within the tarsal tunnel. A cadaver study (Mackinnon & Dellon, 1984) demonstrated that this division occurs in 95% of specimens within 2 cm of a line drawn from the center of the medial malleolus to the calcaneus (see Figure 13.3). In 5% of specimens, however, the posterior tibial nerve had divided proximal to entering the tarsal tunnel, so that as it entered the tunnel the volume occupied by neural tissue was about twice as big as normal. This high division of the posterior tibial nerve is similar to the high division of the median nerve that occurs in the upper extremity, often associated with a persistent median artery.

The calcaneal nerve (often termed the medial calcaneal nerve to distinguish it from a lateral calcaneal nerve that arises from the sural nerve) has a great deal of variability in its origin, which explains the variable incidence of complaints of heel numbness in the population of patients with tarsal tunnel syndrome. In one-third of the cadavers studied (Mackinnon & Dellon, 1984), the calcaneal nerve was found to originate from

FIGURE 13.1

(A) The skin distribution of the sensory components of the peripheral nerves of the lower extremity that are most often responsible for clinical problems. (Upper left) Posterior tibial compression is the tarsal tunnel syndrome. (Upper right) Superficial peroneal nerve compression can occur in the anterolateral compartment syndrome. (Lower left) Deep peroneal nerve compression can occur over the dorsum of the foot beneath the extensor halluces brevis tendon giving just sensory symptoms, or more proximal beneath the inferior extensor retinaculum to include motor involvement of the extensor brevis muscle. (Bottom right) Common peroneal nerve can be compressed at the knee level at the fibular head to include the sensory distribution of both the superficial and deep peroneal nerves. (B) Other peripheral nerves that are important clinically are the (Upper left) anterior femoral cutaneous nerve, which may be injured during cardiac catheterizations, (Upper right) the common sural nerve, which is a common donor site for nerve graft material, (Bottom left) the lateral femoral cutaneous nerve, which can be entrapped at this level but present with thigh, knee, or buttock complaints, and is called meralgia paresthetica, and (Bottom right) the saphenous nerve, whose branches are often injured during knee surgery. Drawing by Glenn George Dellon. Reprinted with permission.

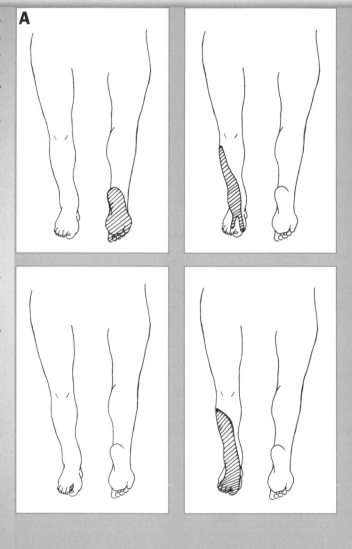

the posterior tibial nerve at a level that was outside the tarsal tunnel. In one-third of the cadavers, it arose from the lateral plantar nerve within the tarsal tunnel, and in the remaining one-third it had a dual origin from the posterial tibial nerve and from the lateral plantar nerve (see Figure 13.4). The calcaneal nerve travels through its own tunnel, called the calcaneal tunnel, to innervate the heel skin. That tunnel is bounded by fibrous septae on its sides, but by the fibrous roof formed from the fascial origins of the abductor halluces brevis muscle from the calcaneus. The calcaneal nerve usually divides into three smaller branches within this tunnel. This tunnel lies along the route most commonly used by surgeons to approach the calcaneus for bone spur removal or for plantar fascial release and is, therefore, at risk for injury during those operations.

The medial and lateral plantar nerves exit the tarsal tunnel, pass through about 1 cm of fat, and then enter into their own separate tunnels, which should be called

FIGURE 13.2

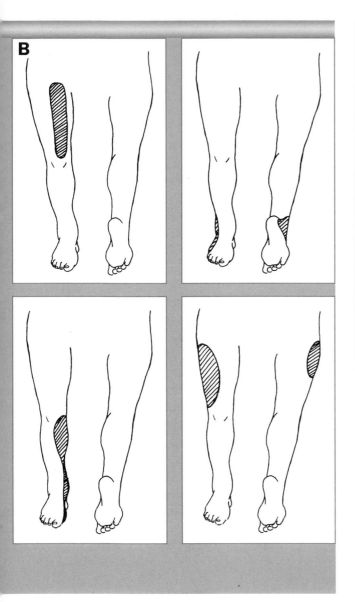

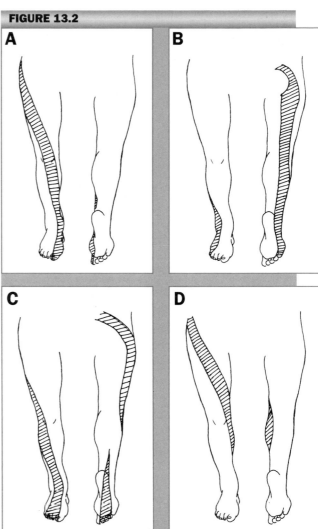

The skin distribution of the spinal nerve roots to the lower extremity. (A) the L4 dermatome, (B) the S1 dermatome, (C) the L5 dermatome, and (D) the L3 dermatome. Drawing by Glenn George Dellon. Reprinted with permission.

the medial and lateral plantar tunnels. These tunnels have as their roof the fascial origin of the abductor halluces brevis muscle, which lies on its deep surface. From this fascia, a septa exists that joins either the calcaneus or the flexor sheaths, or both. This interfascicular septum divides the medial from the lateral plantar tunnels (see Figure 13.5). These tunnels must be considered an integral part of the compression sites that give rise to the symptoms of numbness and tingling in the toes. Therefore, they need to be released during surgery for the treatment of tarsal tunnel syndrome. The homologies between these tunnels and those of the forearm and hand are given in Table 13.1.

FIGURE 13.3

Variation in the site of division of the posterior tibial nerve in the tarsal tunnel. Note that 5% of posterior tibial nerves will divide into the medial and lateral plantar nerve more than 2 cm proximal to a line drawn from the medial malleolus to the calcaneus. Patients, with a high division of the posterior tibial nerve are at increased risk for developing tarsal tunnel syndrome because the nerve occupies a greater volume as it enters the tunnel. From "Tibial Nerve Branching in the Tarsal Tunnel," by S. E. Mackinnon & A. L. Dellon, 1984, Archives of Neurology 41:645-646. Reprinted with permission of the authors.

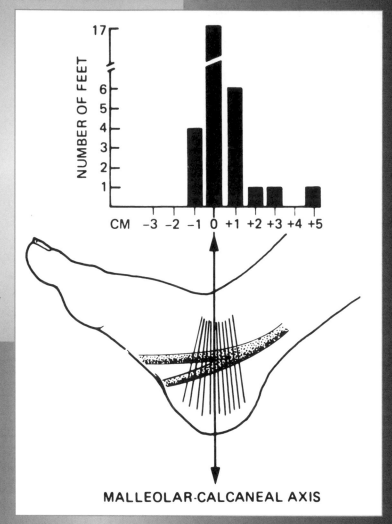

MALLEOLAR-CALCANEAL AXIS

FIGURE 13.4

Variation in the origin of the calcaneal nerve. Note that in one-third of patients the calcaneal nerve may arise proximal to the tarsal tunnel and, therefore, avoids significant compression. This explains the variability in symptoms related to the heel in patients with tarsal tunnel syndrome. From "Tibial Nerve Branching in the Tarsal Tunnel," by S. E. Mackinnon & A. L. Dellon, 1984, Archives of Neurology 41:645-646. Reprinted with permission of the authors.

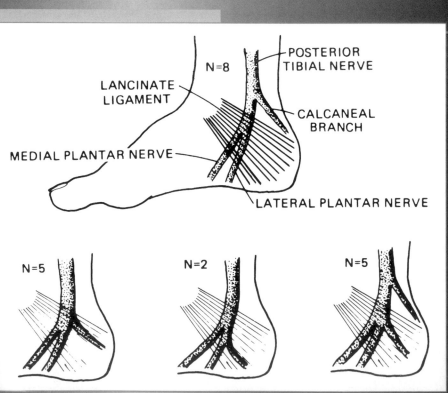

FIGURE 13.5

The medial and lateral plantar nerves each travel through their own separate tunnel after they exit from the tarsal tunnel. The roof of the medial and lateral plantar tunnel is the fascial origin of the abductor halluces brevis. The division between the medial and lateral plantar tunnels is the interfascicular septum, joining the fascia beneath the abductor halluces brevis with the flexor sheath or the calcaneus. From "Tarsal Tunnel Syndrome," by S. E. Mackinnon & A. L. Dellon, 1988, in Surgery of the Peripheral Nerve, *New York: Thieme Publishing. Reprinted with permission of the authors.*

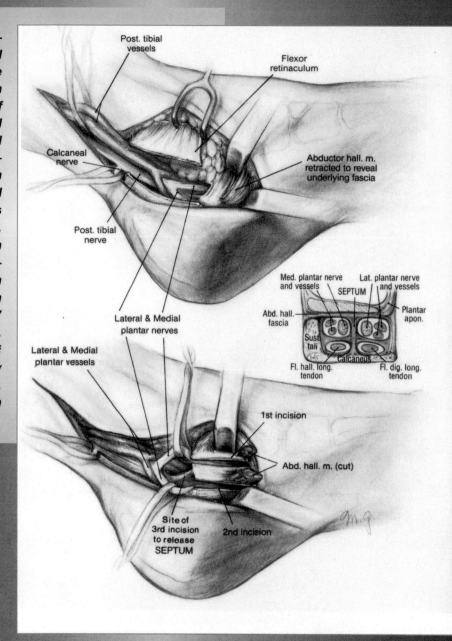

TABLE 13.1 ANATOMIC HOMOLOGIES BETWEEN THE UPPER AND LOWER EXTREMITIES RELATED TO PERIPHERAL NERVE PROBLEMS

Upper Extremity	Lower Extremity
Distal forearm	Tarsal tunnel (tarsal tunnel syndrome)
Carpal tunnel (carpal tunnel syndrome)	Medial plantar tunnel
Median nerve	Medial plantar nerve
Ulnar nerve at wrist level	Lateral plantar nerve
Guyon's canal	Lateral plantar tunnel
Palmar cutaneous branch of the median nerve	Calcaneal branch of the medial plantar nerve
Calcaneal nerve	Hypothenar branches of ulnar nerve
Hamate	Interfascicular septum
Posterior branch of saphenous nerve (medial malleolus)	Lateral antebrachial cutaneous nerve
Common peroneal nerve at fibular head	Radial nerve in the radial tunnel
Deep peroneal nerve, motor	Posterior interosseous nerve
Deep peroneal nerve, sensory (anterior tarsal tunnel syndrome)	Radial sensory nerve entrapment
Dorsal cutaneous branch of ulnar nerve	Sural nerve

THE COMMON PERONEAL NERVE

The common peroneal nerve is one of the two divisions of the sciatic nerve in the thigh. In the popliteal fossa, the common peroneal nerve turns laterally and crosses the fibular head beneath the peroneus longus muscle. This muscle is surrounded by a thickened fascia. At this point, the common peroneal nerve divides into the superficial and deep peroneal nerves, and in doing so doubles its number of fascicles and doubles its amount of connective tissue. Just after crossing the fibular head the deep peroneal nerve innervates the tibialis anterior muscle, and in so doing fixes the nerve at this point, limiting its excursion. All of these anatomic features combine to render the common peroneal nerve at risk for acute and chronic nerve compression and for stretch/traction injuries (see Figure 13.7). In 84% of people, just prior to crossing the fibular head, the common peroneal nerve gives off a lateral sural nerve that is responsible for innervating the lateral calf (the lateral cutaneous nerve of the calf, which may be used as the innervated sensory component to a free fibular flap) and the lateral aspect of the foot (which may be used in nerve grafting). This lateral sural nerve joins the medial sural nerve (a branch from the posterior tibial nerve in the popliteal fossa) to become the common sural nerve, which goes on to innervate the lateral aspect of the heel and dorsum of the foot (see Figure 13.6) (Coert & Dellon, 1994). These two may join anywhere from the popliteal fossa to just above the malleolus. As the common peroneal nerve crosses the fibular head it will give off first several small twigs that innervate the proximal tibio-fibular joint, and then divide into its deep and superficial branches. The deep branch innervates the tibialis anterior and the foot everters, the peronei, and will end with its sensory branch.

The sensory branch can become entrapped beneath the inferior extensor retinaculum to give a clinical syndrome known as anterior tarsal tunnel syndrome (Borges, Hallet, Selkoe, & Welch, 1981). At this level there is still one small motor branch associated with this nerve, the one that innervates the extensor digitorum brevis muscle, permitting electromyography to assist in making this diagnosis. Just down at the mid-foot level, the deep peroneal nerve can become compressed as it travels beneath the tendon of the extensor halluces brevis and over the juncture of

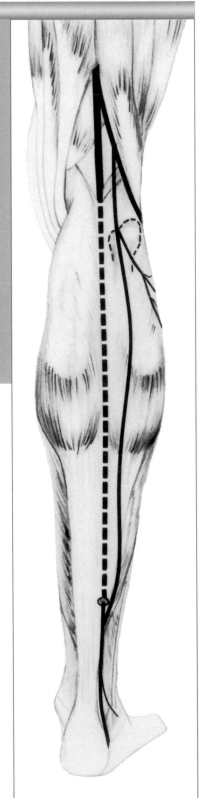

FIGURE 13.6

The anatomy of the sural nerve. This pattern occurs in 84% of people. The medial sural nerve (originating from the posterior tibial nerve) joins with the lateral sural nerve (originating from the common peroneal nerve) to form the common sural nerve just above the ankle. From "Clinical Implications of the Anatomy of the Sural Nerve," by H. Coert & A. L. Dellon, 1994, Plastic and Reconstructive Surgery 94:*850-855. Reprinted with permission of the authors. Note: See preliminary normative sural nerve cutaneous pressure thresholds in Table 13.9.*

the first and second metatarsal with the cuneiforms (see Figure 13.8) (Dellon, 1990). There is an unknown entrapment site for the superficial sensory branch of the peroneal nerve, although it can be a source of pain mimicking anterolateral compartment syndrome if it becomes compressed where it exits the fascia, about 16 cm proximal to the malleolus. This type of problem is most often observed in young athletes and dancers, whose symptoms come on after physical activity, and which can be associated with a small muscle bulge through the fascial window through which the superficial peroneal nerve exits.

FIGURE 13.7

Clinical example of the value of computer-assisted sensory testing using the Pressure-Specified Sensory Device™ in a man 50 years of age with diabetic neuropathy. He is shown here 9 months after surgical decompression of the left posterior tibial and common peroneal nerves. Note: Cutaneous pressure thresholds and two-point discrimination are improved on the left (operated) side. A. L. Dellon, MD, unpublished observations, 1997.

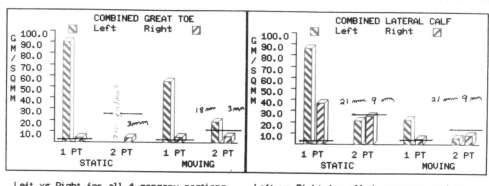

Left vs Right for all 4 sensory postions   Left vs Right for all 4 sensory postions

99 % CONFIDENCE LIMIT

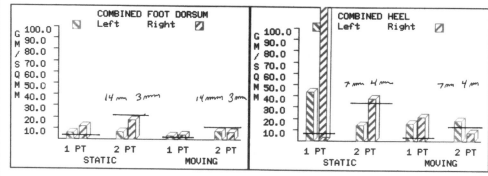

Left vs Right for all 4 sensory postions   Left vs Right for all 4 sensory postions

TABLE 13.2 PRESSURE-SPECIFIED SENSORY DEVICE™: NORMATIVE DATA LATERAL DORSAL FOOT (SURAL NERVE)

	Pressure Perception Threshold					
	(g/mm²)		(mm)	(g/mm²)		(mm)
	1PS	2PS	2PS	1PM	2PM	2PM
< 45 years of age[+]						
mean	0.6	0.5	9.0	1.0	0.4	9.0
s.d.	0.3	0.4	5.0	1.2	0.2	5.0
> 45 years of age[♦]						
mean	1.6	12.5	22.1	na	na	na
s.d.	2.1	15.2	2.8	na	na	na

Note:
[+] n = 3, mean age 32 years, range 10 to 43 years, data for the right hand.
[♦] n = 3, mean age 54.3 years, range 46 to 62 years, data for the right hand.
From V. L. Muse & A. L. Dellon, unpublished data, 1995.

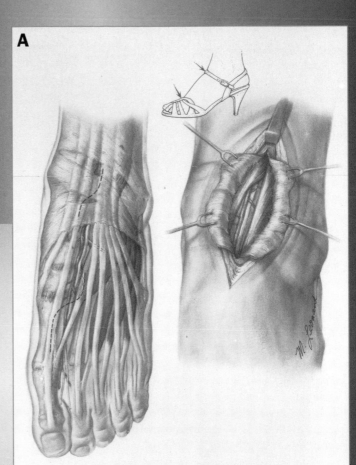

FIGURE 13.8
Entrapment of the deep peroneal nerve over the dorsum of the foot. (A) Relationship of footwear to the deep peroneal nerve. (B) Operative approach to decompression of the deep peroneal nerve beneath the extensor halluces brevis tendon. From "Entrapment of the Deep Peroneal Nerve on the Dorsum of the Foot," by A. L. Dellon, 1990, Foot and Ankle 11:73-80. *Reprinted with permission of the author.*

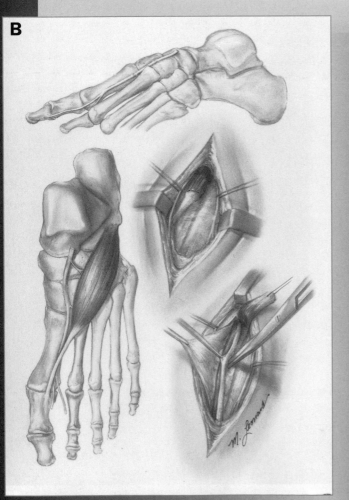

• THE SAPHENOUS NERVE •

The saphenous nerve sends a branch posterior to the medial malleolus that innervates the skin that is anterior to the usual tarsal tunnel incision. If the incision is placed too close to the medial malleolus, this cutaneous branch may become injured during the operation or adherent to the incision, giving rise to a postoperative pain problem. Depending on the extent of innervation in a given individual, the branch of the saphenous nerve that passes anterior to the malleolus may provide sensation to the dorsum of the big toe.

• TARSAL TUNNEL SYNDROME •

CLINICAL DESCRIPTION

Tarsal tunnel syndrome is the commonest nerve entrapment syndrome in the lower extremity. It was described relatively recently in the history of chronic nerve compressions. While median nerve compression at the wrist, in the carpal tunnel, and ulnar nerve compression at the elbow, in the cubital tunnel, were described as nerve entrapment syndromes in the 1830s, it was not until 1962 that chronic compression of the posterior tibial nerve in the tarsal tunnel was described (Mackinnon & Dellon, 1988). The presenting complaints of the patient with tarsal tunnel syndrome include sensory disturbances, most commonly in the region of the metatarsal heads and the toes, followed thereafter by complaints of sensory disturbances in the arch and the heel. These sensory disturbances are most often described as numbness or tingling, or a buzzing (paresthesia), less commonly as unpleasantness or burning (dysesthesia), and least commonly as pain. Patients may complain that they feel as if there were a band around their ankle. Sensory complaints may include the perception of coldness, and the complaints are usually worsened by activities that include standing or walking, and often are perceived to be worse in the evening when the patient goes to bed. Tarsal tunnel syndrome does not include complaints about numbness in the top of the foot, the outside of the foot, or pain when pressure is placed on the foot during walking. The diagnosis of tarsal tunnel syndrome requires that there be a symptom complex and physical examination findings compatible with compression of the posterior tibial nerve in the tarsal tunnel. This definition includes compression of the calcaneal nerve in its tunnel and the medial and lateral plantar nerves in their respective tunnels, although certainly localized anatomic changes and injuries may involve just one of these branches.

DIAGNOSIS

The clinician interested in the care of patients with foot problems must undertake the responsibility to examine the patient's foot, and have confidence in the physical examination. It is simply not proper to obtain a history and then, almost reflexively, refer the patient for electrodiagnostic testing. Electrodiagnostic testing is expensive and painful (see Chapter 8). However, the physical examination, as is all sensory testing, is subjective. If you believe your patient may be less than honest with you, for example, if he or she is involved in litigation or is being examined for a financial award such as a workmen's compensation claim, then electrodiagnostic testing offers a truly objective method of examination. Electrodiagnostic testing is also critical in evaluating the presence or absence of a lumbar radiculopathy, a myopathy, or a diffuse peripheral neuropathy if you clinically suspect that these conditions may be present.

The most conservative, most traditional diagnosis of tarsal tunnel syndrome is to have a patient with symptoms consistent with tarsal tunnel syndrome who has also had electrodiagnostic testing demonstrate a delay in either the distal sensory or motor latency of either the medial or lateral plantar nerves, or denervation of the medial or lateral plantar-innervated intrinsic muscles. Ideally, the electrodiagnostic testing should demonstrate that the observed distal deficits are not due either to an L4 or L5 nerve root problem or to the presence of a generalized peripheral neuropathy. Unfortunately, there is a group of patients with symptoms of tarsal tunnel syndrome in whom the electrodiagnostic testing is interpreted as being within normal limits, or in whom the advanced degree of the neuropathy is such that electrodiagnostic testing is not technically capable of demonstrating a superimposed nerve compression. The reverse situation, a "false positive," occurs as well; that is, a patient may have no symptoms, yet there may be electrodiagnostic evidence of diminished posterior tibial nerve function (Kaplan & Kernahan, 1981).

In a routine clinical situation in which a patient comes to see you for relief of symptoms, the clinical examination is a reproducible technique to use for the diagnosis of chronic nerve compression. The physical examination must demonstrate a positive Tinel sign over the posterior tibial nerve in the tarsal tunnel or the medial plantar nerve in the medial plantar tunnel, or the lateral plantar nerve in the lateral plantar tunnel. The presence of a positive Tinel sign (tapping over the known site of anatomic narrowing produces a sensation of tingling along the distal distribution of the nerve) indicates the presence in that location of demyelination, or of regenerating unmyelinated or myelinated fibers (Dellon, 1984). The physical examination must demonstrate a decrease in sensibility in the distribution of the posterior tibial nerve's branches, with the exception of the calcaneal nerve (which may arise proximal to the retinacular ligament (see above, Relevant Neuroanatomy).

The earliest signs of sensory change that can be tested easily and quickly in the clinical setting are changes in perception of a vibratory stimulus delivered with a tuning fork (Dellon, 1980). The late signs, related to loss of nerve fibers, can be tested easily and quickly with two-point discrimination testing. Theoretically, early changes in pressure threshold should be able to be detected with the Semmes-Weinstein nylon monofilaments. The only available data with these filaments for the lower extremity, however, is that of Holewski, Stess, Graff, and Grunfeld (1988), which was obtained from 20 asymptomatic subjects with a mean age of 63 years (range 47-76 years). The data is given in Table 13.2. Holewski et al. did not evaluate patients with tarsal tunnel syndrome. With the exception of vibratory threshold and thermal sensitivity information, there is very little information available other than this with regard to sensibility in the lower extremity (Dellon, 1981; Mackinnon & Dellon, 1988). The theoretical and practical objections to the use of the nylon monofilaments are given in Table 13.3, but they can be summarized by stating that the nylon monofilaments give an estimate of the range of the pressure threshold, they do not make an exact measurement (see Chapter 6). This implies that the range of pressure thresholds that exists between a given pair of filaments may conceal clinically significant worsening or improvement that would otherwise indicate a change in treatment.

As the degree of compression of the peripheral nerve progresses, the symptom complex will worsen correspondingly. For example, the motor component of the medial plantar nerve can be evaluated by manual muscle testing of the strength of the abductor hallucis brevis, which will become weaker and weaker. At some point in the natural history of tarsal tunnel syndrome, the muscle will have been sufficiently denervated for a sufficiently long period of time that

TABLE 13.3 CUTANEOUS PRESSURE THRESHOLD IN THE FOOT: SEMMES-WEINSTEIN RESULTS

Anatomic site	Sensitivity threshold level[+]
Plantar	
1st metatarsal head	4.40 ± .07
2nd metatarsal head	4.56 ± .08
3rd metatarsal head	4.58 ± .07
4th metatarsal head	4.58 ± .07
5th metatarsal head	4.49 ± .07
Tip of big toe	4.28 ± .09
Heel	5.12 ± .13
Dorsal	
1st/2nd web space	3.87 ± .07
Base of 3rd toe	3.81 ± .07
Base of 5th toe	3.73 ± .06

Note:

[+] Force = log10 (0.1mg) + standard deviation.
From "Aesthesiometry: Quantification of Cutaneous Pressure Sensation in Diabetic Peripheral Neuropathy," by J. Holewski, R. M. Stess, P. M. Graff, & C. Grunfeld, 1988, *Journal of Rehabilitation Research and Development* 25:1-10. Reprinted with permission of the authors.

muscle wasting (atrophy) begins. For the lateral plantar nerve, such weakness and subsequent wasting of the interossei muscles will result in clawing of the toes. The sensory component of the plantar nerves will first demonstrate compression by elevated thresholds to touch stimuli, such as vibration and pressure. Even before axonal loss occurs, there will be an increase in the pressure threshold required to distinguish one from two points at the normal distance of about 6 mm. Once axonal loss begins, the degree of compression is manifested by abnormal two-point discrimination distance as well as by an abnormal pressure threshold. Two-point discrimination is measured most easily with a Disk-Criminator™ (see Chapter 7). This plastic, hand-held instrument may be rotated to bring a series of paired, fixed-distance metal prongs to the skin surface. While inexpensive, efficient, and easy to use, traditional two-point discrimination testing suffers from the inability to specify the pressure required for the subject to make the distinction of one from two points.

The recent application of computer-assisted sensibility testing with the Pressure-Specified Sensory Device™ (see Chapter 7) to the lower extremity has demonstrated its ability to document sensation on the plantar aspect of the toes and on the heel (see Tables 13.4 & 13.5, and Figure 13.9), and to document the presence of tarsal tunnel syndrome (see Table 13.6) (Tassler & Dellon, 1996). The Pressure-Specified Sensory Device™ not only correlates well with electrodiagnostic studies in the diagnosis of tarsal tunnel syndrome, but also documents the existence of tarsal tunnel syndrome in the symptomatic patient with normal electrodiagnostic test results (see Table 13.6). For example, in a study directly comparing the diagnostic accuracy of electrodiagnostic testing and the Pressure-Specified Sensory Device™, there was 81% agreement between these two testing procedures. However, in each of the patients in whom the electrodiagnostic testing was interpreted as normal, the Pressure-Specified Sen-

TABLE 13.4 COMPARISON OF TOUCH SENSIBILITY TESTING INSTRUMENTS

Characteristics	Semmes-Weinstein Nylon Monofilaments	Pressure-Specified Sensory Device™	Disk-Criminator™
Traceable to NIST[+]	no	yes	no
Makes a measurement[*]	no	yes	yes
One probe diameter	no	yes	yes
Data reported as	log10 (0.1mg) force	g/mm² or mm pressure or distance	mm distance
Correlates with nerve conduction testing	no	yes	no
Clinical data available for tarsal tunnel syndrome	no	yes	no

Note:
[+] The numerical value obtained with the instrument is traceable to the National Institute of Standards and Technology.
[*] The set of filaments provides only an estimate of the range of the pressure threshold.

sory Device™ was abnormal, demonstrating increased sensitivity of quantitative sensory testing over electro-diagnostic testing (see Table 13.7). Clinical examples of the value of computer-assisted sensory testing are given in Figures 13.10 through 13.12, with the pressure thresholds and two-point discrimination values obtained with the Pressure-Specified Sensory Device™.

An example of elevated pressure thresholds for the big toe with normal thresholds over the dorsum of the foot, and the presence of a positive Tinel sign over the posterior tibial nerve, documents the presence of tarsal tunnel syndrome even in the patient with normal electrodiagnostic studies (see Figure 13.10). The presence of abnormal pressure thresholds over the dorsum of the foot and the lateral calf in the patient with a poor result from a previous tarsal tunnel release, in the presence of bilateral abnormal pressure thresholds for the big toe,

documents a peripheral neuropathy. The appropriate course of action is referral to a neurologist for further evaluation and possible systemic treatment of the neuropathy instead of reoperating on the tarsal tunnel (see Figure 13.11). The documentation of a decrease in the pressure thresholds along with improved two-point discrimination in the foot of a diabetic who had a tarsal tunnel release demonstrates that the heightened sensations now occurring

TABLE 13.5 PRESSURE-SPECIFIED SENSORY DEVICE™: NORMATIVE DATA FOR INDIVIDUALS LESS THAN 45 YEARS OF AGE

	Big Toe	Foot Dorsum	Heel	Calf
1PS Threshold				
Mean (g/mm^2)	.58	.49	.82	1.0
Stand. deviation	.34	.22	.44	0.7
99% conf. limit	1.0	1.0	1.0	2.0
1PM Threshold				
Mean (g/mm^2)	.63	.42	.76	.70
Stand. deviation	.35	.22	.41	.36
99% conf. limit	1.0	1.0	1.0	1.0
2PS Threshold				
Mean (g/mm^2)	3.9	4.6	8.0	8.0
Stand. deviation	4.3	4.9	8.0	12.6
99% conf. limit	6.7	8.1	13.7	24.0
Mean (mm)	3.8	4.3	4.1	4.8
Stand. deviation	1.0	1.3	1.7	2.6
99% conf. limit	.67	.89	1.2	1.8
2PM Threshold				
Mean (g/mm^2)	3.2	3.3	3.7	2.8
Stand. deviation	2.3	3.7	2.7	3.2
99% conf. limit	4.7	5.6	5.9	12.3
Mean (mm)	3.1	3.2	3.3	3.4
Stand. deviation	1.0	.75	0.5	1.0
99% conf. limit	.69	.53	.37	.71

Note: From "Pressure Perception in the Normal Lower Extremity and in the Tarsal Tunnel Syndrome," by P. L. Tassler & A. L. Dellon, *Muscle and Nerve, 19:*285-289, 1996. Reprinted with permission of the authors.

TABLE 13.6 PRESSURE-SPECIFIED SENSORY DEVICE™: NORMATIVE DATA FOR INDIVIDUALS 45 YEARS OF AGE OR OLDER

	Big Toe	Foot Dorsum	Heel	Calf
1PS Threshold				
Mean (g/mm²)	1.0	1.5	2.7	2.5
Stand. deviation	.76	2.2	2.5	2.5
99% conf. limit	1.6	3.3	5.0	6.0
1PM Threshold				
Mean (g/mm²)	.67	.57	1.7	1.3
Stand. deviation	.23	.37	1.2	.58
99% conf. limit	1.0	1.0	2.8	3.0
2PS Threshold				
Mean (g/mm²)	16.3	16.8	20.4	18.5
Stand. deviation	11.1	11.9	10.1	8.3
99% conf. limit	25.7	26.4	30.0	31.0
Mean (mm)	5.7	6.3	5.7	6.5
Stand. deviation	2.4	2.5	1.4	2.1
99% conf. limit	2.1	2.0	1.4	1.8
2PM Threshold				
Mean (g/mm²)	8.6	6.8	8.0	8.9
Stand. deviation	5.0	5.3	3.7	6.4
99% conf. limit	12.8	11.0	11.1	15.4
Mean (mm)	4.3	4.4	4.5	4.4
Stand. deviation	2.7	2.5	1.3	2.1
99% conf. limit	2.3	2.0	1.2	1.8

Note: From "Pressure Perception in the Normal Lower Extremity and in the Tarsal Tunnel Syndrome," by P. L. Tassler & A. L. Dellon, *Muscle and Nerve, 19:*285-289,1996. Reprinted with permission of the authors.

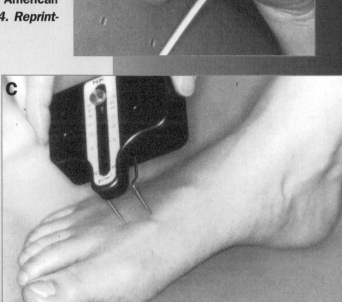

FIGURE 13.9

The Pressure-Specified Sensory Device™ being used to measure sensibility of the medial plantar nerve (A), the calcaneal nerve (B), the deep peroneal nerve (C), and the lateral cutaneous nerve of the calf (D). As described in Chapter 7, this hand-held equipment can be used to test any body surface, with the equipment being "zeroed" for the effect of gravity just prior to use in each new position. The computer-assisted measurements can be done with a connection to any IBM-compatible hardware, and is portable through the use of a laptop computer. From "Cutaneous Pressure Thresholds in Diabetics With and Without Foot Ulceration," by P. L. Tassler, A. L. Dellon, & N. M. Scheffler, 1995, Journal of American Podiatric Medical Association 85:679-684. Reprinted with permission of the authors.

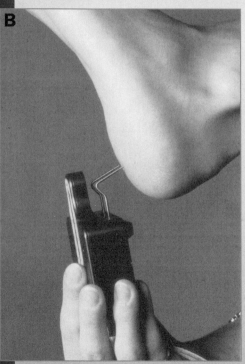

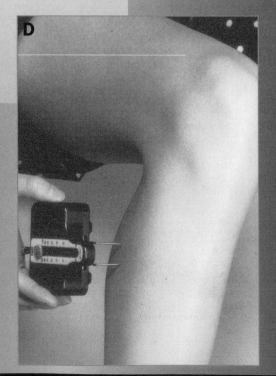

	All TTS	TTS[+] EDT +	TTS[+] EDT –
TABLE 13.7 PRESSURE THRESHOLDS IN THE TARSAL TUNNEL SYNDROME			
1PS Threshold			
Mean (g/mm²)	10.9	15.0*	4.7*
Stand. deviation	17.5	21.1	6.7
1PM Threshold			
Mean (g/mm²)	7.6	11.2◇	2.0◇
Stand. deviation	16.9	21.0	2.7
2PS Threshold			
Mean (g/mm²)	31.1	42.1*	16.4*
Stand. deviation	17.3	13.5	9.0
Mean (mm)	10.7	12.1◇	8.8◇
Stand. deviation	3.3	3.3	2.3
2PM Threshold			
Mean (g/mm²)	23.3	27.3	18.5
Stand. deviation	17.1	18.1	15.5
Mean (mm)	10.0	11.0	8.9
Stand. deviation	3.5	3.0	3.3

Note:
[+] EDT: electrodiagnostic testing; (+) abnormal, (-) normal
* $p < .05$
◇ $p < .001$
From "Pressure Perception in the Normal Lower Extremity and in the Tarsal Tunnel Syndrome," by P. L. Tassler & A. L. Dellon, *Muscle and Nerve, 19:*285-289, 1996. Reprinted with permission of the authors.

TABLE 13.8 COMPARISON OF ELECTRODIAGNOSTIC TESTING AND PRESSURE-SPECIFIED SENSORY DEVICE™ TESTING IN DIAGNOSIS OF LOWER EXTREMITY NERVE ENTRAPMENTS*

			Demographics				
	# Compared Right Left		# Total	# Both Tests Normal	# Disagree	# Agree	% Agreement
Posterior Tibial	9	7	16	0	3	13	81.3
Common Peroneal	5	5	10	1	2	8	80.0

Specificity and Sensitivity of EDT AND PSSD Using Clinical Diagnosis as "Gold Standard"

Tarsal Tunnel Syndrome

	CLIN+	CLIN−	SPEC	SENS
PSSD+	16	0	*	100%
PSSD−	0	0		
EDT+	13	0	*	81%
EDT−	3	0		

Common Peroneal Nerve Entrapment

	CLIN+	CLIN−	SPEC	SENS
PSSD+	9	0	*	90%
PSSD−	1	0		
EDT+	7	0	*	70%
EDT−	3	0		

Note:

+ Disease present

− Disease absent

* Statistically undefined

From "Correlation of Measurements of Pressure Perception Using the Pressure-Specified Sensory Device with Electrodiagnostic Testing," by P. L. Tassler & A. L. Dellon, *Journal of Occupational Medicine* 37:862-866, 1995. Reprinted with permission of the authors.

FIGURE 13.10

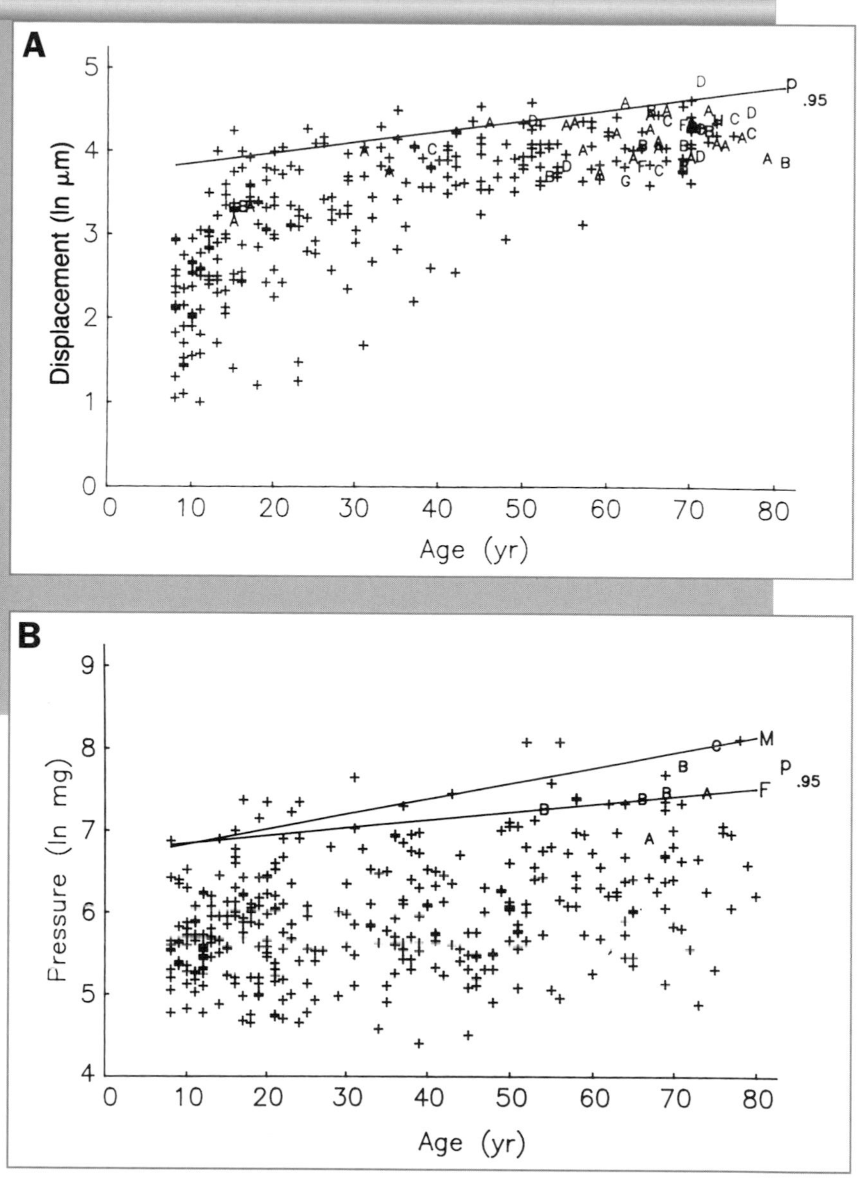

Normative data obtained with the CASE IV System for the big toe dorsum (see Chapter 7 for description). (A) Cutaneous vibratory threshold. (B) Cutaneous pressure threshold. Age-matched. From "Detection Thresholds of Cutaneous Sensation in Humans," by P. J. Dyck, J. L. Karnes, P. C. O'Brien, & I. R. Zimmerman, 1993, in Peripheral Neuropathy, Third Edition, P. J. Dyck, P. K. Thomas, J. W. Griffin, P. A. Low, & J. F. Poduslo, Editors, Philadelphia: W. B. Saunders Company, 1993. Reprinted with permission of the authors.

three months after surgery are the result of neural regeneration and are not due to a worsening of the neuropathy or a complication of the surgery (see Figure 13.12).

The symptom complex for tarsal tunnel syndrome is unique and should not be confused with other clinical problems. However, quantitative sensory testing is crucial in the differential diagnosis. For example, chronic compression of a common plantar digital nerve to the 4th/5th web space by the metatarsal heads, in the absence of shooting pains, may cause symptoms of numbness of the lateral toes, causing confusion between a Morton's "neuroma" and lateral plantar nerve compression. The patient with a Morton's neuroma would have no sensory abnormalities except in the webspace innervated by the common plantar digital nerve. There are two sources of aching or pain in the ankle that may present with symptoms confused with tarsal tunnel syndrome. They are compression of the deep peroneal at the ankle, beneath the inferior extensor retinaculum, the anterior tarsal tunnel syndrome, and compression of the deep peroneal nerve beneath the extensor halluces brevis tendon at the level of the juncture of the cuneiforms with the first and second metatarsals. Each of these syndromes has in com-

FIGURE 13.11

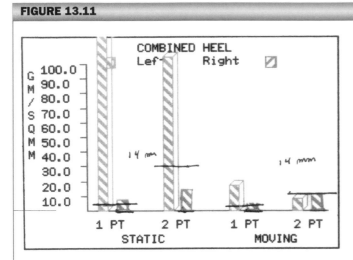

99 % CONFIDENCE LIMIT

Left vs Right for all 4 sensory postions

Clinical example of the value of computer-assisted sensory testing using the Pressure-Specified Sensory Device™. The presence of abnormal pressure thresholds over the heel in the left foot of a patient with heel pain suggests that calcaneal nerve entrapment is the source of the pain, rather than plantar fascitis or a bone spur (even if the spur is present on the X ray). The appropriate treatment is a neurolysis of the calcaneal nerve rather than a plantar fasciectomy. A. L. Dellon, MD, unpublished observations, 1997.

mon a decrease or loss of sensibility in the web space between the first and second metatarsals, dorsally, with the anterior tarsal tunnel syndrome including weakness or wasting of the extensor digitorum brevis muscle. There will be a Tinel sign over the site of compression of each of these nerve entrapments, dorsally.

Common peroneal nerve entrapment will demonstrate abnormal sensibility both in the webspace between the first and second toes as well as over the lateral aspect of the foot, and a Tinel sign over the fibular head. It has been shown in a small group of patients with common peroneal nerve entrapment that quantitative sensory testing with the Pressure-Specified Sensory Device™ is more sensitive than electrodiagnostic testing (see Table 13.7) (Tassler & Dellon, 1995). In my experience, tarsal tunnel syndrome is often misdiagnosed when in association with lower extremity trauma. For example, it is common to see patients who have previously broken their ankle. Regardless of whether they have been treated by an open or closed technique, and re-

gardless of whether they have hardware present or not, they all have in common an episode during which the posterior tibial nerve may have been directly contused following which it was immobilized in an environment of protein-rich edema. It is reasonable for the posterior tibial nerve to be entrapped along its path to the toes, with the time course for the presentation of symptoms being related to the degree of compression on the nerve and the severity of associated lower extremity complaints. This mechanism can occur after metatarsal fractures or after navicular fractures. This same mechanism applies to the patient who had a severe ankle sprain but in whom there was no fracture. A patient may have abnormal sensation documented over the posterior tibial

FIGURE 13.12

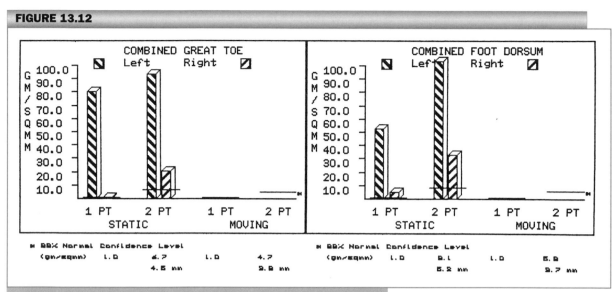

Clinical example of the value of using the Pressure-Specified Sensory Device™ to measure sensory changes in the lower extremity. This 40-year-old man broke his left fibula and distal tibia 2 years ago and has good radiographic healing of the bones, but complains of numbness in his entire left foot. Nerve conduction studies are normal. Due to pain when he walks, he shifts his weight to his opposite (right) foot. Note that the cutaneous pressure thresholds are markedly elevated above the 99% normal confidence limit (horizontal line) for the injured left foot, documenting peroneal (dorsum) and posterior tibial nerve (great toe) compression. Note, too, that the contralateral foot it demonstrating abnormal pressures due to the increased load it has been carrying. The indicated treatment is to surgically decompress the nerves at the left knee and left ankle. A. L. Dellon, MD, unpublished observations, 1997.

that has been injured due to overuse (Tassler & Dellon, 1996). These symptoms may improve following successful treatment of the injured foot, or progress to the point where they, too, need treatment. Quantitative sensory testing and documentation must be directed to the contralateral foot to permit proper diagnosis and assessment of these problems.

nerve and the common peroneal nerve due to a stretch/traction injury associated with an ankle or knee injury. In this situation, the presence of a neuropathy is eliminated if the opposite foot has normal sensibility.

The next most common misdiagnosis that I see is the presence of tarsal tunnel syndrome associated with a systemic disease, especially

when the disease can produce a peripheral neuropathy. Examples of such systemic diseases are diabetes, alcoholic neuropathy, hypothyroidism, collagen vascular disease, and lead poisoning. The relationship between neuropathy and chronic nerve compression is reviewed extensively in Chapter 14. Tarsal tunnel symptoms may occur in the foot contralateral to a foot

REHABILITATION

At one week the patient is seen in the office, the dressing is removed, and they are put into some form of supportive splint, such as an air cast, to minimize ankle motion. They may begin to wash the wound. They are kept non-weight-bearing the second week. The third week they are allowed to begin weight bearing while standing and taking a few steps, attempting to keep the ankle still while lifting the foot from the hip. At the third week following surgery the sutures are removed and full weight bearing is begun. This regimen may require modification if the patient is on steroids or chemotherapy (e.g., methotrexate for rheumatoid arthritis), or if they have diabetes. The patient is instructed in edema control and encouraged to wear elastic support panty hose or stockings while ambulatory. At the sixth postoperative week they are begun on scar massage with a steroid-containing cream.

At the follow-up office visits, evaluation of the posterior nerve is done with screening-type instruments, such as a tuning fork. Often the patient reports increased sensation from the vibratory stimulus. If the degree of nerve compression has caused abnormal two-point discrimination, two-point discrimination is checked with a Disk-Criminator™ and may be found to have become a small distance (improved discrimination). These findings give the patient encouragement that the nerve decompression has been successful. At the sixth or twelfth postoperative visit quantitative sensory testing can be repeated with the Pressure-Specified Sensory Device™ and the results of surgery documented.

Desensitization may be necessary if one of the cutaneous nerves becomes adherent to the incision and is a source of pain. The same desensitization techniques used for the hand may be employed for the foot (see Chapter 4). Desensitization may also be required if the neural regeneration after decompression and internal neurolysis create discomfort. A technique that has been helpful with these types of problems is to have the patient put the foot into a whirlpool, which can be one at the therapist's office or a home bathtub attachment. The swirling water gives good sensory distraction to the foot. A variation of this is to send the patient to a gym with a pool for water therapy. Walking in the pool not only lifts some of the weight from the obese patient, but the swirling water is a good form of desensitization. Another technique is to place something between the hypersensitive surface of the foot and the hand that is touching the foot, like a towel or a thick

sock. Finally, wearing a support stocking can be a good form of desensitization in that the pressure applied will stimulate the slowly-adapting fiber-receptor system, which is often better tolerated than moving-touch stimuli.

Sensory reeducation may be necessary in the patient with tarsal tunnel syndrome if two-point discrimination was abnormal preoperatively. The disturbing sensations that may accompany neural regeneration can at first be treated with desensitization techniques, but will finally be best helped by early and late phase sensory reeducation. A technique that has been helpful in this type of rehabilitation has been to have the patient go to a carpet store and pick up a series of different remnants that differ in pile height, firmness, and material type. The patient can sit and rub the toes back and forth over the different textures, attempting to discriminate among them.

• NERVE RECONSTRUCTION •

Nerve repair and nerve reconstruction is not done as commonly in the lower extremity as it is in the upper extremity. The same concepts regarding neural regeneration apply to the lower extremity nerves as to the upper extremity nerves. The strategy for nerve reconstruction in the lower extremity is a little different, however, in that reconstruction of the posterior tibial nerve is considered worthwhile in an attempt to provide at least protective sensation to the plantar aspect of the foot, but not for recovery of intrinsic muscle function. This will be discussed in more detail in the section below on innervated tissue transfer. An example of recovery following reconstruction of the posterior tibial nerve is given in Chapter 7 (see Figure 7.25).

Injury to the common peroneal nerve is often associated with knee injuries, or may be the unfortunate consequence of joint replacement for the hip or knee. While it is accepted practice to observe the patient clinically and with electrodiagnostic testing, this is a painful method and one that does not detect the earliest sensory changes. The therapist is already involved early in the care of these patients to make the orthotic for the foot drop. In the future, therapists using quantitative sensory testing will have an increased role in management of this problem. The sensory evaluation can be done monthly with little cost and no pain. The common peroneal nerve may be reconstructed to restore tibialis anterior nerve function, but not sensory function to the dorsum of the foot. Indeed, in my approach to common peroneal nerve reconstruction, I use the sensory nerve component of the superficial and deep peroneal nerve as donor nerve graft material.

When the sural nerve is used for nerve grafting in the upper extremity, the adjacent intact superficial peroneal nerve will begin to provide sensation through the phenomenon of collateral sprouting (see Chapter 4). This may cause a disturbing tingling perception in the patient, a problem which will benefit from desensitization techniques. Measurement of the area of sensory loss over time will demonstrate a decrease in this area. Techniques for quantitating sensory recovery after nerve repair are discussed and documented in detail in Chapter 12 on the upper extremity.

• INNERVATED FREE-TISSUE • TRANSFERS

Reconstruction of foot defects is now reliably done using microsurgical transfer of tissue. The goal of such reconstruction is to preserve a functioning foot. It has been debated as to whether such a reconstruction requires providing sensation. Obtaining quantitative information to resolve this issue remains a problem. Scientific resolution of this issue is difficult because
(a) it is known that a high percentage of patients with insensitive feet due to diabetes continue with good foot function if they are meticulous regarding foot hygiene and footwear; (b) foot reconstruction may be done with muscle flaps covered with skin grafts or with various types of flaps; (c) some flaps have a generous fat layer which may give the foot increased shear forces against the shoes compared to the skin-grafted muscle surface which may produce less shear; (d) local flaps, such as the dorsalis pedis, are innervated at the time of transfer; (e) noninnervated free tissue transfers, that is, a transferred free flap in which its original sensory nerve is not neurotized by an existing foot sensory nerve (the sural or calcaneal), will usually become reinnervated to some de-gree from the adjacent in-tact nerves; and (f) many different methods of sensibility examination have been used in the past for the different reported studies. Clearly, the role of the therapist in obtaining reliable and valid measurements of sensibility for this type of clinical outcome study is critical.

A study by May, Halls, and Simon (1985), of the Plastic Surgery Department at Harvard University, has suggested that sensibility is not necessary for stability in foot reconstruction. They studied skin-grafted latissimus muscle transfers and used traditional clinical testing to determine that there was no sensation recovered in these feet. Of importance is that they demonstrated use of the reconstructed surface in ambulation by gait analysis. This study is important because just a single surgical type of reconstruction was used, but the methods of testing sensibility were not as quantitative as is now possible.

A better example of the type of evaluation that has

TABLE 13.9 SENSORY RECOVERY IN INNERVATED FREE-TISSUE TRANSFERS TO THE FOOT

Author/Year	Area Reconstr	Flap Used	Donor Nerve	Recipient Nerve	Result
Chang et al., 1986	heel	lat. dorsi	motor br.	sural	4.73 Swmonofil.
	heel	1st web	deep peron.	sural	17 mm s2PD
	heel	tensor f.l.	lat. fem. cut	calc.	35 mm s2PD
	heel	gracilis	motor br.	sural	5.60 SWmonofil.
Chicarilli et al., 1986	plantar	rad. forearm	med.antebrach	sural	pinprick
Noever, et al., 1988	heel	rad. forearm	lat. antebrach	sural	light touch
Sinha,[+] et al., 1989	plantar	tensor f.l.	lat. fem. cut.	?med.plant	20 mm s2PD
	plantar	dorsalis ped	superf.peron	?med.plant	> 20 mm s2PD
	plantar	rad. forearm	lat.antebrach	?med.plant	> 20 mm s2PD

Note:

[+]The only study to compare ulcerations, which occurred in 3 of 21 noninnervated flaps but in none of the 7 innervated flaps to the foot.

From "Sensory Recovery in Innervated Free-tissue Transfers," by B. Graham & A. L. Dellon, 1995, *Journal of Reconstructive Microsurgery 11:*157-166.

been done to evaluate the role of sensibility in the reconstructed foot is that of Rautio, Kekoni, Hamalainen, Harma, and Asko-Seljavaara (1989) of the Department of Plastic Surgery at the University of Helsinki, Finland. They used vibratory perception thresholds with the Bruel and Kjaer vibrometer at 20, 80, and 240 Hz to study 24 foot reconstructions, comparing areas of the flap with contralateral normal values. They compared, finally, the degree of recovered sensibility (which they called the relative threshold increases, and which divided into three distinct groups) to the stability of the foot reconstructions (which divided into four distinct groups). Four of their flaps were innervated dorsalis pedis local flaps and 20 were noninnervated free-tissue transfers from the shoulder (deltoid), back (parascapular), side (latissimus dorsi), thigh (gluteal thigh), or forearm (radial forearm).

Their conclusion was that the degree of sensibility may have contributed to, but was not essential for, good soft-tissue stability of the reconstruction. As can be seen from the statistical analysis, there was no correlation ($r = .06$, $p = .77$) between degree of recovered sensibility and flap stability. The r value means that the observed data accounts for very little of the results. As described above, there are so many factors to control that this study, one of the best available, still does not prove the degree, if any, to which sensibility is of benefit. This study would have been more appropriate if just one type of foot reconstruction were used. If we look at the results they achieved with just the innervated island dorsalis pedis flaps, all four of their transfers had excellent sensibility and stability. Another criticism of this study is the choice of vibration as the critical sensibility to test. If foot ulceration develops in response to pressure gradients and shear forces, which are functions of the slowly-adapting fiber-receptor systems, then perhaps the measurement of pressure thresholds would be a better choice.

A review of the degree of sensory recovery in innervated free-tissue transfers provides an insight into the type of sensibility that can be recovered in the foot. Graham and Dellon (1995) reviewed all available reports of the degree of sensibility recovered in foot reconstructions, subdivided into the type of free-flap and the donor and recipient nerves (see Table 13.8). No formal sensory reeducation program was used for these foot reconstructions, but it is likely that simply walking and wearing different footwear may not be sufficient therapy. Yet, even without such a program, none of the reported innervated free-tissue transfers developed an ulceration while, in at least one study, 3 of 21 non-sensory-innervated foot reconstructions did develop an ulceration. In gen-

eral, the literature supports the view that in a reconstructed foot in which the flap is well-contoured to the underlying defect, provision of sensory function is not a prerequisite either to achieve good gait or to prevent ulceration, even if the muscle flap is covered with a skin graft.

PRESSURE-SPECIFIED SENSORY DEVICE™: FOOT TESTING PROTOCOL

The Pressure-Specified Sensory Device™ is an instrument designed to measure the threshold for the perception of pressure stimuli on the surface of the human body. Since the position of the testing instrument will vary with respect to gravity, the instrument must be zeroed by touching the appropriate function key on the computer to correct for this force at the start of each testing procedure for each different body surface.

The instrument consists of two metal prongs, each with an identical hemispherical-shaped tip. If just one of these prongs is used as the testing stimulus, the test is called "one point," accompanied by the adjectives "static" or "moving." The adjective used depends on whether the examiner positions the prong so that there is no movement with respect to the skin surface other than increasing the depth of skin indentation (static touch), or whether the examiner moves the prong from proximal to distal along the surface of the skin while increasing the depth of skin indentation (moving touch). If both prongs are used simultaneously as the testing stimulus, the test is called "two point," accompanied by the adjectives "static" or "moving." The adjective used depends on whether the examiner moves the prongs parallel to each other and from proximal to distal along the surface of the skin while increasing the depth of skin indentation (moving two-point discrimination), or does not move them. The threshold is the pressure at which the subject can first detect the given stimulus. The stimuli are, therefore, designated as 1PS (one-point static touch), 2PS (static two-point discrimination), 1PM (one-point moving touch), and 2PM (moving two-point discrimination).

The Pressure-Specified Sensory Device™ provides a threshold measurement throughout a continuous range of applied pressures, and this threshold is reported in grams per square millimeter, or g/mm^2. The distance at which the perception of two points being pressed against the skin surface can be distinguished from one point is called two point discrimination. When the Pressure-Specified Sensory Device™ is used for this measurement, the distance, as is traditional, is expressed in millimeters.

In contrast, the Pressure-Specified Sensory Device™ permits the specification of the minimum pressure required for the discrimination of two points from one point. That pressure threshold is also reported in g/mm². While the Pressure-Specified Sensory Device™ itself may be used to determine the smallest distance for two-point discrimination (by turning the knob at the side that controls interprong distance which is reflected on the computer screen), it is more practical in terms of efficiency for this distance to be approximated first with a Disk-Criminator™, using as much pressure as required to be sure that the patient is receiving a supramaximal pressure stimulus. This distance will be taken as the starting point at which the pressure threshold for two-point discrimination testing will begin.

A complete test of any given surface area using the Pressure-Specified Sensory Device™ will, therefore, be reported in terms of six different values. The value for 1PS and for 1PM will be given as a single number, the pressure threshold, expressed as g/mm². The value of both 2PS and 2PM will be expressed as two separate numbers for each test, one in millimeters and one in g/mm². Thus, a report may state that 1PS is 0.5 g/mm², whereas 2PS is 6 mm at 0.5 g/mm². Such preliminary normative data for the sural nerve is given in Table 13.9.

GENERAL SEQUENCE OF TESTING

The patient must be seated in a comfortable manner. A recliner-type chair is suggested as this brings the feet up into a comfortable position for testing. Both the body surface to be tested and the tester's arm and hand must be placed in a supported position. The examiner must be seated in a comfortable position. The location of the room in which the testing is to be done must be quiet and distraction free. The tester must have confidence that the patient is (a) intelligent enough to understand the testing procedure, (b) not mentally impaired by pain medication or alcohol, and (c) cooperative and not primarily motivated by workmen's compensation or other legal issues that preclude him or her from giving an honest response to the testing. Otherwise, the testing should be discontinued or the causes for the tester's concern listed on the report so that anyone interpreting the testing results will be able to make the correct interpretation. This information will become apparent during the entering of the demographic data at the start of the session and during the familiarization period prior to obtaining data.

A period of familiarization with the testing procedure must be given to the patient, and the first set of measurements obtained should not be used as definitive test results. The testing routine should be done on a body surface presumed to be normal so that the patient will know what type of touch response is caused by the one- and two-point static and moving stimuli. During the familiarization period the subject may see the computer screen, but the view of the screen must be blocked during the testing sequence. As indicated above, the Pressure-Specified Sensory Device™ must be zeroed against gravity and for each new stimulus at each new test site, but not between every trial for each stimulus.

There will be 5 trials recorded for a given test site and a given stimulus. Each trial consists of the examiner bringing the prong into contact with the skin surface, the subject perceiving that a stimulus was delivered, and the subject making a response to the stimulus (by pressing a hand-held button). In general, these 5 data points will be displayed on the screen for the examiner to review. The examiner will select the 3 data points listed on the computer screen that are most closely grouped as representing the data to be averaged and saved. This is done by eliminating the highest and lowest values recorded. If the examiner jams the prong onto the test area, the response measured will be falsely high. If the subject anticipates the touch sequence and presses the button too soon, the response measured will be falsely low. The examiner must be aware of these testing errors and correct for them by administering another test trial. These errors may occur without the examiner being aware of them, in which case they will become apparent when the time comes to average the responses. For example, if the 5 responses obtained for 1PS were, in g/mm², 2.2, 0.5, 0.7, 0.1, and 0.6, then the 3 data points chosen for averaging should be 0.5, 0.7 and 0.6, with the reported 1PS pressure threshold being 0.6 g/mm².

MEASURING THE ONE-POINT TOUCH PRESSURE THRESHOLD

The patient is instructed to respond to the stimulus by pressing the hand-held response button. The examiner selects the appropriate computer screens (moving or static) for which the one-point touch stimulus is to be delivered, and to which body surface the stimulus is to be given. If the one-point static touch threshold is being measured, the patient is then instructed "to make the response at the first detection of the prong touching the skin," followed by, "as soon as you know you are being touched, press the button." If the one-point moving touch threshold is being measured, the verbal instruction is "to make the response at the first detection of the prong moving along the surface of the skin," followed by "do not press the button as soon as you are touched, but only when you can tell that something is moving."

The testing sequence then begins with the examiner alerting the subject that the stimulus is coming by saying, "Shut your eyes and get ready, the test is beginning now." The examiner then slowly brings the prong of the Pressure-Specified Sensory Device™ into contact with the surface to be tested. The examiner must directly observe the prong's approach to, and its contact with, the skin surface to get visual feedback of the testing procedure. The examiner uses visual cues related to the degree of skin indentation and tactile cues related to the feeling in the examiner's own hand as the Pressure-Specified Sensory Device™ is guided onto the test site. These cues permit the examiner to slowly increase the pressure of stimulus application until the subject perceives the stimulus and presses the response button. Subjects may open their eyes between each test. The examiner should check the subject's eyes and realert the subject at the start of each test by saying, "Get ready, shut your eyes, the test is beginning again." After 5 satisfactory trials, the 1PS test sequence is stopped and the data is averaged by the examiner, while the subject is instructed to open his or her eyes and relax. Reassure the subject that the procedures were followed appropriately, if they were, and correct the subject's understanding of the procedures if they were not followed correctly.

MEASURING THE DISTANCE THRESHOLD FOR DETECTION OF TWO POINTS

The uniqueness of the Pressure-Specified Sensory Device™ is its ability to record the pressure threshold and the distance. It is easier to revolve the Disk-Criminator™ through the examiner's fingers than it is to adjust the interprong distance on the Pressure-Specified Sensory Device™, so the Disk-Criminator™ is used to estimate the actual distance measurement. In the absence of a Disk-Criminator™, the Pressure-Specified Sensory Device™ certainly can be used to make the final determination of distance to within less than 1 mm (the limit of resolution of the Disk-Criminator™, if this degree of precision is required).

The patient is first shown the Disk-Criminator™ to alleviate any fears of pain and is informed that he or she is to give a verbal response (not press a button) when the touch stimulus is perceived as either one or two points. The subject is then instructed to shut their eyes. The examiner begins first by touching one prong to the big toe pulp, pressing it moderately hard into the surface to be sure that the test is above the pressure threshold. The examiner asks, "Is that one or two?" The patient should say "One," following which the examiner should provide positive reinforcement by saying, "That is correct, now what is this, one or two?", at which time the examiner does the next test with the Disk-Criminator at a distance of 8 mm. If the patient says "Two," the examiner goes on to a 6 mm distance. If the subject incorrectly identifies the 8 mm stimulus as one point, the examiner must increase the distance to 10 mm and repeat the sequence entirely from the beginning. On the way down to smaller distances, the examiner may proceed from 6 mm, to 5 mm, and then to 4 mm. If the subject gives quick and correct responses, then the examiner has confi-

dence that, in fact, the stimulus is being correctly perceived and may continue down to smaller distances without requiring "7 out of 10" correct responses. As the two-point threshold is approached, the patient's responses will become slower and more thoughtful.

At this time, the one-prong stimulus should be alternated with the two-prong to be sure that the patient can still correctly detect one from two. At the distance selected for the "end-point," the subject must get 2 out of 3 trials correct with the answer of "Two." If the subject incorrectly identifies the two prongs as one, or as a single broad one, the distance selected for the Pressure-Specified Sensory Device™ test should be the next millimeter higher or wider spacing; that is, if the 4 mm distance is not identified as two, set the Pressure-Specified Sensory Device™ at 5 mm for testing. For routine testing it is sufficient to set the Pressure-Specified Sensory Device™ interprong spacing to the nearest whole number, for example, 5 mm rather than 5.5 mm. If the computer electronically records the distance as 5.1 mm or 4.9 mm, that is acceptable and not statistically or clinically significantly different from 5.0 mm, and the examiner should not be concerned about that difference in distance. For routine clinical testing, the final distance

threshold may be accepted as 2 of 3 correct responses, whereas for an outcome study, a research protocol, or repeat of an abnormal screening examination, more strict criteria, such as 3 of 5 or 7 of 10, may be required.

MEASURING THE TWO-POINT DISCRIMINATION PRESSURE THRESHOLD

Once the distance has been entered into the computer by setting the interprong distance with the knob at the undersurface of the Pressure-Specified Sensory Device™, and the desired distance is checked by the examiner by observing the distance displayed on the computer screen's viewing window, the subject must be instructed again. If 2PS is being tested, the examiner says, "You are to press the button when you first detect that two points are touching you. Do not push the button as soon as you feel something touch you. Be sure that you can distinguish two separate points. I may sometimes touch you with just one point to be sure that you are responding to the correct stimulus." If 2PM is being tested the examiner says, "You are to press the button when you first detect that two points are moving along the surface of your skin, for example, the fingertip. Do not push the button as soon as you feel something touch you. Do not push the button as soon as you feel two different points touch you, but be sure that you feel two points moving. I may sometimes touch you with just one point or not move the two points just to be sure that you are responding to the correct stimulus."

The testing sequence then begins with the examiner alerting the subject that the stimulus is coming by saying, "Shut your eyes and get ready, the test is beginning now." The examiner then slowly brings the prongs of the Pressure-Specified Sensory Device™ into contact with the surface to be tested, striving to touch the skin surface with both prongs simultaneously. The examiner must directly observe the prong's approach to, and contact with, the skin surface to get visual feedback of the testing procedure. The examiner uses visual cues related to the degree of skin indentation and tactile cues related to the feeling in the examiner's own hand as the Pressure-Specified Sensory Device™ is guided onto the test site. These cues permit the examiner to slowly increase the pressure of stimulus application until the subject presses the response button.

In contrast to testing 1PS or 1PM, the examiner should also view the computer screen once the prongs have contacted the skin surface, as the test must deliver as close to the same pressure as possible with each of the two prongs. This goal is monitored visually on the computer screen, where each prong's applied pressure is displayed as the height of the bar. The examiner's goal is to keep the two bars at the same height as the Pressure-Specified Sensory Device™ is slowly applied to the test skin site with increasing pressure. The subject may open his or her eyes between each test. The examiner should check the subject's eyes and realert him or her at the start of each test by saying, "Get ready, shut your eyes, the test is beginning again." After 5 satisfactory trials, the 2PS or 2PM test sequence is stopped and the subject is instructed to open his or her eyes and relax. The data is then averaged by the examiner in the same manner as described above, that is, by discarding the highest and lowest pressure values. Reassure the subject that the procedures were followed appropriately, if they were, and correct the subject's understanding of the procedures if they were not followed correctly.

● ● ●

● REFERENCES ●

Borges, L. F., Hallett, M., Selkoe, D. J., & Welch, K. The anterior tarsal tunnel syndrome. *Journal of Neurosurgery* *54*:89-92, 1981.

Coert, H. J., & Dellon, A. L. Clinical implications of the anatomy of the sural nerve. *Plastic and Reconstructive Surgery* *94*:850-855, 1994.

Dellon, A. L. Clinical use of vibratory stimuli to evaluate peripheral nerve injury and compression neuropathy. *Plastic and Reconstructive Surgery* *65*:466-476, 1980.

Dellon, A. L. Entrapment of the deep peroneal nerve on the dorsum of the foot. *Foot and Ankle* *11*:73-80, 1990.

Dellon, A. L. *Evaluation of Sensibility and Re-Education of Sensation in the Hand*. Baltimore: Williams & Wilkins, 1981.

Dellon, A. L. Tinel or not Tinel? *Journal of Hand Surgery (British)* *9*:216, 1984.

Dyck, P. J., Karnes, J. L., O'Brien, P. C., & Zimmerman, I. R. Detection thresholds of cutaneous sensation in humans. In *Peripheral Neuropathy,* 3rd Edition, P. J. Dyck, P. K. Thomas, J. W. Griffin, P. A. Low, & J. F. Poduslo, Editors. Philadelphia: W. B. Saunders Company, 1993.

Graham, B., & Dellon, A. L. Sensory recovery in innervated free-tissue transfers. *Journal of Reconstructive Microsurgery* *11*:157-166, 1995.

Holewski, J., Stess, R. M., Graff, P. M., & Grunfeld, C. Aesthesiometry: Quantification of cutaneous pressure sensation in diabetic peripheral neuropathy. *Journal of Rehabilitation Research and Development 25*:1-10, 1988.

Kaplan, P. E., & Kernahan, W. T. Tarsal tunnel syndrome: An electrodiagnostic and surgical correlation. *Journal of Bone and Joint Surgery 63A*:96-99, 1981.

Mackinnon, S. E., & Dellon, A. L. Tarsal Tunnel Syndrome. *In Surgery of the Peripheral Nerve,* New York: Thieme, 1988.

Mackinnon, S. E., & Dellon, A. L. Tibial nerve branching in the tarsal tunnel. *Archives of Neurology 41*:645-646, 1984.

May, J. W., Halls, M. J., & Simon, S. R. Free microvascular muscle flaps with skin graft reconstruction of extensive defects of the foot: A clinical and gait analysis study. *Plastic and Reconstructive Surgery 75*:627-632, 1985.

Rautio, J., Kekoni, J., Hamalainen, H., Harma, M., & Asko-Seljavaara, S. Mechanical sensibility in free and island flaps of the foot. *Journal of Reconstructive Microsurgery 5*:119-125, 1989.

Tassler, P. L., & Dellon, A. L. Correlation of measurements of pressure perception using the Pressure-Specified Sensory Device with Electrodiagnostic Testing. *Journal of Occupational Medicine 37*:862-866, 1995.

Tassler, P. L., & Dellon, A. L. Pressure perception in the normal lower extremity and in the tarsal tunnel syndrome. *Muscle and Nerve 19*:285-289 ,1996.

Tassler, P. L., Dellon, A. L., & Scheffler, N. M. Cutaneous pressure thresholds in diabetics with and without foot ulceration: Evaluation of sensibility with the Pressure-Specified Sensory Device. *Journal of the American Podiatric Medical Association 85*:679-684, 1995.

Association. *Neurology 43*:1050-1052, 1993.

Asbury, A. K., & Porte, D., Jr. Standardized measures in diabetic neuropathy. *Diabetes Care 18*:59-82, 1995.

Dellon, A. L. Treatment of symptoms of diabetic neuropathy by peripheral nerve decompression. *Plastic and Reconstructive Surgery 89*:689-697, 1992.

Dellon, A. L. *Advances in Podiatry 2:*17-40. 1996. Computer-assisted sensibility evaluation and surgical treatment of tarsal tunnel syndrome.

Dellon, A. L., Tassler, P. L., & Kress, K. Compensatory contralateral change; abnormal pressure perception in the non-injured foot. *Journal of Podiatric Medicine and Surgery*, submitted 1996.

Goodgold, J., Koeppel, H. P., & Sprelholz, N. I. The tarsal tunnel syndrome: Objective diagnostic criteria. *New England Journal of Medicine 173*:742-745, 1965.

Mackinnon, S. E., & Dellon, A. L. Homologies between the tarsal and carpal tunnels: Implications for surgical treatment in the tarsal tunnel syndrome. *Contemporary Orthopedics 14*:75-78, 1987.

• • •

• ADDITIONAL READINGS •

Arezzo, J. C., Bolton, C. F., & Boulton, A. Quantitative sensory testing: A consensus report from the Peripheral Neuropathy

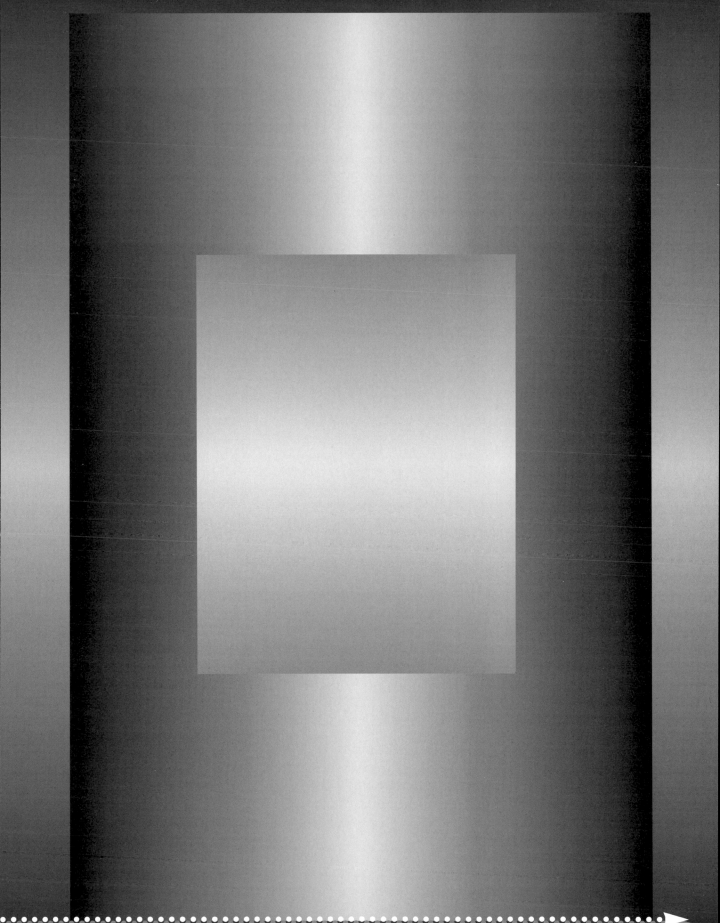

neuropathy

• • •

*N*europathy is damage to the nerves...Neuropathy affects nerves that connect the spinal cord to muscles, skin, blood vessels, and organs. Although neuropathy can affect many parts of the body, it most often affects the feet and the legs...The most common symptoms of neuropathy are numbness, tingling, weakness, burning, or pain. These sensations often start in the fingers or toes and move up the arms or legs. The pain is usually worse at night. It may ease in the morning. Symptoms of neuropathy depend on which nerves are affected. If the nerves of the leg muscles are affected, the result may be difficulty walking. Damage to other nerves may result in frequent diarrhea or constipation, difficult urination, bladder infections, impotence, or poor balance. The person may not feel heat or cold or pressure. This can be dangerous. They might feel no pain when the feet are injured, frozen, or burned. Or a stone in the shoe could cause a blister or ulcer. This could lead to serious foot problems...Infections can be very serious problems...An injury that might not be noticed may cause infection, gangrene, or even amputation. Today there are no cures for neuropathy. But health-care practitioners may prescribe drugs to treat pain, depression, and the loss of sleep that neuropathy often brings...Unfortunately, experts do not know how to prevent neuropathy...

Nerve Complications (Neuropathy),
American Diabetes Association,
Basic Information Series #15, 1989

• • •

• SUSCEPTIBILITY TO •
COMPRESSION

The symptoms of neuropathy are very similar to those of chronic nerve compression. For example, the patient with carpal tunnel syndrome has numbness and tingling in the fingers, and so does the patient with a neuropathy. The difference, classically, is that the patient with a neuropathy has numbness in all the fingers and on both sides of the hand, while the patient with carpal tunnel syndrome has numbness in just the radial three (and-a-half) digits, and primarily over the palmar aspect of the hand. However, if a patient had compression of the median nerve at the wrist level, the ulnar nerve at the elbow level, and the radial sensory nerve in the forearm, then that patient would have a glove-like distribution of numbness, and have the same symptoms as the patient with a neuropathy.

If the pathophysiologic mechanism of the neuropathy causes a condition in the peripheral nerve that made that nerve susceptible to nerve compression, then it would be possible for the patient with a neuropathy to have chronic nerve compression superimposed on the underlying neuropathy. The patient's symptoms might, therefore, be due to the superimposed nerve compression instead of from, or in addition to, the underlying neuropathy. If this susceptibility to compression were to exist in neuropathy, then it may be possible to treat the patient's symptoms by decompression of peripheral nerves. This hypothesis creates a cause for optimism in the patient with neuropathy (Dellon, 1988). Documentation of the condition of the peripheral nerve by the therapist, and rehabilitation of the patient with neuropathy, would become a standard part of the therapist's practice.

There are several known mechanisms that can render a peripheral nerve susceptible to compression. For example, it is known that the diabetic nerve has an increased water content (Jakobsen, 1978). In diabetes, the elevated blood glucose is taken directly into the nerve and is metabolized to fructose and then to sorbitol, a sugar that contains many hydroxyl groups and is, therefore, hydrophilic; that is, it attracts water molecules. A similar mechanism exists in the patient with lead poisoning. Lead has been demonstrated to cause a loosening of the "tight" junctions between the endothelial cells in the blood vessels of the nerve, resulting in an increased endoneurial water content (Ohnishi, et al., 1977; Windebank & Dyck, 1984). Histologic examples of this increase in endoneurial edema are given in Figure 14.1. If a nerve swells in an anatomically narrow space, like the carpal, cubital, or tarsal tunnel, there will be increased pressure on the nerve, resulting in decreased blood flow in the nerve, which results in numbness and tingling.

Another type of mechanism that increases the susceptibility of the peripheral nerve to compression is a decrease in the slow component of axoplasmic flow. This results in the decreased delivery of the proteins required to repair the cell membranes in the axon. Compression of the nerve results in increased need to repair the axon. In diabetes, there is a well-documented decreased axoplasmic transport, although its exact cause is unknown (Jakobsen & Sidenius, 1980). In patients receiving chemotherapy, drugs such as vincristine, cisplatin, and taxol each affect the microtubules that are required for the slow component of axoplasmic transport (Gottschalk, Dyck, & Kiely, 1968; Mollman, 1990; Rowinsky & Donnehower, 1995). Decreasing the slow component of axoplasmic transport decreases the ability of the peripheral nerve to repair itself in these regions of anatomic narrowing, where chronic nerve compression occurs.

The concept that the peripheral nerve can have a site of compression, and that this site of compression can render the rest of the nerve increasingly susceptible to other sites of compression, is critically important in understanding the role of the therapist and the possibility of therapeutic intervention for patients suffering from neuropathy. This concept

FIGURE 14.1

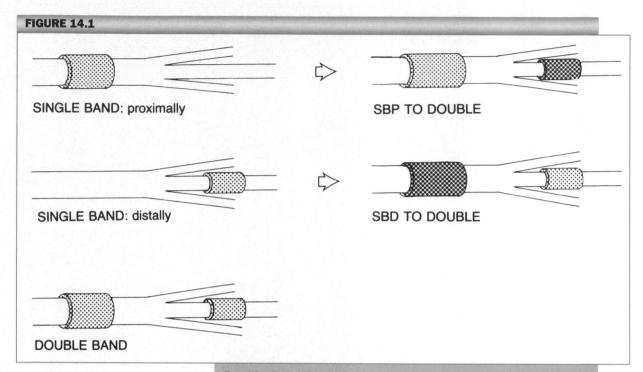

SINGLE BAND: proximally

SBP TO DOUBLE

SINGLE BAND: distally

SBD TO DOUBLE

DOUBLE BAND

Double Crush Hypothesis. The concept that a proximal site of nerve compression will render the distal portion of the peripheral nerve more susceptible to chronic nerve compression was put forth by Upton and McComas in 1973. In this illustration, the sciatic nerve of the rat is shown on the right with a single site of compression produced by a silicone band. After a period of time, a second band could be placed distally. The change in electrophysiologic function of the sciatic nerve could be compared between a group that had a single site of compression, a group that had two sites of compression contemporaneously, and a group that had a second site of compression added after a period of proximal compression. The results of this study demonstrated that a single site of compression did increase the susceptibility of the distal portion of the nerve to compression, thereby confirming the double crush hypothesis. From Surgery of the Peripheral Nerve, *by S. E. Mackinnon & A. L. Dellon, 1988, New York: Thieme Publishing. Reprinted with permission of the authors.*

was first described by Upton and McComas (1973) to explain the frequent occurrence in patients of both a cervical radiculopathy and carpal tunnel syndrome, or both thoracic outlet syndrome and cubital tunnel syndrome. They called this phenomenon the *double crush*, for the two sites of compression along the length of a single peripheral nerve. Figure 14.1 is an illustration from a study that confirmed the double crush hypothesis in the experimental model (Seiler, Schlegel, Mackinnon, & Dellon, 1983). Upton and McComas extended their hypothesis to include the concept that a systemic disease, such as diabetes, could serve as one site of compression, that is, as one of the "crush-

es." This model stated that each site of compression, in and of itself, might not be sufficient to produce symptoms, but that the two sites could summate to produce symptoms.

It followed from this hypothesis that both sites of compression might not need to be corrected to relieve symptoms if this surgical intervention occurred before irreversible changes oc-

FIGURE 14.2

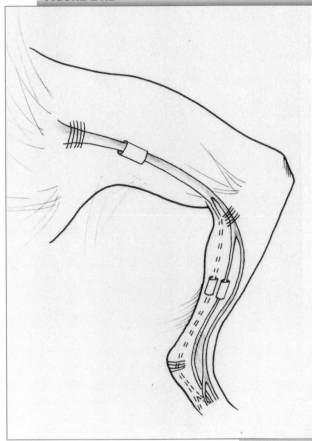

Multiple Crush Syndrome. An experimental model using the monkey was designed that incorporated a silicone tube to create a site of compression along the sciatic nerve in the mid-thigh, and the posterior tibial nerve in the mid-calf, with the tarsal tunnel providing the third site of compression along this single nerve. For the peroneal nerve, the site of narrowing at the fibular head was the most proximal site, with distal sites being created by banding the deep peroneal nerve in the mid-calf, and considering the anatomic site over the dorsum of the foot as the fourth site. Three months later, the peripheral nerves were biopsied and morphometric analysis done. The group of biopsies along the peroneal nerve demonstrated neural degeneration. The group of biopsies along the posterior tibial nerve demonstrated progressive demyelination; that is, mean nerve fiber diameter at the sciatic band level was 5.4 μ, at the mid-calf it was 3.9 μ, and at the tarsal tunnel it was 3.2 μ. In contrast, the mean nerve fiber diameter of the myelinated fibers at the same level in the opposite limb were 7.9 μ, 8.0 μ, and 6.4 μ, respectively, in the one monkey available for this analysis. Thus, the proximal site of nerve compression resulted in the distal nerve demonstrating a progressive increase in the degree of chronic nerve compression compared with the opposite side. Unpublished observations, S. E. Mackinnon, D. A. Hunter, & A. L. Dellon, 1989. Printed with permission of the authors.

curred. This model was then applied to diabetic rats, and demonstrated that a rat with diabetes was more susceptible to nerve compression than a nondiabetic rat (Dellon, Mackinnon, & Seiler, 1988). It was not clear how many sites of nerve compression would be required to create a loss of function of the nerve. This was investigated in a preliminary study in monkeys in which two sites of banding were created along the length of a nerve in the lower extremity. The nerve fiber counts were obtained at each site (see Figure 14.2). This study demon-strated that three sites of compression along the length of a single nerve could create a loss of nerve fibers consistent with a neuropathy; that is, there was a sequential increase in the loss of fibers, being worse distally. This occurred within three months of banding the nerve (Mackinnon & Dellon, unpublished observations, 1991). Nerve fiber loss took at least 1 year to occur when there was just one site of banding (Mackinnon & Dellon, 1988).

Based on the observed changes in electrodiagnostic measurements in the rat model of the double crush, a mathematical model could be developed. Figure 14.3 represents the concept that each site of nerve compression creates a certain degree of electrophysiologic dysfunction of the peripheral

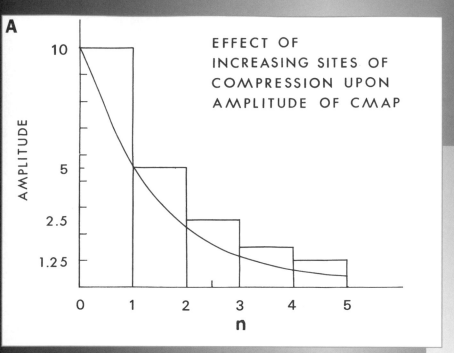

A

EFFECT OF INCREASING SITES OF COMPRESSION UPON AMPLITUDE OF CMAP

AMPLITUDE

10
5
2.5
1.25

0   1   2   3   4   5

n

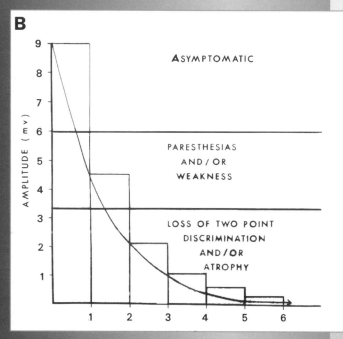

B

AMPLITUDE (m v)

9
8
7
6
5
4
3
2
1

ASYMPTOMATIC

PARESTHESIAS AND / OR WEAKNESS

LOSS OF TWO POINT DISCRIMINATION AND / OR ATROPHY

1   2   3   4   5   6

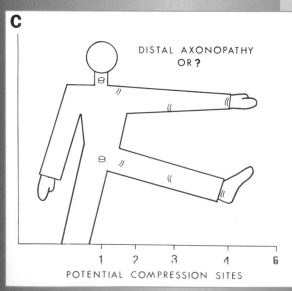

C

DISTAL AXONOPATHY OR ?

1   2   3   4   5

POTENTIAL COMPRESSION SITES

FIGURE 14.3
Mathematical Model of the Multiple Crush Concept. Based on the observed electrophysiologic changes (CMAP is the compound motor action potential) in the rat sciatic nerve subjected to single and double crush, and based on the observed phenomenon in electrical changes in human diabetic neuropathy, a mathematical model incorporating a decay curve was developed. (A) This suggests that each successive site ("M") of banding of the peripheral nerve creates a further decrement in nerve function. (B) This concept is extended to clinical symptoms. It suggests that as long as an irreversible change has not yet occurred in the nerve, removal of any given band can result in improved nerve function. (C) Illustrates potential sites of compression, which can create the electrical appearance of axonopathy if present simultaneously. Unpublished observations of E. M. Nicholas, A. L. Dellon, & E. Rechthand, 1992. Printed with permission of the authors.

nerve, which can be quantified. If it is assumed that each subsequent site along the length of the nerve induces a similar degree of nerve dysfunction, a "decay curve" of that nerve's function can be created. In this theoretical model, removal of any site of compression shifts the nerve function curve backward toward normal.

The applications of these concepts to the treatment of the symptoms of neuropathy are that the basic cause of the neuropathy predisposes the nerve to more distal compression; that is, the neuropathy equals the first crush. Thereafter, known sites of anatomic narrowing, like the vertebral foramina, the "thoracic outlet," the cubital tunnel, the forearm fibrous arches, and the tunnels of the wrist, like Guyon's canal and carpal tunnel, each can provide a separate site of "crush." According to this hypothesis, the therapist can document the degree of sensorimotor dysfunction and, once the underlying neuropathy is receiving maximal medical care, the surgeon may be able to release individual distal entrapment sites, relieving symptoms. The therapist can document these sensorimotor changes.

The commonest causes of peripheral neuropathy in the United States are diabetes, alcoholism, thyroid dysfunction, and collagen vascular diseases (rheumatoid arthritis, lupus). Other known causes are complications of chemotherapy, vitamin deficiency, lead poisoning, and, on a worldwide level, leprosy. Leprosy will be described below as related to an infectious etiology, and may be very variable in presentation depending on which fascicles of the nerves are involved in the infection. The treatment of alcoholic neuropathy is to stop drinking, in which case the neuropathy usually improves. The treatment for the neuropathies related to thyroid problems and to collagen vascular disease usually respond to medical management, as would that related to a vitamin B6 deficiency.

In contrast, the accepted natural history of diabetic neuropathy is for it to progress and to be irreversible, often even in patients under good glycemic control. The prognosis for the patient with a neuropathy related to lead poisoning or chemotherapy is also poor, with no accepted treatment available. These patients have a symmetrical polyneuropathy, usually worse for sensory function then for motor, and usually presenting first in the lower extremities, proceeding from distal to proximal. These are usually axonopathies, with loss of nerve fibers, in contrast to chronic nerve compression which presents first as demyelination, and only in the advanced degree with axonal loss (Dyck, Thomas, Lambert, & Bunge, 1984; Mackinnon & Dellon, 1988). Examples of documentation of a symmetrical polyneuropathy are given in Figure 14.4, using computer-assisted sensibility testing for someone with a severe degree of neuropathy in the lower extremity, and for someone in whom the lower extremity is affected more than the upper extremity.

• DIABETES •

Diabetes affects at least 4% of the United States population. At the time of diagnosis, up to 25% of the diabetic population may have neuropathy present as determined by electrodiagnostic testing. By the time the patient has had diabetes for 25 years, between 50% and 75% of the patients will have a detectable neuropathy. While there are a wide number of different neuropathies present in this population, the most common is a diffuse, symmetrical polyneuropathy affecting sensory and motor function and, in many patients, also autonomic function. The less common types of neuropathies affect (a) an isolated cranial nerve; (b) the proximal peripheral nerves associated with pain and weakness (dia-

FIGURE 14.4

Documentation of symmetrical polyneuropathy with computer-assisted sensory testing using the Pressure-Specified Sensory Device™. (A) This 50-year-old man had a left tarsal tunnel release which was ineffective in relieving his symptoms. Clinically, there was a sensory loss on both the dorsum and the plantar surface of both feet, suggesting a neuropathy. Quantitative sensory testing demonstrates abnormal sensibility in the peroneal, the posterior tibial, and the sural nerve, with the loss being symmetrical, consistent with the type of neuropathy seen in diabetes. The absence of two-point discrimination is consistent with severe axonal loss. The upper extremity examination was normal. Further workup failed to demonstrate a definitive etiology for this neuropathy, and the patient's symptoms were treated with neuropathic pain medication. (B) This 34-year-old woman complained of heel pain. Her clinical examination suggested that she might have upper extremity problems as well. Her primary care physician had obtained nerve conduction studies, which were normal. Quantitative sensory testing demonstrates abnormalities of the median and ulnar nerves in the upper extremity, and the peroneal and posterior tibial nerves in the lower extremities. The two-point discrimination is abnormal, suggesting that this is an axonopathy. The lower extremities are more affected than the upper extremities. A definitive cause for this neuropathy has not been identified. Note that in both patients, the quantitative sensory testing was done as a screening examination, and only one-point static and two-point static testing was done. A. L. Dellon, MD, unpublished observations.

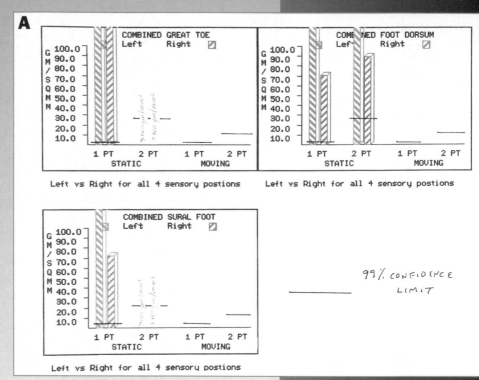

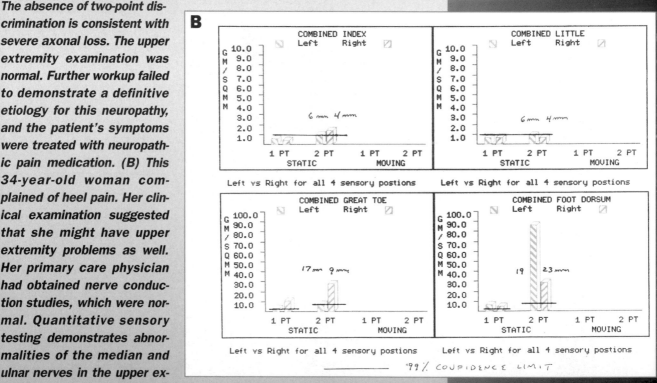

betic amyotrophy); (c) a burning, painful neuropathy which may not be associated with sensory and motor changes; (d) asymmetrical peripheral nerve compressions (mononeuritis multiplex); and (e) individual nerve compressions, like carpal tunnel syndrome (Dyck, Thomas, Asbury, Winegrad, & Porte, 1987).

There is no accepted explanation for the presence of any of these types of neuropathies. The theories for the commonest form have ranged from the presence of atherosclerosis of the large blood vessels of the extremities, to biochemical abnormalities (increased activity of aldose reductase and decreased concentration of myoinositol). While narrowing of the large vessel does exist, this is no longer accepted as the etiology of neuropathy. Specific clinical trials to alter the biochemical abnormalities have not been successful. At present, a leading theory is that the neuropathy is due to narrowing of the small blood vessels that supply the peripheral nerves.

The result of the neuropathy in the lower extremity is loss of sensibility in the feet, collapse of the tarsal arches, and loss of sweating, all resulting in increased susceptibility to infection, skin breakdown and, ultimately, loss of tissue. Diabetes is the leading cause of amputation in the United States, and about 30% of the patients with one amputated limb will have the other limb amputated (Siitonen, Niskanen, & Laakso, 1993).

• FOOT ULCERATION •

This section will deal with the measurement of peripheral neuropathy as it relates to foot ulceration, and as it relates to the theory that the symptoms of the neuropathy may be treated by decompression of multiple peripheral nerves.

Foot ulceration in the diabetic continues to be a problem of worldwide proportions. While new nonoperative and operative treatment options continue to be described, it is clear that prevention of foot ulceration is the ideal goal to be pursued (Dellon, 1992; Siitonen, et al., 1993; Clark & Lee, 1995). Prevention requires identification of the population at risk. Tests for cardiac autonomic function, and electrodiagnostic measurement of motor and sensory nerve conduction, do not distinguish between groups of diabetics with and without foot ulceration. However, peripheral sympathetic nerve function, as determined by venous occlusion plethysmography, was significantly worse in the diabetic neuropathy group that had foot ulceration (Gilmore, Allen, & Hayes, 1993).

While impaired sympathetic innervation decreases sweating and may contribute to stiffening of the plantar skin, it is possible that the impaired sympathetic innervation occurs parallel with impairment of sensibility in diabetic neuropathy in the lower extremity. The cutaneous pressure threshold, as estimated with the Semmes-Weinstein nylon monofilaments, has been reported to correlate with the presence of foot ulcers, but the range over which this can occur as recorded with this instrument is large (Holewski, 1988; Sosenko, Kato, & Soto, 1990). Abnormal vibratory perception has been correlated with foot ulceration in patients with diabetic neuropathy for a decade (Boulton, Kubrusly, & Bowker, 1986), but has not come into widespread use. It is of interest, therefore, that computer-assisted sensibility testing with the Pressure-Specified Sensory Device™ is capable of quantifying the human pressure perception threshold in the foot.

Computer-assisted measurement of sensibility was done at four anatomic sites of the foot of nondiabetics, and in diabetics with and without foot ulceration (Tassler, Dellon, & Schiffler, 1995; Tassler & Dellon, 1996). The patients were able to differentiate the pressure stimulus of this testing instrument from the paresthesias of the neuropathy, and the stimulus

TABLE 14.1 NORMATIVE LOWER EXTREMITY PRESSURE THRESHOLDS (> THAN 45 YEARS OF AGE)				
Pressure (g/mm²)	**Great Toe**	**Foot Dorsum**	**Lateral Calf**	**Heel**
One-point static touch	1.0	1.5	2.5	2.7
One-point moving touch	0.6	0.6	1.3	1.7
Two-point static touch	16.3	16.8	18.5	20.4
Two-point moving touch	8.6	6.8	8.9	9.1
Distance (mm)				
Two-point static discrimination	5.7	6.3	6.5	5.7
Two-point moving discrimination	4.3	4.4	4.4	4.5

Note: From "Quantitative Sensory Testing: Normative Data in the Lower Extremity," by P. L. Tassler & A. L. Dellon, *Muscle and Nerve 19*:285-289, 1996. Reprinted with permission of the authors.

was not perceived as painful. (This distinction may be difficult to make for the patient with neuropathy if a vibratory or electrical stimulus is used for threshold testing.)

The cutaneous pressure threshold measurements of the diabetics were compared to measurements on 30 non-diabetic, nonulcerated feet (see Tables 14.1 & 14.2). The results of this study demonstrate that the mean one-point static pressure threshold for all four lower extremity anatomic areas tested was significantly higher (indicating decreased sensation) for diabetics without ulceration than in nondiabetic, age-matched normal subjects (p < .001). There were also significant differ-

ences in one-point static pressure thresholds for the great toe and the dorsum of the foot in diabetics with foot ulcerations compared to diabetics without ulceration (p < .001). Computer-assisted sensibility testing also demonstrated significantly higher pressure thresholds for one-point moving touch and two-point discrimination in the ulcerated compared to the nonulcerated diabetic foot (see Figure 14.5).

The lowest thresholds at which a patient with diabetic neuropathy was found to have a foot ulcer were one-point static threshold 9.1 g/mm², and two-point static threshold 32.9 g/mm², at a distance of 9 mm on the great toe. This set of sensory

measurements falls clearly within the range of those patients with neuropathy and no ulcerations. Therefore, the presence of only minimally elevated thresholds does not imply that a patient will not develop foot ulceration. In addition, the presence of markedly elevated thresholds does not imply that a patient will develop foot ulceration, if they have been paying attention to their daily foot hygiene. However, the presence of an ulceration in a patient with this set of measurements helps to establish a limit at which an ulceration may develop. Based on the results of this cross-sectional study, the cutaneous pressure threshold above which there

TABLE 14.2 PRESSURE THRESHOLDS IN DIABETICS

| | Without Ulcer | | | |
	Great Toe	Foot Dorsum	Lateral Calf	Heel
Pressure (g/mm²)				
One-point static touch	30.5	25.6	18.0	15.0
One-point moving touch	19.2	13.2	3.2	16.4
Two-point static touch	23.6	16.8	28.2	33.7
Two-point moving touch	20.2	12.0	22.3	24.1
Distance (mm)				
Two-point static discrimination	7.5	5.8	5.5	4.8
Two-point moving discrimination	8.1	4.3	6.4	3.0
	With Ulcer			
	Great Toe	Foot Dorsum	Lateral Calf	Heel
Pressure (g/mm²)				
One-point static touch	60.7	44.2	20.7	34.6
One-point moving touch	49.6	18.5	12.1	38.0
Two-point static touch	41.3	33.7	39.4	53.1
Two-point moving touch	47.6	25.8	28.0	52.2
Distance (mm)				
Two-point static discrimination	11.0	10.0	7.9	8.4
Two-point moving discrimination	8.3	9.1	7.1	6.0

Note: From "Cutaneous Pressure Threshold in Diabetics with and without Foot Ulceration: Evaluation of Sensibility with the Pressure-Specified Sensory Device," by P. L. Tassler, A. L. Dellon, & N. M. Scheffler, 1995. *Journal of the American Podiatric Medical Association, 85:*679-684. Reprinted with permission of the authors.

is an increased likelihood of ulceration is 30 g/mm². (See Chapters 7 and 13 for descriptions of the relative merits of the different instruments for measurement of sensibility in the foot, and the protocol for use of the Pressure-Specified Sensory Device™ in the lower extremity.)

These observations have relevance for the development of a program to monitor sensibility with quantitative sensory testing, as recommended by the American Diabetes Association and the American Society for Peripheral Neuropathy (Asbury & Porte, 1988; Arezzo, Bolton,

FIGURE 14.5

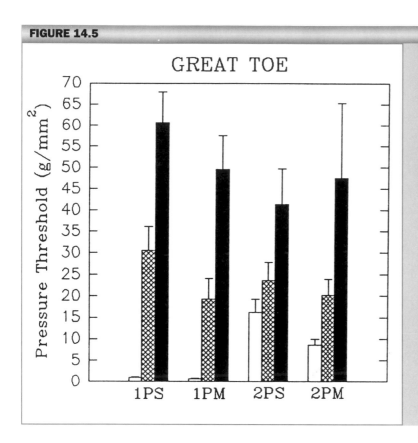

GREAT TOE

Foot ulceration present in diabetics with neuropathy represents a degree of sensory loss which is significantly worse than is present in diabetics without ulceration. The measurements of sensibility were made with the Pressure- Specified Sensory Device™. The presence of neuropathy gives a degree of sensibility that is significantly worse than in the normal population. From "Cutaneous Pressure Threshold in Diabetics with and without Foot Ulceration: Evaluation of Sensibility with the Pressure-Specified Sensory Device," by P. L. Tassler, A. L. Dellon, & N. M. Scheffler, Journal of the American Podiatric Medical Association 85: 679-684, 1995. Reprinted with permission of the authors.

& Boulton, 1993). It has been concluded that computer-assisted sensibility testing of the touch threshold in the foot in the diabetic is valid for documenting diminished sensation in the foot, and for identifying those individuals whose feet should be protected with customized, molded footwear. Computer-assisted sensibility testing can document the need for these shoes for third-party insurance carriers.

TREATMENT OF
• **SYMPTOMS BY NERVE** •
DECOMPRESSION

Diabetic neuropathy is generally believed to be a progressive and irreversible problem (Dyck, et al., 1987; Clark & Lee, 1995). The hypothesis that the symptoms of the neuropathy may be due to superimposed nerve compressions along the length of the peripheral nerve, combined with the observation that the compression of more than one peripheral nerve (median, radial sensory, and ulnar nerves) at the same time can create a glove pattern of sensory loss, suggested that decompression of multiple peripheral nerves

may be able to treat the symptoms of the patient with diabetic neuropathy (Dellon, 1988).

The ideal candidate for decompression of peripheral nerves would be the diabetic who, despite good glycemic control, develops symptoms of numbness and tingling in the hands or feet. In addition, there may be weakness in the hands or feet. The degree of numbness is usually the same in both feet and in both hands, with the feet usually becoming affected before the hands, and with the feet usually being worse than the hands. This may be uncomfortable, but is not the severe burning sensation present in the primarily painful form of diabetic neuropathy, and the weakness, if present, is distal, not proximal. Therefore, the ideal candidate has a diffuse, symmetrical, distal, sensorimotor neuropathy. The surgical decompression should be done before there is muscle wasting, ulceration, and loss of two-point discrimination (see Figures 14.6 & 14.7). The physical examination will demonstrate a positive Tinel sign over the site of nerve compression in patients in whom a good result from the surgery may be anticipated.

The results in the first 50 patients, who had a total of 154 nerves decompressed, was reported in 1992 (Dellon, 1992). The results demonstrated, by any of 6 different end-assessment techniques, that 80% of the patients could expect good to excellent results. Figure 14.8 illustrates the results plotted for each individual nerve when the patients with Type I diabetes were asked whether they were satisfied with the outcome of their surgery. In that study, the mean follow-up was about 3½ years, with the longest follow-up being 7 years. None of the patients during the time of observation had a loss of function in the decompressed nerve. It was

FIGURE 14.6

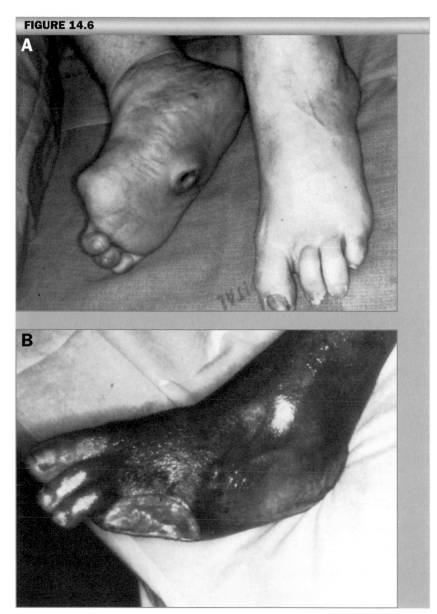

possible to obtain follow-up electrodiagnostic studies in a subgroup of these patients. Even this end-result assessment demonstrated that 68% of the patients had improvement following decompression of peripheral nerves. In contrast, 50% of the patients had progression of the neuropathy in an unoperated extremity during

this same period of observation (see Figure 14.8), suggesting that decompression of peripheral nerves can change the natural history of diabetic neuropathy.

Subsequently, experimental work with a rat model of progressive diabetic neuropathy (Dellon, A. L., Dellon, E. S., & Seiler, 1994) demonstrated that decompression

FIGURE 14.6 (CONTINUED)

Treatment of the symptoms of diabetic neuropathy by decompression of multiple peripheral nerves. and In the past, patients have not been referred to the surgeon unless they have required (A) drainage of infection, amputation of toes, or (B) closure of ulceration. Even if the referral comes at a time when the sensory loss is severe, if the patient is having reconstructive surgery (C) it may be worthwhile to attempt (D), decompression of the posterior tibial nerve in the tarsal tunnel, as in this patient. At 3 years following the surgery (E), there has been sufficient protective sensibility recovered that the remaining toes have been preserved. A. L. Dellon, MD, unpublished observations.

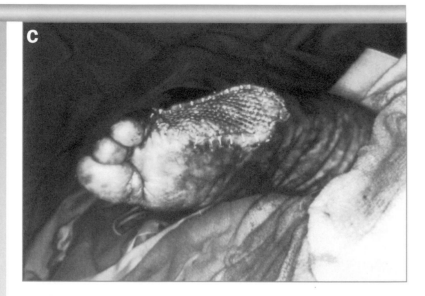

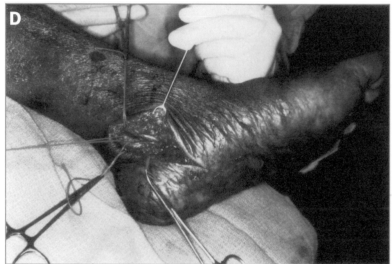

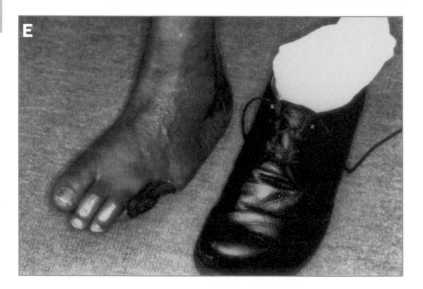

of the tarsal tunnel at the time of onset of the diabetes would prevent the neuropathic walking track pattern from occurring.

I continue to provide this surgical procedure for patients referred to me with diabetes, and they continue to recover sensibility. Now, however, it is possible to obtain documentation of the

FIGURE 14.7

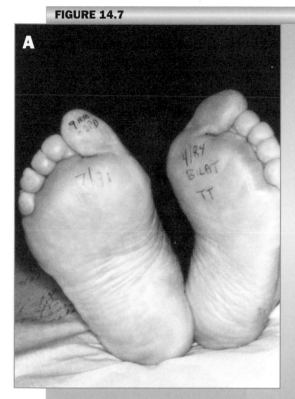

A

Treatment of the symptoms of diabetic neuropathy by decompression of multiple peripheral nerves. (A) If the patient is referred at a time when there has been no soft tissue loss, there is the possibility for neural re-generation, such as in this patient who is 7 years after decompression of the posterior tibial nerve and its branches, bilaterally. There is now 9 mm moving two-point discrimination. This patient is 55 years of age and had Type II diabetes for 10 years prior to surgery. (B) The results of this surgical approach in a series of patients evaluated through 1989. This group is com-posed of Type I diabetics. Each symbol on the chart is a different nerve. The years on the x-axis represent years of diabetes. The mean follow-up after surgery for this group is 3½ years. These patients evaluated their own outcome from the decompression in terms of symptomatic relief, and 80% rated themselves as hav-ing good or excellent results. From "Treatment of Symptoms of Diabetic Neuropathy by Peripheral Nerve Decompression," by A. L. Dellon, 1992, Plastic and Reconstructive Surgery 89:689-697. Reprinted with permission of the author.

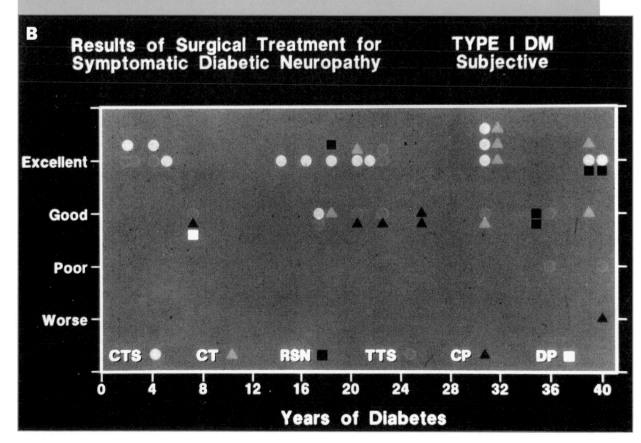

B

Results of Surgical Treatment for Symptomatic Diabetic Neuropathy   TYPE I DM Subjective

FIGURE 14.8

Treatment of the symptoms of diabetic neuropathy by decompression of multiple peripheral nerves. (A) Detailed assessment comparing before and after for the decompression of the median nerve in the carpal tunnel and the posterior tibial nerve in the tarsal tunnel. Note that for each measure there was improvement. (B) Detailed assessment in this same patient comparing two lower extremity nerves that were not decompressed. Note that these nerves not only did not improve but they became progressively worse, as expected for untreated diabetic neuropathy. These results, all in the same patient over the same time period, with the same degree of glycemic control, suggest that the decompression of the peripheral nerves altered the natural history of the neuropathy in the surgically treated nerves. A. L. Dellon, MD, unpublished observations.

A   NO SURGERY

L.M.   59   TYPE I DIABETES, 2 years

Carpal tunnel syndrome	symptoms	electrical
R sural		3.6 mse ↓ no response
11/81	persistent	
8/85	persistent	
R peroneal		4.7 msec ↓ no response
11/81	persistent	
8/85	persistent	

B   SURGERY

L.M.   59   TYPE I DIABETES, 2 years

Carpal tunnel syndrome	m2PD	symptoms	grading clinical	electrical
2/84	3	persistent	Good ⌐ Good	4.9 msec ↓
4/86	3	gone	Excellent ⌐	4.5
Tarsal tunnel syndrome				
5/84	10	persistent	Fair ⌐ Excellent	5.2 msec ↓
4/86	5	gone	Excellent ⌐	3.9

degree of sensory recovery with computer-assisted sensory testing. Examples of this are illustrated in Figures 14.9 and 14.10.

It is clear that the therapist increasingly will be called on to provide documentation of the degree of sensibility present in the hands and feet of diabetics because it will be required for preoperative counseling and postoperative evaluation of the results of the treatment of the neuropathy. Even if some form of medical therapy becomes available for the treatment of diabetic neuropathy, such as the use of an insulin-like growth factor, this documentation by the therapist will still be required.

The initial assessment of the diabetic for neuropathy will include an electrodiagnostic evaluation, which will probably have been ordered by the primary care physician or the endocrinologist prior to the patient's being referred to the therapist. The therapist's initial evaluation should include the measurement of one-point moving and static pressure thresh-

A

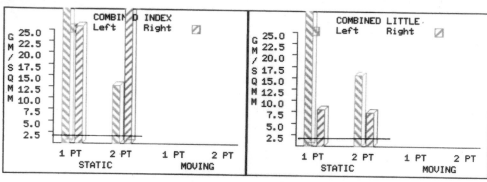

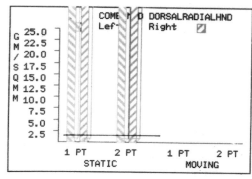

99 % CONFIDENCE
LIMIT

FIGURE 14.9

Treatment of the symptoms of diabetic neuropathy by decompression of multiple peripheral nerves. (A) and (B) Computer-assisted sensory testing of 2 patients with diabetic neuropathy in the upper extremity. In (A) the patient is a 56-year-old Type II diabetic of 10 years duration, while in (B) the patient is a 30-year-old Type I diabetic of 12 years duration.

Note the generally symmetrical nature of the sensory loss. In (C) the sensory testing is done 6 months after decompression of the left median nerve at the wrist and in the forearm, and the ulnar nerve at the elbow. This patient is a 40-year-old man with Type I diabetes of 18 years duration. Note that the sensory thresholds for each nerve are lower in the side that had the surgical decompression. Figure 14.9 continued on following page. A. L. Dellon MD, unpublished observations.

FIGURE 14.9 CONTINUED

B

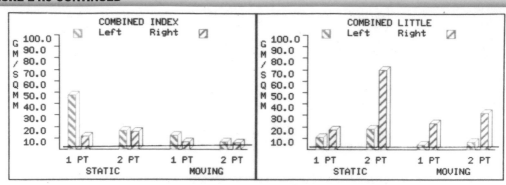

Left vs Right for all 4 sensory postions   Left vs Right for all 4 sensory postions

_____ 99 % CONFIDENCE LIMIT

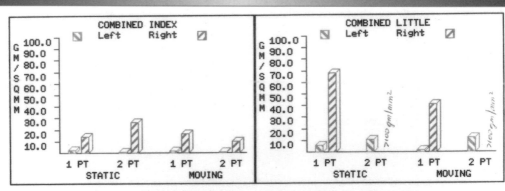

C

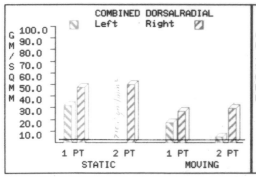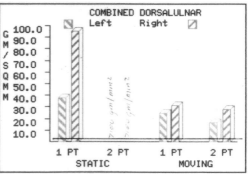

Left vs Right for all 4 sensory postions   Left vs Right for all 4 sensory postions

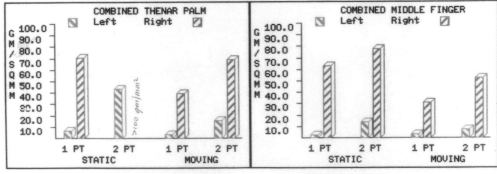

Left vs Right for all 4 sensory postions   Left vs Right for all 4 sensory postions

The PSSD Notepad is printed at the end of the report

A

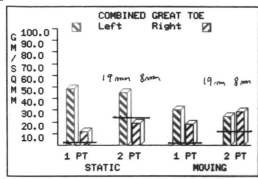

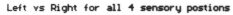

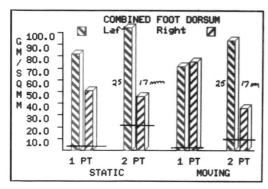

Left vs Right for all 4 sensory postions

99% CONFIDENCE LIMIT
_____

FIGURE 14.10

Treatment of the symptoms of diabetic neuropathy by decompression of multiple peripheral nerves. In the lower extremity, (A) a 70-year-old man with severe neuropathy after 15 years of Type II diabetes. This quantitative sensory testing was done 6 months after the right leg had a decompression of the posterior tibial nerve and the common peroneal nerve. The patient had such increased burning after surgery that he believed he had been made worse. However, the results of the testing demonstrate neural regeneration with both the pressure threshold and the distance at which one could be distinguished from two points being lowered for the medial plantar and calcaneal branches of the posterior tibial nerve and for the deep peroneal branch of the common peroneal nerve. (B) and (C) are the preoperative and postoperative results of quantitative sensory testing with the Pressure-Specified Sensory Device™ for a 35-year-old woman with a 20-year history of Type I diabetes. Her degree of neuropathy is more severe than the patient in (A), as noted by the loss of axons such that she has almost completely lost two-point discrimination in all regions of her foot. In (C), 6 months after decompression of the left posterior tibial and the common peroneal and the deep peroneal nerves, she has regained one-point moving and static touch on the left, while at the same time she has had progression of the neuropathy on the right with loss of one-point moving touch from the big toe, and loss of moving two-point discrimination on the dorsum of the foot, and from the lateral calf. This is similar to the patient in Figure 14.9, who had improvement in the decompressed nerves while over the same period of observation had progression of the neuropathy in nerves that had not been decompressed. Figure 14.10 continued on following page. A. L. Dellon, MD, unpublished observations.

FIGURE 14.10 CONTINUED

B

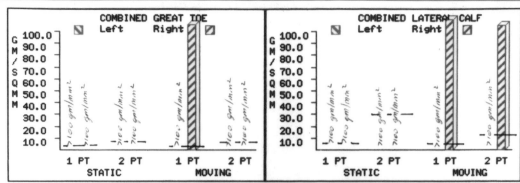

Left vs Right for all 4 sensory postions   Left vs Right for all 4 sensory postions

99% CONFIDENCE LIMIT

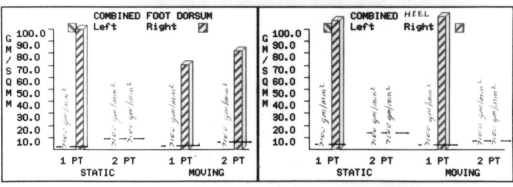

Left vs Right for all 4 sensory postions   Left vs Right for all 4 sensory postions

C

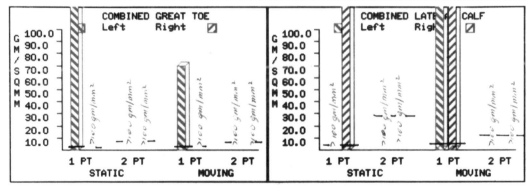

Left vs Right for all 4 sensory postions   Left vs Right for all 4 sensory postions

99% CONFIDENCE LIMIT

Left vs Right for all 4 sensory postions   Left vs Right for all 4 sensory postions

FIGURE 14.11

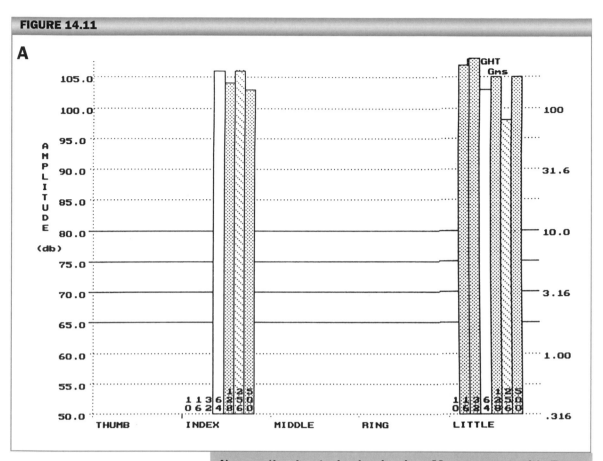

Neuropathy due to lead poisoning. Measurement with Force-Defined Vibrometer™, which tests at 10, 16, 32, 64, 128, 256, and 500 Hz (frequency noted at bottom of each bar, see Chapter 7 for further description of this instrument). The right (A) and left (B) hand of a painter 7 years after exposure to lead, with a severe symmetrical neuropathy involving the median (index finger) and ulnar (little finger) nerves. Note that the perception of the low-frequency vibratory stimuli is the first to be lost. The normal threshold for this young man should be below 70 decibels (3.16 microns of amplitude). Both feet of a man who was sandblasting a bridge 6 years ago when he developed lead poisoning. (See also Figure 14.11 (B) – (D) on the following pages.) A. L. Dellon, MD, unpublished observations.

olds, and both moving and static two-point discrimination thresholds, noting both the distance at which the two-points can be distinguished and the pressure required to make that distinction.

All of these measurements are essential because in diabetic neuropathy, in contrast to chronic nerve compression alone, there is an underlying axonopathy, which results in loss of nerve fibers, plus a susceptibility to compression, which results in demyelination. Thus, there will be a loss of two-point discrimination in terms of both the distance and the pressure required to make this distinction. Once the nerves have been decompressed, neural regeneration will occur. To monitor this, the values of one-point moving touch must be measured because this will be the first threshold to improve, followed by one-point static touch, and then by moving two-point discrimination, and finally by improvement in static two-point discrimination (Dellon & Azman, unpublished observations, 1995).

FIGURE 14.11 (CONTINUED)

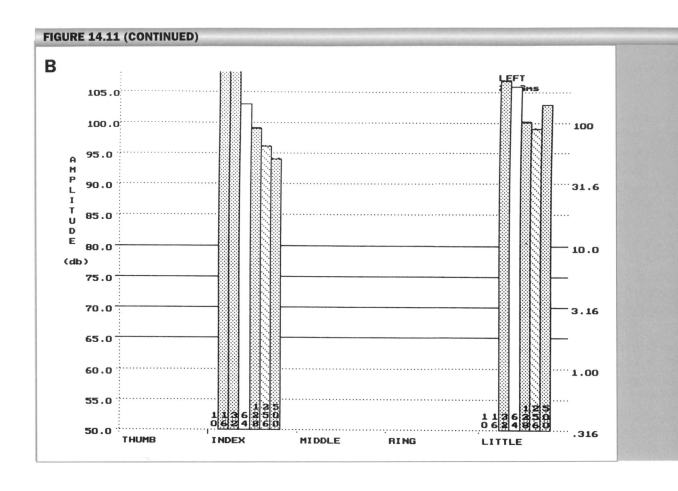

• LEAD POISONING •

The toxic effect of lead on the peripheral nerve was demonstrated more than 100 years ago in guinea pigs (Gombault, 1880). Chronic lead ingestion has been demonstrated experimentally to cause Schwann cell dysfunction consisting of segmental demyelination, and this evidence has been extensively reviewed (Windebank & Dyck, 1984). The clinically observed variability in electrophysiologic evaluation (Catton, Harrison, Fullerton, & Kazantzis, 1970) may be due to variability in the extent of this demyelination, and the degree to which axonal function is secondarily altered.

While this line of evidence would not be supportive of surgical intervention in lead neuropathy, the experimental models of chronic lead intoxication also demonstrate that lead induces a breakdown of the blood-nerve barrier (Ohnishi et al., 1977) (see Figure 14.1B). With the perineurial microvessels contributing to endoneurial edema, each fascicle of the peripheral nerve may increase to twice its normal area. It is possible that the presence of a swollen nerve in known areas of anatomic narrowing, such as the carpal and cubital tunnel, or the radial sensory nerve in the forearm, will decrease blood flow in the nerve sufficient to cause paresthesias. Over time, this increased pressure may result in chronic nerve compression leading to sensorimotor symptoms.

There are only rare reports of neuropathy due to lead poisoning (Loi, Battista, & Malentacchi, 1981; Antonini, Palmieri, Spagnoli, & Millefiorini, 1989). These patients' symptoms did improve with chelation therapy. The most recent extensive

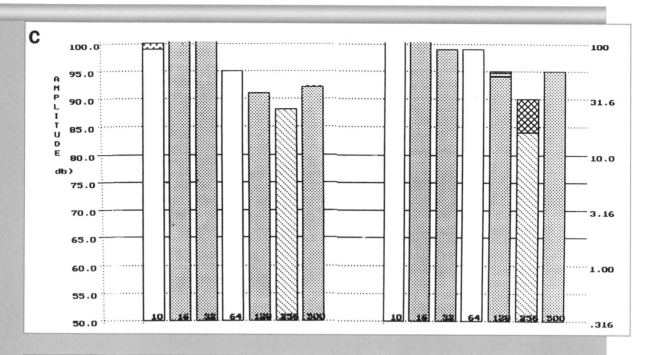

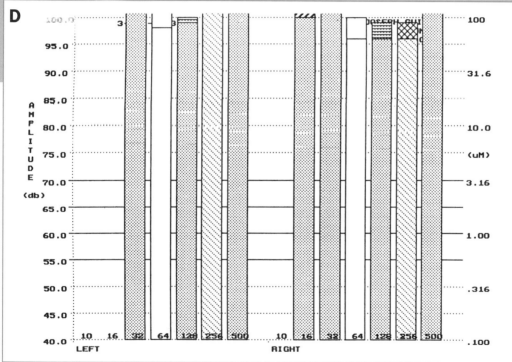

Neuropathy due to lead poisoning. In (C), note that the thresholds are higher for the lower frequencies. In (D), 11 months later, with progressive neuropathy, note that there is a loss of perception in the lower frequencies, while the threshold for perception of the higher frequencies is increased. From unpublished observations, A. L. Dellon, 1991-1993.

review of lead neuropathy (Windebank & Dyck, 1984) does not mention the possibility of surgical treatment. Recently, we have had the opportunity to extend the hypothesis applied to patients with symptoms of diabetic neuropathy to those with lead neuropathy, namely that the susceptibility to nerve compression induced by the metabolic neuropathy creates the situation in which the symptoms are generated by the nerve compression (Dellon & Keough, 1996).

These patients were a minimum of 2 years after lead exposure, with most of them being either 4 or 6 years after exposure. Each patient was symptomatic despite maximum chelation therapy, and in 3 patients the lead levels were at acceptable levels at the time of the surgical decompression. To date, 4 patients have had decompression of multiple peripheral nerves in each extremity, with 2 patients having completed the sequence of having all four extremities decompressed. The quantitative sensory testing done on these patients is given in Figures 14.11 and 14.12. These examples demonstrate the use of many different computer-assisted sensory testing devices, including the Neurometer™, the Force-Defined Vibrometer™, and the Pressure-Specified Sensory Device™.

This report documents the first patients to have improvement in sensorimotor upper extremity symptoms of lead neuropathy by surgical decompression of peripheral nerves. It is emphasized that each of these patients had a long therapeutic trial of chelation prior to surgical intervention. It is clear that the therapist will play a critical role in screening patients of lead poisoning for neuropathy, and in the documentation of the progression of that neuropathy during chelation or surgical therapy.

• LEPROSY •

Leprosy is a disease known and described since biblical times. In general, it remains misunderstood by the majority of people, and perhaps by medical personnel as well. For example, the loss of fingers and toes is not the inevitable result of leprosy. Rather, it is the result of improper care of the insensitive digits that results from the neuropathy associated with the disease. Leprosy is caused by a bacteria that is similar to the one that causes tuberculosis. Leprosy is, therefore, treatable by taking an antibiotic that can be administered orally. The bacteria prefer to live in an environment that is relatively cool; therefore, it infects the skin and the peripheral nerves. The most superficial peripheral nerves are the ones that are most affected, and these are the common peroneal nerve, the ulnar nerve, and the facial nerve.

Worldwide, leprosy is probably the commonest cause of facial paralysis. It is the anesthesia that attends the infection of the peripheral nerves that creates the possibility of soft tissue loss. Just as the diabetic will develop ulceration and soft tissue loss in the feet if proper attention is not given to hygiene and footwear, so too will the leper develop these problems. In ancient times, when the leper was isolated and impoverished, the rat-infested camps would provide the nighttime setting for these rodents to eat the anesthetic digits (van Brakel, 1994).

Today, programs to monitor lepers for peripheral nerve involvement provide the basis for identifying patients with neuropathy who might benefit from surgical intervention. Mapping of sensory defects in the leper is essential, since the bacteria may infect just a few fascicles with the peripheral nerve, giving a pattern of sensory loss that is not typical of any given peripheral nerve (Narita & Aoki, 1986; Birke & Sims, 1986) (see Figure 14.13). Sensory testing can include any measure of touch, such as vibration, Semmes-Weinstein nylon monofilaments, and two-point discrimination (see Figures 14.14 & 14.15). Because lepers often live in outlying vil-

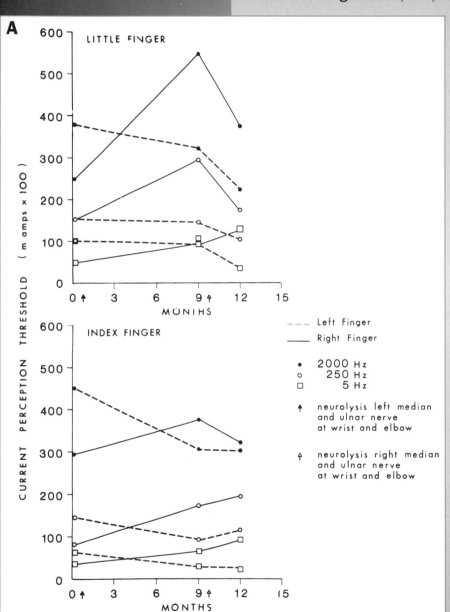

FIGURE 14.12

Neuropathy due to lead poisoning. (A) Measurement with the Neurometer™ (see Chapter 7 for further description of this instrument). This man is 7 years after exposure to lead from painting a bridge. The left and right hand are depicted in both the top and bottom panels in which the Neurometer™ was used to obtain the threshold for the perception of an electric current oscillating at 2000, 250, and 5 Hz. The perception of the 2000 Hz stimulus is believed to be due to the function of the large myelinated fibers, while the perception of the 5 Hz stimulus is believed to be due to the function of the unmyelinated fibers. Note that the left hand had a neurolysis of the median (index finger) and the ulnar (little finger) nerves at the beginning of the clinical study, and the patient's symptomatic improvement is reflected in the progressive decline in the thresholds for these fingers. In contrast, the untreated left hand has a slowly progressive neuropathy manifested by increasing thresholds, until about 9 months into the study, when the nerves in the right hand are decompressed. (B) and (C) Serial measurements of cutaneous pressure threshold made with the Pressure-Specified Sensory Device™ in a different man with lead neuropathy. In (B) note steady decrease in pressure thresholds (improvement in sensation) for both index fingers following bilateral carpal tunnel release. During this

B

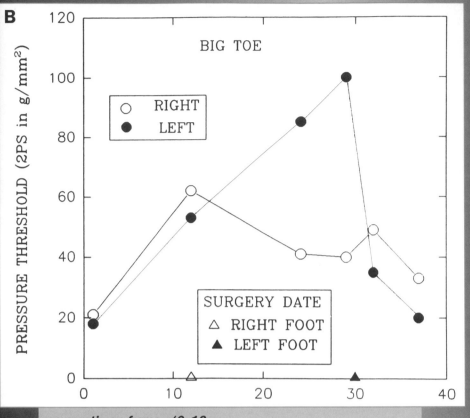

same time frame (0–10 months) the feet became worse as noted in (C). Note the progressive improvement in thresholds that correlated with clinical improvement in the right big toe (medial plantar nerve) following neurolysis of the posterior tibial nerve and its branches at the ankle on the right, while the unoperated left foot progressively got worse until it, too, had a tarsal tunnel decompression. From "Lead Neuropathy: Improvement in Symptoms by Decompression of Multiple Peripheral Nerves," by A. L. Dellon & J. Keough, unpublished observations.

C

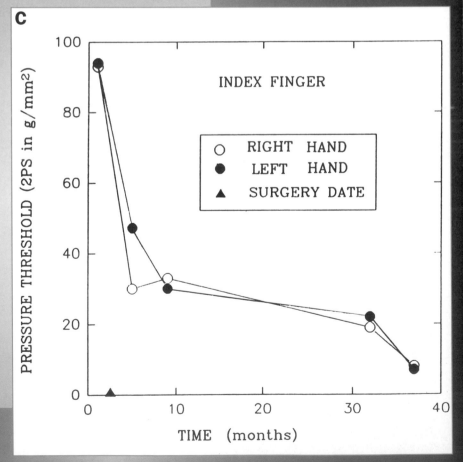

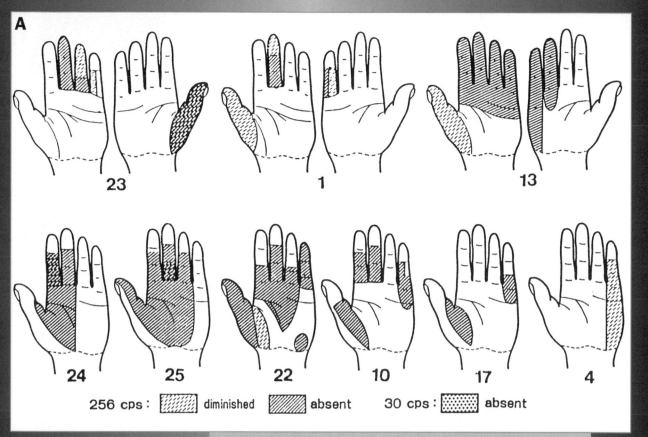

A

23   1   13

24   25   22   10   17   4

256 cps : ▨ diminished ▨ absent   30 cps : ▦ absent

FIGURE 14.13
Leprosy. Sensory testing demonstrating patterns of sensory loss that are most often not in the distribution of a complete peripheral nerve lesion. (A) Sensory testing with vibratory stimuli. (B) Sensory testing with the Semmes-Weinstein nylon monofilaments. The bold numbers beneath each hand refer to the patient number in the series of patients reported. Note that while patients 4 and 13 in (A), and 21, 14, and 2 in (B) may be considered to have sensory loss in the distribution of the ulnar nerve, and that patients 13, 24, 25, and 10 in (A), and 21 and 14 in (B) may be considered to have sensory loss in the distribution of the median nerve, patients 23, 1, 10, and 17 in (A), and 8 and 7 in (B) do not fit into any classic peripheral nerve territory. Even the patients whose pattern fits the median or ulnar nerves have distal phalangeal regions that appear to have been "skipped." This pattern is clearly that of a distal axonopathy, like diabetes, in which the involvement is always worse distally, and is not the classic appearance of chronic nerve compression, in which the sensory loss is usually uniform throughout the distribution of the nerve, and also includes the distal fingertips. This involvement demonstrates the invasion of individual nerve fascicles by the leprosy bacteria. From "Clinical Study on Sensibility Disturbance of the Hand in Leprosy," by M. Narita & M. Aoki, 1986, Japanese Journal of Leprosy 55:1-12. Reprinted with permission of the authors. (See also Figure 14.13 (B) on following page.

B

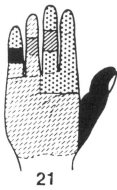

21

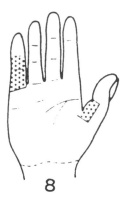

8

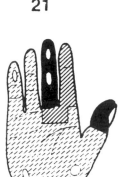

14

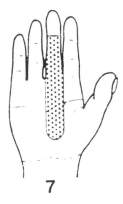

7

Semmes-Weinstein monofilament

□	3.22~3.61
▓	3.84~4.31
▨	4.56~6.45
▨	6.65
■	over 6.65

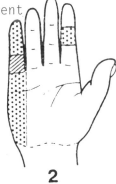

2

FIGURE 14.14

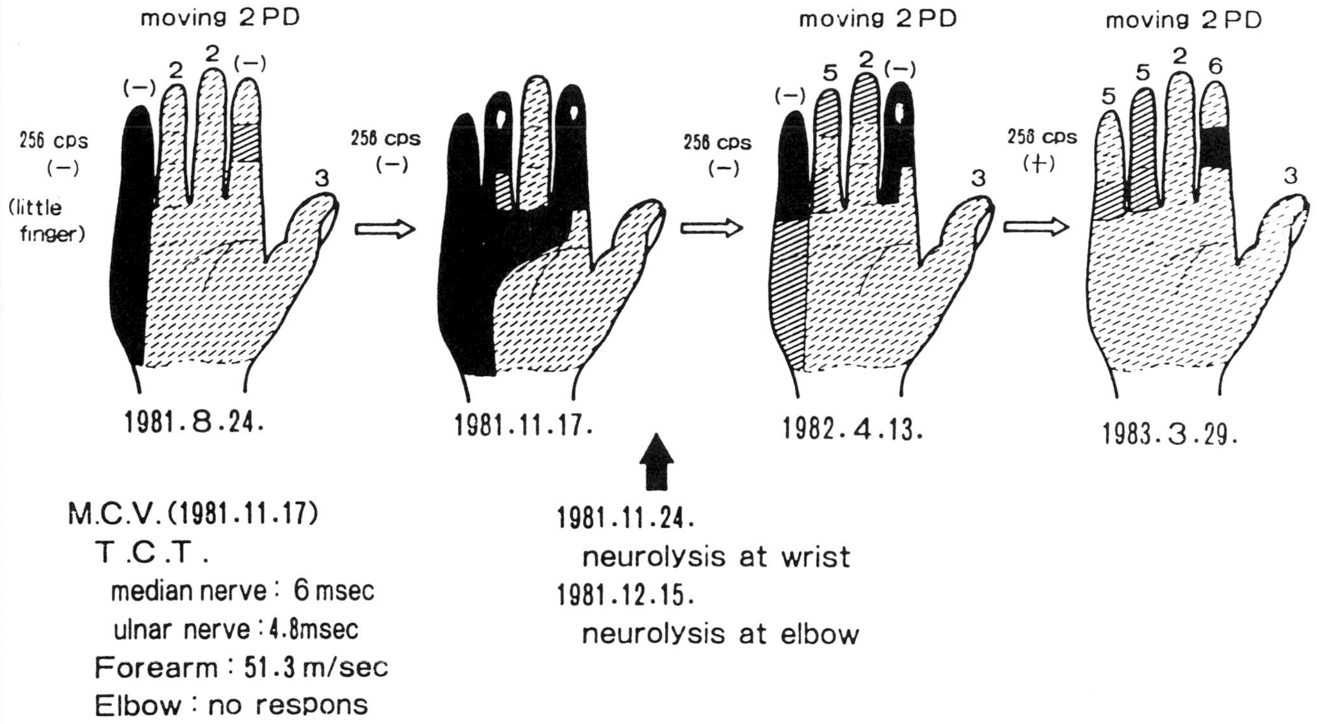

moving 2 PD

256 cps
(−)
(little finger)

(−) 2 2 (−)
3

1981.8.24.

M.C.V.(1981.11.17)
T.C.T.
  median nerve : 6 msec
  ulnar nerve :4.8msec
Forearm : 51.3 m/sec
Elbow : no respons

moving 2 PD

256 cps
(−)

1981.11.17.

1981.11.24.
  neurolysis at wrist
1981.12.15.
  neurolysis at elbow

moving 2 PD

256 cps
(−)

(−) 5 2 (−)
3

1982.4.13.

moving 2 PD

256 cps
(+)

5 5 2 6
3

1983.3.29.

Leprosy. Documentation of sensory recovery following neurolysis of peripheral nerves. Two separate evaluations of sensibilities were done prior to surgery, and these documented progressive loss of moving two-point discrimination (the "(-)" indicates no two-point discrimination is present, while the numbers 2 through 6 indicate distance in millimeters at which one point can be distinguished from two. In this author's grading system, a 6 indicates normal sensibility, and a zero or no score indicates absence of sensibility). The sensory abnormalities implicate both the median and ulnar nerves, and a separate neurolysis was done of each nerve at the wrist and elbow level. By 15 months following surgery, two-point discrimination had improved in all fingers except the thumb. Refer to the legend in the photograph of Figure 14.14 for the definition of the shaded areas, tested by Semmes-Weinstein nylon monofilaments. Neurolysis resulted in a lowering of pressure thresholds throughout the surface of the hand. Vibratory perception to the 256 Hz stimuli was absent preoperatively, and was recovered by the time of the last sensibility testing. From "Clinical Study on Sensibility Disturbance of the Hand in Leprosy," by M. Narita & M. Aoki, 1986, Japanese Journal of Leprosy 55:1-12. Reprinted with permission of the authors.

lages, these simple testing tools have been used to practical advantage (see Table 14.3).

Once an appropriate period of medical treatment has been instituted, if the infection still results in increased pressure within the peripheral nerve, especially in anatomic areas of known tightness, such as the cubital tunnel and the fibular head, then surgical decompression, or decompression plus internal neurolysis, may be effective in relieving symptoms and in recovery of function (Enna, 1974; Pandya, 1976; Chaise & Roger, 1985). If abscess formation has occurred with destruction of neural tissue, interposition nerve grafting has been found to be useful (McLeod, Hargrave, Gye, & Sedal, 1975). During surgical exploration of the peripheral nerves, sites of infection outside the known areas of compression may exist, and recent use of intraoperative spinal root stimulation may prove of value in locating these regions, so they may be adequately treated as well (Turkof, Tambwekar, Mansukhani, Millesi, & Mayr, 1994).

The role of the therapist in the treatment of leprosy must be defined to include evaluation sensibility in addition to the splinting of contractures that result from the motor paralysis, and therapy directed at the use of tendon transfers. The computer-assisted sensorimotor testing devices will be of benefit in this regard. One-point static testing can replace the Semmes-Weinstein monofilaments as a reliable measurement of sites over the skin surface that can screen for fascicular involvement of the leprosy bacillus. Battery-powered laptop computer models will permit the introduction of this equipment into the remotest villages.

FIGURE 14. 15

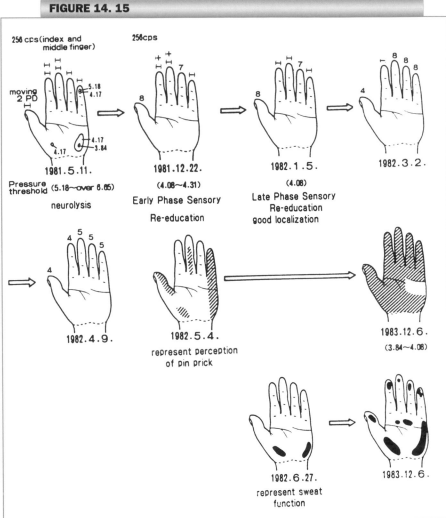

Leprosy: Documentation of sensory recovery following neurolysis of peripheral nerves. Detailed sensibility evaluation on the day of surgery demonstrated absent two-point discrimination, absent vibratory perception to the 256 Hz stimuli, and abnormal Semmes-Weinstein pressure threshold measurements. Postoperatively, this patient received sensory reeducation. By 7 months after surgery vibratory perception had recovered, and the thumb and ring finger had recovered moving two-point discrimination. By 10 months after surgery, moving two-point discrimination had recovered in all fingers except the index finger, and continued to improve thereafter. Perception of pain by pinprick also returned, as did sweating. This time frame for recovery fits with neural regeneration, rather than with recovery from a neuropraxia. From "Clinical Study on Sensibility Disturbance of the Hand in Leprosy," by M. Narita & M. Aoki, 1986, Japanese Journal of Leprosy 55:1-12. Reprinted with permission of the authors.

TABLE 14.3 TOUCH THRESHOLDS IN HEALTHY NEPAL VOLUNTEERS

	Semmes-Weinstein Nylon Monofilaments	
	Confidence Limit	
	95%	99%
Index finger	70 mg	200 mg
Thumb	70 mg	200 mg
Little finger	70 mg	200 mg
Metacarpal phalangeal	70 mg	200 mg
Hypothenar	70 mg	200 mg
Big toe		2000 mg
Metatarsal head 1		2000 mg
Metatarsal head 5		2000 mg
Heel		2000 mg

	Moving Two-point Discrimination (Disk-Criminator™)	
	Confidence Limit	
	95%	99%
Index finger	3 mm	4 mm
Little finger	3 mm	4 mm
Big toe	6 mm	8 mm
Heel	6 mm	8 mm

Note: From "Evaluation of Sensibility in Leprosy—Comparison of Various Clinical Methods," by W. H. van Brakel, J. Shute, J. A. Dixon, & H. Arzet, *Leprosy Review,* in press: 1995.

• CHEMOTHERAPY •

The side effects of *chemotherapy* are generally well known, such as hair loss, nausea and vomiting, and decrease in the bone marrow-derived white blood cells and platelets. These side effects are generally accepted in order to treat cancer. Less known is the side affect related to the peripheral nerves, a sensory neuropathy. Unfortunately, while the other side effects resolve in time, the sensory neuropathy usually persists. In the patient cured of cancer, or in the patient in remission, the sensory neuropathy can be signifi-cantly disabling.

The first class of drugs to have a sensory neuropathy associated with their use was the vinca alkaloids, including vincristine and vinblastine (Gottschalk, Dyck, Kiely, & Vinca, 1968). These drugs are still in use today, primarily for the treatment of

Hodgkin's disease and other types of lymphomas. The next class of drugs to cause a sensory neuropathy and to enter widespread use was the group containing the metal platinum, including cisplatinum and carboplatin. These platinum-containing drugs are used to treat ovarian and testicular cancer, and metastatic cancer to the head and neck area (Mollman, 1990). The newest chemotherapy drug causing a sensory neuropathy is taxol, a drug derived from a fungus that was found growing on the leaves of the Pacific Yew tree (Rowinsky & Donehower, 1995). This drug can now be synthesized artificially and was released in 1994 for general use in the United States. It is effective against many types of cancer, including breast cancer. Each of these drugs produces a dose-dependent and dose-limiting peripheral neuropathy in cancer patients.

The clinical problem related to the sensory neuropathy induced by cisplatin has been the most well described (Roelofs, Hrushessky, & Roghn, 1984; Thompson, Davis, & Kornfeld, 1984; Riggs, Ashraf, Snyder, & Gutmann, 1988; Siegal & Haim, 1990). Cisplatin, like vincristine and taxol, affects the protein tubulin, which is essential in the formation of the microtubules. The microtubules, in the axoplasm of the peripheral nerve, are required for the slow compo-

nent of axoplasmic transport, the system that delivers the protein building blocks necessary to repair the membrane of the axon. Since the early 1980s, a dose-dependent peripheral neuropathy has been recognized as a major dose-limiting toxicity of cisplatin chemotherapy. This neuropathy is primarily sensory and is almost universal in patients receiving more than 300 mg/m^2 of cisplatin. Signs and symptoms of this clinical disorder worsen with increasing doses of cisplatin and, in perhaps one-third of patients, tend to gradually resolve when this chemotherapy is discontinued. The pathogenesis of the neuropathy is incompletely understood. The only accepted treatment for this uncomfortable and disabling toxicity is to discontinue the cisplatin and wait for the symptoms to resolve.

A peripheral neuropathy can be induced in rats treated with cisplatin. This has been quantified using nerve conduction testing to demonstrate impaired function of the sciatic nerve in the thigh following cisplatin chemotherapy. This animal model has been used to study compounds designed to reduce the neurotoxicity of cisplatin. The potential utility of decompressive surgery in cisplatin neuropathy has not been studied in patients, but has been studied recently in the rat model

(Tassler, Dellon, Lesser, & Grossman, 1996).

In the rat model, the study was designed to test the hypothesis that the neuropathy results from the repetitive mechanical compression of the peripheral nerve rendered susceptible to injury because of cisplatin-induced microtubular dysfunction. Tarsal tunnel decompression was performed prior to cisplatin treatment, at the conclusion of cisplatin treatment, and 6 weeks after completion of cisplatin treatment. A neuropathic walking track pattern, characterized by an increase in print length, developed in treated animals after 8 weeks of cisplatin. The neuropathy progressed for 6 weeks after cisplatin was stopped and then reversed slowly over the next 3 months. The neuropathy was completely prevented by early tarsal tunnel decompression. The neuropathy was reversed by decompression of the tarsal tunnel at the completion of therapy, but did not alter the natural history of the neuropathy once the neuropathy was well established.

This model provides insight into the etiology and possible therapeutic approaches to cisplatin neuropathy. The results support the hypothesis that microtubular dysfunction induced by cisplatin renders peripheral nerves susceptible to compression injury in areas of anatomic tightness. This

FIGURE 14.16

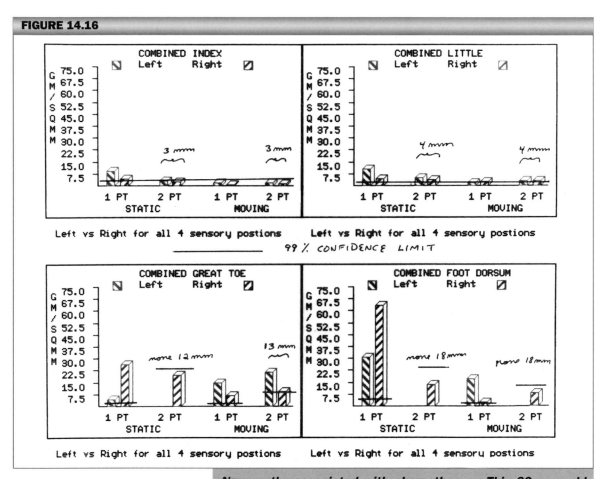

Neuropathy associated with chemotherapy. This 60- year-old woman is 10 years after chemotherapy for the treatment of cancer. Cisplatin was included in the chemotherapy regimen. She has complaints of paresthesias in the fingers, and when directly questioned admits that the toes have numbness as well. The quantitative sensory testing with the Pressure-Specified Sensory Device™ demonstrates that the thresholds in the upper extremity are above borderline for the little finger, and approaching the 99% confidence level for normal for the index finger, while at the same time there is axonal loss in the lower extremity nerves in addition to the abnormally high cutaneous pressure thresholds. This is consistent with a distal axonopathy related to the chemotherapy. A. L. Dellon, unpublished observations.

data also suggests that patients with preexisting compression of peripheral nerves, such as carpal tunnel syndrome, may be at high risk to develop severe peripheral neuropathies without a decompressive procedure.

It is likely that therapists will be asked to quantitate the degree of neuropathy, and follow patients with sequential monitoring during chemotherapy (see Figure 14.16). It is possible that the mechanism by which the chemotherapeutic agent induces the symptoms of the neuropathy is related to the double crush hypothesis. If this is true, then relief of these symptoms by decompression of peripheral nerves may be possible. In the future, therefore, thera-pists will become involved in all aspects of this relatively underappreciated clinical problem.

• • •

• REFERENCES •

Antonini, G., Palmieri, G., Spagnoli, L. G., & Millefiorini, M. Lead brachial neuropathy in heroin addiction: A case report. *Clinical Neurology and Neurosurgery 91*:167-170, 1989.

Arezzo, J. C., Bolton, C. F., Boulton, A., & Dyck, P. J. Quantitative sensory testing: A consensus report from the Peripheral Neuropathy Association. *Neurology 43*:1050-1052, 1993.

Asbury A. K., & Porte D., Jr. Diabetic neuropathy: Consensus statement. *Diabetes 37*:1000-1010, 1988.

Birke, J. A., & Sims, D. S. Plantar sensory threshold in the ulcerative foot. *Leprosy Review 57*:261-267, 1986.

Boulton A. J. M., Kubrusly, D. B., & Bowker, J. G. Impaired vibratory perception and diabetic foot ulceration. *Diabetes Medicine 3*:192, 1986.

Catton, M. J., Harrison, M. J. G., Fullerton, P. M., & Kazantzis, G. Subclinical neuropathy in lead workers. *British Medical Journal 2*:80-82, 1970.

Chaise, F., & Roger, B. Neurolysis of the common peroneal nerve in leprosy. *Journal of Bone and Joint Surgery 67B*:426-429, 1985.

Clark, C. M., Jr., & Lee, A. Prevention and treatment of the complications of diabetes mellitus. *New England Journal of Medicine 332*:1210-1217, 1995.

Dellon, A. L. A cause for optimism in diabetic neuropathy. *Annals of Plastic Surgery 20*:103-105, 1988.

Dellon, A. L. Treatment of symptoms of diabetic neuropathy by peripheral nerve decompression. *Plastic and Reconstructive Surgery 89*:689-697, 1992.

Dellon, A. L., Dellon, E. S., & Seiler, W. A., IV. The effect of tarsal tunnel decompression in the streptozotocin-induced diabetic rat. *Microsurgery 15*:265-268, 1994.

Dellon, A. L., & Keough, J. Lead neuropathy: Improvement in symptoms by decompression of multiple peripheral nerves. *Journal of Hand Surgery,* submitted: 1997.

Dellon, A. L., Mackinnon, S. E., & Seiler, W. A., IV. Susceptibility of the diabetic nerve to chronic compression. *Annals of Plastic Surgery 20*:117-119, 1988.

Dyck, P. J., Thomas, P. K., Asbury, A. K., Winegrad, A. I., & Porte, D. J., Jr. *Diabetic Neuropathy.* Philadelphia: W. B. Saunders Company, 1987.

Dyck, P. J., Thomas, P. K., Lambert, E. H., & Bunge, R., Editors, *Peripheral Neuropathy,* 2nd edition. Philadelphia: W. B. Saunders Company, 1984.

Enna, C. D. Neurolysis and transposition of the ulnar nerve in leprosy. *Journal of Neurosurgery 40:*734-737, 1974.

Gilmore, J. E., Allen J. A., & Hayes, J. R. Autonomic function in neuropathic diabetic patients with foot ulceration. *Diabetes Care 16*:61, 1993.

Gombault, A. Contribution á l'étude anatomique de la névrite parenchymateuse subaigue et chronique-névrite segmentaire peri-axile. *Archives of Neurology (Paris) 1*:11, 1880.

Gottschalk, P. G., Dyck, P. J., & Kiely, J. M. Vinca alkaloid neuropathy: Nerve biopsy studies in rats and in man. *Neurology 18*:875-882, 1968.

Holewski, J. Aesthesiometry: Quantification of cutaneous pressure sensation in diabetic peripheral neuropathy. *Journal of Rehabilitation Research and Development 25*:1, 1988.

Jakobsen, J. Peripheral nerves in early experimental diabetes: Expansion of the endoneurial space as a cause of increased water content. *Diabetologia 14*:113-119, 1978.

Jakobsen, J., & Sidenius, P. Decrease in axonal transport of structural proteins in streptozotocin diabetic rats. *Journal of Clinical Investigation 66*:292-296, 1980.

Loi, F., Battista, G., & Malentacchi, G. M. Familial lead poisoning from contaminated wine. *Italian Journal of Neurological Sciences 3*:283-290, 1981.

Mackinnon, S. E., & Dellon, A. L. *Surgery of the Peripheral Nerve.* New York: Thieme, 1988.

McLeod, J. G., Hargrave, J. C., Gye, R. S., & Sedal, L. Nerve grafting in leprosy. *Brain* 98:203-212, 1975.

Mollman, J. E. Cisplatin neurotoxicity. *New England Journal of Medicine 322*:126-127, 1990.

Narita, M., & Aoki, M. Clinical study on sensibility disturbance of the hand in leprosy. *Japanese Journal of Leprosy 55*:1-12, 1986.

Ohnishi, A., Schilling, K., Brimijoin, W. S., Lambert, E. H., Fairbanks, V. F., & Dyck, P. J. Lead neuropathy. 1. Morphometry, nerve conduction and choline acetyltransferase transport: New finding of endoneurial edema associated with segmental demyelination. *Journal of Neuropathology and Experimental Neurology 36*:499, 1977.

Pandya, J. N. Surgical decompression of nerves in leprosy. An attempt at prevention of deformity: A clinical, electrophysiologic, histopathologic and surgical study. *International Journal of Leprosy 46*:47-55, 1976.

Riggs, J. E., Ashraf, M., Snyder, R. D., & Gutmann, L. Prospective nerve conduction studies in cisplatin therapy. *Annals of Neurology 23*:92-94, 1988.

Roelofs, R. I., Hrushessky, W., & Roghn, J. Peripheral sensory neuropathy and cisplatin chemotherapy. *Neurology 34*:934-938, 1984.

Rowinsky, E. K., & Donnehower, E. C. Paclitaxel (Taxol). *New England Journal of Medicine 332*:1004-1014, 1995.

Seiler, W. A., Schlegel, R., Mackinnon, S. E., & Dellon, A. L. The double crush syndrome: Development of a model. *Surgical Forum 34*:596-598, 1983.

Siegal, T., & Haim, N. Cisplatin-Induced Peripheral Neuropathy. *Cancer 66*:1117-1123, 1990.

Siitonen, O. I., Niskanen L. K., & Laakso, M. Lower extremity amputations in diabetic and nondiabetic patients. *Diabetes Care 16*:16, 1993.

Sosenko, J. M., Kato, M., & Soto, R. Comparison of quantitative sensory threshold measures for their association with foot ulceration in diabetic patients. *Diabetes Care 13*:1057, 1990.

Tassler, P. L., & Dellon, A. L. Quantitative sensory testing: Normative data in the lower extremity. *Muscle and Nerve 19*:285-289, 1996.

Tassler, P. L., Dellon, A. L., Lesser, G., & Grossman, S. Cisplatin neuropathy: Prevention and treatment of neuropathy by tarsal tunnel decompression in the rat model. *Journal of Neurosurgery*, submitted: 1996.

Tassler, P. L., Dellon, A. L., & Scheffler, N. M. Cutaneous pressure threshold in diabetics with and without foot ulceration: Evaluation of sensibility with the Pressure-Specified Sensory Device. *Journal of the American Podiatric Medical Association 85:* 679-684 ,1995.

Thompson, S. W., Davis, L. E., & Kornfeld, M. Cisplatin neuropathy, clinical, electrophysiologic, morphologic, and toxicologic studies. *Cancer 54*:1269-1275, 1984.

Turkof, E., Tambwekar, S., Mansukhani, K., Millesi, H., & Mayr, N. Intraoperative spinal root stimulation to detect most proximal site of leprous ulnar neuritis. *Lancet 343*:1604-1605, 1994.

Upton, A. R. M., & McComas, A. J. The double crush in nerve entrapment syndromes. *Lancet 2*:359-362, 1973.

van Brakel, W. H. Peripheral neuropathy in leprosy: The continuing challenge. *CIP-Gegevens Koninklijke Bibliotheek*. The Hague, The Netherlands, 1994.

van Brakel, W. H., Shute, J., Dixon, J. A., & Arzet, H. Evaluation of sensibility in leprosy—Comparison of various clinical methods. *Leprosy Review*, in press: 1995.

Windebank, A. J., & Dyck, P. J. Lead intoxication as a model of primary segmental demyelination. In *Peripheral Neuropathy*, Second Edition, P. J. Dyck, P. K. Thomas, E. H. Lambert, & E. Bunge, Editors. Philadelphia: W. B. Saunders Company, 1984.

• ADDITIONAL READINGS •

Dellon, A. L. Computer-assisted sensibility evaluation and surgical treatment of tarsal tunnel syndrome. *Adv. Podiatry 2:* 17-40. 1996.

Lampert, P. W., & Schochet, S. S., Jr. Demyelination and remyelination in lead neuropathy. *Journal of Neuropathology and Experimental Neurology 27*:527, 1968.

Schoumburg, H. H., Spencer, P. S., & Thomas, P. K. Toxic neuropathy: Occupational biological and environmental agents. *In Disorders of Peripheral Nerves*, H. H. Schoumburg, P. S. Spencer, & P. K. Thomas, Editors. Philadelphia: F. A. Davis Company, 1983.

Sunderland, S. The internal anatomy of nerve trunks in relation to the neuronal lesions of leprosy—Observations on pathology, symptomatology and treatment. *Brain 96*:865-868, 1973.

• • •

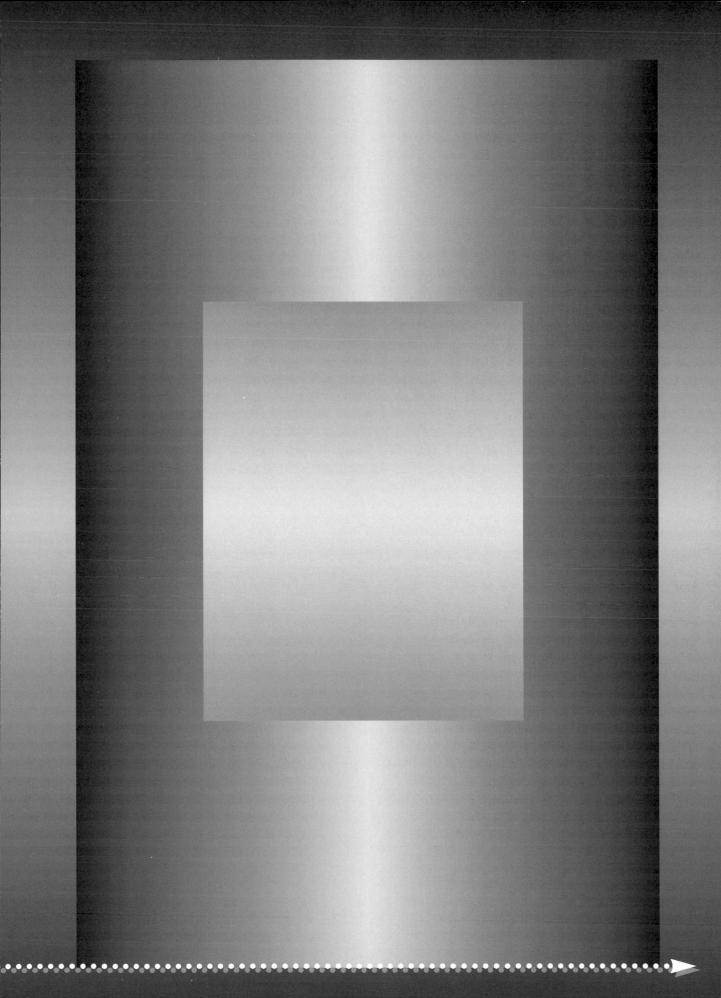

the head & neck

• • •

The nervous system, hitherto the most unsatisfactory part of a physiologist's studies, has assumed a new character. The intricacies of that system have been unravelled, and the peculiar structure and functions of the individual nerves ascertained; so that the absolute confusion in which this department was involved has disappeared, and the natural and single order discovered.

Sir Charles Bell, lecture to the Royal Society of London, July 12, 1821

• • •

• RELEVANT NEUROANATOMY •

Sir Charles Bell began to understand the complicated neuroanatomy of the head and neck region through his experiments. He divided the nerve in front of the ear of an awake donkey and noted that, thereafter, the nostrils no longer flared, and the lips no longer moved on that side, whereas when he cut the nerve beneath the lower eyelid on the opposite side of the face, the donkey gave a great bellow of pain and the face contin-

ued to move.
He thus established that the
trigeminal
nerve (the
fifth cranial
nerve) was responsible for
sensation of
the face, while
the facial
nerve (the seventh cranial
nerve) was responsible for
movement.

The *trigeminal nerve* has
three separate
divisions that
are responsible for areas
of facial sensibility. The *ophthalmic division*
innervates the
cornea
through one
set of branches within the orbit, and then
innervates the forehead
through the supratrochlear
nerves, and the upper eyelid
and portions of the nose
through its infratraochlear
nerves. The *maxillary division*
innervates the cheek, lower
eyelid, and side of the nose
and upper lip through its infraorbital branch. The
mandibular division innervates the upper and lower
teeth through its alveolar
nerves, and then the inferior
alveolar nerve continues distally to innervate the chin
and the lower lip through its
terminal branch, mental

FIGURE 15.1

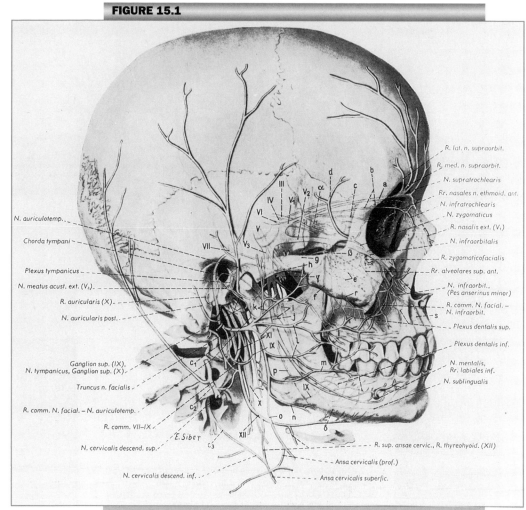

Sensory innervation of the face. From **Pernkopf's Atlas of Topographical and Applied Human Anatomy,** *Philadelphia:* **W.B. Saunders Company, 1963. Reprinted with permission of the publisher.**

nerve. The neck, scalp, and
ear are innervated through
the cervical plexus, C1-4.
The ear is innervated
through the cervical plexus
by its greater auricular
branch, as well as some by
innervation in the concha
from small branches of cranial nerves 9 and 10 (see
Figure 15.1).

The oral cavity is inner-

vated by the branches of cranial nerves nine, the *glossopharyngeal*, and 10, the *vagus*. Furthermore, the
tongue is innervated by special sensory nerves for taste,
which originate from cranial
nerves (see Figure 15.2). The
tongue is innervated by cranial nerve 12, the *hypoglossal*,
which is the motor nerve to
the tongue. The lingual

FIGURE 15.2

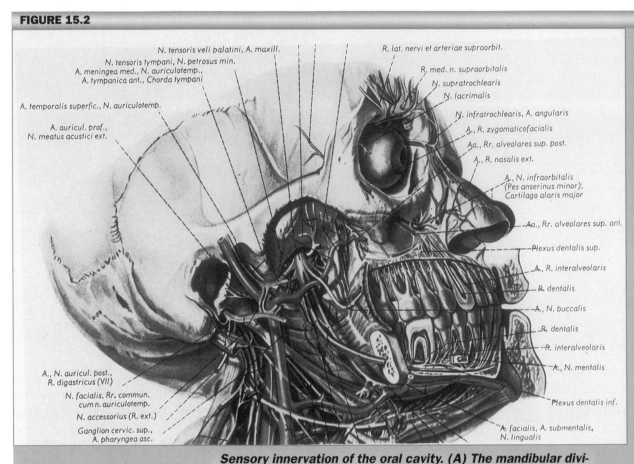

Sensory innervation of the oral cavity. (A) The mandibular division of the trigeminal nerve exits the base of the skull to give rise to the inferior alveolar nerve, which enters the mandible to innervate the teeth. In this location it is near the roots of the molars. It will terminate in the mental nerve, innervating the lip. (B) The other branch of the mandibular division, the lingual nerve, enters the oral cavity to innervate the anterior two-thirds of the tongue, and the floor of the mouth. From Pernkopf's Atlas of Topographical and Applied Human Anatomy, Philadelphia: W.B. Saunders Company, 1963. Reprinted with permission of the publisher.

nerve carries primarily taste fibers to the anterior two-thirds of the tongue, while the glossopharyngeal nerve supplies the taste fibers to the posterior one-third of the tongue, where the *circumvallate papillae* are located. These nerves have been well understood for more than a century and formed the basis of many early investigations into neural regeneration. For example, the glossopharyngeal nerve of the frog was used to demonstrate the effect of nerve transection on the distal nerve (see Chapter 1), and Vulpian used these nerves for the first nerve graft experiments (Dellon & Dellon, 1993).

The myelinated nerve fiber population of the branches of the trigeminal nerve have been counted and the results are given in Table 15.1, with the nerve fiber histogram given in Figure 15.3. The sensory receptors of the human face are primarily free nerve endings and innervated hair follicles.

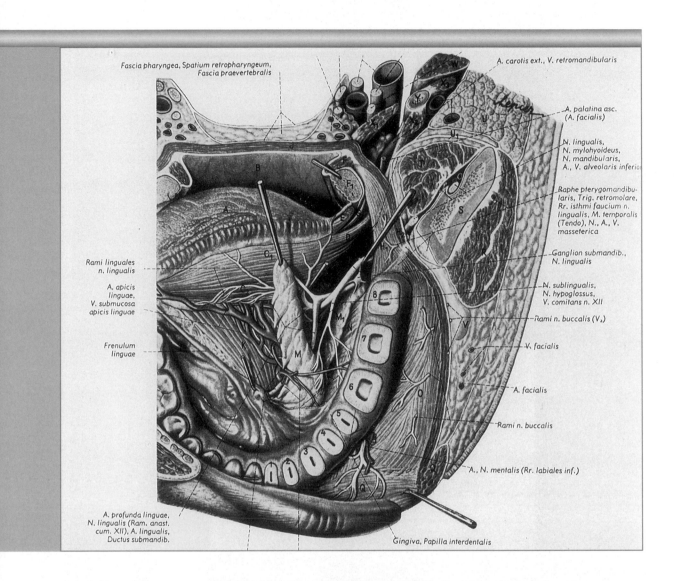

Fascia pharyngea, Spatium retropharyngeum,
Fascia praevertebralis

A. carotis ext., V. retromandibularis

A. palatina asc.
(A. facialis)

N. lingualis,
N. mylohyoideus,
N. mandibularis,
A., V. alveolaris inferior

Raphe pterygomandibu-
laris, Trig. retromolare,
Rr. isthmi faucium n.
lingualis, M. temporalis
(Tendo), N., A., V.
masseterica

Ganglion submandib.,
N. lingualis

N. sublingualis,
N. hypoglossus,
V. comitans n. XII

Rami n. buccalis (V₃)

V. facialis

A. facialis

Rami n. buccalis

A., N. mentalis (Rr. labiales inf.)

Gingiva, Papilla interdentalis

Rami linguales
n. lingualis

A. apicis
linguae,
V. submucosa
apicis linguae

Frenulum
linguae

A. profunda linguae,
N. lingualis (Ram. anast.
cum. XII), A. lingualis,
Ductus submandib.

TABLE 15.1 HISTOMORPHOMETRY OF THE TRIGEMINAL NERVE

Division of Trigeminal Nerve	Total Area (mm^2)	Number of Fascicles	Number of Fibers	Fiber Density (n/mm^2)
Ophthalmic	2.2	29	26,000	11,700
Maxillary	4.2	27	50,000	11,800
Mandibular	8.0	22	78,000	12,300

Note: Adapted from "Histometric Study of Myelinated Fibers in the Human Trigeminal Nerve," by E. Pennisi, G. Cruccu, M. Manfredi, & G. Palladini, 1991. *Journal of Neurological Science 105*:22-28. Reprinted with permission of the authors and with kind permission of Elsevier Science-NL.

FIGURE 15.3

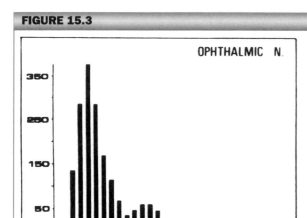

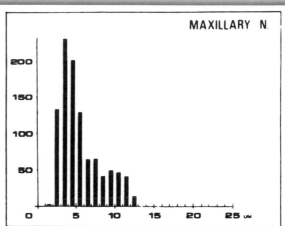

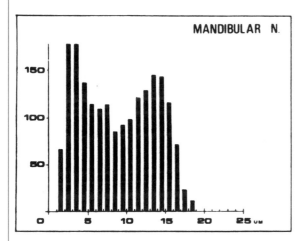

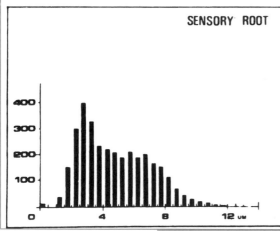

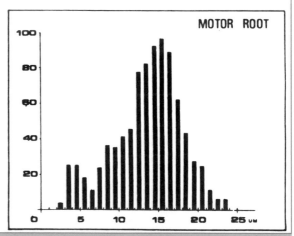

Histogram of external diameter of myelinated nerve fibers of the divisions of the trigeminal nerve from one human specimen. From "Histometric Study of Myelinated Fibers in the Human Trigeminal Nerve," by E. Pennisi, G. Cruccu, M. Manfredi, & G. Palladini, 1991, Journal of Neurological Sciences 105:22-28. Reprinted with permission of the authors and with the kind permission of Elsevier Science-NL.

FIGURE 15.4

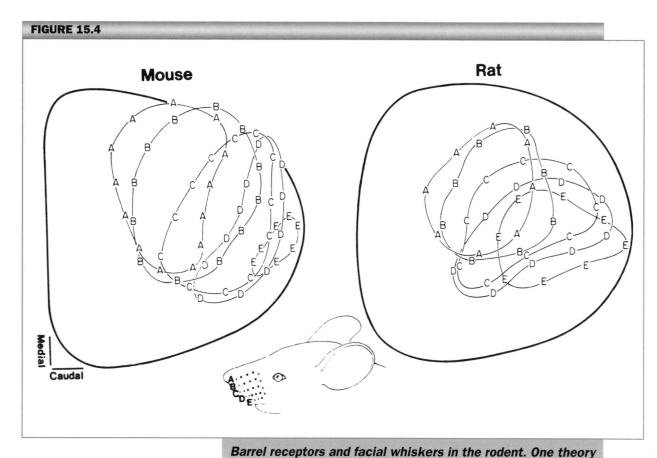

Mouse **Rat**

Medial

Caudal

Barrel receptors and facial whiskers in the rodent. One theory holds that during evolution whiskers became useful for transmitting information about the environment. This information was sensory, such as touch, but also could be used for defense or for withdrawing from the environment. Therefore, information regarding pain and temperature was important. Loss of whiskers results in disadvantages to the rodent in fighting and swimming, and in loss of attentive and orienting behavior. The sensory receptors around the base of the facial hair (vibrissae or whiskers) are linked in spatial orientation and overlapping with visual receptor fields in the brain's superior colliculus. A through E (from dorsal to ventral), are represented (from medial to lateral) primarily in the rostral-lateral quadrant of the superior colliculus. From Barry E. Stein & M. Alex Meredith, The Merging of the Senses, Cambridge, MA: The MIT Press, 1993.

In animals with whiskers, such as the rat and cat, there is an extensive innervation that links the follicles of the whiskers with the sensory cortex. The cortical receptors are called *barrel receptors*, and because of their unique topographical arrangement they have permitted much detailed research into the function of these facial hairs (see Figure 15.4). These receptors are no different from those described in Chapter 2 for the hairy skin of the hand. The innervation of the oral mucosa is again similar to the skin, but is devoid of the Pacinian corpuscle and the Merkel cell neurite complex. The mucosa contains nerve networks and free intraepithelial nerve endings, as well as the mucocutaneous end-organ, best thought of as the Meissner corpuscle of this specialized surface covering (see Figure 15.5).

FIGURE 15.5

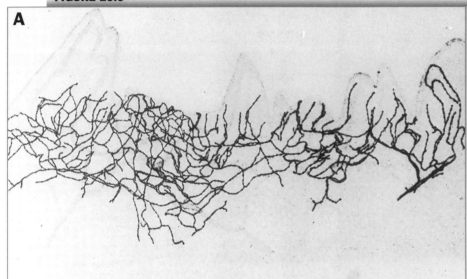

A

Sensory receptors of the oral cavity. (A) A network of nonmyelinated nerve fibers in the subpapillary layer of the inner lip mucosa. (B) Intraepithelial fiber transition zone of lip, 350x. (C) Two glomerular terminations, mucocutaneous end-organs, arising from a thick stem myelinated nerve fiber in the transition zone of the lip, 350x. (D) Fine nonmyelinated mass of a mucocutaneous end-organ near the epithelium of the lip, 230 x. From Symposium on Oral Perception and Sensation, *by J. Bosma, 1967, Springfield, IL: Charles C. Thomas, Publisher. Reprinted with permission of the author.*

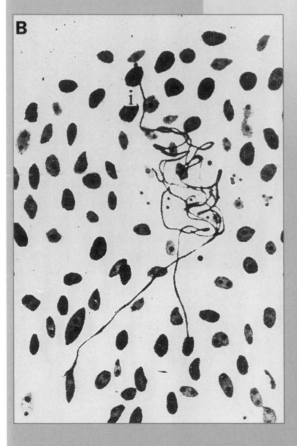

B

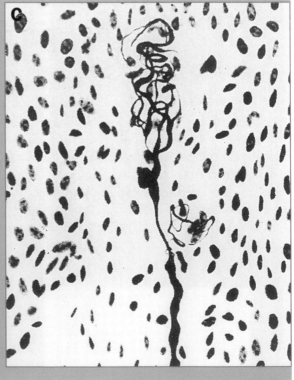

C

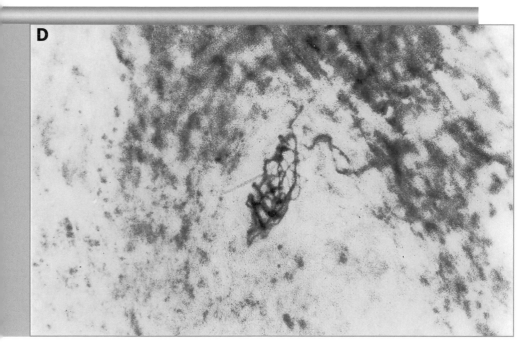

D

NORMAL HEAD AND NECK SENSIBILITY

The measurement of sensibility of the head and neck region has gone relatively neglected compared to that of the hand. However, as has been reviewed by Dellon (1981), it has been recognized from the earliest measurements of Weber (1835) and von Fry (1908) that the lip and tongue possess an ability to discriminate that is at least comparable to that of the fingertips. Penfield's "homunculus," the little figure of a man laid out on the somatosensory cortex (see Figure 10.1), has a surface area of the brain devoted to the tongue that is probably larger relative to its actual anatomical size than does the hand. The ability of the tongue to give information that permits magnitude judgements for vibratory stimulation has been compared to the hand (thenar eminence) (Fucci, Harrison, & Petrosino, 1984).

That study, using a 250 Hz stimulus with magnitudes ranging from 2 to 40 decibels, demonstrated that the tongue and the thenar eminence have a very similar ability to provide information related to vibratory stimuli. So it is clear that the ability of certain regions of the head and neck to perceive sensation other than sight, smell, and taste received early attention. It is appropriate, then, that as measurement devices passed beyond those used in the 1960s to give information about oral stereognosis (identification of shapes placed within the oral cavity; see Figure 15.6), atten-

tion has been directed to the cutaneous nerves of the head and neck region (see Figure 15.7) and, finally, inward to oral cavity reconstruction. The normative data also will permit evaluation of patients undergoing facial reconstruction for congenital problems, and of patients after facial injury. This chapter will not discuss the evaluation of taste.

The beginning of comprehensive sensibility evaluation for the head and neck region was built on the concepts developed for evaluating sensibility of the hand (Dellon, 1981). These concepts are that sensibility for touch should be measured with devices to evaluate both the quickly- and slowly-adapting large myelinated nerve fiber populations, and to measure both the thresholds for stimulation and for distinguishing one from two points. Phillip Robinson, Professor of Oral and Maxillofacial Surgery at the School of Dentistry in Sheffield, England has been a consistent contributor on the subject of sensibility testing in the head and neck region (Robinson, Smith, Johnson, & Coppins, 1992). His suggestions are to use a test of pressure, such as the British version of the von Fry hairs

FIGURE 15.6

A

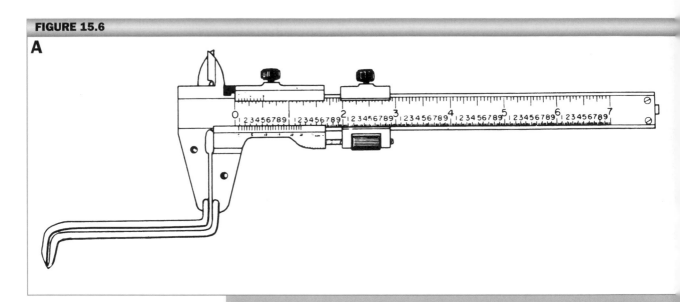

B

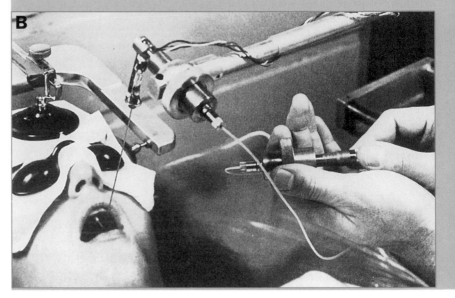

(which reports force in milliNewtons), a test of pain, such as his own torsion spring-loaded needle (a modification of Sunderland's spring-loaded device), and two-point discrimination testing. Robinson's group did not report normative data. Mackinnon's group (then at Sunnybrook Hospital, University of Toronto, Department of Plastic Surgery, and now at the Department of Plastic Surgery, Washington University, in St. Louis) was the first to report normative data using the approach that had been developed for sensibility testing in the hand (Kesarwani, et al., 1989).

This approach has since been followed by others. They include Posnick, Zimbler, and Grossman (1990), (at Sick Children's Hospital in Toronto and New York University's Department of Plastic Surgery), Costas,

Heatley, and Seckel (1994) (at the Lahey Clinic at Burlington, Massachusetts's Plastic Surgery Department), and Vriens, Moos, and Scott (1994) (at the Plastic Surgery and Maxillofacial Surgery Unit at Canniesburn Hospital, Glasgow, Scotland). These studies have largely been consistent in their findings. They used the Biothesiometer™, the Semmes-

Weinstein nylon monofilaments, and the Disk-Criminator™ (see Chapter 7 for detailed explanation of instrumentation). These four studies, reporting normative data, included 60, 32, 116, and 100 normal subjects, respectively. The agreement between the absolute values they found for the thresholds, the similar conclusions with regard to age-related

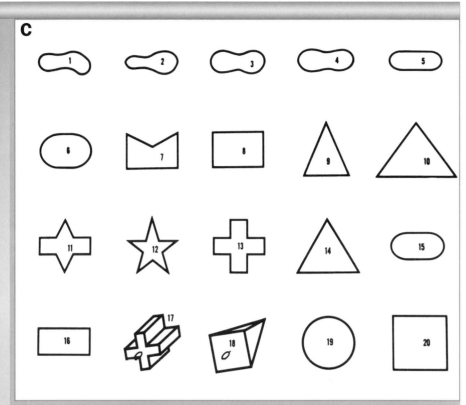

Instruments for examining intraoral sensibility. (A) Extensions applied to an engineer's sliding ruler are helpful in obtaining intraoral examination. (B) Close up view of transducer positioning mechanism attached to stereotactic device for localizing touch stimuli. (C) Twenty-five test instruments that may be placed into the oral cavity to test for stereognosis. (D) Instruments similar to those in (C), but attached to rods. From Symposium on Oral Perception and Sensation, by J. Bosma, 1967, Springfield, IL: Charles C Thomas, Publisher. Reprinted with permission of the author.

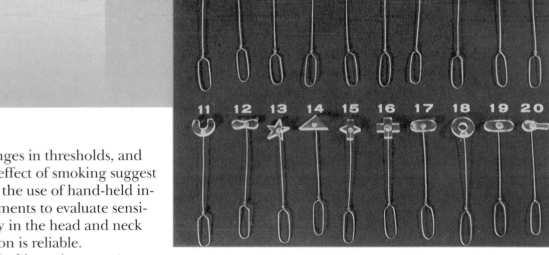

changes in thresholds, and the effect of smoking suggest that the use of hand-held instruments to evaluate sensibility in the head and neck region is reliable.

Mackinnon's group (see Kesarwani et al., 1989) was the first to record moving two-point discrimination for the head and neck region (see Figure 15.7). Their results for the forehead, cheek, chin, and lip were 9 mm, 8 mm, 7 mm, and 3 mm, respectively. These values were about 2 mm less than static two-point discrimination for each of these four sites. Overall, the forehead had the highest sensibility thresholds, and the lower lip the lowest (most sensitive)

FIGURE 15.7

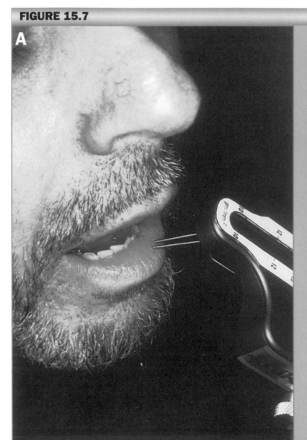

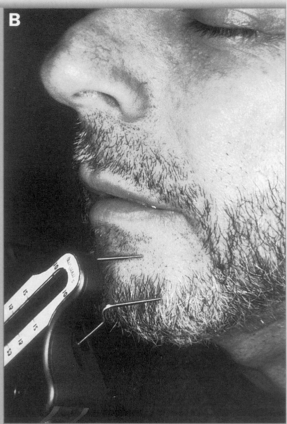

Measurement of cutaneous pressure threshold of the (A) lip and (B) chin with the NK Pressure-Specified Sensory Device™. This device can be zeroed (corrected) for gravity and can, therefore, be used in any position. The length of the prongs can be increased for intraoral use. Both one- and two-point static and moving touch can be measured with this device. Illustrations (A) and (B) copyright A. Lee Dellon. Reprinted with permission.

thresholds. With regard to age-related changes, they found that the threshold increases significantly above 50 years of age for all modalities tested (see Figure 15.8). There was no difference in sensibility between the left and right side of the face. With regard to sex, the thresholds were consistently lower for females than for males, but these differences did not reach a level of statistical significance. Mackinnon's group was the only one that compared the normative measurements in these regions to those found in 20 patients with facial trauma. Therefore,

their normative data is given in Figures 15.13 and 15.14 in the section on facial trauma.

The study of normal sensibility in the head and neck region by Posnick, Zimbler, and Grossman (1990) included many more anatomic sites than did the Kesarwani et al. (1989) study. These sites are illustrated in Figure 15.9 and the data combined and presented in Table 15.2.

Posnick et al. also found no difference between the left and right side of the face. They had an insufficient number of subjects to evaluate the difference in thresholds between males and females (23 women and 13 men in the study), or any age-related changes (range 20 to 50 years of age, mean not given). Of interest is their measurement of the sensibility of the index fin-

FIGURE 15.8

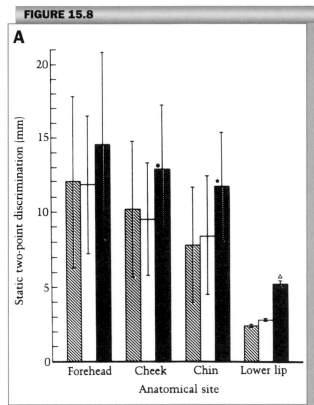

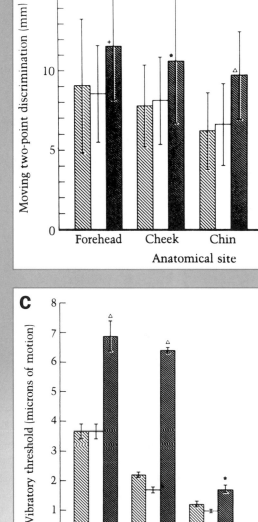

Changes in normal facial sensibility related to age. (A) Static two-point discrimination. (B) Moving two-point discrimination. (C) Vibratory threshold to 120 Hz stimuli. For each graph, the grey bar represents the mean for 22 normal subjects ≤ 30 years old, the clear bar represents the mean for 21 normal subjects 31 to 50 years of age, and the black bar represents the mean for 17 patients ≥ 51 years of age. For each graph, the statistical significance between the age groups is indicated to be p < .05 by the black dot, p < .01 by the asterisk, and p < .001 by the clear triangle. From "Facial Sensibility Testing in the Normal and Posttraumatic Population," by A. Kesarwani, O. Antonyshyn, S. E. Mackinnon, J. S. Gruss, C. Novak, & L. Kelly, 1989, Annals of Plastic Surgery 22:416-425. Reprinted with permission of the authors.

gertip with each sensory submodality tested. The fingertip value is given in Figure 15.9 for comparison to the facial sensibility threshold.

The same trend of higher thresholds for the forehead, and lowest thresholds (most sensitive) for the lip, was confirmed.

The study of normal sensibility in the head and neck region by Costas, Heatley, and Seckel (1994) included the greatest number of anatomical sites, as illustrated in Figure 15.10. The distribution of the Semmes-Weinstein nylon monofilament data is given in Table 15.3.

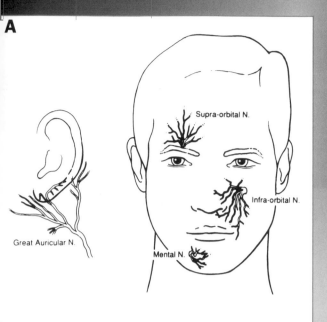

A

Supra-orbital N.

Infra-orbital N.

Great Auricular N.

Mental N.

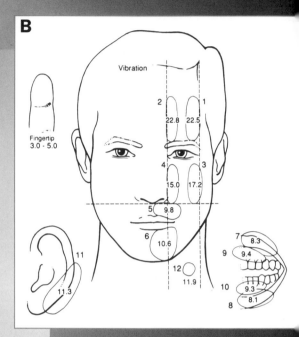

B

Vibration

Fingertip
3.0 - 5.0

2   1
22.8 22.5

4   3
15.0 17.2

5   9.8

6   10.6

11

12
11.9

11.3

7   8.3

9   9.4

10   9.3

8   8.1

FIGURE 15.9

Normative values for sensibility in the head and neck region. (A) The four major sensory nerves include the supraorbital, the infraorbital, the inferior alveolar-mental, and the greater auricular. For the next three diagrams, the numbers 1 through 12 refer to the anatomical sites tested (see Table 15.1). (B) The mean cutaneous thresholds obtained with the Biothesiometer™ (120 Hz stimulus reported in millivolts, however, instead of microns of motion). (C) Static two-point discrimination. (D) Moving two-point discrimination (reported in mm). From "Normal Cutaneous Sensibility of the Face," by J. C. Posnick, A. G. Zimbler, & J. A. Grossman, 1990, Plastic and Reconstructive Surgery *86:429-433. Reprinted with permission of the authors.*

C

Static 2 point
discrimination

Fingertip
2.0 - 4.0

2   1
12.7 13.4

4   3
7.4   9.0

5   4.3

6   5.4

11

12
13.7

13.2

7   7.0

9   5.2

10   4.6

8   6.1

D

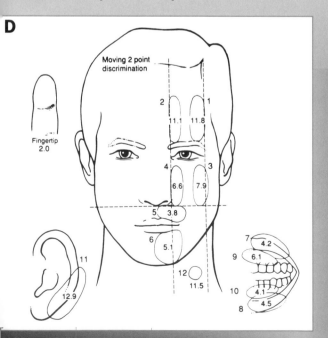

Moving 2 point
discrimination

Fingertip
2.0

2   1
11.1 11.8

4   3
6.6   7.9

5   3.8

6   5.1

11

12
11.5

12.9

7   4.2

9   6.1

10   4.1

8   4.5

TABLE 15.2 NORMAL CUTANEOUS SENSIBILITY OF THE HEAD AND NECK

Anatomic site	Semmes-Weinstein[+]	Vibratory[◆]	Static 2PD[★]	Moving 2 PD[★]
1. Lateral forehead	1.95	22.5	13.4	11.8
2. Medial forehead	1.93	22.8	12.7	11.1
3. Anterior cheek	1.84	17.2	9.0	7.9
4. Nasolabial	1.75	15.0	7.4	6.6
5. Upper white lip	1.81	9.8	4.3	3.8
6. Chin	1.95	10.6	5.4	5.1
7. Upper red lip	2.38	8.3	7.0	4.2
8. Lower red lip	2.26	8.1	6.1	4.5
9. Upper lip mucosa	2.80	9.4	5.2	6.1
10. Lower lip mucosa	2.91	9.3	4.6	4.1
11. Ear lobe	1.99	11.3	13.2	12.9
12. Neck	2.13	11.9	13.7	11.5

Note:

[+] The mean of the log values listed on the filament for each patient. (Note that this is mathematically not a proper statistical value but is a frequent reporting mistake. The correct method is to take the mean of value obtained when the logarithm to the base 10 of the force in tenths of milligrams is divided by the area of the filament to give pressure, that is, g/mm^2 (see Chapter 7).

[◆] The mean of the voltage applied in millivolts. (Note that a better reporting technique is microns of displacement of the probe tip; see Chapter 7).

[★] Mean of the distance in mm required to distinguish one from two points.

From "Normal Cutaneous Sensibility of the Face," by J. C. Posnick, A. G. Zimbler, & J. A. I. Grossman, 1990, *Plastic and Reconstructive Surgery 86:*429-433. Reprinted with permission of the authors.

This study did not include vibratory thresholds or measurement of moving two-point discrimination. This study again demonstrated no difference in sensibility between the left and right side of the face, or between individuals who were left or right-handed. The study found women to be significantly more sensitive than men only at the tip of the nose. It found that static two-point discrimination was significantly higher (less sensitive) for subjects over age 50 and for those with a cigarette smoking history of > 10 pack years.

The study of normal sensibility in the head and neck region by Vriens, Moos, and Scott (1994) measured both static and moving two-point discrimination. It confirmed the observations made previously that there was no significant difference between the left and right side, and that moving two-point discrimination was 2 mm to 3 mm less for any given test

FIGURE 15.10

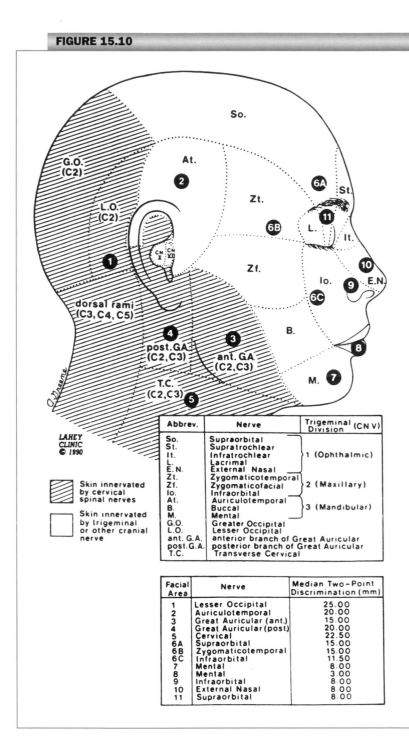

Abbrev.	Nerve	Trigeminal Division (CN V)
So.	Supraorbital	
St.	Supratrochlear	
It.	Infratrochlear	1 (Ophthalmic)
L.	Lacrimal	
E.N.	External Nasal	
Zt.	Zygomaticotemporal	
Zf.	Zygomaticofacial	2 (Maxillary)
Io.	Infraorbital	
At.	Auriculotemporal	
B.	Buccal	3 (Mandibular)
M.	Mental	
G.O.	Greater Occipital	
L.O.	Lesser Occipital	
ant. G.A.	anterior branch of Great Auricular	
post.G.A.	posterior branch of Great Auricular	
T.C.	Transverse Cervical	

Facial Area	Nerve	Median Two-Point Discrimination (mm)
1	Lesser Occipital	25.00
2	Auriculotemporal	20.00
3	Great Auricular (ant.)	15.00
4	Great Auricular (post)	20.00
5	Cervical	22.50
6A	Supraorbital	15.00
6B	Zygomaticotemporal	15.00
6C	Infraorbital	11.50
7	Mental	8.00
8	Mental	3.00
9	Infraorbital	8.00
10	External Nasal	8.00
11	Supraorbital	8.00

Normative values for sensibility in the head and neck region. Detailed illustration of cutaneous nerves with anatomic sites numbered to correspond to values in Table 15.3. Note that numbered pairs 6A and 11, 7 and 8, and 6C and 9 are ambiguous, and have been renamed in Table 15.3 for clarity. From "Normal Sensation of the Human Face and Neck," by P. D. Costas, G. Heatley, & B. R. Seckel, 1994, Plastic and Reconstructive Surgery *93: 1141-1145.*

trend for females to have slightly lower thresholds than males, but this difference was not statistically significant. The order of magnitude of the threshold values is similar to the earlier studies; therefore, the data is not included in this chapter.

The normative data for the Neurometer™, which uses an electric current stimulus, is available for the trigeminal nerve. The electrode for this measurement is placed in front of the ear, in the pre-auricular region. The normative data is given in Chapter 7, in which this device is described. This data was collected with the concept that facial sensibility would be compared to sensibility of the hand and the foot in establishing the diagnosis of a peripheral neu-

site. For two-point discrimination and for the pressure threshold measured with the Semmes-Weinstein nylon monofilaments, this study confirmed that smokers had significantly higher (p < .01) thresholds than nonsmokers (pack years not defined), as did those above 50 years of age than did those below 50 years of age. There was a

TABLE 15.3 NORMAL CUTANEOUS SENSIBILITY OF THE HEAD AND NECK

Distribution of Cutaneous Pressure Thresholds

	SW Nylon Marking	1.65	2.36	2.4	42.83
	Pressure (g/mm²)	0.25	3.3	4.3	6.3[+]

Anatomic site

1.	Lesser occipital	79%	17%	3%	1%
2.	Auriculotemporal	82%	13%	3%	2%
3.	Greater auricular (ant)	70%	20%	7%	3%
4.	Greater auricular (post)	68%	25%	6%	1%
5.	Cervical	73%	17%	8%	2%
6A.	Supraorbital	88%	10%	2%	0%
6B.	Zygomaticotemporal	85%	13%	2%	0%
6C.	Infraorbital (near cheek)	80%	15%	3%	2%
7.	Mental (chin)	78%	10%	10%	2%
8.	Mental (lower lip)	89%	9%	2%	0%
9.	Infraorbital (at alar rim)	97%	3%	0%	0%
10.	Nasal	97%	3%	0%	0%
11.	Infratrochlear	78%	14%	7%	1%

Note:
[+] The pressure values given in the original paper are listed here, but they do not agree with the ones calculated by Levin, Pearsall, & Ruderman (1978) (see Table 7.3). The correct pressure recordings for these four filaments would be 1.45, 5.20, 3.25, and 4.86 g/mm².
From "Normal Cutaneous Sensibility of the Face," by J. C. Posnick, A. G. Zimbler, & J. A. I. Grossman, 1990, *Plastic and Reconstructive Surgery 86:*429-433. The names of anatomic sites 7-11 have been altered to reflect their location. Adapted with permission of the authors.

ropathy, and not really to diagnose problems with facial sensibility. The electrode system is sufficiently large that this device is probably not suitable for testing specific regions of trigeminal nerve innervation after facial injury.

The introduction of computer-assisted sensory testing adds another set of measurements for head and neck normative data. The first to be reported was that obtained with the CASE IV system (see Chapter 7) from the Mayo Clinic. Figure

15.11 gives the touch-pressure and vibratory thresholds on more than 300 subjects, arranged by age (Dyck, Karnes, O'Brien, & Zimmerman, 1993). Table 15.4 has the few available data points obtained over the last 2 years with the Pressure-Specified Sensory Device™ on patients I have seen in my office for evaluation of clinical problems in this anatomic region. One of these patients, who had a nerve graft to reconstruct the inferior alveolar nerve, has been reported recently and is discussed in detail in the next section (Evans, Crawley, & Dellon, 1994; and see Figure 15.12). Peter Grime, a surgeon from England, while doing a microsurgical fellowship in Taiwan with Fu-Chan Wei at Chang Gung Memorial Hospital, studied 16 normal Chinese subjects to evaluate their lower lip sensibility. Their data is given in Table 15.5 and suggests that the lip is the most sensitive body surface for the detection of static pressure (Grime & Wei, unpublished observations, 1994).

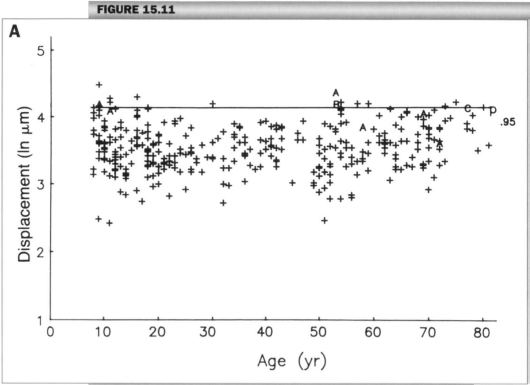

FIGURE 15.11

Normative values for the lip obtained with the CASE IV system, a computer-assisted sensory examination. (A) Vibratory threshold expressed in microns of displacement. (B) Touch-pressure threshold expressed in milligrams of force. Data is for 326 normal subjects in (A), and 380 normal subjects in (B), arranged by age. The line at .95 represents the 95% upper confidence interval. From "Detection Thresholds of Cutaneous Sensation in Humans," by P. J. Dyck, J. Karnes, P. C. O'Brien, & I. R. Zimmerman, 1993 in Peripheral Neuropathy, P. J. Dyck, P. K. Thomas, J. W. Griffin, P. A. Low, & J. F. Poduslo, Editors, Philadelphia: W. B. Saunders Company. Reprinted with permission of the authors.

• CRITICAL ANALYSIS OF NORMATIVE SENSIBILITY TESTING • IN THE HEAD AND NECK REGION

The strategy of applying the neurophysiologic basis of sensibility of the fingertip to the head and neck region has been successful in producing consistent observations about the cutaneous sensibility of the face. It is clear that the confusing aspects of reporting thresholds in values that are both scientifically and clinically meaningful is a problem. For example, some of the normative data is still reported in

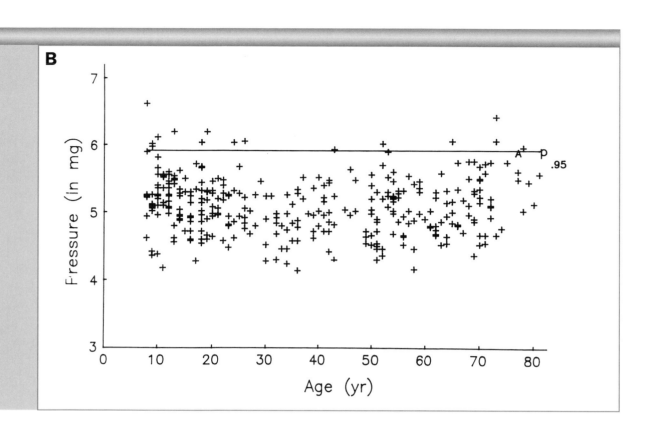

TABLE 15.4 NORMATIVE DATA FOR CUTANEOUS PRESSURE THRESHOLD OF THE LIP OBTAINED WITH THE PRESSURE-SPECIFIED SENSORY DEVICE™

	Lower Lip Cutaneous Pressure Threshold					
	1PS g/mm^2	2PS g/mm^2	2PS mm	1PM g/mm^2	2PM g/mm^2	2PM mm
Patient						
S.H.	0.1	0.3	2.6	0.1	0.4	2.5
L.G.	0.4	0.4	3.0	0.3	0.3	2.6
P.S.	0.4	0.6	4.0	0.3	0.5	4.0
	Chin					
S.H.	0.2	*	*	0.2	*	*
L.G.	0.5	*	*	0.8	*	*
P.S.	0.6	0.6	4.0	0.6	0.4	4.0

Note: *Data point not obtained at time of examination.
From unpublished data obtained by A. L. Dellon.

FIGURE 15.12

Inferior Alveolar Nerve

Date	Grafted Side (Right)						Normal Side (Left)					
	1PS	2PS[a]	2PS[b]	1PM	2PM[c]	2PM[d]	1PS	2PS[a]	2PS[b]	1PM	2PM[c]	2PM[d]
Vermilion												
01/27/93	21.0	—	—	4.0	—	—	0.1	0.3	2.5	0.1	0.4	2.5
03/23/93	17.0	—	—	6.0	—	—	0.1	0.1	2.6	0.1	0.2	2.5
08/03/93	0.7	0.6	2.6	0.2	0.5	2.6	0.1	0.4	2.6	0.1	0.2	2.6
12/29/93	1.0	0.8	3.0	0.2	0.3	2.9	0.2	0.2	2.9	0.3	0.2	2.9

Date	Grafted Side (Right)		Normal Side (Left)	
	1PS	1PM	1PS	1PM
Chin				
01/27/93	71.0	12.0	0.2	0.2
03/23/93	54.0	6.0	0.2	0.2
08/03/93	0.5	0.5	0.3	0.3
12/29/93	0.3	0.4	0.2	0.4

Pressure-Specified Sensory Device™ (see also Figure 15.7) made serial measurements after grafting to reconstruct the inferior alveolar nerve. This nerve was injured during extraction of a third molar. The success of the nerve graft may be judged by the sensibility recovered on the grafted side in contrast to the normal side. (The superscripts in the table a and c are two-point discrimination thresholds reported in g/mm², while b and d are the thresholds reported in mm.) 1PS and 1PM are one-point static and moving touch thresholds. 2PS and 2PM are two-point static and moving discrimination thresholds. From "Inferior Alveolar Nerve Grafting: An Approach Without Intermaxillary Fixation," by G. R. D. Evans, W. Crawley, & A. L. Dellon, (1994), Annals of Plastic Surgery 33:221-224. Reprinted with permission of the authors.

microvolts for vibratory threshold, and as log values, which are the markings on the Semmes-Weinstein nylon monofilaments. The correct reporting technique for these observations should be *microns of motion* (displacement of the vibrating probe tip), and g/mm², which is pressure. Applying hand-held measuring instruments to measure facial sensibility has been demonstrated to be reliable, since several different studies reporting normative data from different centers have produced a series of observations that are internally consistent, and which have similar magnitudes of thresholds. It is clear that the lip has the highest sensitivity, that is, the lowest thresholds, and that the forehead has the lowest sensitivity, that is, the highest thresholds, and that the cheek is somewhere in between. It is also clear that all thresholds are significantly elevated in subjects older than 50 years of age, and in smokers.

Considering the results of the studies described above, it is recommended that evaluation of facial sensibility be done using a quantitative approach. It is not clear that measuring the vibratory threshold in the face adds any additional information to the observations that would be made by measuring cutaneous pressure threshold. This is true especially if the moving-touch thresholds are measured, because they also use the same quickly-adapting fiber receptor system as do vibratory stimuli. To evaluate facial sensibility in a person with a neuropathy, the present recommendation would be to use the Neurometer™ to test the current perception threshold. The reason is that this device offers the possibility, through neuroselective stimulation, to evaluate nerve fiber systems of varying fiber diameters, which may reflect the underlying neuropathy. Furthermore, the statistical evaluation package of the Neurometer™ relates the trigeminal threshold to that of the media.

The quantitative approach to evaluating facial sensibility implies that the preferred instrument should be one capable of measuring both the pressure and the distance at which one from two points can be distinguished, as well as the static and moving one-point touch thresholds. The only equipment capable of doing this is the Pressure-Specified Sensory Device™. The CASE IV system can measure the one-point static threshold. The Disk-Criminator™ can mea-

sure the distance at which two points can be distinguished, but not the pressure at which this measurement is made. In the hand, with peripheral nerve compression, it is this pressure threshold which changes first and, therefore, it is this pressure which will most likely be the first parameter to be altered in a trigeminal nerve injury (see Chapter 12). In the absence of a Pressure-Specified Sensory Device™, the Semmes-

Weinstein nylon monofilaments will give an approximation or estimate, but not a true measurement, of the cutaneous pressure threshold for one-point static stimuli. It remains, however, for normative data to be collected for the head and neck area with the Pressure-Specified Sensory Device™. Testing instruments are still not adequate to properly test intraoral sensibility, and this, too, represents an area for future improvement.

• DENTAL EXTRACTIONS •

Two different nerves may be injured during a dental extraction—the *inferior alveolar nerve* and the *lingual nerve*. The inferior alveolar nerve, a branch of the mandibular, or the third division of the trigeminal nerve, enters the mandibular canal at the mandibular foramen at the lingual aspect of the ramus of the mandible. Just before it enters the bony canal it gives off its motor branch to the mylohyoid muscle and the anterior belly of the digastric muscle. Within this motor branch are the sympathetic fibers to the submandibular gland, and a few terminal sensory fibers to the mental protuberance. The sensory branches of the inferior alveolar nerve are the dental nerves and the terminal fibers (three small branches) that will become the mental nerve, innervating the chin (one branch) and the lower lip and mucous membrane adjacent to the lip (two branches). The mental nerves exits the mandible between the incisor and the bicuspid (see Figure 15.2). It is the close relationship of the inferior

TABLE 15.5 NORMATIVE DATA FOR CUTANEOUS PRESSURE THRESHOLD OF THE LIP OBTAINED WITH THE PRESSURE-SPECIFIED SENSORY DEVICE™

One-point Static Pressure Threshold (g/mm²)

Anatomic site	Right	Left
Upper lip (white)	0.28 ± 0.20	0.40 ± 0.13
Upper lip (red)	0.20 ± 0.12	0.32 ± 0.12
Lower lip (red)	0.37 ± 0.17	0.36 ± 0.14
Chin	$0.28 \pm .017$	0.41 ± 0.15

Note: From unpublished observations on 34 normal subjects, in "Human Perception Values for the Lip," by P. Grime & F. C. Wei, 1994.

alveolar nerve to the roots of the third molar that put it at risk for injury during dental extraction. Unless the dental canal carrying this nerve is located near the upper third or middle third of the root, there is increased risk of the nerve being injured. The molar's root may indent the dental canal, or the nerve may pierce through the root.

In contrast, the lingual nerve, at its origin, also branches off the mandibular division of the trigeminal (V cranial) nerve, and runs parallel to the inferior alveolar nerve, but on the inside, or lingual side, of the mandible, deep to the lateral pterygoid muscle. It is here joined by the special sensory branch of the facial (VII cranial) nerve carrying taste fibers to the anterior two-thirds of the tongue and the sympathetic fibers to the sublingual glands. The lingual nerve will enter the oral cavity on the way toward the tongue, innervating the mucous membranes along the floor of the mouth (see Figure 15.2). It is in this portion of its course that the lingual nerve may lie directly on the medial bone plate of the mandible overlying the third molar's buccal roots, placing the lingual nerve at risk for injury during dental extraction. During the extraction of impacted third molars, a bone flap may need to be elevated, a broken root removed, or the canal burred, all of which may place both

the inferior alveolar nerve and the lingual nerve at risk for injury.

While there have been many reports of injury of these nerves due to dental extraction, and while this problem is well known, there have been only a few comprehensive studies that permit a comment on the incidence of the problem and the prognosis for recovery of lip and tongue sensation after injury. One prospective study was reported by Rood (1983) of the Maxillofacial Department of the University of Manchester, England. By stroking the lip and chin with his fingertip, and in some patients supplementing this exam with cotton wisp stroking and a pin, he noted areas of sensory loss in 105 cases of third molar extraction from a series of 1,400 such extractions (7.5% incidence). He noted that most cases recovered completely by 3 months, and that only 5 of these cases failed to recover completely (permanent sensory loss in the lip of 0.4%).

Wofford and Miller (1987) prospectively studied 315 subjects having their third molar removed at the Oral and Maxillofacial Department of the United States Air Force Medical Center in Keesler, Mississippi. Sensory loss following the extraction was studied by moving a cotton wisp over the lip and chin and mapping the area of decreased sensibility.

There were 19 cases of sensory change in 576 extractions for an overall incidence rate per patient of 6.0%, and per extracted tooth of 3.3%. Fifteen (79%) of these 19 sensory losses were for the lip, and 4 (21%) were for the tongue. All but one of the 19 patients had recovery of the sensory loss by 6 months after the extraction, while the one remaining area of sensory loss, the tip of the tongue, remained numb at the last time of follow up, 13 months after the extraction.

Another prospective study was reported by Masson (1988), of the Oral and Maxillofacial Surgery Department at St. Luke's Hospital in England. Masson reported that 120 cases of loss of tongue sensibility occurred in 1,040 dental extractions (11.5%) in 602 patients. The sensory exam included a cotton wisp, sharp and dull testing, two-point discrimination testing with blunt dividers, and pain perception with a probe. All but 6 cases of sensory loss recovered within 6 months. The remaining 6 cases (5%) each had complete loss of sensibility in the distribution of the lingual nerve, whereas the ones that recovered all had incomplete sensory loss. The common factors noted at surgery during the cases that developed lingual sensory loss were deep impaction of the third molar, necessity for the surgeon to elevate a lingual mucosal or bone flap, and the length of the operation. Seniority of the surgeon did not have a significant effect on outcome.

The pattern of recovery is of interest in that it raises the question of the source of the regenerating axons and the possibility of collateral sprouting. The lower lip receives innervation primarily from the ipsilateral mental branch of the inferior alveolar nerve. But, as discussed above with respect to using anesthetic blocks to identify the source of the innervation after recovery of sensibility, it is possible that recovered sensation might occur from the ipsilateral buccal nerve, the ipsilateral cervical plexus, the terminal branch of the mylohyoid nerve, or even the contralateral equivalents of these nerves. Rood (1983) observed two patterns of decrease in the area of sensory loss after third molar extraction that injured the inferior alveolar nerve. The most common involved a shrinkage of the area in a distal direction, that is, the proximal area, which is that area closest to the mental nerve (the chin), suggesting regeneration from the proximal ipsilateral inferior alveolar nerve. But there were patients (he did not indicate the percentage) who, in addition to having this proximal evidence of expected regeneration, had a shrinkage of the distal area too, suggesting collateral sprouting from the adjacent, normally

innervated contralateral lip and ipsilateral mucous membrane and skin. This observation is one that may be used in sensory rehabilitation, both to facilitate desensitization and to promote recovery. It may also provide a clue to the potential to reinnervate an anesthetic lower lip.

The treatment of the patient with loss of sensibility of the tongue or lip following extraction of a third molar should be based on the principles of nerve injury and recovery outlined in Chapter 4. The most common mechanism of injury will be that the nerves and fascicles are still intact, and that recovery within a few months can be expected. Evaluation of sensibility quantitatively is critical to prognosis and management decisions. The ideal instruments to do this are computerized sensory testing equipment (see Table 15.6). Pain relief with analgesics and desensitization exercises by the therapist will be helpful, as well as cautions not to further injure the dysethestic or anesthetic skin or mucosa with hot or pointed food. If,

after 6 months, sensory loss is persistent, with or without attendant pain, nerve reconstruction is the appropriate consideration.

Techniques for reconstruction of the inferior alveolar nerve have been reported by Dellon & Crawley (1992) using the bioabsorbable Neurotube™ (a conduit made from polyglycolic acid which is absorbed within 3 months after the nerve has regenerated through the tube), or a traditional autogenous nerve graft (Evans et al., 1994). In both of these cases complete pain relief and close to normal sensibility was documented by 1 year after neural regeneration. The recovery sensibility to the lip and chin was documented with the Pressure-Specified Sensory Device™ in the Evans et al. report, and is illustrated in Figure 15.12. Many of the reports on recovery of tongue sensibility indicate less complete recovery, probably due to the lateness of the attempt at nerve reconstruction and because of the use of repair instead of nerve grafting techniques.

• MANDIBULAR AND MAXILLARY OSTEOTOMY •

Orthognathic surgery attempts to reestablish the normal relationship between the upper and lower jaw, that is, between the maxilla and the mandible. This relationship is essential for proper occlusion, which is the appropriate meshing of the teeth. Improper occlusion can be the source of jaw or facial pain. An imbalance in the relationship between the maxilla and the mandible can also be the source

TABLE 15.6 CUTANEOUS PRESSURE THRESHOLD OF THE LIP AND CHIN: UNILATERAL INFERIOR ALVE-OLAR NERVE DYSFUNCTION OBTAINED WITH THE PRESSURE-SPECIFIED SENSORY DEVICE™

Patient	1PS g/mm^2	2PS g/mm^2	2PS mm	1PM g/mm^2	2PM g/mm^2	2PM mm
		Lower Lip Cutaneous Pressure Threshold				
S.H.[+]	21.0			3.7		
L.G.[♦]	96.0			96.0		
P.S.[*]	0.4	0.6	4.0	0.3	0.5	4.0
		Chin				
S.H.[+]	71.0			11.5		
L.G.[♦]	41.0			18.6		
P.S.[*]	5.4	8.2	6.1	0.6	1.6	5.1

Note:
[+] This patient had pain and numbness develop after a third molar was extracted.
[♦] This patient had a unilateral cerebrovascular accident, loosing the trigeminal nerve.
[*] This patient had a sliding genioplasty that resulted in numbness of just one side of the chin.
(These three patients have their normal side listed in Table 15.3.)
From unpublished data obtained by A. L. Dellon.

of considerable distress to a person because of the way it affects their appearance, either by causing a protruding or receding chin, or a prominent upper lip with protruding incisors. The correction of these skeletal imbalances is possible through surgery that requires saw cuts through the facial skeleton at precise locations, and then realignment of the facial bones by sliding them. The repositioned bones are then held in place either by wiring the jaws together (intermaxillary fixation), by placing bone grafts to prevent the bones from sliding back into their original positions, or by placing metal plates and screws. Sometimes, of course, a combination of techniques is used. Clearly, this approach to facial bones puts the cutaneous nerves, and particularly the inferior alveolar nerve, at risk for injury.

The only published material available on the *maxillary osteotomy* is from Posnick, Al-Qattan, and Pron (1994) in which sensibility testing was done with a vibrometer (Biothesiometer), Semmes-Weinstein nylon monofilaments, and two-point discrimination testing with the Disk-Criminator™. The infraorbital nerve was tested bilaterally in 59 patients who had cleft lip and palate repairs, and who also had a LeForte I maxillary osteotomy. These nerves were also tested in a group of 17 patients with developmental jaw abnormalities who had a LeForte I maxillary osteotomy. No postoperative sensory complaints were present subjectively, and there were no significant sensory changes documented by the testing. The authors concluded that "it appears permanent functional sensory alteration of the soft tissues supplied by the infraorbital nerve is rare after the LeForte I osteotomy." The explanation for this appears to be that the saw cut through the maxillary is sufficiently below the anatomic course of the infraorbital branch of the maxillary division of the trigeminal nerve that the nerve is not injured.

In contrast to maxillary osteotomies, *mandibular osteotomies* carry a high risk of nerve injury. The most recent review of this subject, by Posnick, Al-Qattan, and Stepner (in press, 1996), includes an extensive bibliography that documents injury to the inferior alveolar nerve during mandibular osteotomies, where the nerve was subjected to direct injury by the saw, by traction or stretch injury, or by compression by the hardware, with the incidence of these nerve problems approaching 30%. An incidence of chin numbness after sliding genioplasty, designed to lengthen the chin when the dental occlusion is normal, approaches 20%.

Posnick's group evaluated 14 nerves in adolescents 1 year after sagittal split osteotomies of the mandible for mandibular advancement, 40 nerves in adolescents 1 year after a genioplasty alone, and 42 nerves in adolescents 1 year after a combined mandibular osteotomy and genioplasty. They evaluated sensibility in the lip and chin with Semmes-Weinstein nylon monofilaments, static and moving two-point discrimination, and vibrometry. They compared their postoperative surgical groups with a normal population. They found an incidence of persistent sensory change present in 29% of the patients having a bilateral sagittal split mandibular osteotomy, a 10% incidence in the patients having a sliding genioplasty, and a 67% incidence in the patients having the combined procedure. This high incidence is similar to the 70% incidence found by two other studies (Nishioka, Zysset, & VanSickels, 1987; Lindquist & Obeid, 1988). Posnick's group found that patients with numbness of the lip and chin had a degree of drooling, lip biting, and lack of awareness of retained food particles on the lower lip that was considered problematic.

From a technical point of view, reconstruction of these patients is difficult. In contrast to the group of patients with numbness and pain after a dental extraction, the exact site of the nerve injury is unknown. After dental extraction, it can be assumed that there is a region near the tooth root that can be identified, excised, and reconstructed. With a group of patients with mandibular split ostomies and genioplasty, there is likely to be injury to the nerve at at least two locations, plus a stretch/traction component, requiring bilateral long nerve grafts for reconstruction.

Sensibility testing for this group of patients has been done in my office with computerized sensory testing using the Pressure-Specified Sensory Device™. The results of those tests in a small group of patients is given in Table 15.7. These test results demonstrate the wide spectrum of sensory changes that occurred in this group of patients. Some have almost complete axonal loss, with no two-point discrimination, while others have just pressure threshold changes. It is difficult to decide whether to do extensive bilateral inferior alveolar nerve grafts for only a moderate degree of sensory loss, as in the case of the first three patients in Table 15.7. However, for pain accompanied by severe sensory loss, as documented in patient 4, it would appear that such a reconstructive effort would be justified. It is clear that quantitative sensory testing will be necessary for the preoperative evaluation of these patients, as well as to document postoperative recovery after nerve grafting.

TABLE 15.7 CUTANEOUS PRESSURE THRESHOLD OF THE LIP AND CHIN: BILATERAL INFERIOR ALVEOLAR NERVE DYSFUNCTION OBTAINED WITH THE PRESSURE-SPECIFIED SENSORY DEVICE™

Lower Lip
Cutaneous Pressure Threshold

	Right						Left					
	1PS g/mm²	2P g/mm²	2PS mm	1PM g/mm²	2PM g/mm²	2PM mm	1PS g/mm²	2PS g/mm²	2PS mm	1PM g/mm²	2PM g/mm²	2PM mm
Patient												
1. MH	0.6	2.7	8.0	0.1	4.2	6.7	0.5	5.5	7.1	0.3	3.4	6.6
2. PT	4.2	none		0.3	2.4	6.6	0.5	4.3	6.2	0.3	3.6	5.0
3. SS	0.3	7.3	5.6	0.1	2.5	4.1	0.3	5.6	5.2	0.6	1.8	4.5
4. WS	38	none		27	none		12	none		17	none	

Chin

	Right						Left					
	1PS g/mm²	2P g/mm²	2PS mm	1PM g/mm²	2PM g/mm²	2PM mm	1PS g/mm²	2PS g/mm²	2PS mm	1PM g/mm²	2PM g/mm²	2PM mm
Patient												
1. MH	0.5	*	*	0.	*	*	0.5	*	*	0.3	*	*
2. PT	0.9	*	*	0.2	*	*	0.2	*	*	0.3	*	*
3. SS	0.8	*	*	0.3	*	*	1.5	*	*	0.6	*	*
4. WS	50	none		87	5	15	12	none		17	13	16

Note: All of these patients had bilateral mandibular advancements requiring sagittal split of the mandibular. Patient WS also had a sliding advancement genioplasty.
From unpublished data obtained by A. L. Dellon.

• CLEFT LIP AND CLEFT PALATE •

Quantitative sensory testing has been used to evaluate the sensibility of the upper lip and cheek in adolescents born with a cleft lip. Posnick et al. (1994) used vibrometry (Biothesiometer), Semmes-Weinstein nylon monofilaments, and the Disk-Criminator™ to evaluate sensibility in a group of 68 adolescents who had undergone cleft lip repair at about 1 year of age. They found no difference in facial sensibility between unilateral and bilateral cleft children, or between cleft and age-matched, non-cleft lip children.

• FACIAL INJURIES •

Facial injury may directly injure the nerves in the head and neck region by the force of a direct contusion, by entrapping or disrupting the nerves within fracture sites, or as a consequence of surgery by directly injuring a nerve with a reconstruction plate. In fact, however, there have been few reported cases of such problems. So unusual do these conditions seem to be that a report of a neuroma of the supraorbital nerve, a complication of a halo fixation frame used to correct a cervical spine injury, was thought worthy of publication as a case report (Friedman, Rohrich, & Finn, 1992). That patient had the neuroma of the supraorbital nerve resected and a nerve repair done, relieving the pain and restoring sensibility. A neuroma of the supraorbital or supratrochlear nerves was reported to occur in only 3 of 179 pin-related halo frame complications previously reported (Grafin, Botte, & Waters, 1986).

Clearly, there must be a greater incidence of nerve injury associated with head and neck injury, but most likely the injuries themselves are often so devastating that the residual numbness or discomfort that occurs from them go unreported. The only study to systematically evaluate a group of patients after pan-facial fractures is that reported by Kesarwani, et al. (1989). Among 20 patients injured from 2 to 6 years previously, they found that 12 had subjective sensory complaints when directly asked about them. These included dysesthesia (6 patients), cold intolerance (4 patients), anesthesia (2 patients), and hyperalgesia (1 patient). When compared statistically, every one of the sensibility tests demonstrated that posttraumatic facial measurements, as a group, were significantly abnormal (see Figures 15.13 &15.14).

The availability of computer-assisted sensory testing techniques should provide useful information about a variety of subjects related to facial trauma (see Figure 15.12). For example, following a mandibular fracture, what percent of the patients lose sensibility in their lip? What percent recover? Once recovery has occurred, can it be assumed to come from regeneration of the inferior alveolar nerve on the injured side, or might sensation have been recovered from collateral sprouting from the ipsilateral buccal nerve or cervical plexus, or from the contralateral inferior alveolar nerve growing across the midline? Use of local anesthetic blocks could provide the answer, followed by repeat sensory testing. Understanding the nature of this regeneration may provide us with alternative reconstructive possibilities following facial injuries.

• ORAL CAVITY RECONSTRUCTION •

The results of the studies that have been done with recovery of sensation in noninnervated flaps (by in-growth of adjacent nerves) and in reinnervated flaps (by microsurgical reconstruction) will be reviewed below (see Table 15.8 & 15.9). The enormous surgical effort given to reconstruct sensation in the oral cavity presupposes that the restored sensibility will provide some functional benefit; yet, in fact, this has not been demonstrated. It seems intuitive that a person who has intraoral sensibility will be better able to position food, swallow, and avoid aspiration. It is also within all of our experience, following a trip to the dentist, to realize the value of having sensibility in the lip with regard to drinking, eating, and speaking. It is also clear after being with a patient who has lost this sensibility due to a stroke or tumor surgery, that their oral function is restricted in many ways. At the very least they bite the inside of their cheek and lip, and they may drool. As with the replantation of fingers, the early effort was directed first at achieving the technical goal of revascularization, with attention to hand function following, finally, in time.

The first pioneering attempts to reconstruct the oral cavity began with the need to provide extensive lining, and free-tissue transfer was used. As with the replantation of digits, the earliest, and even some of the most recent, papers on free-flap reconstruction of the oral cavity (Soutar & McGregor, 1986; Schusterman et al., 1994) are primarily concerned with the percent of the flaps that survive, the percent requiring re-exploration for salvage, and the percent of complications. Oral cavity function is generally not mentioned. It was only thereafter that the possibility of reinnervating these transfers was considered and done, and recovery of sensibility quantitated (Dubner & Heller, 1992). Dubner and Heller demonstrated that 4 mm static two-point discrimination was

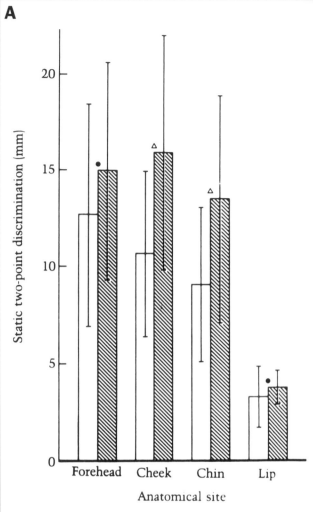

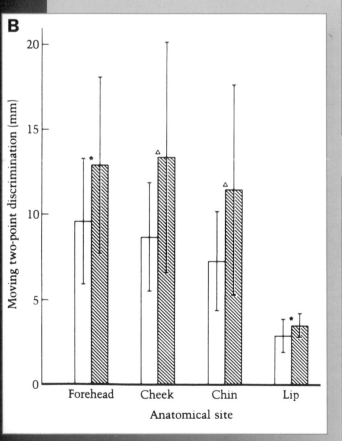

FIGURE 15.13

Changes in facial sensibility following panfacial fractures. (A) Static two-point discrimination. (B) Moving two-point discrimination. (C) Vibratory threshold to 120 Hz stimuli. For each graph, the clear bars represent the mean for 60 normal subjects, while the filled-in bars represent the mean for 20 patients 2 to 6 years after facial trauma. For each graph, the statistical significance between the normal and the facial injury group is indicated to be p < .05 by the black dot, p < .01 by the triangle, and p < .005 by the asterisk. From "Facial Sensibility Testing in the Normal and Posttaumatic Population," by A. Kesarwani, O. Antonyshyn, S. E. Mackinnon, J. S. Gruss, C. Novak, & L. Kelly, 1989, Annals of Plastic Surgery 22:416-425. Reprinted with permission of the authors and with permission of Little, Brown & Co., Inc.

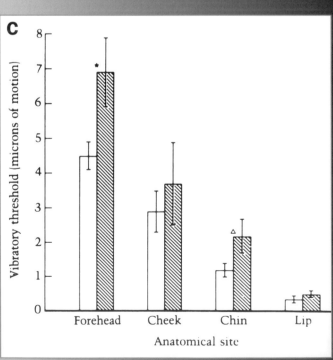

recovered in all three patients they studied, and as the patients recovered sensibility they indicated that they had a better ability to manipulate food intraorally. Studies are underway to assess oral cavity function with respect to swallowing, food handling ability, and aspiration, all functions which can be measured.

There is some support for the value of providing sensibility within the oral cavity for speech. The hearing and speech therapy community has been far in advance of the hand surgery community in designing studies to evaluate function, and in providing rehabilitation. For example, McCroskey (1958) did a very clever experiment to evaluate the relationship between auditory and tactile feedback and speech. A group of 6 normal subjects had a speech sample evaluated by a panel of experts. The subjects received auditory blocking of the normal instantaneous feedback by an imposed delay of 0.18 seconds. At a separate time, they had a block done of the inferior alveolar, the buccal and lingual nerves. The results demonstrated that the rate at which speech progressed was significantly retarded when the auditory feedback was altered, while the loss of oral sensibility caused articulation errors and a significant decrease in speech intelligibility.

This study was repeated

FIGURE 15.14

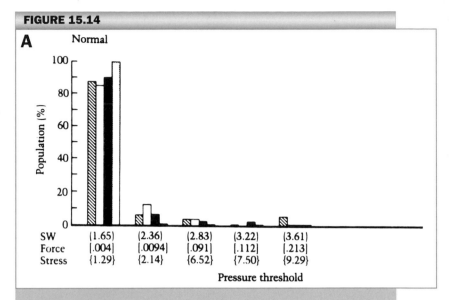

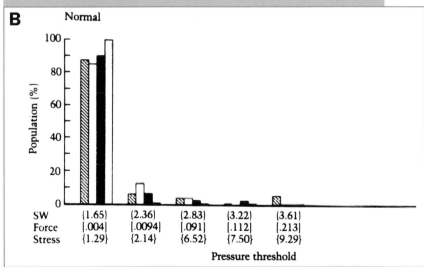

Changes in facial sensibility following pan-facial fractures as estimated with the Semmes-Weinstein nylon monofilaments. The normal group consists of 60 healthy subjects while the posttraumatic group consists of 20 patients 2 to 6 years after facial fracture. The four areas of facial sensibility that are compared are the forehead (diagonal bar to the left), cheek (empty bar), chin (diagonal almost black bar to the right), and lip (grey bar). Force is reported as grams, and stress (pressure) as g/mm². The shift to the right (toward higher cutaneous pressure thresholds) is evident in the posttraumatic group. From "Facial Sensibility Testing in the Normal and Posttraumatic Population," by A. Kesarwani, O. Antonyshyn, S. E. Mackinnon, J. S. Gruss, C. Novak, & L. Kelly, 1989, Annals of Plastic Surgery 22:416-425. Reprinted with permission of the authors and with permission of Little, Brown & Co., Inc.

TABLE 15.8 INTRA-ORAL SENSIBILITY OF INNERVATED AND NONINNERVATED FLAPS, COMPARED TO THE CONTRALATERAL TONGUE

	Intra-Oral Surface			
Sensory Test:	Contralateral (Normal) Tongue	Innervated Radial Forearm Flap	Noninnervated Radial Forearm Flap	Pectoralis (Noninnervated) Flap
Pinprick	100%	100%	10%	0%
Hot/cold	100%	100%	45%	30%
Semmes-Weinstein	7 g/mm^2	14 g/mm^2	27 g/mm^2	430 g/mm^2
Static two-point	4 mm	4 mm	28 mm	30 mm
Moving two-point	3 mm	3 mm	12 mm	> 30 mm

Note: From "Reinnervated Lateral Antebrachial Cutaneous Neurosome Flaps in Oral Reconstruction: Are We Making Sense?" by B. Boyd, S. Mulholland, P. Gullane, & L. Kelly, 1994. *Plastic and Reconstructive Surgery 93:*1350-1359. Reprinted with permission of the authors.

with some methodologic alterations by Ringel and Steer (1963) using 13 normal subjects. They used a topical anesthetic, and also local blocks, and then used them in combination. They found that loss of sensibility caused a significant alteration in mean peak level, articulation and rate variability, mean syllable duration, and mean phonation/time ratio variables, and that these trends were increased; that is, they were made worse by multiple sensory defects. While the definitions of these terms is beyond the scope of this chapter, the conclusion is clear: Impaired oral sensibility results in impaired speech.

One study measured intraoral sensibility in a group of age-stratified healthy subjects and in a group of patients radiated for squamous cell carcinoma of the floor of the mouth and tongue. Aviv, Hecht, Wineberg, Dalton, and Urken (1992) measured static and moving two-point discrimination by cutting a plastic Disk-Criminator™ into 8 triangles and inserting the appropriate distance probe toward the floor of the mouth and the tongue. This normative data is given in Tables 15.10 and 15.11. The irradiated patients are statistically significantly less able to discriminate one from two points, but the mean difference

between the groups is just 1.0 mm. Similarly, the healthy subjects over 61 years of age are statistically significantly less able to discriminate one from two points, but the mean difference is just 1.0 mm. My view of this is that the continual use of the tongue during speech and eating serves to rehabilitate or reeducate the somatosensory cortex, so that the effect of irradiation and aging on the sensory receptors is minimized. The Pressure-Specified Sensory Device™ has been modified for Urken's group to permit better measurement of the oral cavity. In one study, Vriens, Acosta, Soutar, & Webster (1995), at the Plastic

TABLE 15.9 INNERVATED FREE-TISSUE TRANSFERS IN THE ORAL CAVITY

Author/date	Reconstructed Area	Flap Utilized	Cases Nerve	Donor Nerve	Recipient Recovery	Sensory
Matloub, et al., 1989	pharynx	lateral forearm	2	post. cut.	not given	not measured
Urken et al., 1990	pharynx	radial forearm	1	lateral antebr	greater auricular	25 mm 2 pt.static
Sadove, et al., 1991	lower lip & chin	radial	3	lateral forearm	mental antebr	light touch
Urken, et al., 1992	tongue	radial forearm	9	lateral antebr.	lingual	light touch
Dubner, et al., 1992	tongue	radial forearm	3	lateral antebr.	lingual	3 mm 2 pt.static
Boyd, et al., 1994	tongue	radial forearm	8	lateral antebr.	lingual	3 mm 2 pt. moving

Note: From "Sensory Recovery in Innervated Free-tissue Transfers," by B. Graham & A. L. Dellon, 1995, *Journal of Reconstructive Microsurgery 11:*157-166. Reprinted with permission of the authors.

TABLE 15.10 TWO-POINT DISCRIMINATION IN THE ORAL CAVITY: HEALTHY CONTROLS

Region	Mean two-point Discrimination*	
	Static (mm)	Moving (mm)
Tongue tip	2.6 ± 0.6	2.4 ± 0.5
Lateral dorsal tongue	4.5 ± 1.4	3.7 ± 1.1
Lateral ventral tongue	6.4 ± 2.0	4.9 ± 1.6
Floor of mouth	7.3 ± 2.3	6.6 ± 1.6

Note:
*n=60 healthy subjects 20-80 years of age.
From "Surface Sensibility of the Floor of the Mouth and Tongue in Healthy Controls and in Radiated Patients," by J. E. Aviv, C. Hecht, H. Wineberg, J. F. Dalton, & M. L. Urken, 1992, *Otolaryngology and Head and Neck Surgery 107:*418-422. Reprinted with permission of the authors.

TABLE 15.11 TWO-POINT DISCRIMINATION IN THE ORAL CAVITY: IRRADIATED PATIENTS		
	Mean two-point Discrimination*	
Region	**Static (mm)**	**Moving (mm)**
Tongue tip	2.9	2.9
Lateral dorsal tongue	5.7	5.4
Lateral ventral tongue	6.7	6.4
Floor of mouth	8.7	7.9

Note:

*$n=20$ cancer patients, mean age 50. These values are each significantly greater than the age-matched values from Table 15.10, $p < .05$.

From "Surface Sensibility of the Floor of the Mouth and Tongue in Healthy Controls and in Radiated Patients," by J. E. Aviv, C. Hecht, H. Wineberg, J. F. Dalton, & M. L. Urken, 1992, *Otolaryngology and Head and Neck Surgery 107:*418-422. Reprinted with permission of the authors.

and Oral Surgery Unit at Canniesburn Hospital, Glasgow, Scotland, evaluated the recovery of sensation in 40 radial forearm flaps transferred by microvascular technique into the oral cavity. None of these flaps was reinnervated by direct microneurosurgical techniques. Sensibility was evaluated by light moving touch, two-point discrimination, pain perception, and temperature perception between 6 months and 11 years after tissue transfer. Four (10%) of the flaps were anesthetic, 21 flaps (53%) recovered partly, and 15 flaps (37%) had perception of all sensory modalities tested in at least two-thirds of the flap area. All patients who had good sensibility in the area surrounding the area reconstructed with the flap recovered good sensation in the flap. This suggests that these flaps can be reinnervated by the surrounding tissues, just as has been shown for flaps placed into other areas of the body.

While there have been encouraging reports of innervated flaps used for intraoral reconstruction, for example, from Urken and Biller's Otorhinolaryngology Department at Mount Sinai Hospital in New York City (Urken & Biller, 1994), the most exciting report with regard to evaluation of sensibility in the oral cavity is that from Boyd, Mulholland, and Gullane (1994) of the Plastic Surgery Department at the University of Toronto. Their therapist, Louis Kelly, evalu-ated 8 innervated radial forearm flaps that had their lateral antebrachial cutaneous nerve repaired to the lingual nerve, 10 noninnervated radial forearm flaps, and 10 pectoralis major flaps that had been used for intraoral reconstruction. In each flap, and in the contralateral (normal) tongue, the cutaneous pressure threshold was estimated with the Semmes-Weinstein nylon monofilaments, static and moving two-point discrimination were measured with the Disk-Criminator™, the perception of pain was tested with a needle, and the perception of hot and cold was tested.

Table 15.8 gives the results of this study, which demonstrated that in all modalities examined, the reinnervated radial forearm flap proved statistically significantly superior to the noninnervated radial forearm flap and to the (noninnervated) pectoralis flap, and proved to be not significantly different from the contralateral tongue. The sensibility recovered in the innervated flaps in the oral cavity was significantly better than the normal sensibility in that flap in its normal location on the forearm. The ability to chew food was rated subjectively by the patients against the value of 10 for the normal side of their mouth, with the finding that the reinnervated flap scored a 7 versus the noninnervated flap which scored a 3, and the pectoralis flap which scored a 2. The authors concluded that the degree of sensibility recovered was related to the degree of cortical importance given to the area of innervated skin rather then to the innervation density of the skin, since the innervated flap had developed better sensibility and function as a sensory flap intraorally than it had on the forearm.

A review of sensory recovery in innervated free tissue transfers to the oral cavity (Graham & Dellon, 1995) demonstrates that the best results have been achieved when the flap donor nerve is neurotized by the lingual nerve, at least for the anterior floor of mouth and

tongue reconstruction (see Table 15.9).

• • •

*N*ow with our ability to determine true sensory loss, disability can be assessed and then surgical or medical treatment initiated and assessed. The objective evaluation of treatment that is now available should result in improved rehabilitation.

Posnick, Zimbler, & Grossman, 1994

• • •

• REHABILITATION •

The principles that guide sensory rehabilitation elsewhere in the body may be applied to the head and neck region, as well. As evident from the discussion about loss of inferior alveolar nerve function after injury from dental extraction or panfacial fractures, or after stretch/traction injuries during orthognathic surgery, if the injury by its nature permits neural regeneration, this will occur with the dysesthesias that occur in the extremities. If the injury by its nature results in loss of neural integrity, then pain results from the neuroma, and pain relief and restoration of function can occur through nerve reconstruction. The intraoral application of these principles is now at the level where reconstruction of the oral cavity with free flaps can be done so as to reinnervate these flaps with the goal of restoring oral function.

Particular rehabilitation goals, as always, will require ingenuity on the part of the therapist. To desensitize the lip, it may be appropriate, in addition to gentle massage techniques, to suck on straws of different textures, blow on a whistle, or blow bubbles. For a woman, putting on lipstick may be a useful technique. For the intraoral sensory rehabilitation, simply speaking, eating, and swallowing provide a huge amount of stimulation. Additional stimulation may be possible by chewing gum and practicing identification of different intraoral shapes or foods of differing textures.

• • •

• REFERENCES •

Aviv, J. E., Hecht, C., Wineberg, H., Dalton, J. F., & Urken, M. L. Surface sensibility of the floor of the mouth and tongue in healthy controls and in radiated patients. *Otolaryngology and Head and Neck Surgery* 107:418-422, 1992.

Bosma, J. F. *Symposium on Oral Sensation and Perception.* Springfield, IL: Charles C Thomas, Publisher, 1967.

Boyd, B., Mulholland, S., Gullane, P., & Kelly, L. Reinnervated lateral antebrachial cutaneous neurosome flaps in oral reconstruction: Are we making sense? *Plastic and Reconstructive Surgery* 93:1350-1359, 1994.

Costas, P. D., Heatley, G., & Seckel, B. R. Normal sensation of the human face and neck. *Plastic and Reconstructive Surgery* 93:1141-1145, 1994.

Dellon, A. L. *Evaluation of Sensibility and Re-Education of Sensation in the Hand.* Baltimore: Williams & Wilkins, 1981.

Dellon, A. L., & Crawley, W. A. Nerve reconstruction with alloplastic material in the head and neck region. *Oral Maxillofacial Surgery Clinics - North America* 4:527-533, 1992.

Dellon, E. S., & Dellon, A. L. The first nerve graft, Vulpian and the 19th century neural regeneration controversy. *Journal of Hand Surgery* 4:1993.

Dubner, S., & Heller, K. S. Re-innervated radial forearm free flaps in head and neck reconstruction. *Journal of Reconstructive Microsurgery* 8:467-468, 1992.

Dyck, P. J., Karnes, J., O'Brien, P. C., & Zimmerman, I. R. Detection thresholds of cutaneous sensation in humans. In *Peripheral Neuropathy,* P. J. Dyck, P. K. Thomas, J. W. Griffin, P. A. Low, & J. F. Poduslo, Editors. Philadelphia: W. B. Saunders Company, 1993.

Evans, G. R. D., Crawley, W., & Dellon, A. L. Inferior alveolar nerve reconstruction. *Annals of Plastic Surgery* 33:221-224, 1994.

Friedman, R. M., Rohrich, R. J., & Finn, S. S. Management of traumatic supraorbital neuroma. *Annals of Plastic Surgery* 28:573-574, 1992.

Fucci, D., Harris, D., & Petrosino, L. Sensation magnitude scales for vibrotactile stimulation of the tongue and thenar eminence. *Perception and Motor Skills* 58:843-848, 1984.

Grafin, S. R., Botte, M. J., & Waters, R. L. Complications associated with the use of the halo fixation device. *Journal of Bone and Joint Surgery* 68:320-325, 1986.

Graham, B., & Dellon, A. L. Sensory recovery in innervated free-tissue transfers. *Journal of Reconstructive Microsurgery* 11:157-166, 1995.

Kesarwani, A., Antonyshyn, O., Mackinnon, S. E., Gruss, J. S., Novak, C., & Kelly, L. Facial sensibility testing in the normal and posttraumatic population. *Annals of Plastic Surgery* 22:416-421, 1989.

Levin, S., Pearsall, G., & Ruderman, R. S. von Fry's method of measuring pressure sensibility in the hand: An engineering analysis of the Weinstein-Semmes Pressure Aesthisiometer. *Journal of Hand Surgery* 3:211-216, 1978.

Lindquist, C. C., & Obeid, G. Complications of genioplasty done alone or in combination with sagittal split ramus osteotomy. *Journal of Oral Surgery* 66:13-17, 1988.

Masson, D. A. Lingual nerve damage following lower third molar surgery. *International Journal of Oral Maxillofacial Surgery* 17:290-294, 1988.

McCroskey, R. L., Jr. The relative contribution of auditory and tactile cues to certain aspects of speech. *Southern Speech Journal* 24:84-90, 1958.

Nishioka, G. J., Zysset, M. K., & VanSickels, J. E. Neurosensory disturbances with rigid fixation of the bilateral sagittal split osteotomy. *Journal of Oral Maxillofacial Surgery* 45:20-24, 1987.

Pennisi, E., Cruccu, G., Manfredi, M., & Palladini, G. Histometric study of myelinated fibers in the human trigeminal nerve. *Journal of Neurological Sciences* 105:22-28, 1991.

Pernkopf, Eduard. *Eduard Pernkopf's Atlas of Topographical and Applied Human Anatomy,*

Helmut Ferner, Editor. Philadelphia: W. B. Saunders Company, 1964.

Posnick, J. C., Al-Qattan, M. M., & Pron, G. Facial sensibility in adolescents with and without clefts one year after undergoing LeForte I osteotomy. *Plastic and Reconstructive Surgery 94*:431-435, 1994.

Posnick, J. C., Al-Qattan, M. M., & Stepner, N. M. Facial sensibility in adolescents one year after undergoing sagittal split and chin osteotomies of the mandible. *Plastic and Reconstructive Surgery,* in press: 1996.

Posnick, J. C., Zimbler, A. G., & Grossman, J. A. I. Normal cutaneous sensibility of the face. *Plastic and Reconstructive Surgery 86*:429-433, 1990.

Ringel, R. L., & Steer, M. D. Some effects of tactile and auditory alterations on speech output. *Journal of Speech and Hearing Research 6*:369-378, 1963.

Robinson, P. P., Smith, K. G., Johnson, F. P., & Coppins, D. A. Equipment and methods for simple sensory testing. *British Journal of Oral Maxillofacial Surgery 30*:387-389, 1992.

Rood, J. P. Degrees of injury to the inferior alveolar nerve sustained during the removal of impacted mandibular third molars by the lingual split technique. *British Journal of Oral Surgery 21*:103-116, 1983.

Schusterman, M. A., Miller, M. J., Reece, G. P., Kroll, S. S., Marchi, M., & Goepfert, H. A single center's experience with 308 free flaps for repair of head and neck cancer defects. *Plastic and Reconstructive Surgery 93*:472-478, 1994.

Soutar, D. S., & McGregor, I. A. The radial forearm flap in intraoral reconstruction: The experience of 60 consecutive cases. *Plastic and Reconstructive Surgery 78*:1-8, 1986.

Stein, B. E., & Meredith, M. A. *The Merging of the Senses*. Cambridge, MA: MIT Press, 1993.

Urken, M. L., & Biller, H. F. A new bilobed design for the sensate radial forearm flap to preserve tongue mobility following significant glossectomy. *Archives of Otolaryngological Head and Neck Surgery 120*:26-29, 1994.

von Fry, M. The distribution of afferent nerves in the skin. *Journal of the American Medical Association 47*:645-648, 1908.

Vriens, J. P. M., Acosta, R., Soutar, D. S., & Webster, M. H. C. Recovery of sensation in the radial forearm free flap in oral reconstruction. *Journal of Reconstructive Microsurgery,* submitted:1995.

Vriens, J. P. M., Moos, M. B., & Scott, E. M. Evaluation of normal values for static and dynamic two-point discrimination and for static light touch sensation in the face. *Plastic and Reconstructive Surgery*, submitted: 1994.

Weber, E. Ueber den Tatsinn. Archive fur Anatomy und Physiology. *Wissenshaft Medical Muller's Archives 1*:152-159, 1835.

Wofford, D. T., & Miller, R. I. Prospective study of dysesthesia following odontectomy of impacted mandibular third molars. *Journal of Oral Maxillofacial Surgery 45*:15-19, 1987.

• ADDITIONAL READINGS •

Dellon, A. L. Management of peripheral nerve injuries: Basic principles of microneurosurgical repair. *Oral Maxillofacial Surgery Clinics - North America 4*:393-403, 1992.

Dellon, A. L. Testing for facial sensibility. *Plastic and Reconstructive Surgery 87*:1140-1141, 1991.

Merrill, R. G. Prevention, treatment and prognosis for nerve injury related to the difficult impaction. *Dental Clinics — North America 23*:471-488, 1979.

Posnick, J. C., Al-Qattan, M. M., Pron, G. E., & Grossman, J. A. I. Facial sensibility in adolescents born with cleft lip after undergoing repair in infancy. *Plastic and Reconstructive Surgery 93*:682-689, 1994.

Smith, K. G., & Robinson, P. P. Does a delay prior to lingual nerve repair prejudice the outcome? *British Journal of Oral Maxillofacial Surgery 31*:57, 1993.

• • •

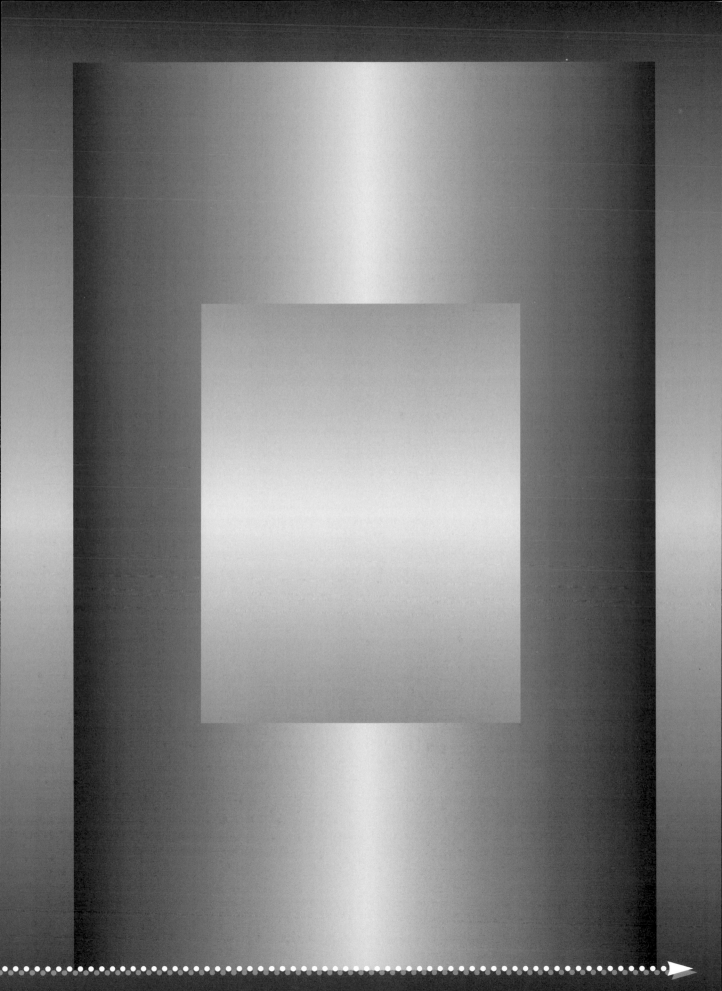

the breast

• RELEVANT NEUROANATOMY •

There is agreement that the breast is a modified sweat gland and, as such, is innervated by the cutaneous nerves. Located on the anterior chest wall, the breast is innervated by the intercostal nerves that go to this region of skin. The cervical plexus, by means of its supraclavicular branches (C4-5), also extends on to the anterior chest wall and provides sensation to the superior and central quadrant of the breast skin (see Figure 16.1). The basic anatomical plan for the intercostal nerve to the breast is given in Figure 16.2. The skin of the breast that is not innervated by the supraclavicular nerve is innervated by the 2nd through the 6th intercostal nerves. The intercostal nerve has a lateral branch that exists in the anterior axillary line and is, therefore, called its lateral branch. This branch then goes both posterior and anterior. The anterior branch will innervate the lateral aspect of the breast, and is called the lateral ramus. The terminal branch of the intercostal nerve turns up to innervate the medial chest skin at the sternum, and is called the medial ramus.

The final termination of the intercostal nerves into the skin of the breast and the nipple/areolar complex has been evaluated. There are few intraepithelial endings. Only a few corpuscular endings have been observed, and they appear to be similar to the mucocutaneous end organ. Definite

Meissner and Pacinian corpuscles have not been observed. Rather, innervated hair follicles and a rich plexus of nonmyelinated nerve fibers in the dermis are found. The muscle fibers that create nipple erection are innervated. It is probably the hair follicles in the nipple/areolar region that give rise to sensory organization, more like hairy than glabrous skin.

Several anatomic studies have determined that it is the lateral ramus of the 4th intercostal nerve that innervates the nipple/areolar complex, and that it enters this complex at the 4 o'clock position for the left breast, and the 8 o'clock position for the right breast. However, there is still no clear description of the exact pathway through the soft tissues that the lateral ramus takes to reach this destination. For example, it has been described as reaching the nipple/areolar complex from "the depth of the breast," or as remaining deep until midway to the nipple/ areolar complex and then becoming superficial. From my own clinical observations during surgery, I have never seen intercostal nerve branches entering the breast on its deep surface, that is, going upward or superficial from the surface of the pectoralis fascia. This plane is totally open all the time during a subglandular breast augmentation, when the implant is placed between the breast and the pectoralis muscle.

FIGURE 16.1

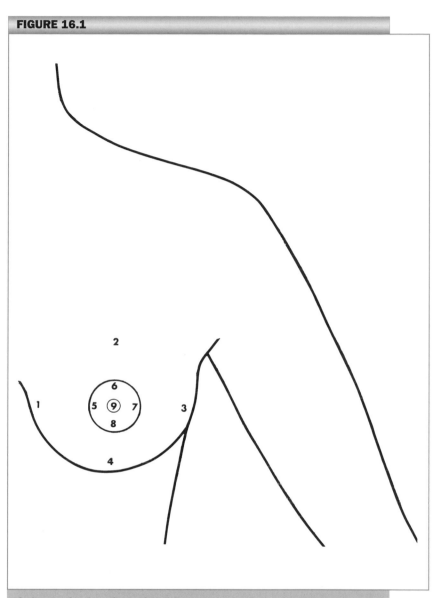

Schematic drawing of the breast to indicate regions of sensibility testing as they are referred to in the text. Region 2 is innervated by the supraclavicular nerves of the cervical plexus, originating in C 4 and 5. The rest of the breast is innervated by branches of the 2nd through 6th intercostal nerves. Region 1 is innervated by the medial ramus of the anterior cutaneous branch of the intercostal. Regions 3, 4, 7, and 8 are innervated by the lateral ramus of the lateral cutaneous branch of the intercostal. It is unclear which nerve innervates regions 5 and 6. From "The Sensational Transverse Rectus Abdominous Musculocutaneous Flap: Return of Sensation After TRAM Breast Reconstruction," by S. Slezak, B. McGibbon, & A. L. Dellon, 1992, Annals of Plastic Surgery 28:210-217. Reprinted with permission of the authors and with permission of Little, Brown & Co., Inc.

FIGURE 16.2

Schematic drawing of the basic intercostal nerve plan as it relates to the breast. The exact anatomic course of the terminal branches of the nerve into the nipple/areolar complex remains to be determined. From "The Sensational Transverse Rectus Abdominous Musculocutaneous Flap: Return of Sensation After TRAM Breast Reconstruction," by S. Slezak, B. McGibbon, & A. L. Dellon, 1992, Annals of Plastic Surgery 28:210-217. Reprinted with permission of the authors.

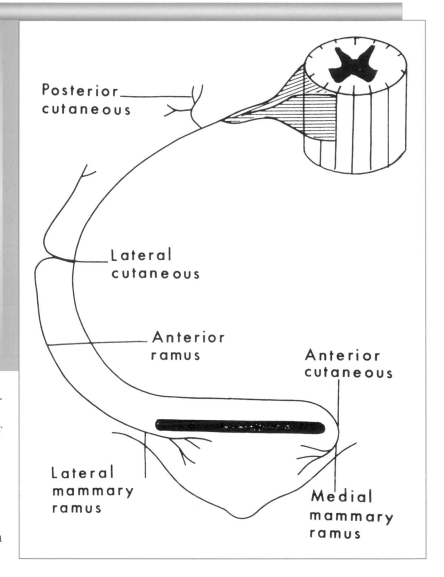

I have never seen the intercostal nerve branches entering directly into the dermis of the nipple/areolar complex. The entire nipple/areolar complex is removed during a breast reduction, in which the breast is amputated and the nipple/areolar is removed as a full thickness graft to be used in the breast reconstruction. I also have not seen nerves going into the substance of the breast during any of the techniques used for breast excision during reduction mammaplasty. Certainly, these intercostal nerves do innervate the breast, but there is a need for further studies to determine the exact anatomic pathway so we might better appreciate the design of flaps for breast surgery, and to enable us to reinnervate the breast during reconstruction.

• NORMATIVE DATA •

Based on neuroanatomy and common experience, it is reasonable to assume that the breast is capable of transmitting the same perceptions as other regions of skin, with the added physiological requirement of neuroendocrine function for lactation, and the added psychological function of erotic sensation. Erotic sensation cannot be directly measured, but may be assessed subjectively by questionnaire. Pain perception has been studied with the Vitapulp™, a dental electrical stimulator for nerve root viability, and the Staodyn™, another electrical stimulator. Temperature sensibility has been tested with metal probes heated in hot water to 115°F, or cooled in ice water to 32°F. It is clear that pain and temperature perception are critical for protective sensibility (see Figure 16.3), and that the breast without protective sensibility is at risk for injury. Vibration has been tested with a 30 Hz and 256 Hz tuning fork, and with the Biothesiometer™ at 120 Hz. Pressure perception has been tested with the Semmes-Weinstein nylon monofilaments. Two-point discrimination has been tested with the Disk-Criminator™.

Available normative data for eleven women (22 breasts) between 20 and 60 years of age, bra size not specified, and for ten women (20 breasts) between 23 and 35 years of age, bra size either A or B, are given in Tables 16.1 and 16.2, respectively. Another group of 27 normal breasts (8 normal and 10 masotpexied breasts) in women whose ages were not stated was evaluated by Shaw, Orringer, Ratto, and Mersmann (1989). These values are given in Table 16.3. Sensibility in breasts that are exceptionally large, bra size of at least D, is discussed in the section on breast reduction because breasts of this size probably should not be considered as always having normal sensibility.

The quickly-adapting and slowly-adapting fiber systems are present, as evidenced by the thresholds for vibratory perception and pressure perception, but their thresholds are higher than for the fin-

FIGURE 16.3

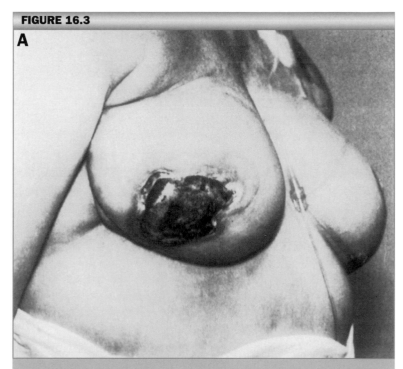

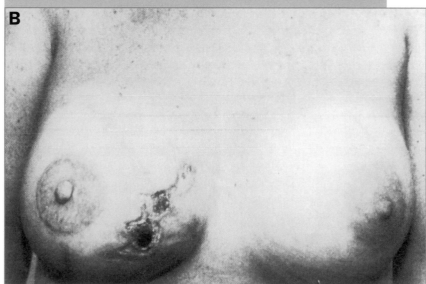

The reconstructed breast after mastectomy may be devoid of protective sensation. Without the ability to perceive pain or temperature stimuli, the reconstructed breast is at risk of injury, as exemplified by these patients who sustained burns from a heating pad in a breast reconstructed with a latissimus dorsi flap (A) and a transverse rectus abdominous flap (B). From "Second and Third-degree Burns as a Complication in Breast Reconstruction," by G. P. Maxwell & R. Tornambe, 1989, Annals of Plastic Surgery 22:386-390. Reprinted with permission of the authors.

gertip or the lip. These thresholds are appropriate to measure when evaluating breast sensibility. Innervation density, as judged by the ability to discriminate one from two points, is poor, and therefore static and moving two-point discrimination are not appropriate sensibility testing measurements to apply to the breast. The pain perception threshold in the nipple and breast skin is the highest, with the most sensitive region for pain being the areola.

Nipple erectility has also been measured (Terzis, Vincent, Wilkins, Rutledge, & Deane, 1987). The mean time to achieve nipple erec-

tion after squeezing the nipple was 21.8 seconds (range 6 to 45 seconds).

It appears, therefore, that the best tests of sensibility for evaluating the breast are the vibratory and static pressure perception thresholds, and that it is inappropriate to measure two-point discrimination. While it is possible to measure the perception of temperature and pain, these perceptions appear to be unrelated to breast function. Breast function, in terms of being an organ for lactation, requires relative insensitivity to pressure, pain, and temperature, and relative sensitivity to oscillating motion. That oscil-

lating motion may be measured by the vibratory threshold, as has been done in the past, or with the Pressure-Specified Sensory Device™ in the future, as this device can measure the moving-touch threshold. The moving-touch threshold should evaluate the same quickly-adapting nerve fiber population as the vibratory perception threshold, but the moving-touch threshold is probably easier to obtain and more reliable. The currently available vibrometers are force-dependent, meaning that if the examiner presses too hard on the breast with the vibrating probe, the probe's oscillation

TABLE 16.1 BREAST SENSIBILITY THRESHOLDS

Region of Breast	Semmes-Weinstein g/mm² (mean ±)*	Biothesiometer μm (mean ±)*	Pain mamps	Temperature % hot	% cold
Nipple	3.4 ± 0.1	8.3 ± .06	255	100	100
Areola	3.8 ± 0.1	9.0 ± .39	123	75	84
Skin	3.3 ± 0.1	10.7 ± .49	261	91	97

Note: *There appears to be a significant discrepancy between the absolute values for the thresholds for pressure and vibration obtained by the two different investigators when Table 16.1 is compared to Table 16.2. The most reasonable explanation for this is that while the heading of Table 16.1 indicates that the pressure threshold was recorded as g/mm², it was probably calculated as the nylon filament marking; that is, a filament marking of 3.8 generates a pressure of 19.3 g/mm², which is of the same order of magnitude as the value in Table 16.2. Similarly, while the heading for Table 16.1 indicates that the vibratory threshold is in microns, it was probably read from the Biothesiometer as volts; that is, a voltage of 8 correlates with .66 microns of motion, which is then of the same order of magnitude as the value in Table 16.2. From "Breast Sensibility: A Neurophysiologic Appraisal in the Normal Breast," by J. K. Terzis, M. P. Vincent, L. M. Wilkins, K. Rutledge, & L. M. Deane, 1987, *Annals of Plastic Surgery 19:*318-322. Reprinted with permission of the authors.

TABLE 16.2 BREAST SENSIBILITY THRESHOLDS

Region of breast	Semmes-Weinstein` g/mm² (mean ±)	Biothesiometer μm (mean ±)
Nipple	28.5 ± 7	0.3 ± .2
Areola	31.6 ± 4	0.1 ± .1
Skin	23.1 ± 13	0.4 ± .3

Note: From "The Sensational Transverse Rectus Abdominous Musculocutaneous Flap: Return of Sensation After TRAM Breast Reconstruction," by S. Slezak, B. McGibbon & A. L. Dellon, 1992, *Annals of Plastic Surgery 28*:210-217, 1992. Reprinted with permission of the authors.

is damped. The dial on the vibrometer is still reading the amount of current or voltage that is going into the vibrating device, and converting that voltage into microns of displacement or motion. The vibrometer was calibrated against air, and not against the pressure of breast skin. Thus, pressing the probe into the breast damps the vibration and gives an inaccurate reading. This is probably the basis for the difference in vibratory perception found between Tables 16.1 and 16.2 for different areas of the breast. The future will see studies identical to those referred to below but with the cutaneous thresholds being obtained with the Pressure-Specified Sensory Device™. Because this device reads out directly in units of pressure, that is, g/mm², its use will prevent the confusion that continues to be associated with the

TABLE 16.3 BREAST SENSIBILITY THRESHOLDS

Region of breast	Semmes-Weinstein g/mm² (mean ±)*
Nipple/areola	1.28 ± .48

Note: *There appears to be a significant discrepancy between the absolute values for the thresholds for pressure obtained by the two different investigators when Table 16.3 is compared to 16.2. The most reasonable explanation for this is that while the heading of Table 16.3 indicates that the pressure threshold was recorded as g/mm², it was probably calculated as the milligrams of force; that is, a filament marking of 4.08 generates a force of 1.20 mg which, after correction for the cross-sectional area of the filament, gives a pressure of 29.3 g/mm², which is then of the same order of magnitude as the value in Table 16.2.
From data presented at the 68th annual meeting of the American Association of Plastic Surgeons, by W. W. Shaw, J. S. Orringer, L. L. Ratto, & C. A. Mersmann, Scottsdale, AZ, May 10, 1989. Reprinted with permission of Dr. Shaw.

Semmes-Weinstein nylon monofilaments, such as the differences in the normal pressure threshold for the breast reported in three different studies (see Tables 16.1, 16.2, and 16.3).

One final interpretation of the normative breast sensibility data is required. There is a difference in the volume between a breast that is a bra size A, and a breast that is a bra size D. The difference in volume is directly related to a difference in the surface area of the breast, that is, the amount of skin required to cover it. There are only a given number of axons in every intercostal nerve. It follows, therefore, that the innervation density of a bra size A breast will be different from that of a bra size B breast. By definition, therefore, there may be expected to be a difference in sensibility between a woman with mammary hypertrophy and one with a "normal" size breast (Slezak & Dellon, 1993).

A confounding variable in this concept of breast sensation is the erotic nature of the breast. In this context, sensibility is related to breast function. All the psychological factors from childhood through adulthood that are related to the female breast and to self-image may impact on the neural impulses generated when the breast is physically stimulated. Clearly, the interpretation of the neural impulses depends on many factors other than the simplistic notion of the number of nerve fiber types and the amount of skin available for those endings. Availability of quantitative sensory testing may provide data to explore these different relationships.

• BREAST AUGMENTATION *

The majority of writing about breast augmentation is related to surgical technique, such as the type of implant (silicone gel-filled or saline-filled), the location of the implant (subglandular or subpectoral), the location of the incision for the surgery (inframammary, periareolar, axillary), or now even endoscopic (through the umbilicus). A second major focus of writing about breast augmentation is related to its potential complications, such as capsular contracture (the implant feeling harder due to encapsulation by fibrous tissue), leakage of silicone outside the breast implant, implant rupture, breast cancer related to the implant, host immune response to the implant, and more routine possibilities for complications like bleeding and infection.

When breast augmentation is done for the purpose of simply increasing the size of the normal female breast, that is, not for breast reconstruction, then any complications are almost intolerable. It is interesting, therefore, to look at what the literature has to say about the risk of sensory changes after breast augmentation. In fact, changes in breast sensation are reported to occur in more than 40% of patients (see Table 16.4). These changes may range in degree from a permanent loss of all sensation to temporary loss of some sensation. Some patients even report heightened sensation after breast augmentation. Most importantly for the purposes of this book, it is important to note that none of the studies that have reported sensory changes in the breast after breast augmentation have documented those changes with quantitative sensory testing. The reports have relied on interviewing techniques and questionnaires to gain information retrospectively. It would be meaningful to obtain baseline sensory measurements in women prior to, at 1 month after, and at 6 months after breast augmentation. The Pressure-Specified Sensory Device™ provides the measurements necessary for such a study.

Computer-assisted measurements can also be used to analyze the confounding variable of breast hardness related to capsular contracture. Up to 40% of women believe that their breast implants are too hard. In reality, the implant itself does not change; rather, the body generates a fibrous capsule around the breast implant, just as it does around an ar-

TABLE 16.4 SENSORY CHANGES AFTER BREAST AUGMENTATION

| Date of report | Anesthesia | Percentage of Patients With | | Normal |
		Hypesthesia	Hyperesthesia	
1979		49%		
1985		33%	8%	
1993	4%	23%	11%	48%

Note: Subjective response of patients to questionnaire, not quantitative sensory testing. From questionnaire devised by W. W. Shaw, J. S. Orringer, L. L. Ratto, & C. A. Mersmann, presented at the 68th annual meeting of the American Association of Plastic Surgeons, Scottsdale, AZ, May 10, 1989. Reprinted with permission of Dr. Shaw.

tificial joint. The degree of capsular hardness can be modified by such techniques as (a) minimizing postoperative bleeding and infection, which would increase scarring; (b) placing the implant into a subpectoral location instead of subglandular, which puts the implant into a muscle environment with its better blood supply and frequent massaging effect of the underlying implant; (c) adding steroid to the inside of the implant or the wound pocket, which will biochemically alter scar formation; and (d) giving the patient a postoperative exercise regimen, which will apply a force counter to that of the spherical contracture.

At present, the only accepted grading system for the degree of capsular contracture, or breast hardness, is the Baker Classification which, simply stated, is that Class I is a normal appearing and feeling breast, while

a Class IV is a rounded, hard, physically contracted breast. Class II looks normal but feels slightly harder than normal. Class III appears abnormal and is clearly more firm than normal. A classification that was based on some measure of breast compliance, or on how breast compliance was altered by the capsule formed around the implant, would be ideal. The computer-assisted Breast Compliance Device™ (see Figure 16.4) can obtain measurements of the breast in four quadrants and over the nipple, so that the development of capsular contracture may be followed over time. This device is similar to the device to measure skin compliance (see Chapter 7), but has been modified to give its probe a larger surface area and a greater depth of displacement to make it appropriate to measure the breast versus the fingertip.

The device in my office has proven to be sensitive enough to detect changes in breast hardness. Hardness is the inverse of compliance (softness). In women with mammary hypoplasia who desire a breast augmentation, the Breast Compliance Device™ is capable of measuring changes associated with capsular contracture (see Figure 16.5) and implant rupture (see Figure 16.6). A disadvantage of this device has been observed in the large breast that is augmented. There may be a capsular contracture around the implant, but the large amount of overlying soft breast tissue gives a Breast Compliance Device™ measurement that is low, instead of measuring the region deep within the breast that has the hardness associated with it.

Areas for future investigation by the therapist in association with the plastic surgeon (in addition to those

FIGURE 16.4

Breast Compliance Device™. This device measures the skin compliance of the breast. (A) The device is held against the breast quadrant being measured, and (B) pressed in until the base of the device touches the skin. The more resistance met, the higher the pressure needed to depress the probe. These measurements are useful to follow the development, or lack thereof, of capsular contracture. In (C), the pre-op and 3-month post-op pressure measurements (skin hardness) are recorded. (Hardness is the inverse of compliance.) Note the increase in hardness, representing the presence of a modest capsular contracture in these normal-appearing breasts. Breast quadrants are labelled upper and lower, inner and outer (UO, UI, LO, LI).

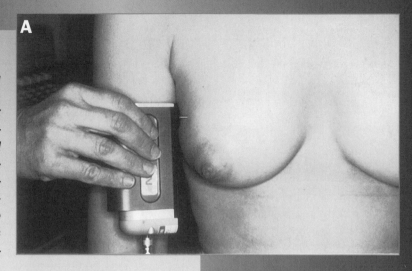

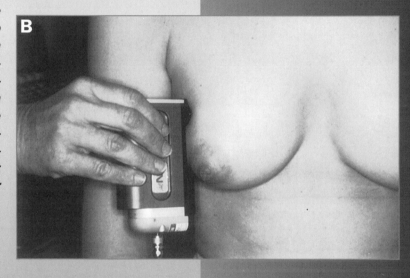

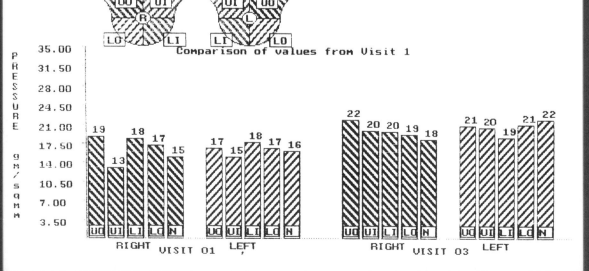

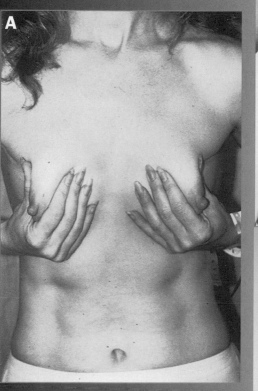

A

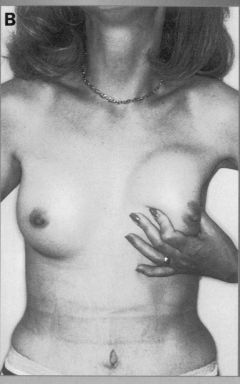

B

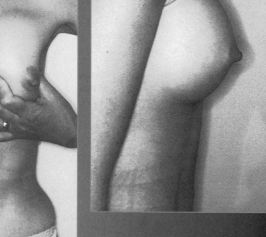

C

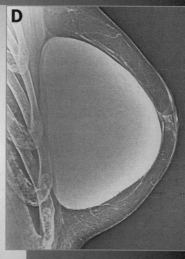

D

FIGURE 16.5
Breast compliance device. (A) Preoperative illustrating softness of breasts. (B) One year postoperatively there are marked capsular contractures as noted by loss of compressibility. (C) and (D) Lateral views 1 year postoperatively with capsular contracture evident visually and on mammogram. Implant is located submuscularly. (E) The pre-op versus post-op breast hardness measurements document the increased pressure required to compress the breast. (The N measurement is the nipple.)

E

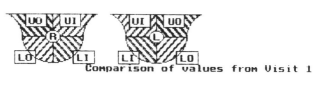

Comparison of values from Visit 1

PRESSURE gm/sqmm

		70.00
		63.00
		56.00
		49.00
		42.00
		35.00
		28.00
		21.00
		14.00
		7.00

RIGHT — VISIT 01 — LEFT

UO 12, UI 11, LI 11, LO 10, N 12 (RIGHT)
UO 11, UI 12, LI 10, LO 11, N 11 (LEFT)

RIGHT — VISIT 03 — LEFT

UO 42, UI 40, LI 38, LO 38, N 40 (RIGHT)
UO 41, UI 41, LI 37, LO 38, N 39 (LEFT)

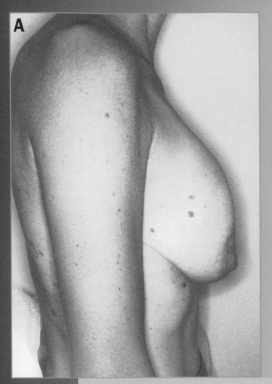

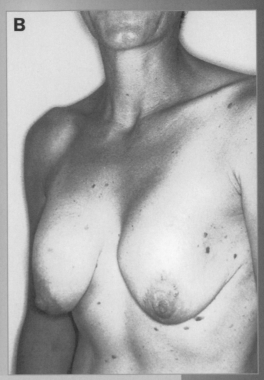

FIGURE 16.6

Breast Compliance Device™. (A) This 43-year-old woman is 7 years after bilateral breast augmentation. During those 7 years breast ptosis has developed so that the nipple-areolar complex has descended below the implant, as noted in this right lateral view. (B) The left three-quarter oblique view demonstrates a ruptured left breast implant, with silicone having migrated upward and laterally. (C) The superior view of the left breast demonstrates the implant rupture as the lateral bulge. (D) The breast harness measurements demonstrate the firmness of the right breast and the increased harness over the upper outer and upper inner left breast in the region of the rupture. Note that the ptotic, hanging nipple-areolar complex (N) is the softest area of each breast.

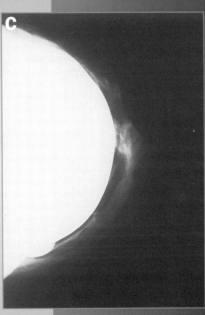

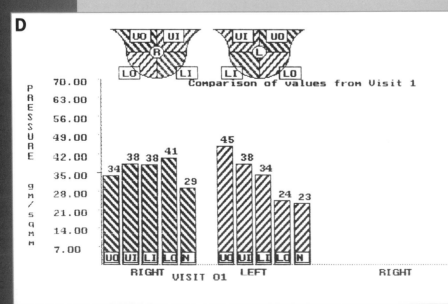

in Chapter 20), would be to evaluate with quantitative sensory testing the sensory changes associated with different surgical incisions, the sensory changes associated with different implant locations, and the sensory changes associated with capsular contracture. With regard to the latter problem, many patients with capsular contracture have breast pain. It is possible that this is due to the intercostal nerves becoming adherent in the capsular scarring, and this may be detected by quantitative sensory testing with the Pressure-Specified Sensory Device™ as a chronic nerve compression.

● BREAST REDUCTION ●

During residency training in plastic surgery, I was taught to inform patients who were seeking a consultation regarding breast reduction that one of its possible complications was the loss of sensation in the breast. This was most likely to occur in the breast reduction technique in which the nipple/areolar complex is totally excised from a very large breast, the breast is then amputated, and the nipple/areola is repositioned as a free, full thickness graft. This is in contrast to techniques for large, but not enormous, breasts in which the nipple/areolar complex is left attached to the breast, and is transposed to its new location by a pedicle of breast tissue.

To my surprise, this potential complication posed little concern to most patients seeking breast reduction because, as they often indicated, they had "little sensation" in their breasts anyway. Furthermore, postoperatively, many patients indicated that they had better feeling in their breasts than they did before surgery. In fact, patients who had a free nipple/areola graft would tell me they had sensation in the graft at the time the sutures were removed. While many of these observations might be explained by the patient's psychological unhappiness with their large breasts preoperatively, and their happiness with them following surgery, there was an alternative explanation: that there was a real neurophysiologic basis for decreased sensation in the very large breast. This hypothesis was investigated in 1989 in collaboration with Sheri Slezak, who at that time was the Chief Resident in Plastic Surgery at the Johns Hopkins Hospital, and who now is on the full-time faculty of the Johns Hopkins-University of Maryland Plastic Surgery training program.

The previous studies of breast sensibility following breast reduction were most often qualitative. The most frequently quoted study, that of Courtiss and Goldwyn (1976), comprehensively reviewed the previous literature, comprising some 15 studies. Just one study had attempted to quantitate sensibility. Conclusions from earlier studies ranged from recovery of normal sensation to recovery of abnormal sensation in 50% of patients. Courtiss and Goldwyn used a pain stimulus, the Vitapulp™, to give a painful electrical stimulus to the breast. They found that after 2 years, pain perception had returned to normal levels in only 65% of the breasts. They noted that no breast, even as long as 2 years after surgery, had normal sensation in the nipple and areola. With regard to free nipple/areola grafting, conclusions of earlier studies essentially agreed that free nipple graft nerve grafts rarely regain anything but poor sensibility.

In contrast, however, Townsend (1974) evaluated 46 breasts 1 year after they had been reduced with the amputation/free nipple graft technique. He compared the results of those patients' sensory testing with those of 14 patients who were evaluated at the time of their preoperative visit for breast reduction surgery. His testing used stroking of the skin with cotton wool, pin prick, two-point discrimination, and testing of nipple erectility. There was little difference between those patients who were 1 year after their grafting and those who were preop. For example, both groups of patients had the same perception of cotton wool (93% and 80% for the pre-ops versus the post-ops), and the same perception of two-point discrimination at one inch or less (38% versus 39%). Whereas 100% of the pre-op group could perceive the pin prick and had nipple erectility, within the postoperative group of patients just 65% had perception of pin prick, and just 72% had nipple erectility.

Using the quantitative sensory testing instruments available in 1989, 13 prospective breast reduction candidates, bra cup size of at least D, were tested with Semmes-Weinstein monofilaments and the Biothesiometer™ to quantitate cutaneous pressure and vibratory perception thresholds. Nine patients had surgery and were available for postoperative testing 6 to 12 months after surgery. Of these 9, 6 had an amputation/free nipple grafting technique and 3 had a McKissock, double verticle pedicle nipple/areola transposition technique. The mean weight of breast tissue resected was 1,096 g per breast (range 522 g to 2100 g), and the average bra size was 42DD (range 36D to 46 DD+). The results of the quantitative sensory testing are given in Table 16.5.

This study demonstrated that women who are candidates for breast reduction have significantly higher vibratory perception thresholds ($p < .001$) and significantly higher pressure perception thresholds ($p < .04$) than do women with smaller breasts. Furthermore, this study demonstrated that breast reduction, whether done by an amputation and free nipple/areola grafting technique or by a pedicle transposition technique, does

TABLE 16.5 BREAST SENSIBILITY THRESHOLDS RELATED TO BREAST REDUCTION

	Pre-operative Semmes-Weinstein mean g/mm²	Biothesiometer mean μm	Post-operative Semmes-Weinstein mean g/mm²	Biothesiometer mean μm
Nipple Graft				
Nipple	4.6	3	6.9	30
Areola	5.1	39	5.5	30
Skin	6.2	63	2.4	22
Nipple Pedicle				
Nipple	11	34	4.0	38
Areola	11	34	4.9	38
Skin	12	32	3.1	32

Note: Compared to the values in Table 16.2, for normal size breasts, the values for women who are candidates for breast reduction have a significantly higher vibratory perception threshold ($p < .001$) and a significantly higher pressure perception threshold ($p < .04$).

From "Quantitation of Sensibility in Gigantomastia and Alteration Following Reduction Mammaplasty," by S. Slezak, & A. L. Dellon, 1993, *Plastic and Reconstructive Surgery* 91:1265-1269. Reprinted with permission of the authors.

not decrease sensation in the breast as determined by these measurement techniques. Analysis of this data in view of the normal neural anatomy presented in the opening paragraph of this chapter suggests the following explanation for these observations: The large breast skin envelope of women with large breasts is innervated by the same number of intercostal sensory nerve fibers, resulting in a decreased innervation density for these large breasts. Furthermore, over many years, the weight of the large breasts may create a stretch/ traction injury to the intercostal nerves. These two factors combine to cause abnormal sensibility in the large female breast.

During free nipple grafting, the nipple/areolar complex is placed onto a dermal bed containing the non-stretched, normal innervation density nerve fibers of the superior chest skin, providing an immediate source of postoperative sensation to this graft, and to the source of graft reinnervation. During the pedicle transposition techniques, the transposed nipple/areola may still contain some of its original innervation, depending on the location and size of the pedicle, and the nipple/areolar complex can be reinnervated from the dermal nerve net of the normally innervated medial and lateral skin flaps into whose environment it is placed.

The conclusions from the Slezak and Dellon (1993) study were confirmed by the study of Gonzalez, Brown, Gold, Walton, and Schafer (1993). These authors used a "central parenchymal pedicle technique." They found that in women with up to 550 gms resected from each breast, 90% of preoperative sensibility was preserved (as measured with Semmes-Weinstein monofilaments), and that if greater than 550 gms were resected, still 85% of preoperative sensibility was preserved. In their comparison of macromastic breasts (84 breasts) with sizes A and B bra cup (12 breasts), they noted that there was better, that is, lower, pressure threshold sensibility in the smaller breasts, p < .01. (They correctly converted the logarithmic values of the monofilament markings to pressure measurements before doing their statistical analysis.)

Quantitative sensory testing now available with the Pressure-Specified Sensory Device™ will provide the measurements necessary to analyze different breast reduction techniques to determine which pedicle will provide the best postoperative sensibility, in addition to the most pleasing shape. By substituting the threshold for moving touch for the threshold for vibratory perception, the quickly-adapting fiber system can still be tested without concern for the force of application of the Biothesiometer™ into the breast tissue damping the actual oscillation.

• BREAST RECONSTRUCTION •

The most common indication for breast reconstruction is correction of the deformity created by mastectomy for the treatment of breast cancer. The radical mastectomy that was practiced through the 1970s was initiated because many of the breast tumors were sufficiently large at the time of diagnosis that mastectomy with the resection of the underlying pectoralis muscle, and an axillary lymph node dissection, were required. Radiation therapy was often added to this regimen. Over the past two decades, earlier diagnosis of breast cancer, facilitated by public awareness programs, breast self-examination programs, and mammography have combined to generate a group of women whose breast cancer at the time of diagnosis can be treated successfully by a variety of techniques that do not require radical mastectomy.

Many women today will be treated by a lumpectomy (partial mastectomy) and radiation therapy to the breast, a so-called breast conservation approach. Lymph node dissection is still usually done to determine the stage of the cancer, and the majority of women get chemotherapy, as an adjunct, even if they have no lymph node metastases. For those women who do have a mastectomy, breast reconstruction has gone through a similar evolution. That evolution has gone from the earliest days in which no reconstruction was available, to the use of the latissimus dorsi myocutaneous flap plus an implant (1970s), to the use of an implant beneath a preserved pectoralis muscle (1970s), to the use of the pedicled transverse rectus abdominous (TRAM) flap (1980s) and, finally, to the free, microvascular transfer of either the rectus or the gluteus myocutaneous flap (1990s). A variety of techniques developed to create the nipple/areolar complex, either with grafts or tattooing, also exist to complete breast reconstruction.

Traditionally, rehabilitation has been a part of the treatment for the mastectomy patient because of the frequent development of a stiff shoulder or lymphedema. Protocols for the treatment of each of these conditions are well accepted and have been proven to be effective. These protocols are beyond the scope of this book. However, as the patients illustrated in Figure 16.3 demonstrate, lack of sensibility can provide problems ranging from burns to the pain syndromes associated with the phantom breast.

A prospective study of 120 women in Denmark, reported by Kroner, Krebs, Skov, and Jorgensen (1989) considered the incidence and relationships of the pain associated with an absent breast and its phantom sensations. These women did not have breast reconstruction. The incidence of phantom pain and nonpainful phantom sensations was 13.3% and 15%, respectively, at 3 weeks after surgery, and 12.7% and 11.8% at 1 year after surgery. These pains were different from the pain of the operation itself (cicatrix pain), which occurred in another 35% of the patients at 3 weeks, and was still present in 22.7% of the patients at 1 year after surgery. The only correlation these authors found was a significant correlation between preoperative cancer pain and postoperative painful phantom breast syndrome. I have never seen a patient with phantom breast pain, although 1 patient has shared with me that after her mastectomy she still perceived that her (absent) nipple would become erect whenever she walked past the frozen food section of the supermarket. Of interest is that a paper reported by Houpt, Dikstra, and van Leeuwen (1988), from the Netherlands, did not report even one case of phantom breast problems in 109 patients who had breast reconstruction after mastectomy.

It became of interest to investigate the degree of sensory recovery in patients reconstructed with TRAM flaps after Bernard McGibbon, a plastic surgeon in Baltimore, shared his observation with me that when he attempted to tatoo an areola onto what he assumed would be an anesthetic abdominal flap now located on the chest, the patients, to his surprise, would complain of pain from the tatoo needles. This observation was made at the time that Sheri Slezak was doing her plastic surgery residency and, in conjunction with the study reported above on the patients with gigantomastia, provided her the opportunity to apply quantitative sensory testing techniques to this population of patients.

Figure 16.7 outlines the regions tested on the TRAM flap for 10 patients varying in time of reconstruction from 1 to 7 years. Eight of the 10 patients evaluated did recover sensation in the TRAM flap. The results of this study are given in Table 16.6 and demonstrate that the sensory thresholds for vibration and pressure in these 8 reconstructed breasts were significantly higher than normal. However, when the vibratory thresholds are plotted over time, it is clearly seen in Figure 16.8 that there is gradual improvement in these thresholds toward the normal values. The best sensibility was recovered

FIGURE 16.7

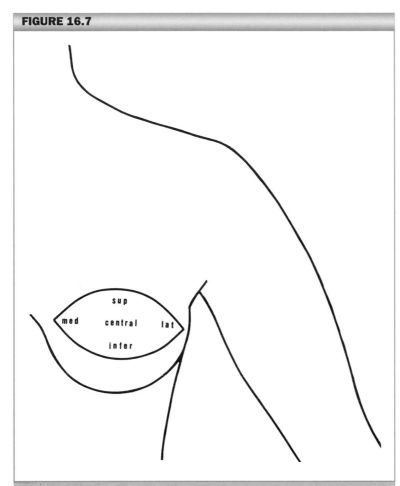

Schematic drawing of the regions of the transverse abdominal flap in location on the chest wall following breast reconstruction. These areas correspond to the regions of sensibility testing described in the text. From "The Sensational Transverse Rectus Abdominous Musculocutaneous Flap: Return of Sensation After TRAM Breast Reconstruction," by S. Slezak, B. McGibbon, & A. L. Dellon, 1992, Annals of Plastic Surgery 28:210-217. Reprinted with permission of the authors.

in the superior, medial, and inferior quadrants of the TRAM flap, suggesting that reinnervation of the TRAM occurs from the medial ramus of the 3rd to 5th intercostal nerves, the lateral ramus of the 7th intercostal nerve, and the supraclavicular nerves. The region with the poorest recovery was, on average, the central region of the TRAM flap, suggesting that reinnervation proceeded from the periphery. It is likely that the lateral ramus of the intercostal nerves becomes entrapped in the interface between the flap and chest wall, or is already suffi-ciently scarred from the mastectomy. Careful palpation of the lateral chest wall in many of these patients revealed tender sites that could be neuromas of these lateral rami.

Based on these observations in patients with TRAM flap reconstructions, it was hypothesized that it may be possible to directly neurotize the TRAM flap. Figure 16.10 demonstrates two potential nerves within the rectus muscle that may be used for neurotization. There are the intercostal nerves that provide innervation of the rectus muscle itself (see Chapter 3 regarding proprioception and the reinnervation of a "motor" nerve by a cutaneous nerve), and the intercostals to the skin of the TRAM flap itself. Slezak, therefore, tried in 2 patients to innervate the TRAM flap by suturing the 4th intercostal nerve's lateral ramus to the nerve to the rectus muscle. The two patients had bilateral TRAM flaps, and one side was reinnervated while the other side was not. At the 6- and 9-month postoperative sensibility evaluation of these patients, vibratory perception was recovering earlier than in the noninnervated side.

Reconstruction with free, microvascular transfer of tissue was reported in 1989 at the 68th annual meeting of the American Association of Plastic Surgeons by Shaw, Orringer, Ratto, and Mers-

TABLE 16.6 BREAST SENSIBILITY THRESHOLDS RELATED TO BREAST RECONSTRUCTION WITH THE TRAM FLAP

Flap Test Area	Post-operative Semmes-Weinstein mean g/mm²	Biothesiometer mean μm
Medial	211	4.4
Superior	267	4.0
Inferior	213	4.6
Lateral	323	6.9
Central	383	8.3

Note: Compared to the values in Table 16.2, for normal size breasts, the values for women who had breast reconstruction with a TRAM flap have a significantly higher vibratory perception threshold (p < .0001) and a significantly higher pressure perception threshold (p < .0001).

From "The Sensational Transverse Rectus Abdominous Musculocutaneous Flap: Return of Sensation After TRAM Breast Reconstruction," by S. Slezak, B. McGibbon, & A. L. Dellon, 1992, *Annals of Plastic Surgery 28:*210-217. Reprinted with permission of the authors.

FIGURE 16.8

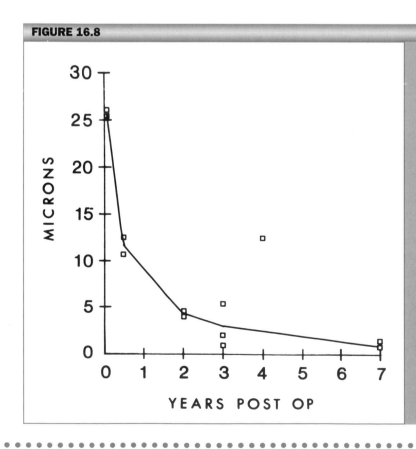

Recovery of vibratory threshold in breasts reconstructed with a TRAM flap related to postoperative time interval. From "The Sensational Transverse Rectus Abdominous Musculocutaneous Flap: Return of Sensation After TRAM Breast Reconstruction," by S. Slezak, B. McGibbon, & A. L. Dellon, 1992, Annals of Plastic Surgery 28:210-217. Reprinted with permission of the authors.

FIGURE 16.9

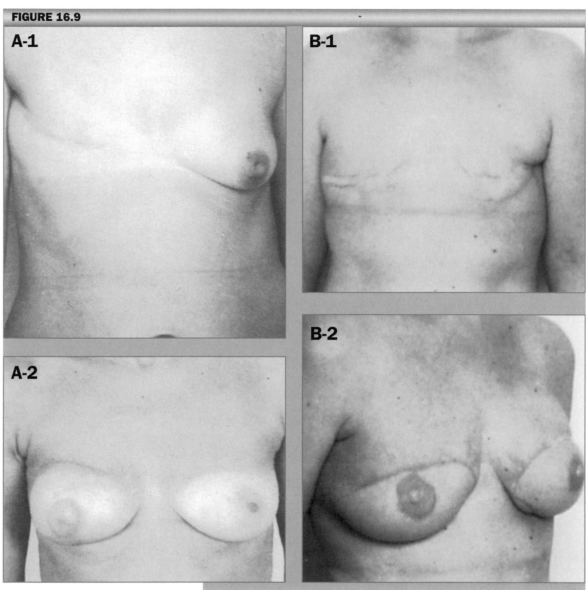

Example of a (A-1, A-2) unilateral and (B-1, B-2) bilateral breast reconstruction with the transverse abdominal myocutaneous flap (TRAM flap). Note top is pre-op, bottom is post-op. Photos reprinted with permission of Serpa Aljaselavarra, MD, Chief of Plastic Surgery, University of Helsinki, Finland.

mann. Their study involved 33 breast reconstructions using 20 free gluteal flaps, 8 free TRAM flaps, and 5 pedicled TRAM flaps. The data was pooled for all flaps and is given in Table 16.7. This data was interpreted as demonstrating that these free flaps were reinnervated, and that the periphery of the free flap was reinnervated before the central region.

It was also noted that the pressure perception threshold improved over time (see Figure 16.11). Furthermore, a questionnaire was administered to these patients regarding their subjective

views of their reconstruction. With regard to the subject of phantom pain, described above, it is interesting to note one observation made by these patients: 94% considered their chest to be

FIGURE 16.10

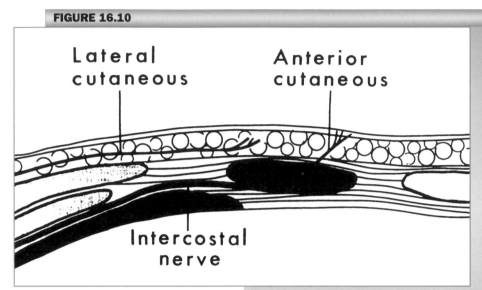

Lateral cutaneous

Anterior cutaneous

Intercostal nerve

Schematic drawing of the intercostal nerve in the region of the umbilicus, from which the transverse abdominous myocutaneous flap originates. Two branches of the intercostal nerve exist in this region and, theoretically, may be transferred with the flap to provide target end organs for reinnervation during breast reconstruction. From "The Sensational Transverse Rectus Abdominous Musculocutaneous Flap: Return of Sensation After TRAM Breast Reconstruction," by S. Slezak, B. McGibbon, & A. L. Dellon, 1992, Annals of Plastic Surgery 28:210-217. Reprinted with permission of the authors.

comfortable to touch following reconstruction, whereas only 34% would make this statement prior to reconstruction. It was also noted that 82% of the patients recovered the ability to perceive cold, and 64% recovered the ability to perceive heat. All patients recovered the ability to perceive a 30 Hz and a 256 Hz tuning fork stimulus.

● REHABILITATION ●

Rehabilitation of the patient after breast reduction or breast reconstruction should concentrate first on scar massage to minimize any painful incisions, and then on sensory reeducation techniques to help the patient focus on the new flow of neural impulses that will represent the new location of the breast mound and the nipple/areolar complex. Previously, for a breast reduction patient, touching the superior chest skin had a certain location/meaning, but now that the nipple is located in this area, 21 cm instead of 36 cm from the suprasternal notch, reeducation techniques will enable the patient to make the new identification. In this regard, even though many breast reduction patients have had a breast amputation, they do not go through a phantom breast syndrome or pain syndrome. This must be because immediately after surgery the cerebral cortex has the ability to begin to receive neural impulses that can be reintegrated. The cortex never experiences a prolonged period of loss, but rather experiences an immediate relocation of impulses.

With primary breast reconstruction being done in conjunction with mastectomy for breast cancer, this same concept holds true. For the patient who has a delayed breast reconstruction, there will be a period of time when the cerebral cortex experiences a decrease in neural impulses from the amputated breast. If the cutaneous nerves become entrapped in scar and become painful, this may set up the conditions necessary for the painful phantom breast syndrome. These observations may suggest to the reconstructive surgeon that the original wound be explored

TABLE 16.7 BREAST SENSIBILITY THRESHOLDS RELATED TO BREAST RECONSTRUCTION WITH FREE, MICROVASCULAR, TISSUE TRANSFER

Region of flap	Semmes-Weinstein g/mm^2 (mean ±)*
Central	66 ± 91
Periphery	35 ± 42

Note: *There appears to be a significant discrepancy between the absolute values for the thresholds for pressure obtained by the two different investigators when Table 16.7 is compared to Table 16.2. The most reasonable explanation for this is that while the heading of Table 16.7 indicates that the pressure threshold was recorded as g/mm^2, it was probably calculated as milligrams of force; that is, a filament marking of 5.46 generates a force of 28 g which, after correction for the cross-sectional area of the filament, gives a pressure of 107 g/mm^2, which is the same correction made for Table 16.3. Similarly, filament marking 5.88 generates a force of 76 g which, after correction for the cross-sectional area of the filament, gives a pressure of 181 g/mm^2. These values for pressure are of the same order of magnitude as the values found in Table 16.6. From data presented at the 68th annual meeting of the American Association of Plastic Surgeons, by W. W. Shaw, J. S. Orringer, L. L. Ratto, & C. A. Mersmann, Scottsdale, AZ, May 10, 1989. Reprinted with permission of Dr. Shaw.

to identify these painful neuromas at the time of reconstruction. Certainly, prior to reconstruction the patient should be sent for rehabilitation, where the same desensitization techniques that are useful in the extremities can be tried for the chest wall. Often the pain will be related to the second intercostobrachial nerve, which becomes stretched or divided during the axillary node dissection. This painful neuroma may be surgically treated by excision. The observation that the reconstructed breast does not appear to develop the painful phantom breast syndrome may be useful in devising strategies for lower extremity amputation, and for preventing the phantom limb syndrome that can be so devastating.

The concept of attempting to help reinnervate the breast reconstructed by leading the intercostal nerves beneath the reconstructed breast, (for the nerves to reinnervate the flap, rather than becoming trapped at the periphery in scar), or by directly suturing the intercostal nerves to the motor nerves of the flap, should become part of surgical teaching. Rehabilitation of these patients should include simple reeducation techniques that include self-massage in the shower, massage with skin cream to soften the scars, massage while directly observing the activity in the mirror, and massage while simultaneously massaging the contralateral breast. All these techniques are designed to send a stream of neural impulses to the cerebral cortex to facilitate cortical reorganization.

Finally, the relationship between macromastia and loss of sensibility in the hand should be mentioned. Women who request breast reduction may complain of numbness in the little and ring fingers. This was first illustrated by Kaye in 1972. The presumed mechanism is pressure by the bra strap

FIGURE 16.11

Recovery of pressure threshold in breasts reconstructed with a free flap related to postoperative time interval. From data presented at the 68th annual meeting of the American Association of Plastic Surgeons, by W. W. Shaw, J. S. Orringer, L. L. Ratto, & C. A. Mersmann, Scottsdale, AZ, May 10, 1989. Reprinted with permission of Dr. Shaw.

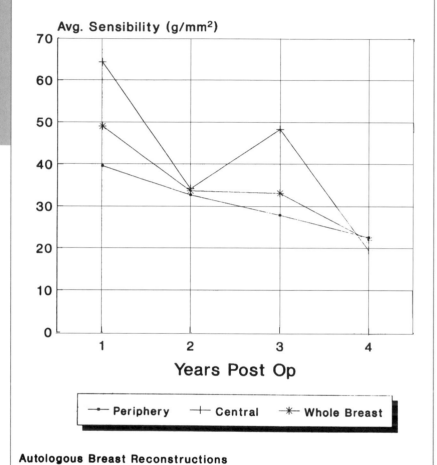

Years Post-Op Versus Average Sensibility

Avg. Sensibility (g/mm²)

Years Post Op

—•— Periphery   —+— Central   —*— Whole Breast

Autologous Breast Reconstructions

transmitted onto the brachial plexus, with compression at the C8 or lower trunk or medial cord resulting in "ulnar nerve" patterns of sensory loss (see Figure 16.12). These symptoms are improved following reduction mammoplasty. The therapist may be asked to document these sensory changes prior to surgery (Gonzalez, Schafer, Walton, & Bora, 1993).

• • •

• REFERENCES •

Courtiss, E. H., & Goldwyn, R. M. Breast sensation before and after plastic surgery. *Plastic and Reconstructive Surgery 58*:1-10, 1976.

Gonzalez, F., Brown, F. E., Gold, M. E., Walton, R. L., & Schafer, B. Pre-operative and post-operative nipple-areola sensibility in patients undergoing reduction mammoplasty. *Plastic and Reconstructive Surgery 92*:809-814, 1993.

Gonzalez, F., Schafer, B., Walton, R. L., & Bora, G. Reduction mammoplasty improves the symptoms of macromastia. *Plastic and Reconstructive Surgery 91*:1265-1270, 1993.

Houpt, P., Dikstra, R., & van Leeuwen, J. B. S. The result of breast reconstruction after mastectomy for breast cancer in 109 patients. *Annals of Plastic Surgery 21*:517-525, 1988.

Kaye, B. L. Neurologic changes associated

FIGURE 16.12

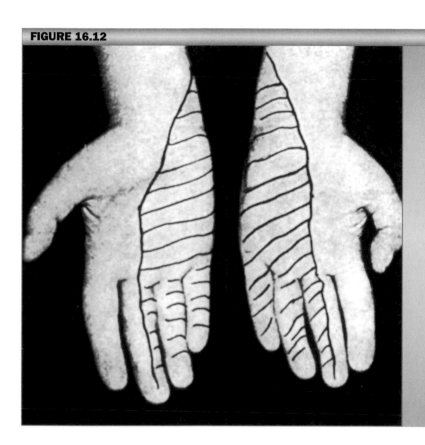

Pattern of sensory loss in hands associated with brachial plexus compression by weight of large breasts hanging from bra straps. From "Neurologic Changes Associated with Macromastia," by B. L. Kaye, 1972, Southern Medical Journal 65: 177-180. Reprinted with permission of the author.

with macromastia. *Southern Medical Journal 65*:177-180, 1972.

Kroner, K., Krebs, B., Skov, J., & Jorgensen, H. S. Immediate and long-term phantom breast syndrome after mastectomy: Incidence, clinical characteristics, and relationship to pre-mastectomy breast pain. *Pain 36*:327-324, 1989.

Maxwell, G. P., & Tornambe, R. Second- and third-degree burns as a complication in breast reconstruction. *Annals of Plastic Surgery 22*:386-390, 1989.

Shaw, W. W., Orringer, J. S., Ratto, L. L., & Mersmann, C. A. Data presented at the 68th annual meeting of the American Association of Plastic Surgeons, Scottsdale, AZ, May 10, 1989.

Slezak, S., & Dellon, A. L. Quantitation of sensibility in gigantomastia and alteration following reduction mammaplasty. *Plastic and Reconstructive Surgery 91*:1265-1269, 1993.

Slezak, S., McGibbon, B., & Dellon, A. L.

The sensational transverse rectus abdominous myocutaneous (TRAM) flap: Return of sensibility after TRAM reconstruction. *Annals of Plastic Surgery 28*:210-217, 1992.

Terzis, J. K., Vincent, M. P., Wilkins, L. M., Rutledge, K., & Deane, L. M. Breast sensibility: A neurophysiologic appraisal in the normal breast. *Annals of Plastic Surgery 19*:318-322, 1987.

Townsend, P. L. G. Nipple sensation following breast reduction and free nipple transplantation. *British Journal of Plastic Surgery 27*:308-310, 1974.

• ADDITIONAL READINGS •

Beale, S., Hambert, G., & Lisper, H. O. Augmentation mammaplasty: The surgical and psychological effects of the operation and prediction of the results. *Annals of Plastic Surgery 14*:473-493, 1985.

Caffee, H. H. Measurement of implant capsules. *Annals of Plastic Surgery 11*:412-415, 1983.

Craig, R. D. P., & Sykes, P. A. Nipple sensitivity following reduction mammoplasty. *British Journal of Plastic Surgery 23*:165-168, 1970.

Dellon, A. L. *Evaluation of Sensibility and Re-Education of Sensation in the Hand*. Baltimore: Williams & Wilkins, 1981.

Dellon, A. L. The vibrometer. *Plastic and Reconstructive Surgery 71*:427-431, 1983.

Dellon, A. L., Mackinnon, S. E., & Brandt, K. E. The Semmes-Weinstein nylon filaments' markings. *Journal of Hand Surgery 18A:*756-757, 1993.

Edwards, E. A. Surgical anatomy of the breast. In *Plastic and Reconstructive Surgery of the Breast*, R. M. Goldwyn, Editor. Boston: Little, Brown & Company, Inc., 1976.

Farina, M. A., Newby, B. G., & Alani, H. M. Innervation of the nipple-areola complex. *Plastic and Reconstructive Surgery 66*:497-501, 1980.

Fiala, T. G. S., Lee, W. P. A., & May, J. W., Jr. Augmentation mammoplasty: Results of a patient survey. *Annals of Plastic Surgery 30*:503-509, 1993.

Freilinger, G., Holle, J., & Sulzgruber, S. C. Distribution of motor and sensory fibers in the intercostal nerves: Significance in reconstructive surgery. *Plastic and Reconstructive Surgery 62*:240-244, 1978.

Hetter, G. P. Satisfactions and dissatisfactions of patients with augmentation mammaplasty. *Plastic and Reconstructive Surgery 64*:151-154, 1979.

Levin, S., Pearsall, G., & Ruderman, R. J. von Fry's method of measuring pressure sensibility in the hand: An engineering analysis of the Weinstein-Semmes pressure aesthesiometer. *Journal of Hand Surgery 3*:211-216, 1978.

Markowski, J., Wilcox, J. P., & Helm, P. A. Lymphedema incidence after specific postmastectomy therapy. *Archives of Physical Medicine and Rehabilitation 62*:449-452, 1981.

Peterson, R. D., Bowen, D., Netscher, D. T., & Wigoda, P. Capsular compliance: A measure of a "hard" prosthesis. *Annals of Plastic Surgery 32*:237-341, 1994.

Terzis, J. K., & Dykes, R. W. Reinnervation of glabrous skin in baboons: Properties of cutaneous mechanoreceptors subsequent to nerve transection. *Journal of Neurophysiology 44*:1214-1219, 1980.

Wingate, L., Croghan, I., Natarajan, N., & Michalek, R. Rehabilitation of the mastectomy patient: A randomized, blind, prospective study. *Archives of Physical Medicine and Rehabilitation 70*:21-24, 1989.

Winkelman, R. K. *Nerve Endings in Normal and Pathologic Skin: Contributions to the Anatomy of Sensation*. Springfield, IL: Charles C. Thomas, Publisher, 1960.

• • •

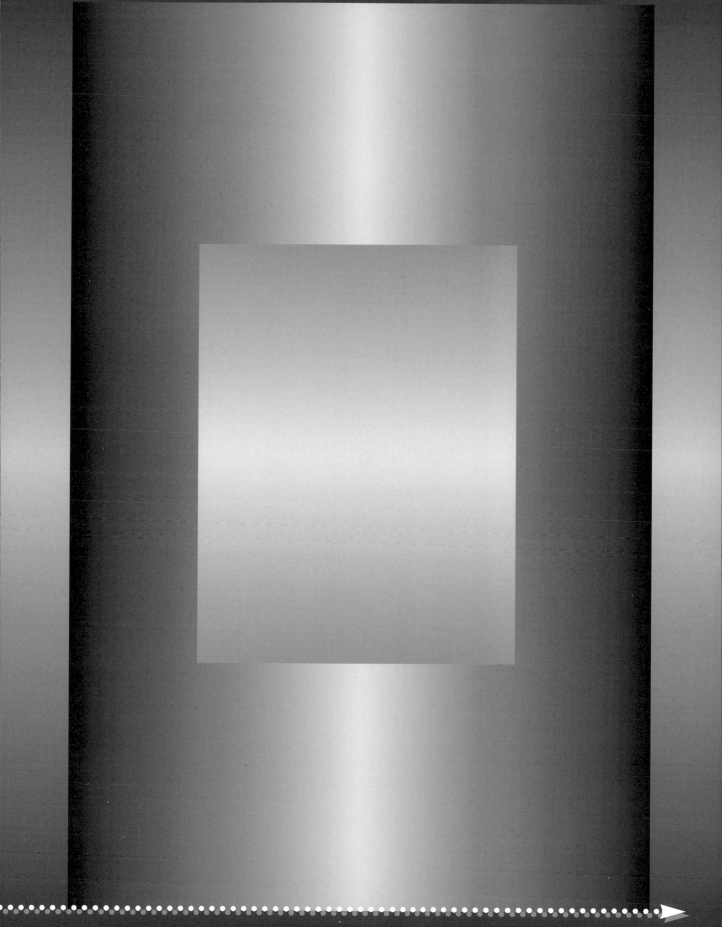

the penis

This chapter will focus on the measurement of penile sensibility in normal and abnormal physiologic conditions. That penile sensibility underlies the perception that sensation is erotic is taken for granted, until that perception is lost. It has only been since the advent of *phalloplasty*, penile reconstruction, that reconstructive microsurgery has attempted to provide innervation appropriate for the sensory function of the penis. Such clinical information as we have comes from (a) the evaluation of transsexual surgery, the attempt to create external male genitalia on a biologic female; (b) the evaluation of men whose penis has been surgically amputated for the treatment of carcinoma; and (c) the evaluation of men whose penis has been amputated during trauma. It was only as recently as 1985 that the innervation of the reconstructed penis was connected to the *internal pudendal nerve*, giving the correct pathway for sensation.

It is important to recognize that there is innervation to the penis that does not concern the perception of touch stimuli. That innervation must accomplish changes in blood flow necessary for erection (the parasympathetic nerves), transmission of environmental sensory stimuli such as pain and temperature (the group A-delta and group C-fibers), and ejaculation (the sympathetic fibers). Clearly, the afferent innervation related to touch (the group A-beta fibers) is linked to the efferent parasympathetic and sympathetic fibers through spinal cord reflex pathways (a paraplegic can achieve an erection even though he may not be conscious that this has occurred), as well as through cortical associative pathways that can supervene over spinal reflexes (an erection can occur as the result of the stimulation of visual imagery, without the penis being physically stimulated).

It is increasingly apparent that techniques to evaluate penile sensibility and techniques to rehabilitate sensation are becoming increasingly important as reconstructive microsurgery accomplishes the task of penile reconstruction, and urologists delve deeper into the mechanisms of impotence.

base. From the symphysis, the dorsal nerve of the penis is finally dorsal. It travels parallel with its twin from the contralateral side toward the glans, sending branches ventral to innervate the rest of the shaft (see Figure 17.1).

• RELEVANT NEUROANATOMY •

PERIPHERAL NERVOUS SYSTEM

The *glans* of the penis, the *penile corona*, and the *penile shaft* are all innervated by the dorsal nerve of the penis. This is a sensory nerve, and is the terminal branch of the pudendal nerve. The pudendal nerve arises from ventral branches of S2, S3, and S4, travels through the greater sciatic notch medial to the sciatic nerve, curves around the sacrospinous ligament to enter the lesser sciatic notch, and then travels through the ischiorectal fossa and alongside the inferior pubic ramus. During its course along the ischium and the inferior pubic ramus, the nerve is covered by the obturator fascia in the space described by the Irish anatomist Alcock, in about 1801, also called the pudendal canal. Thus, the pudendal nerve enters the perineum without having gone across the pelvic floor. Motor branches of the internal pudendal nerve are given off as it exists this canal, and are distributed via the inferior rectal nerve to the anal sphincter. Sensory branches from the inferior rectal nerve innervate the anus. The internal pudendal nerve then divides to form the *perineal nerve* and *dorsal nerve* of the penis.

The perineal nerve contains motor fibers that innervate the *ischiocavernosus* and the *bulbocavernosus* (the muscle involved in the bulbocavernosus reflex), as well as the sensory fibers that innervate the skin of the perineum in both sexes, the labia in women and the scrotum in men. The terminal branch of the internal pudendal nerve in women is the nerve to the clitoris. In men, the terminal branch of the internal pudendal nerve is the dorsal nerve to the penis. This nerve travels from the perineal body, at the base of the scrotum, anterolaterally toward the corpora cavernosa to reach the dorsal root of the penis, near the pubic symphysis. The dorsal nerve to the penis gives off a branch to the corpora at its

AUTONOMIC NERVOUS SYSTEM

While it was known that at the level of the sacral sympathetic ganglia chain some autonomic nerves enter the anterior branches of S2-S4 that are destined to become the internal pudendal nerve, the precise anatomic pathway by which the sympathetic and parasympathetic nerves travel across the pelvis to the *corpora cavernosa* and *corpus spongiosis* were elucidated precisely only in the 1980s. This information is the result of dissections done by urologists Walsh and Donker (1982) at the Johns Hopkins University School of Medicine (in the fetus), and by Lue, Zeineh, Schmidt, and Tanagho (1984) at the University of California, San Francisco (in dogs, monkeys, and adult humans), designed to elucidate the mechanism of impotence following prostatectomy for cancer. It was found that the major portions of the parasympathetic (from S2-S4) and sympathetic (T11-L2) nerves, after joining the pelvic plexus, travel with the inferior vesical (bladder)

FIGURE 17.1

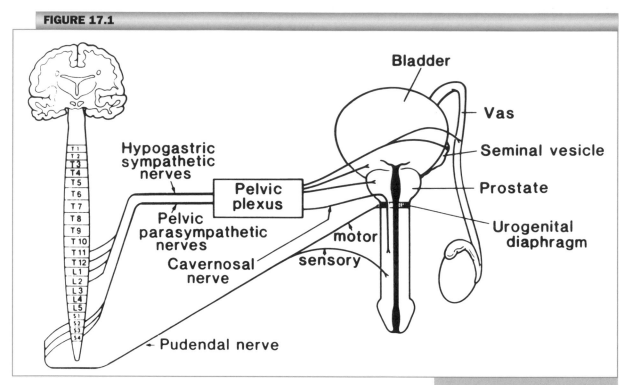

Diagram of interplay of autonomic and somatosensory innervation of the penis. From "Disorders of Male Sexual Function," by D. K. Montague, 1988, Chicago: Year Book Medical Publishers. Reprinted with permission of the author.

artery, lying in a thin connective tissue in the plane alongside and lateral to the rectum, bladder, and prostate.

At the prostate, the autonomic nerves change planes to follow the path of the urethra. The membranous urethra contains these nerves on its lateral borders, or at the 3 and 9 o'clock positions. This is the transition zone, exiting the pelvis, and the membranous urethra, with these nerves, goes through the urogenital diaphragm. This structure is composed of the fascial sheaths of the surrounding muscles and is thicker and more rigid interiorly. The autonomic nerves, after passing through this membrane, move to more anterior positions along the bulbous portion of the ure-

thra, the 1 and 11 o'clock positions. Here they enter the corpus spongiosis and the corpora cavernosa, and then join with the terminal vessels of the pudendal artery (see Figure 17.1).

CENTRAL NERVOUS SYSTEM

The portion of the central nervous system related most to the penis, other than the primary sensory area in the somatosensory cortex of the post-central gyrus, is the *limbic system*. This system appears to be the association center for olfactory (smell), taste, auditory, visual, and tactile input related to sexuality. The limbic center is located near the top of the brain stem and is

comprised of those portions of the brain termed the *hippocampus*, the *cingula*, and regions adjacent to the hippocampus. Subcortical regions that contain clusters of cell bodies, or nuclei, are also related to the limbic system, such as the *amygdala*, the anterior region of the hypothalamus, the *thalamus*, and the *basal ganglia*.

During the conscious state, sensory impulses from the periphery are received in

FIGURE 17.2

Diagram of innervation of the (A) perineal and (B) dorsal penile regions. The internal pudendal nerve enters the perineal region through Alcock's canal medial to the pubic ramus, at which point it gives off perineal branches and then courses dorsally to become the dorsal nerve of the penis. The same nerve innervates the homologous structures in women. From "Phallic Reinnervation Via the Pudendal Nerve," by D. A. Gilbert, M. W. Williams, C. E. Horton, J. P. Terzis, & A. Devine, 1988, Journal of Urology 140:295-299. Reprinted with permission of the authors.

A

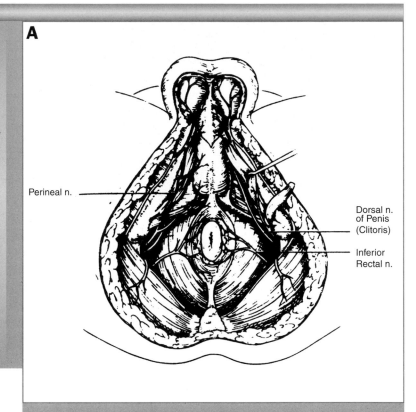

Perineal n.

Dorsal n. of Penis (Clitoris)

Inferior Rectal n.

B

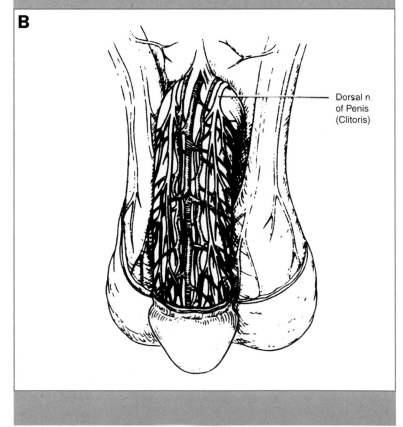

Dorsal n. of Penis (Clitoris)

their primary cortical region and relayed to the limbic system, where they are associated and processed. Appropriate excitatory or inhibitory signals are then generated from a region called the *pre-optic area of the hypothalamus*, down through the *median forebrain bundle*, and ultimately to the sympathetic and parasympathetic nuclei in the *intermediolateral columns* of the spinal cord.

In the unconscious or sleeping state, stimuli through this system occur in the absence of peripheral stimulation, causing *nocturnal penile tumescence* (NPT), or penile swelling. NPT may occur up to four times per night, and may be measured in the sleep lab in coordination with cortical recordings of the alpha-waves, as a measure of sexual dysfunction. Men who are impotent but who still have NPT may be diagnosed as having psychogenic impotence, where the central nervous system, through the limbic system, inhibits sexual arousal during the conscious state.

HISTOLOGY

The nerve terminals and corpuscular end-organs in the penis have been studied with modern histologic techniques by Halata and Munger (1986), and provide a basis for comparison of the sensibility of the penis with that of the finger. The skin of the glans differs from that of the glabrous (non-hairy) skin of the finger in that there are no papillary ridges (fingerprints), and the *rete ridges* of the dermis are fewer and less well developed. The skin of the penis has been found to have few true Meissner corpuscles and Merkel cell neurite complexes, although there are many so-called *genital end-bulbs*. The density of these genital end-bulbs per area of dermis is about the same as the density of Meissner corpuscles.

In my view, the genital end-bulb is the neurophysiologic correlate of the Meissner corpuscle in the fingertip, and the mucocutaneous end-organ in the lip. Thus, whereas in the skin of the

finger the myelinated nerve grows up into the dermal papillae to become ensheathed in Schwann cell processes, or *lamellae*, to form the Meissner corpuscle, the myelinated nerve fiber in the dermis of the penis does not find a papillae, and so forms a similar, but simpler, structure. In the hairy skin, these same nerve fibers form ring-like, or lanceollate endings around a hair follicle. These corpuscular endings in the penis should be the receptors for the quickly-adapting nerve fibers, and subserve the perception of moving touch and vibration.

A few Pacinian corpuscles have been identified, and these represent the receptors for the quickly-adapting fibers most responsive to high-frequency vibratory stimuli. The receptors for pressure, and the slowly-adapting fibers, are represented by the few Merkel-like cells identified, and by a few Rufinni-corpuscles in the deepest dermis, or *Dartos fascia*. There are abundant free nerve endings, the small fiber population being related to the perception of pain and temperature, and to the diffuse perception of touch.

METHODS OF SENSIBILITY TESTING

GENERAL CONSIDERATIONS

During the process of sensibility testing in men who are not impotent, the penis may become erect. One group of investigators, evaluating nerve conduction velocity, taped the penis to a wooden tongue depressor to keep its length from changing! It is not clear what the effect of erection has on the human penile sensory threshold. However, there is evidence from a rat model of impotence developed at the University of Florida at Gainsville that the sensory threshold for stimulation decreases; that is, the penis becomes more sensitive in the erect state. Previous human studies have not commented on whether the sensory data they present is for the penis in the flaccid or erect state. It may be important to note this in future studies. With the advent of pharmacologic treatment of impotence by injection of a vasoactive (dilate) drug like papaverine into the corpora, it is possible to directly test the effect of erection on sensory threshold, if men with psychogenic or vasculogenic impotence (but not neurogenic impotence) are chosen for the subjects. Their sensibility can be tested in the flaccid state, and then tested again about 15 minutes after the pharmacologic agent has taken effect.

VIBRATION

Once it was clear that vibration was a touch sensation and not a separate 6th sense, which some had called pallesthesia, it was appropriate to study penile sensibility with vibratory stimuli. The first to do this was Newman (1970), who noted that "vibration was preferred to touch or pressure (as a method of testing sensibility) purely because the latter are too difficult to measure accurately." His normative data from 100 men, given in Table 17.1, demonstrates a large variability in the normal value for each age group evaluated.

This data was obtained using a hand-held instrument whose probe tip was 0.5 cm and which vibrated at 120 Hz, being a fixed frequency, variable amplitude device. This may have been the forerunner of the Biothesiometer™ popularized for use in the hand by Dellon in 1983, and illustrated in Figure 17.3 for penile sensibility testing (see also Table 17.2). While other vibrometers are available, they usually require the skin area to be tested to be placed on a surface with a small opening, up through which will protrudes the vibrating probe. These are clearly not applicable to sensibility testing for the penis, so I still favor the Biothesiometer™ for this particular body surface. Application of the Biothesiometer™ testing probe to the penis requires careful attention to keeping the penis stabilized so that it does not move away from the stimulus.

Newman's (1970) normative data for penile vibratory perception, as presented in Table 17.1, demonstrates that the vibratory threshold increases gradually with age, becoming markedly elevated after 55 years of age (statistical evaluation was not done). This is similar to findings in general for the fingertip and toe, where vibratory thresholds increase above 45 years of age. Newman found that the threshold was lowest for the corona in 65%, that the corona and the glans had equivalent thresholds in 20%, and that the glans was the more sensitive region of the two in the remaining 15% of normal subjects. The wide variability in his data, however, does not permit us to accept more than the general trend of increasing vibratory threshold with age from this study. In addition,

TABLE 17.1 NORMAL PENILE VIBRATORY THRESHOLD

Age	n	Mean[+]	Range
17–34	12	2.48	0.01–21.16
35–44	14	6.13	0.12–49.00
45–54	12	9.33	0.36–36.00
55–64	14	17.62	0.42–49.00
65–74	31	168.42	0.36–1029.29
75–88	17	284.70	7.02–1296.00

Note:
[+] Force in units of voltage, using a 0.5 cm diameter probe at 120 Hz, where "force was roughly proportional to the square of the applied voltage."
From "Vibratory Sensitivity of the Penis," by H. F. Newman, 1970, *Fertility and Sterility* 21:791-793. Reprinted with permission of the author.

FIGURE 17.3

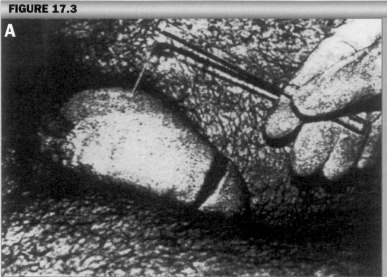

A

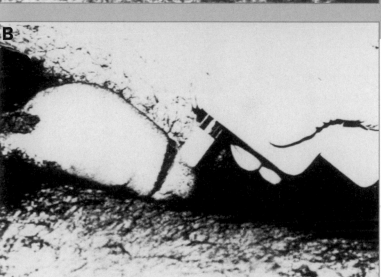

B

Sensibility testing methods for the penis. (A) The cutaneous pressure threshold as measured with a Semmes-Weinstein nylon monofilament. (B) The vibratory threshold as measured with a Biothesiometer, at 120 Hz, 0.5 cm diameter probe. From "Phallic Reinnervation Via the Pudendal Nerve," by D. A. Gilbert, M. W. Williams, C. E. Horton, J. P. Terzis, & A. Devine, 1988, Journal of Urology 140:295-299. Reprinted with permission of the authors.

er side, given the known increase in threshold with age.

PRESSURE

The cutaneous pressure threshold has been measured for the penis using the Semmes-Weinstein nylon monofilaments, and Gilbert et al.'s (1988) data is given in Table 17.4 (see also Figure 17.3). These nylon rods have been the only available instruments with which to test penile pressure thresholds; however, the criticism of this instrument remains valid for the penis as it does for any other test site. The series of filaments vary in diameter, requiring the subject to discriminate both a difference in force as well as a change in the cross-sectional area of the testing instrument. Fur-

since the data was reported in voltage, it is not comparable to subsequent data sets.

Gilbert, Williams, Horton, Terzis, and Devine (1988) studied 30 normal men, 18 to 50 years of age, and observed that all four regions of the penis had the same vibratory threshold. Their data (see Table 17.3) is reported in microns of motion and was obtained with the Biothesiometer™, so it is comparable with other data sets from other areas of the body. Thus, it is possible to conclude that the vibratory threshold of the penis is about the same order of magnitude as is the vibratory threshold of the fingertip. This normative data may be criticized for lacking the standard deviation, and for including subjects above 45 years of age who may have skewed the data to the high-

TABLE 17.2 NORMAL PENILE VIBRATORY THRESHOLD

		(Median Volts)	
Age	n	Index Finger	Glans Penis
17–46	11	5.3	19.2
46–55	10	4.3	18.6
56–71	10	6.9	23.9

Note: From "Comparison of Biothesiometry and Neuro-urophysiological Investigations for the Clinical Evaluation of Patients with Erectile Dysfunction," 1995, by B. L. H. Bemelmans, L. B. P. M. Hendrikx, E. L. Koldewijn, W. A. J. G. Lemmens, F. M. J. Debruyne, & E. J. H. Meueleman. *Journal of Urology 153:*1483-1486, 1995.

TABLE 17.3 NORMAL PENILE VIBRATORY THRESHOLD

		Glans[+]		Shaft[+]	
		Tip	Corona	Dorsal	Ventral
Age	n				
18–50	30	0.20	0.21	0.20	0.20

Note:
[+] Microns of relative motion, using the Biothesiometer™, at 120 Hz, 0.5 cm diameter probe tip.
From "Phallic Reinnervation via the Pudendal Nerve," by D. A. Gilbert, M. W. Williams, C. E. Horton, J. P. Terzis, & A. Devine, 1988, *Journal of Urology 140:*295-299. Reprinted with permission of the authors.

thermore, the markings on the filaments are counterintuitive, being log values of force, not pressure, and force in 0.1 milligrams. Therefore, besides being very difficult to transfer the marking values into statistically usable values, the filaments generate noncontinuous data sets, such that the basic assumptions of the normal distribution of data may not apply.

Gilbert et al. (1988) measured the cutaneous pressure threshold in 30 normal men 18 to 50 years of age with the Semmes-Weinstein nylon monofilaments (see Table 17.4). The values they obtained, though not stratified for age, are comparable to data sets obtained with the nylon monofilaments for other body surfaces. Such a comparison suggests that the penile cutaneous pressure threshold is much higher in the penis than it is in the fingertip by about a factor of 4.

In 1992, Dellon and Dellon described the Pressure-Specified Sensory Device™, which measures the perception of pressure with a single diameter probe, reporting directly through a pressure transducer to a computer. The measured pressure is reported as g/mm^2, the units of pressure, and the device generates continuous data points, satisfying the normal distribution requirement for

TABLE 17.4 NORMAL PENILE PRESSURE THRESHOLD

		Glans[+]		Shaft[+]	
Age	n	Tip	Corona	Dorsal	Ventral
18–50	30	18.5	18.4	19.0	18.8

Note:
[+] g/mm², measured with the Semmes-Weinstein nylon monofilaments.
From "Phallic Reinnervation via the Pudendal Nerve," by D. A. Gilbert, M. W. Williams, C. E. Horton, J. P. Terzis, & A. Devine, 1988, *Journal of Urology 140*:295-299. Reprinted with permission of the authors.

FIGURE 17.4

Penile reconstruction using the one-stage, microneurovascular transfer of the radial forearm flap containing the lateral antebrachial cutaneous nerve. At the time of transfer, a skin graft and catheter are inserted within the flap to permit urethral reconstruction, with the result demonstrated in (A), (B), and (C), the ability to urinate through the tip of the penis. The donor nerve from the flap was connected to the nerve that normally innervates the penis, the internal pudendal nerve, permitting the recovery of sensation with sufficient erotic quality to permit orgasm. The penis has some rigidity from either incorporating a thin piece of the radius (bone) with the flap, or by inserting a silicone rubber rod. The re-

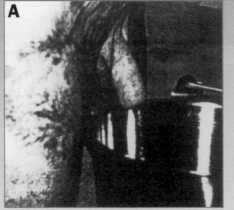
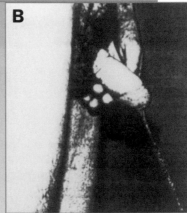
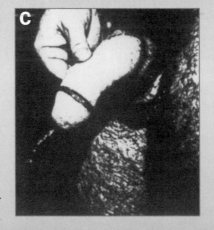
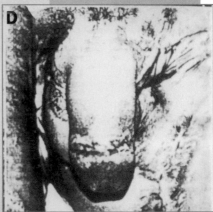

covery of sensation in this type of reconstruction also provides sufficient protection to prevent erosion of the semistiff implant without the patient being aware that too much pressure is being applied. The appearance of the dark ring in the region of the coronal sulcus is achieved by the use of a skin graft. From "Phallic Reinnervation via the Pudendal Nerve," by D. A. Gilbert, M. W. Williams, C. E. Horton, J. P. Terzis, & A. Devine, 1988, Journal of Urology 140:295-299. Reprinted with permission of the authors.

data. This device can record the cutaneous pressure threshold for moving-touch, a touch sensation that may be critical for the perception of touch stimuli as erogenous.

Attempts to use the Pressure-Specified Sensory Device™ to measure sensibility of the penis need to prevent movement of the penis away from the direction of applied pressure. The penis must be supported by a foam cushion. Normative data for penile sensibility is currently being obtained with this device (J. R. Berman and A.L. Dellon, 1997.)

TWO-POINT DISCRIMINATION

Gilbert et al. (1988) made the observation that static and moving two-point discrimination was difficult to perform on the penis, and responses were inconsistent and unreproducible. There is no normative data.

TEMPERATURE

Gilbert et al. (1988) made the observation that "temperature differentiation in various areas of the penis elicited virtually 100% correct responses in all patients (with a reconstructed penis) and, thus, temperature differentiation proved to be relatively insensitive....and an

unsuitable indicator of penile sensibility." There is no normative data.

TOUCH LOCALIZATION

Gilbert et al. (1988) made the same observation for touch localization that they made for temperature differentiation. (See preceding paragraph.)

ELECTRIC CURRENT

The Neurometer™ is designed to deliver electrical stimuli at controlled amounts of amperage, regulated through a feedback circuit that theoretically controls for the thickness (resistance) of the skin. The frequency of the electrical stimulus can be varied from 5 Hz, to 250 Hz, to 2000 Hz, theoretically enabling testing of the thresholds from the smallest diameter nerve fibers (5 Hz) to the largest diameter nerve fibers (2000 Hz). This type of sensibility testing differs conceptually from those for vibration and pressure because the electrical current stimulates the nerve fibers directly, and does not directly stimulate the mechanoreceptors the way a vibrometer or Pressure-Specified Sensory Device™ does. Thus, the current perception threshold cannot be directly compared to the vibratory or pressure

thresholds for penile sensibility.

The Neurometer™ is well-suited for penile testing because it straps into place, permitting a discrete measurement of sensibility for the glans and for the proximal shaft of the penis (see Figure 17.5). Table 17.5 contains the data obtained with this device during a study of men with impotence. While no data is available for non-impotent men from that study, it may be that the data from the men with psychogenic and vasculogenic impotence approximates the normal data.

ELECTRODIAGNOSTIC

The bulbocavernosus reflex is probably the best test available for electrophysiological testing. In this test, an electrical stimulation is given to the glans penis, traveling along the pudendal nerve to the spinal cord where it is transmitted to the cerebral cortex, eliciting the perception of touch or pain, depending on the stimulus intensity. At the spinal cord level, interneurons relay the signal to the motor side of the spinal cord, eliciting a response through motor fibers traveling back through the pudendal nerve to the bulbocavernosus muscle. The motor response is detected with a needle electrode in the bulbocavernosus

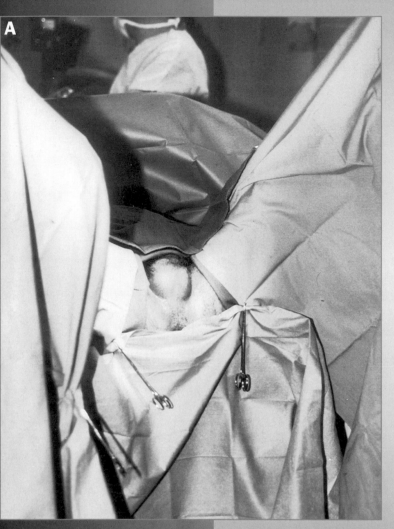

A

C

FIGURE 17.5

Decompression of autonomic and sensory nerves in a 32-year-old juvenile diabetic with advanced complications of diabetes, including neuropathy, retinopathy, nephropathy, and advanced atherosclerosis. (A) Intraoperative lithotomy positioning of the patient. (B) Location for the subscrotal incision. (C) Vessel loop around the internal pudendal artery and nerve as they exit from Alcock's canal after decompression of the nerve. (D) Ruler indicating mild degree of success of correction of impotence after decompression of the parasympathetic nerves. (E) The healing subscrotal incision. Postoperative testing of sensibility with the Neurometer™ demonstrating placement of the electrodes at the (F) glans and the (G) base of the shaft.

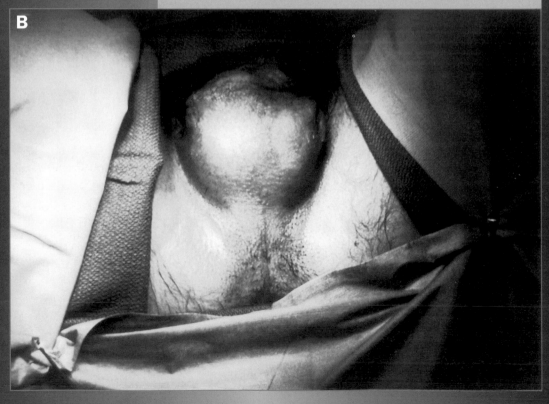

B

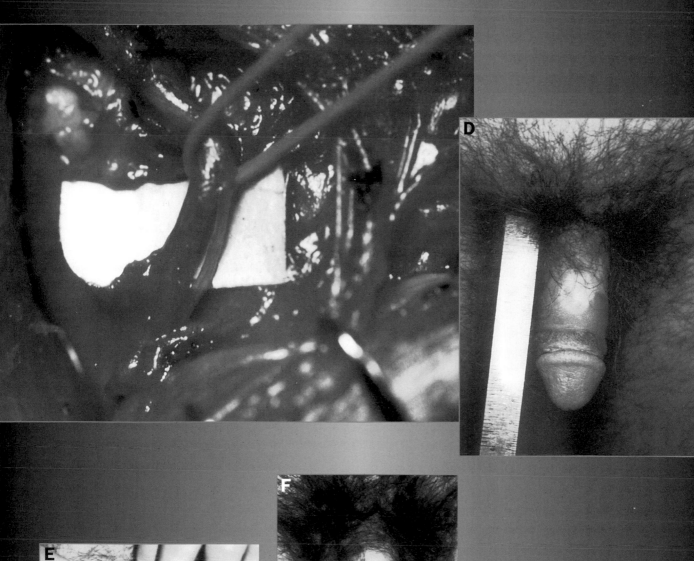

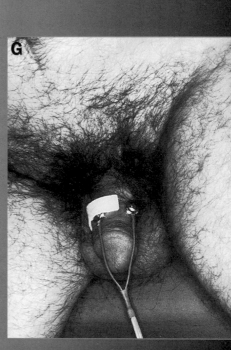

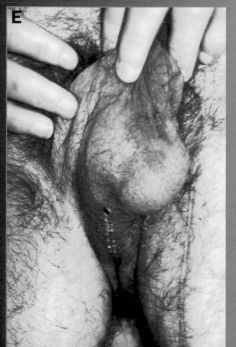

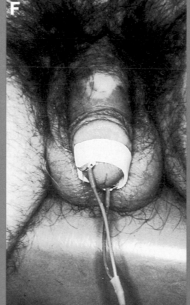

TABLE 17.5 PENILE CURRENT PERCEPTION THRESHOLD IN MEN WITH IMPOTENCE

Etiology of impotence	(n)	Neurometer™ Values[+]		
		5 Hz	250 Hz	2000 Hz
Psychogenic		41	67	218
Vasculogenic		47	84	234
Neurogenic		84	93	312

Note:

[+] Mean current perception threshold.

The difference between the neurogenic and the other two groups is significant at the $p < .05$ level.

From A. L. Dellon, A. L. Scally, & C. Brendler, unpublished data, 1993.

muscle. The normal mean response time for this reflex has been determined by Krane and Siroky (1980) to be 35 m/sec, with a range of 27 to 42 m/sec.

In patients with a spinal cord lesion above the S2 level, these values are unchanged. With a lesion that impinges on the sacral level spinal cord or below, which at this level is called the *cauda equina*, the latency of the reflex is prolonged or absent. In patients with a peripheral neuropathy due to alcoholism or diabetes, in whom the degree of neuropathy is variable, the latency of the reflex is also variable, having a mean response time in 17 patients tested of 42.1 m/sec, with a range of 26.2 to 64 m/sec. Thus, this reflex may be normal in patients who clinically have a peripheral neuropathy in the lower extremities.

In 42 men with impotence on a functional basis, that is, normal vascular studies and no evidence of peripheral neuropathy, the reflex response time was found to be normal, with a mean of 33 m/sec, and a range of 25 to 45 m/sec. This reflex is of particular value in that it may be measured bilaterally, and because the afferent side of the reflex is carried by smaller diameter nerve fibers whose conduction velocity is slower than that for the large diameter motor fibers on the efferent side. Thus, by comparing the components of the response stimulating on one side and recording on the opposite side, inferences can be made as to whether the delay is due to a sensory or motor nerve problem.

Conventional nerve conduction testing has been reported by Gerstenberg and Bradley (1983) for the dorsal nerve of the penis for a

group of 5 normal men, and for a group of 14 men with diabetes-related impotence. Electrical stimulation is applied to the dorsal surface of the glans and the signal is recorded at the dorsal base of the penile shaft. The mean nerve conduction velocity for the normal men was 23.8 m/sec, with a mean for the control sural nerve of 52.4 m/sec. In contrast, for the diabetic men with impotence the mean nerve conduction velocity for the dorsal nerve of the penis was 10.9 m/sec, with a mean for their sural nerve of 38.2 m/sec. The bulbocavernosus reflex correlated well with the readings for these men.

In 1983, Gerstenberg and Bradley extended their study to a group of 23 normal men and 20 diabetic men with impotence. They found that the nerve conduction velocity of the dorsal nerve of the penis demonstrated abnormality at a time when the bulbocavernosus reflex and the somatosensory evoked potential were still normal. This suggests that nerve conduction velocity may be the first electrodiagnostic test to become abnormal in men with impotence related to diabetes.

Most recently, somatosensory evoked potentials have been recorded from the surface of the skull after penile stimulation. This is called the *pudendal evoked response.* Padma-Nathan and Levine (1987) did both vibratory threshold testing and evoked cortical response testing on men with nonpsychogenic impotence. In men who were less than 60 years of age, 93% of those with normal vibrometry had normal evoked responses. The vibrometry was more sensitive than the evoked response in that just 47% of men with abnormal vibrometry also had abnormal evoked responses. Therefore, it appears that the pudendal evoked response is not as good as vibratory threshold testing for screening for neurologic problems related to penile sensibility.

Clinical follow-up found that the men with abnormalities in these tests had impotence related to either diabetic or alcoholic neuropathy. Bemelmans et al. (1991) studied men with reported erectile dysfunction and normal clinical neurological examination, using the pudendal evoked potential as well as the bulbocavernosus reflex. They included 50 normal men in their study, and reported that the 95% confidence intervals for the pudendal evoked response were 36 to 47 sec. In the men with complaints of erectile dysfunction but normal clinical examination, the percentage of patients with abnormal evoked potentials ranged from 33% in those in the 23-39 age group, to 57% in those in the 60-77 age group. When an abnormal tibial evoked potential was combined with the pudendal evoked potential, it was clear that these men had a peripheral neuropathy. These studies, taken together, demonstrate that the pudendal evoked potential can identify sensory abnormalities related to penis function.

• CLINICAL CONDITIONS WITH ALTERED SENSIBILITY •

PENILE RECONSTRUCTION

Reconstruction of the penis may be required after cancer surgery, after a traumatic amputation of the penis, or for the gender reassignment surgery done with transsexuals. The scrotum may require reconstruction as well. Varying amounts of tissue with the potential to transmit erogenous sensation may be present in each of these cases. In the female having gender reassigned to male, the clitoris and labia may be used in the reconstruction in some manner, and new innervation may not be brought into the new penis. If the scrotum or base of the corpora cavernosa or spongiosa remain, they may receive direct mechanical stimulation from the reconstructed penis during intercourse, providing sufficient erogenous sensation that innervation may not need to be brought into the new penis.

Penile reconstruction first used techniques that required multiple stages during which tissue was transferred, usually as a tubed pedicle, from the lower abdomen, thigh, or groin into the pubic region. Urination was usually as a form of *hypospadia,* although if the patient was willing to tolerate the additional stage of reconstruction, a skin graft over a tube could be implanted within the neophallus to form a urethra. Some form of stiffener, such as cartilage, a bone graft, or silicone rod was inserted. Sensibility was not provided, and this not only minimized the erotic sensation recovered, but left the reconstructed penis without even protective sensation. This absence of sensation was often blamed for the erosion of the implant through the skin of the reconstructed penis.

Microsurgical techniques permitted the transfer of a large amount of well-vascularized soft tissue sufficient to provide covering for the penis, lining for a neo-urethra, support for either an implant or a self-contained cartilage or bone strut and, finally, a sensory nerve. And all of this could be accomplished, theoretically, in one operation. The earliest reports of these one-stage microsurgical procedures, from 1984 through 1987, connected the nerve from the transferred flap to the most available cutaneous nerves in the anatomical region, such

as the saphenous and the ilioinguinal nerves. Protective sensibility was recovered, but not erogenous sensation.

The combined plastic surgical and urological efforts of Gilbert, Horton, Terzis, and Devine were the first to connect the flap donor nerve to the internal pudendal nerve. They reported their results in 1988. Their measures of penile sensibility after reconstruction of the penis with an innervated radial forearm flap are given in Table 17.6, and their clinical result is illustrated in Figure 17.4. They reported 7 patients who were past pu-

berty, who indicated that they had recovered erogenous sensation and could masturbate to orgasm. Each of these patients also had reestablished a bulbocavernosus reflex, although the time for the reflex was delayed. They concluded that the connection of the flap nerve to the internal pudendal nerve had restored sensibility sufficient for sexual satisfaction, and that the patient's use of the new penis both for masturbation and sexual intercourse served as a basis for sensory reeducation that permitted cortical reorganization.

TABLE 17.6 COMPARISON OF PENILE VIBRATORY AND PRESSURE THRESHOLDS: PENILE RECONSTRUCTION VERSUS NORMAL

| Threshold | Glans[+] | | Shaft[+] | |
	Tip	Corona	Dorsal	Ventral
Vibration[+]				
Normal	0.20	0.21	0.20	0.20
Phalloplasty	3.3	3.5	1.8	2.9
Pressure[+]				
Normal	18.5	18.4	19.0	18.8
Phalloplasty	23.3	21.4	37.6	32.5

Note:
[+] Microns of relative motion, using the Biothesiometer™, at 120 Hz, 0.5 cm diameter probe tip.
[+] g/mm², measured with the Semmes-Weinstein nylon monofilaments.
From "Phallic Reinnervation via the Pudendal Nerve," by D. A. Gilbert, M. W. Williams, C. E. Horton, J. P. Terzis, & A. Devine, 1988, *Journal of Urology 140*:295-299. Reprinted with permission of the authors.

Gilbert et al. (1988) reported an interesting observation. One patient required closure of the perineal wound prior to what was to be a difficult penile reconstruction. In preparation for that reconstruction, a sural nerve graft was connected to the internal pudendal nerve to bring it into the pubic region. The internal pudendal nerve regenerated down the graft, creating a neuroma at its distal end. Instead of being painful, this neuroma was erogenous.

Replantation of the penis following amputation has been attempted by simply burying the penis within the scrotum while suturing its base back to the original region. Predictably, this leads to varying amounts of necrosis of the glans, the skin, and the shaft, but some degree of preservation was possible. In a review of the literature, Lowe, Chapman, and Berger (1991) found that 2 of the 24 cases (8.5%) they reviewed recovered some degree of sensibility in this type of reconstruction. In contrast, with the development of techniques for microvascular surgery, 5 of the 6 (83%) recovered "good" sensation. In the microvascular replant that these authors report, they found the nerves technically not able to be repaired (they did not try a nerve graft, which would be the indicated option). However, by individually repairing the arteries to each cor-

pora cavernosa they were able to achieve sufficient revascularization that their patient even recovered nocturnal penile tumescence. It was their patient among the microvascular cases that did not recover sensation.

IMPOTENCE

Impotence, the inability to develop and sustain an erection sufficient to have intercourse, is different from the inability to ejaculate. As described in the section above on the autonomic nervous system, the parasympathetics may be affected with or without the sympathetic nerves being affected. For example, in spinal cord-injured men, if the level of the injury is at or below L2, there is no ability to have an erection, and the men are impotent. However, they can still ejaculate, since this is a function of the higher T12-L2 sympathetic nerves. Pharmacologic agents that substitute for the neurotransmitter of the sympathetic nerves, such as the acetylcholinesterase inhibitor physostigmine, can be injected into the penis to give the same result as stimulation of the sympathetic nerves.

Erection requires the relaxation of the smooth muscle cells in the blood vessels of the arteries supplying the corpora, and this is what the parasympathetic innervation does. The increased blood

flow fills the corpora creating tumescence, or swelling. When the pressure from the soft tissues within the corpora gets sufficiently high, the venous valves collapse, preventing outflow of blood and causing the penis to become rigid. Injection of pharmacologic agents such as papaverine, a smooth muscle relaxant, into the corpora, can create an erection, assuming there is sufficient arterial inflow. The stimulus to the autonomic nervous system to carry out the above functions, other than psychic stimuli, comes from tactile stimulation of the penis. This requires an intact and functioning internal pudendal nerve.

It therefore follows that impotence may be due to problems in the central nervous system at the cortical level, called *psychogenic impotence*, or at the arterial inflow level, called *vasculogenic impotence*, or at the autonomic/peripheral nerve level, called neurogenic impotence.

In general, psychogenic impotence is a diagnosis of exclusion, with added help from the sleep lab in which NPT may be demonstrated in the patient with a normal neurological evaluation and normal arterial inflow to the penis. Vasculogenic impotence must be based on a demonstrated decreased arterial inflow to the penis, most usually determined by simply obtaining the blood pressure of the penis, using a doppler and a small blood pressure cuff, and comparing that pressure to the blood pressure obtained in the arm. This ratio is called the *penile-brachial index*, or PBI, and impotence is usually present when this index is less than .75. A patient with a normal PBI who has no NPT would be considered to have neurogenic impotence. Such patients would then be evaluated with further neurologic examinations, such as the bulbocavernosus reflex, nerve conduction of the dorsal penile nerve, or pudendal evoked potential. Most recently, quantitative sensory testing has been evaluated by the neurologic and urologic community. It has been found to be a very sensitive screening test for neurogenic impotence.

The largest population in the United States with neurogenic impotence are men with diabetes. In a classic investigation of this problem, Ellenberg (1971) carried out a survey of 200 diabetic men. Among this group, 59% indicated that they had impotence, and of these, 82% had an associated peripheral neuropathy. Among the 41% of the diabetic men who indicated that they did not have impotence, just 12% had a peripheral neuropathy. The relationship was investigated further on the assumption that the same autonomic nerves that are responsible for erection are those that control function of the urinary bladder. Thus, Ellenberg evaluated bladder function in a group of 45 impotent diabetic men who were an average of 43 years of age. Ellenberg found that 37 of the 45 men had urinary bladder dysfunction, and that 38 of the men also had a peripheral neuropathy. In contrast, in a group of 30 diabetics who were not impotent, and who were an average of 43 years of age, he found that only 3 had bladder involvement and only 6 had a peripheral neuropathy. Importantly, he studied the endocrine function in these men and found that the diabetic men who were impotent had normal levels of testosterone, and that giving them testosterone was of no benefit.

This study demonstrated the causal relationship of the autonomic nervous system in diabetics with impotence, and suggested the possible role of peripheral neuropathy (the internal pudendal nerve) in impotence, since such a high percentage of the men with impotence had an associated peripheral neuropathy. The potential diagnostic role for quantitative sensory testing of the penis in men with impotence is clear from this work. The possibility that compression of these nerves in diabetics, who are susceptible to chronic nerve compression, may now be considered in the therapy of impotence, is discussed below (see Figure 17.5).

NERVE COMPRESSION

Any nerve in the body may become compressed. The most common sites for compression are normal areas of anatomic narrowing, such as the carpal tunnel and cubital tunnel in the upper extremity, and the tarsal tunnel in the lower extremity. The very exit site of the spinal nerve from the vertebra, the vertebral foramen, may be considered as the most proximal of these sites of potential compression. If a basic disease process makes a peripheral nerve more susceptible to compression, it follows that chronic compression of peripheral nerves will become more common in that disease. If a particular occupation or sports activity puts unusual pressure on a peripheral nerve, it follows that symptoms of chronic nerve compression may develop. I believe that these considerations apply to impotence in diabetics and in cyclists.

As previously explained for the nerves of the upper and lower extremities in my 1988 editorial, "A Cause for Optimism in Diabetic Neuropathy," the diabetic nerve contains an increased amount of water due to conversion of glucose to sucrose. This makes the nerve larger in diameter than the normal nerve. Thus, the diabetic nerve is more susceptible to compression in tight anatomic spaces. Furthermore, the diabetic nerve has a decreased slow component to axoplasmic transport due to the basic underlying metabolic disease. This makes the nerve unable to repair distal areas of compression as well as the normal nerve. These two factors combine to render the diabetic nerve susceptible to chronic compression. Support for this hypothesis comes from the 80% success rate of peripheral nerve decompression in the upper and lower extremities in diabetics, as I reported in 1992.

Where might the autonomic and internal pudendal nerves be entrapped in the diabetic? The anatomy review at the beginning of this chapter clearly identifies two areas which, theoretically, could be the sites for compression: the urogenital diaphragm and Alcock's canal. Cadaver dissections (see Figure 17.5) have suggested that an approach through the base of the scrotum would give sufficient exposure to divide the fibrous portion of the urogenital diaphragm, thereby decompressing the autonomic nerves that are passing alongside the bulbous portion of the urethra, and to release the fascia along Alcock's canal, thereby decompressing the sensory fibers in the internal pudendal nerve.

This procedure was attempted in one patient, a man 34 years of age, who had Type I diabetes since he was 4 years old. He was quite advanced in terms of peripheral neuropathy, retinopathy, and nephropathy, and already had had a cardiac bypass. While he recovered sensibility in his penis, as documented by current perception testing with the Neurometer™ (see Table 17.8), he did not recover sufficient penile tumescence to achieve a full erection. Further application of this concept of peripheral nerve decompression appears warranted in diabetics in whom there is a normal brachiopenile index, indicating sufficient vascular inflow potential, and in whom their overall physical condition is stronger than in the first patient illustrated in Figure 17.5.

There are only anecdotal stories among cyclists about problems with erection. However, cyclists' problems with ulnar nerve compression at the wrist in Guyon's canal have been documented, and this repetitive trauma and direct compression causes numbness in the little and ring finger, a sense of coldness in the fingers, and some degree of weakness and loss of coordination. Appropriately padded gloves have been designed, placing gel or padding directly over the hypothenar eminence. With regard to complaints of impotence, typically, after a

25- or 50-mile cycling trip, some cyclists (the incidence is unknown) will experience a problem in achieving an erection. Usually, within 12 to 24 hours this problem is gone. At present, there is not even one reference in the urology literature about this problem, and few urologists have encountered a patient with these complaints. To these superb young athletes this is a disturbing problem, and one often attributed to either pure fatigue or the stress of the race. Could not the problem be due to acute compression of the internal pudendal nerve by the bicycle seat against the pubic ramus, where the nerve is normally in the tight Alcock canal? Would alteration of the cyclists' seat in this critical juncture zone make a difference, or perhaps more padding in this location? The Pressure-Specified Sensory Device™ may offer an excellent way to test this hypothesis by measuring the cutaneous pressure threshold of the glans penis before and after a long cycling trip. For those professional or die-hard amateur cyclists for whom impotence is a persistent problem, decompression of the internal pudendal nerve might be an appropriate therapeutic consideration.

I recently had the opportunity to evaluate a man who had blunt trauma to the perineum. He lost penile sensibility. Preoperative testing with the Neurometer™ documented abnormal sensory thresholds (see Table 17.7). Preoperative somatosensory evoked potentials (see Chapter 8) demonstrated absent brain waves after penile stimulation, all consistent with impaired function of the internal pudendal nerve. Testing with the Pressure-Specified Sensory Device™ was tried, but it was found to be difficult to test the penis. Each time the Pressure-Specified Sensory Device™ was pressed against the penis, the penis would move. Testing with the Neurometer™ was found to be more valid for this skin surface. At surgery, both internal pudendal nerves were decompressed in Alcock's canal. The 6-month post-op Neurometer™ values were improved, and the post-op somatosensory evoked potentials demonstrated were normal.

REHABILITATION

There is not a great deal of material available on rehabilitation of sensation in the penis. The earliest information that I have found can be inferred from Newman's study (1970) on vibratory threshold in the penis. In that study, the vibratory threshold was separated based on the patient's age, and then again on the frequency with which he had sexual intercourse. Frequency was given in terms of an estimate of sexual intercourse over a 1-year period. It is clear from that data (see Table 17.8) that for any given age group, the vibratory threshold was lower in the group that had sexual intercourse. This is in line with the old adage, "use it or lose it." It may be inferred that whereas the vibratory threshold would be expected to increase with age due to the normal physiologic effect of receptor aging or programmed neuronal loss, the perception of vibratory sensation may be kept within younger physiologic limits through more frequent sensory stimulation.

TABLE 17.7 SENSORY CHANGE FOLLOWING DECOMPRESSION OF THE INTERNAL PUDENDAL NERVE

(A) Diabetic with Neurogenic Impotence

	Neurometer™ Values[+]		
	5 Hz	250 Hz	2000 Hz
Pre-op	120	215	400
1 month post-op	100	160	308
3 month post-op	60	75	220
6 month post-op	26	42	139

(B) A Man 2 Years After Blunt Trauma to Perineum

	Neurometer™ Values[+]		
	5 Hz	250 Hz	2000 Hz
Pre-op	34	58	212
6 month post-op	16	34	110

Note:
[+] Mean current perception threshold.
From A. L. Dellon & A. L. Scally, unpublished observations, 1991–1996.

TABLE 17.8 RELATIONSHIP OF PENILE SENSIBILITY AND FREQUENCY OF INTERCOURSE

Age	n	Intercourse Per year	Vibratory Threshold[+]
35-44	2	none	25.48
	12	109	4.90
45-53	2	none	13.62
	10	81	8.40
65-74	17	none	176.15
	13	22	39.40

Note:

[+] Force in units of voltage, using a 0.5 cm diameter probe at 120 Hz, where "force was roughly proportional to the square of the applied voltage."

From "Vibratory Sensitivity of the Penis," by H. F. Newman, 1970, *Fertility and Sterility* *21:*791-793. Reprinted with permission of the author.

The direct implication for rehabilitation of penile sensibility is similar to what has been proven for the upper extremity: that increased sensory stimulation results in better cortical perception of that stimulus and, presumably, better function. There is a role for quantitative sensory testing to document recovery of sensation in men with penile reconstruction, in the diagnosis of neurogenic impotence, and in evaluating the possibility of chronic compression of the internal pudendal nerve. Repeat testing is, in itself, a form of sensory reeducation, as it focuses the patient's attention on perception and understanding of the neural impulses he is receiving. It is unlikely that, with the exception of testing sensibility, the therapist will become involved with what is likely to be the most effective form of sensory reeducation for the penis, the patient's own stimulation of the penis, by rubbing its tip and shaft, by masturbation, and by sexual intercourse.

● SUMMARY ●

The penis is innervated by sensory fibers from the internal pudendal nerve. Penile sensibility is best expressed as the threshold for the perception of pressure and for the perception of vibration, for which some normative data is available. This data suggests that the penis has about the same sensitivity for vibratory stimuli as does the fingertip, while the sensitivity for pressure stimuli is about four-fold higher than for the fingertip.

Reconstructive microsurgery is capable of creating a new penis, and quantitative sensibility testing has demonstrated that the results with the innervated radial forearm flap, connecting the nerve within the flap to the internal pudendal nerve, can regenerate to give sensibility sufficient to provide a basis for orgasm. The recovered sensation is not only protective, but also erotic. New testing devices that are applicable to testing the sensory deficits related to impotence are the Neurometer™ and the Pressure-Specified Sensory Device™. Operative procedures to decompress the autonomic

nerves and the internal pudendal nerve may become an option to treat neurogenic impotence and to relieve chronic compression

of the internal pudendal nerve which may be associated with certain sports activity, such as long-distance cycling.

• • •

• REFERENCES •

Bemelmans, B. L. H., Hendrikx, L. B. P. M., Koldewijn, E. L., Lemmens, W. A. J. G., Debruyne, F. M. J., & Meuleman, E. J. H. Comparison of biothesiometry and neuro-urophysiological investigations for the clinical evaluation of patients with erectile dysfunction. *Journal of Urology 153*:1483-1486, 1995.

Bemelmans, B. L. H., Meuleman, E. J. H., Antem, B. W. M., Doesburg, W. H., Van Kerrebroeck, P. W. V., & Debruyne, F. M. J. Penile sensory disorders in erectile dysfunction: Results of a comprehensive neuro-urophysiological diagnostic evaluation in 123 patients. *Journal of Urology 146*:777-783, 1991.

Dellon, A. L. A cause for optimism in diabetic neuropathy. *Annals of Plastic Surgery 20*:103-105, 1988

Ellenberg, M. Impotence in diabetes: The neurologic factor. *Annals of Internal Medicine 75*:213-219, 1971.

Gerstenberg, T. C., & Bradley, W. E. Nerve conduction velocity measurement of dorsal nerve of penis in normal and impotent males. *Journal of Urology 21*:90-92, 1983.

Gilbert, D. A., Williams, M. W., & Horton, C. E., Terzis, J. P., & Devine, A. Phallic reinnervation via the pudendal nerve. *Journal of Urology 140*:295-299, 1988.

Halata, Z., & Munger, B. L. The neuroanatomical basis for the protopathic sensibility of the human glans penis. *Brain Research 371*:205-230, 1986.

Krane, R. J., & Siroky, M. B. Studies on sacral evoked potentials. *Journal of Urology 124*:872-877, 1980.

Lowe, M. A., Chapman, W., & Berger, R. E. Repair of a traumatically amputated penis with return of erectile function. *Journal of Urology 145*:1267-1270, 1991.

Lue, T. F., Zeineh, S. J., Schmidt, R. A., & Tanagho, E. A. Neuroanatomy of penile erection: Its relevance to iatrogenic impotence. *Journal of Urology 131*:273-280, 1984.

Montague, D. K. *Disorders of Male Sexual Function.* Chicago: Year Book Medical Publishers, 1988.

Newman, H. F. Vibratory sensitivity of the penis. *Fertility and Sterility 21*:791-793, 1970.

Padma-Nathan, H., & Levine, F. Vibration testing of the penis. *Journal of Urology 4*:201-206, 1987.

Walsh, P. C., & Donker, P. J. Impotence following radical prostatectomy: Insight into etiology and prevention. *Journal of Urology 128*:492-497, 1982.

• ADDITIONAL READINGS •

Caine, D. B., & Pallis, C. A. Vibratory sense: A critical review. *Brain 89*:723-733, 1966.

Chapelle, P. A., Roby-Brami, A., Yakovleff, A., & Bussel, B. Journal of Neurology, *Neurosurgery and Psychiatry 51*:197-202, 1988.

Cheng, K-X., Hwang, W-Y., Eid, A. E., Wang, S-L., Chang, T-S., & Fu, K-D. Analysis of 136 cases of reconstructed penis using various methods. *Plastic and Reconstructive Surgery 95*:94-98, 1995.

Dellon, A. L. *Evaluation of Sensibility and Re-Education of Sensation in the Hand.* Baltimore: Williams & Wilkins, 1981.

Dellon, A. L. The vibrometer. *Plastic and Reconstructive Surgery 71*:427-431, 1983.

Dellon, A. L. Treatment of the symptoms of diabetic neuropathy by peripheral nerve decompression. *Plastic and Reconstructive Surgery 89*:689-697, 1992.

Dellon, E. S., Crone, S., Mourey, R., & Dellon, A. L. Comparison of the Semmes-Weinstein monofilaments with the Pressure-Specified Sensory Device. *Restorative Neurology Neuroscience 5*:323-326, 1993.

Dellon, E. S., Mourey, R., & Dellon, A. L. Human pressure perception values for constant and moving one-and two-point discrimination. *Plastic and Reconstructive Surgery 90*:112-117, 1992.

Katims, J. J., Naviasky, E. H., Rendell, M. S., Ng, L. K. Y., & Bleeker, M. I. Constant current sine wave transcutaneous nerve stimulation for the evaluation of peripheral neuropathy. *Archives of Physical Medicine and Rehabilitation 68*:210-213, 1987.

Kuhn, R.A. Functional capacity of the isolated human spinal cord. *Brain 73*:1-6, 1950.

Levin, S., Pearsall, G., & Ruderman, R. J. von Fry's method of measuring pressure sensibility in the hand: An engineering analysis of the Weinstein-Semmes pressure aesthisiometer. *Journal of Hand Surgery 3*:211-216, 1978.

Lin, J. T., & Bradley, W. E. Penile neuropathy in insulin-dependent diabetes mellitus. *Journal of Urology 133*:213-215, 1985.

O'Brien Cofelice, M., Lumpkin, D., & Kerstein, M. D. Penile waveform analysis: Its usefulness in evaluating vasculogenic impotence. *Bruit 10*:242-243, 1986.

Sachs, B. D., & Liu, Y-C. Maintenance of erection of penile glans, but not penile body, after transection of rat cavernous nerves. *Journal of Urology 146:*900-905, 1991.

Wasserman, J. D., Pollack, C. P., & Spielman, A. J. The differential diagnosis of impotence: The measurement of nocturnal penile tumescence. *Journal of the American Medical Association 243*:2038-2042, 1980.

● ● ●

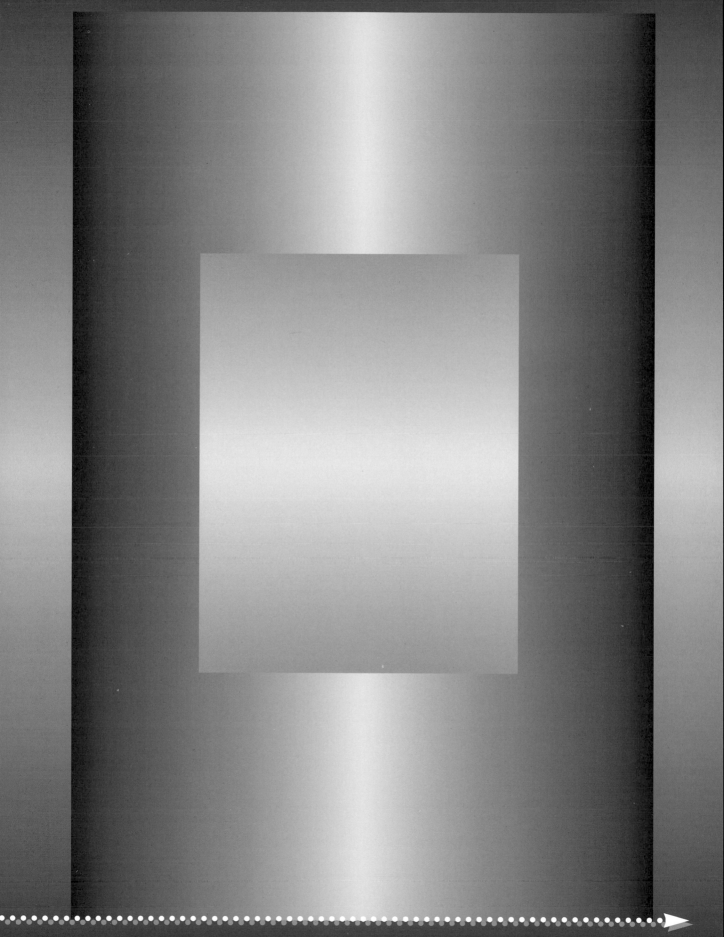

18

cumulative trauma disorders

• • •

What's in a name?
Impairment versus Disability.
Person versus Patient versus Claimant.
Thoracic Outlet Syndrome versus
Brachial Plexus Compression.
Occupational Disease versus Cumulative
Trauma Disorder.

• • •

What we name something can have significant implications. When a worker is injured by a discrete event at work, such as being hit by a piece of steel in a steel mill, there is no doubt that the resultant physical problems are causally related to that event. But can chronic exposure to a work environment produce a problem that is properly called an occupational disease or disorder?

Historically, among the first physical ailments to be thought of in these terms was testicular cancer in chimney sweepers in England. It became accepted that there were carcinogens in the soot in the chimneys that over a period of time could induce cancer in the workers exposed to it. Extension of this type of association has led to acceptance of problems such as pulmonary disease being occupationally caused by working in a coal mine or with asbestos, skin cancer being occupationally caused by exposure to certain substances or conditions, and a disease of the hand being occupationally caused by X ray exposure of the early fluoroscope machines used by radiologists.

Today, we see this type of occupational disease in painters who develop lead poisoning. But will using an extremity repetitively at a job produce an occupational disease or disorder? The answer to this question is still being debated scientifically, even though industry and the U.S. government have, although grudgingly, accepted that repetitive motion activities in the work place can produce, over time, a disorder related to the accumulation of trauma to the musculoskeletal system. The name for this problem is *cumulative trauma disorder*. Papers have been written using the abbreviation CTD for cumulative trauma disorder, but this acronym may be confused with carpal tunnel disease or decompression; therefore, this chapter will not use the abbreviation. *Repetitive motion injury or disorder* would be an acceptable synonym for this problem.

Is there an epidemic of cumulative trauma disorders? Over the past decade, the number of patients seen by physicians and therapists for problems related to their job has increased dramatically. Several textbooks have appeared, including *Occupational Hand and Upper Extremity Injuries and Diseases* (Kasdan, 1991), *Occupational Disorders of the Upper Extremity* (Millender, Louis, & Simmonds, 1992), *Occupational Musculoskeletal Disorders* (Hadler, 1993), and *Occupational Neurology and Clinical Neurotoxicology* (Bleecker, 1994). It seems almost intuitive that jobs that require repetition, working at a fast pace, working with body mechanics that place certain joints at increased stress, working in positions that place nerves under muscle tension, and placement of hands in space that requires continual shoulder girdle muscle function *should* cause biomechanical problems that translate into musculoskeletal complaints and peripheral nerve compressions.

Armstrong (1992) has compiled a list from our descriptive medical language that includes a variety of names of clinical complaints suggesting causality with respect to the work place, sports, or a hobby. Examples are gamekeeper's thumb, washer woman's sprain, drummer's palsy, pipe setter's thumb, reedmaker's elbow, flute player's palsy, tobacco-primer's wrist, wall washer's thumb, bowler's thumb, tennis elbow, and space invader's thumb. Table 18.1 lists a group of industries or jobs in which research has suggested there exists an occupational disorder(s) due to cumulative trauma.

For example, compared with shop assistants who had an incidence of carpal tunnel syndrome of 0.0%, the incidence of carpal tunnel syndrome in garment workers has been reported to be 18%, and in meat packers 15% (Masear, Hayes, & Hyde, 1986). Another example is the demonstrated relationship between jobs requiring high force and high repetitiveness and the incidence of carpal tunnel syndrome. Silverstein, Fine, and Armstrong (1987) found that the prevalence of developing carpal tunnel syndrome was 15.5% for those workers whose jobs required a combination of both high force and high repetitiveness, in contrast to those workers whose jobs required a combination of low force and low repetitiveness, whose prevalence of carpal tunnel syndrome was 1.8%. (This data was based, however, on a small subset of just 12 patients.)

Intuitive as it all seems, there are, nevertheless, those who are quick to point out that patients with occupational disorders may be influenced by a changing work ethic, by the widespread dissemination of information about these problems, by the financial rewards of sickness rather than the financial

TABLE 18.1 REPORTS OF CUMULATIVE TRAUMA DISORDERS IN INDUSTRY

Industry/Occupation	Author(s) of Report/Year of Publication
Gamekeeper's thumb	Campbell, 1955
Electronic assembly workers	Hymovich & Lindholm, 1966
Bowler's thumb	Howell & Leach, 1970
Computer data entry	Spaans, 1970
Factory workers	Jarvinen & Kuorinka, 1979
Tobacco-primer's wrist	Parsons, 1981
Aircraft motor assembly	Cannon, Bernacki, & Walter, 1981
Poultry industry	Armstrong, Foulke, Joseph, & Goldstein, 1982
Sewing machine operators	Vihma, Nurminen, & Mutanen, 1982
Computer data entry	Feldman, Goldman, & Keyserling, 1983
Meat packers	Steib & Sun, 1984
Meat packers	Masear, Hayes, & Hyde, 1986
Electronics industry	Kilbom, Persson, & Jonsson, 1986
Reed-maker's elbow	Dawson, 1986
Electronic assembly workers	Feldman, Travers, Chirico-Post, & Keyserling, 1987
Hardware assembly workers	Arndt, 1987
Supermarket checkers	Margolis & Kraus, 1987
Forestry workers	Brammer, Piercy, Auger, & Nohara, 1987
Casting plant workers	Silverstein, Fine, & Stetson, 1987
Cashiers, computer data entry, assembly line	Hagberg & Wegman, 1987
Automobile assembly	Armstrong, Punnett, & Ketner, 1989
Dental technicians	Hjortsberg, Rosen, & Orbaek, 1989
Shipyard workers	Cherniak, Letz, Gerr, Brammer, & Pace, 1990
Computer data entry	Tadano, 1990
Gold miners	Narini, Novak, Mackinnon, & Coulson-Ross, 1993
Garment industry	McAtamney & Corlett, 1993
Assembly line	Neelam, 1994

benefits of daily work, and by the advertising of lawyers. Furthermore, some people point out that many of the "diseases" that are being identified would occur anyway in the natural process of aging.

Prominent authors writing about this "alternative" etiology are Norton Hadler (1990, 1993) and Peter Nathan (Nathan, Keniston, Myers, & Meadows, 1992). Hadler, for example, has written that a person with a musculoskeletal problem has the following three options: to persist as a person, to choose to be a patient with an illness, or to choose to be a claimant with an illness or injury. There can be no doubt that part of the "epidemic" is not a true increase in incidence of work-related problems, but rather an increased awareness that has led to increased reporting of what are prevalent problems, with possibly some related simply to the aging process itself. Sorting out a person's complaints into those that are related to the normal aging process, to leisure time activities, or perhaps to a preexisting medical problem, such as diabetes, from those that are causally related to his or her job is a difficult problem, the solution to which may change that person into either a patient or a claimant.

While there is increased public and professional attention devoted to cumulative trauma disorders today, it is humbling to read what has been discovered to be probably the very first description of this problem, almost 300 years ago! I am indebted to Dean Louis (1992) for his most complete quote from Ramazzini (1964).

• • •

Various and manifold is the harvest of diseases reaped by certain workers from the crafts and trades that they pursue. All the profit that they get is fatal injury to their health, mostly from two causes. The first and most potent is the harmful character of the materials they handle. The second I ascribe to certain violent and irregular motions and unnatural postures of the body, by reason of which, the natural structure of the vital machine is so impaired that serious disease gradually develops therefrom. [With regard to potters] First their hands become palsied, and then they become paralytic, splenic, lethargic, cachectic, and toothless, so that one rarely sees a patient whose face is not cadaverous, and the color of lead. [They failed to seek help until they were terribly crippled, and when told that they must refrain from their trades, they would refuse to do so because it was their only means of sustenance.]

• • •

Louis (1992) has also given us a rare glimpse into the earliest impairment rating schemes. He notes that under early Arab law

The loss of a portion of a thumb or a great toe was considered to be equivalent to the loss of one-half of a finger. Compensation for the loss of a penis was based upon its length, and for an ear, its surface area was considered. Injuries to the head were compensated in camels...A simple scratch was equivalent to one camel; if the injury involved the dura mater, it was recompensed by 33 camels; if there was brain damage then the recompense was 100 camels. Brain damage was considered to be fatal in those days, so that one life was considered to be worth 100 camels.

• • •

• HYPOTHESIS •

While Hadler and Nathan would have us consider that much of what is termed cumulative trauma disorder is related to the aging process and to financial incentives of the compensation system, other hypotheses related to the pathophysiology of the musculoskeletal system are emerging. In 1988, for example, Edwards put forth a hypothesis based on progressive changes in muscle fibers and the central nervous system control of peripheral motor events. Edwards marshalled a line of reasoning that included observed histopathologic changes in muscle fibers, abnormal electromyographic activity, calcium channel changes leading to susceptibility of the muscle plasma membrane to free radicals, and poorly regulated central nervous system control of muscle activity. Once initiated, these factors can lead to excessive contraction force per muscle fiber, leading to hypoxia, acidosis, and metabolic depletion followed by calcium-mediated cellular damage. A self-perpetuating vicious cycle of cellular damage then ensues. Edwards notes, in support of his theory, that a calcium channel blocker drug has been observed to relieve exercise-induced muscle pain of undetermined cause. Edwards finally suggests that

Occupational muscle pain might be a consequence of a conflict between motor control of the postural muscular activity and that needed for rhythmic movement or skilled manipulations. The important new argument is that rather than the emphasis on the peripheral (muscle) metabolic changes or pathology, the primary cause might be sought in altered central motor control, resulting in imbalance between harmonious motor unit recruitment and relaxation of muscles not directly involved in the activity...It is a popular credence that the more skilled the worker or more proficient the performer the less this occurs, with benefit to the precision of the task or act and with less fatigue or risk of injury....It is noted that peripheral influences or consequences of injury may cause what have hitherto been considered central neurological disturbances, e.g., the induction of involuntary movements (focal dystonia)...Furthermore, the primary disorder underlying "fibrositis" is also a disturbance of central control of postural motor units such that there is failure of proper relaxation of low threshold units between periods of activity during the day and in sleep...Viewed in this light, the industrial worker who depends for his or her livelihood on muscular activity seems singularly poorly prepared, compared with the performers on stage or track, to achieve the desired performance without risk of developing muscle pain or injury.

Another hypothesis for the sequelae of cumulative trauma has been advanced by Mackinnon and Novak (1994). They sought a unifying concept to explain the multiplicity of complaints that patients with cumulative disorders have. Their hypothesis may be put forth in terms that use the neck and shoulder muscles and the brachial plexus as the anatomic substrata. Therefore, the illustrations for this hypothesis, Figures 18.1 and 18.2, will also be applicable to the following section on thoracic outlet syndrome. The Mackinnon-Novak hypothesis has three intertwining elements that must each work in concert to produce symptoms in a patient with cumulative trauma. They are:

Element 1

Particular extremity positions will result in direct increased pressure around specific nerves at various entrapment points, and result in chronic nerve compression...At these entrapment points, edema and subsequent fibrous connective tissue can tether the nerve so that normal neural excursion is decreased. Placing the nerve on stretch will also increase tension on the nerve...[this] tends to be slowly but surely progressive...A motor nerve contains many sensory affer-

FIGURE 18.1

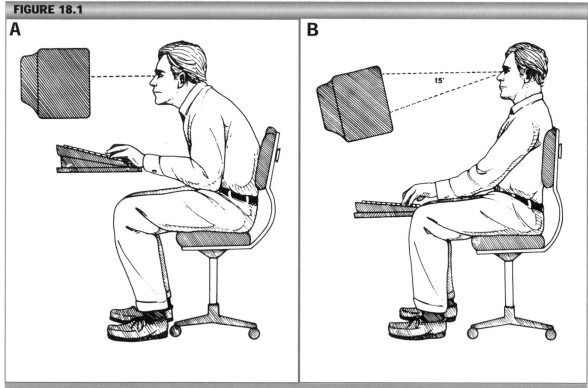

A

B

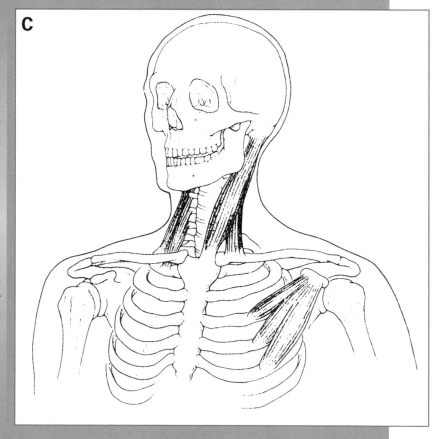

C

Proposed mechanism of cumulative trauma disorder, using brachial plexus compression in the thoracic inlet as an example. Abnormal posturing during work activity, such as the positioning while typing (A) creates a poked- forward position of the head and neck and a flexed forward position of the shoulder. This results in shortening of the scalene, sternocleidomastoid, and pectoralis minor muscles (C). Correction of these abnormal postures, as in (B), will be required as part of the overall rehabilitation. From "Clinical Commentary: Pathogenesis of Cumulative Trauma Disorder," by S. E. Mackinnon & C. B. Novak, 1994, Journal of Hand Surgery 19A:873-883, Churchill Livingstone, New York. Reprinted with permission of the authors.

FIGURE 18.2

Proposed mechanism for cumulative trauma, using brachial plexus compression in the thoracic inlet as an example. (A) In the normal posture, the levator scapulae (LS), rhomboids (R), trapezius (T), and serratus anterior (SA) position the scapula against the thorax. (B) The abnormal posturing demonstrated in Figure 18.1 result in lengthening of the middle and lower trapezius (shaded area), with abduction of the scapula and shortening of the serratus anterior muscle (shaded area). Weakness of these stretched muscles will occur. (C) Compensation for these abnormal muscle tensions occurs by contractions of the upper trapezius, levator scapulae, and rhomboids (dark area), causing hypertrophy due to overuse. From "Clinical Commentary: Pathogenesis of Cumulative Trauma Disorder," by S. E. Mackinnon & C. B. Novak, 1994, Journal of Hand Surgery 19A:873-883, Churchill Livingstone, New York. Reprinted with permission of the authors.

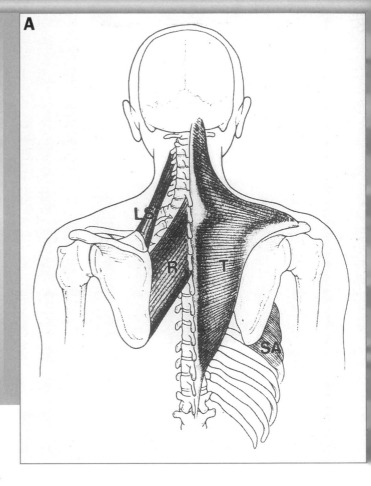

ent fibers and when compressed will produce a dull aching sensation in the location of the muscles innervated by that motor nerve. Finally, nerve compression at one point along the nerve may render both distal and proximal sites less tolerant of the effects of compression, the double crush phenomenon.

Element 2

Abnormal postures can result in a set of muscles being maintained and used in shortened positions. These tight muscles will become painful, especially when stretched. Some muscles, when in a

tightened position, will secondarily compress neurovascular structures... [These shortened muscles] will then reset at even shorter and tighter positions. When the individual attempts to assume a more appropriate...posture, these muscles become stretched and are painful.

Element 3

Abnormal postures will result in some muscles being underused and subsequently weakened. Weakness of one set of muscles will then result in a compensatory

overuse of a second set of muscles, and a cycle of muscle imbalance will be established...This self-perpetuating cycle of tight muscles becoming tighter and weak muscles becoming weaker explains why rest alone will not relieve all of the symptoms of [cumulative trauma disorders]. It also explains why physiotherapy directed at "general strengthening" is likely to result in strengthening of muscles already "too strong" and will be unsuccessful at restoring muscle balance.

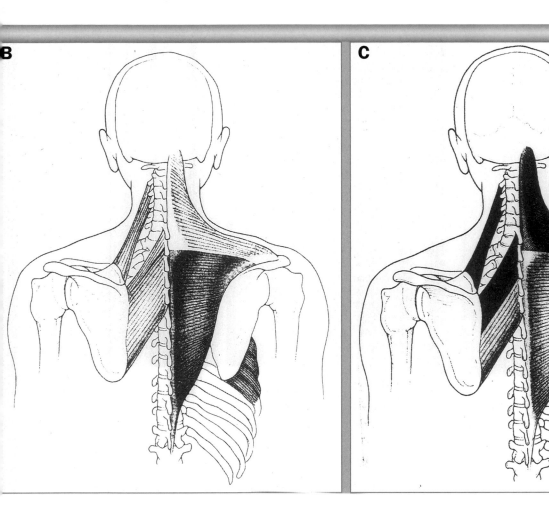

• CRITICAL ANALYSIS • OF CUMULATIVE TRAUMA DISORDERS

The factors concerning the origin and treatment of cumulative trauma disorders are somewhat similar to those of the origin and treatment of diabetic neuropathy. That is, clinicians can agree that patients are suffering from a given problem and can measure the effects of that problem, but the cause of the problem remains unclear. Therefore, treatment remains based on empirical grounds. But medicine's origin is empiric. To the best we are able, today's approaches are based on randomized prospective studies. The above hypotheses regarding cumulative trauma can be tested and in time either confirmed, modified, or replaced. It appears justified for now, therefore, to accept that there will always be a percentage of patients with complaints that may be related to cumulative trauma.

We will need to assess in our own minds, and with the use of appropriate tests for malingering, those whom we believe to be exaggerating or misleading because of the potential rewards of the compensation or tort system, and those whom we believe are "legitimate" patients. For the latter group, who represent the overwhelming majority, in my view, our approach must be based on taking a careful history, doing a careful physical exam, making measurements with the best devices available, and then instituting a treatment plan.

Specific areas related to cumulative trauma will be discussed below to illustrate this approach.

• THORACIC OUTLET • SYNDROME

The symptom complex commonly called the *thoracic outlet syndrome* remains poorly understood and, perhaps for that reason alone, controversial. The book, *Thoracic Outlet Syndrome: A Common Sequela of Neck Injuries* (Sanders, 1991), has an exceptional annotated bibliography reviewing papers from 1821 through 1990. Another source for clarification of this problem is Chapter 14, "Multiple Crush Syndromes," in *Surgery of the Peripheral Nerve* (Mackinnon & Dellon, 1988).

Virtually everything about this syndrome is controversial except the following, about which both neurologists and surgeons agree: (a) The presence of a cervical rib can cause vascular obstruction to either the subclavian artery or vein, resulting in well-defined vascular problems that should be treated surgically; and (b) the presence of intrinsic muscle wasting and numbness of the little finger associated with abnormal electromyography and decreased amplitude of the sensory response to the little finger is due to "true, neurogenic, thoracic outlet syndrome," and should be treated surgically. The reason for this agreement between neurologists and surgeons is that these two subgroups of patients within the larger group of thoracic outlet syndrome patients have uniform complaints, objective physical findings, and an identifiable pathology.

However, the largest group of patients has neurologic and musculoskeletal complaints, and usually no or only a few objective findings on physical examination, while radiographic and electrodiagnostic tests are usually normal (see Table 18.2). The extent to which this clinical problem is controversial may be glimpsed by reading the pro and con exchanges that have graced the scientific literature, most notably between Wilbourn and Urschel (1984) over the use of electrodiagnosis, Roos and Wilbourn (1990) over the prevalence of the syndrome, and Cherington and Cherington's (1992) attribution of financial reward as the main concern of the surgeon in treating these patients.

The names given to this symptom complex (see Table 18.3), the commonest complaints of which are given in Table 18.4, are confusing and have added to the diagnostic and therapeutic problem. Since a name usually suggests an etiology, names such as *scalenus anticus syndrome* or *cervical rib syndrome* have led to resecting the anterior scalene muscle or the cervical rib, or both. Names such as the *costoclavicular syndrome* have led to resecting either the clavicle or the first rib or both, to the exclusion of considering whether any other structures may be responsible for compression of the brachial plexus or the subclavian vessels. The name most currently in use, thoracic outlet syndrome, just compounds the confusion. That is because the name suggests that the diaphragm be resected, because the thoracic outlet is the region between the thorax and the abdomen! I prefer the name

TABLE 18.2 THORACIC OUTLET SYNDROME CLINICAL PRESENTATIONS

Vascular	Up to 10%
Arterial	
Venous	
True Neurogenic	Less than 1%
Neurologic	About 90%

TABLE 18.3 THORACIC OUTLET SYNDROME SYNONYMS

Cervical rib syndrome (Cooper, 1821)

Effort vein thrombosis (von Schroetter, 1884)

Scalenus anticus syndrome (Nafziger, 1938)

Costoclavicular syndrome (Falconer & Weddell, 1943)

Hyperabduction syndrome (Wright, 1945)

Pectoralis minor syndrome (Wright, 1945)

Thoracic outlet syndrome (Peet, Hendrickson, Anderson, & Martin, 1956)

Thoracic outlet compression syndrome (Rob & Standeven, 1958)

Neurogenic thoracic outlet syndrome (Gilliatt, LeQuesne, Logue, & Sumner, 1970)

Upper and lower thoracic outlet syndrome (Roos, 1980)

Fracture clavicle/rib syndrome (Connolly & Dehne, 1986)

Cervico-thoracic outlet syndrome (Narakas et al., 1986)

Brachial plexus compression in the thoracic inlet (Dellon, 1993)

brachial plexus compression in the thoracic inlet (Dellon, 1993). Even though this name is longer, it does not precondition the clinician's mind as to the anatomic structures that may be responsible for the diverse group of neurologic and musculoskeletal complaints that are caused by the compression (see Figure 18.3).

Thus, the therapist directs attention to all structures that might compress or entrap the brachial plexus, and the surgeon will attempt to correct the anatomic problems related to the supraclavicular brachial plexus from the vertebral foramen to the clavicle, and possibly to the infraclavicular brachial plexus, if the pectoralis minor remains tight (see Figure 18.4).

The diagnosis of brachial

TABLE 18.4 SYMPTOMS OF THORACIC OUTLET SYNDROME (BRACHIAL PLEXUS COMPRESSION IN THE THORACIC INLET)

Neurologic
Numbness in the little and ring finger
Numbness in the whole hand
Aching in the shoulder
Aching in the back
Headaches
Aching in the anterior chest
Breast discomfort
Jaw discomfort
Weakness and clumsiness
Shoulder pain
Neck pain
Coldness in the hand

Arterial
Coldness in the hand
Black fingertip

Venous
Swelling of the hand/arm
Pinker/bluish color to hand

Note: Usually all symptoms are aggravated or initiated by elevating the hand above the head.

FIGURE 18.3

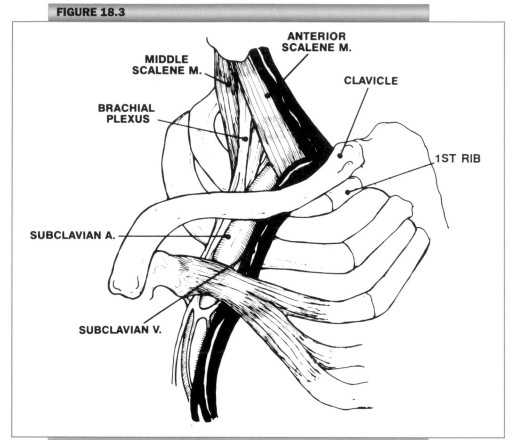

Brachial plexus compression may occur from distal to the vertebral foramen to the coracoid process of the scapula. The most common site for compression is in the thoracic inlet. This schematic anatomic drawing illustrates the brachial plexus emerging between the anterior and middle scalene muscles, with the subclavian vein anterior, and the subclavian artery posterior, to the anterior scalene muscle. The vascular syndromes associated with the thoracic outlet syndrome occur where the subclavian vessels are between the clavicle and first rib in the narrow costoclavicular space. This space may be decompressed by removal of the anterior portion of the first rib, anterior scalenectomy, or removal of the middle third of the clavicle. Clearly, the roots and trunks of the brachial plexus cannot be compressed in this space by normal anatomical structures since they are superior and lateral to the tight region. Indeed, the clavicle bows, or is concave, in the region of the plexus. The infraclavicular plexus can become compressed beneath the pectoralis minor muscle as it inserts into the coracoid. From Thoracic Outlet Syndrome: A Common Sequela of Neck Injuries, *by R. J. Sanders, 1991, Philadelphia: J. B. Lippincott Company. Reprinted with permission of the author.*

plexus compression in the thoracic inlet must begin with a detailed history and a careful physical examination. The history should include questions regarding the usual symptoms that can be related to this problem, as outlined in Table 18.4. Unless the patient has a cervical rib that is the cause of the problem (see Figure 18.5), there is almost always some history of an injury—either a motor vehicle accident, a clavicle fracture or shoulder dislocation, a direct blow to the neck and shoulder area, or some form of repetitive motion—and the history taking must try to elicit this. There are also a few systemic diseases, such as diabetes and collagen vascular disease, that predispose to peripheral nerve entrapments.

The physical examination is almost always negative, except for tenderness over the brachial plexus beneath the scalene muscles and the ability to duplicate the patient's symptoms when either the arm is elevated above the head or the examiner puts a little pressure over the

FIGURE 18.4

A

B

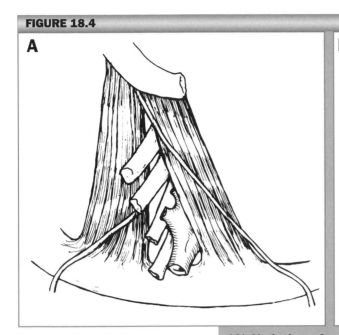
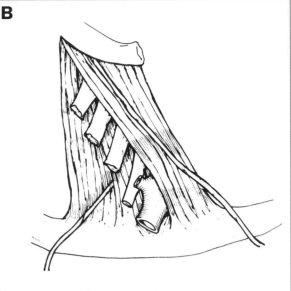

(A) Variations from the normal scalene triangle render the brachial plexus susceptible to compression after injury to the neck region. (B) The common arrangement found in patients with thoracic outlet syndrome. Note that the medial and anterior scalene muscles insert closer to each other, narrowing the base of the triangle. It is also common for scalene muscle slips to emerge between the roots and trunks of the plexus. Patients with this problem often have what appears to be a "long" neck, causing the roots and trunks of the plexus to emerge from higher up in the triangle. From **Thoracic Outlet Syndrome: A Common Sequela of Neck Injuries,** *by R. J. Sanders, 1991, Philadelphia: J. B. Lippincott Company. Reprinted with permission of the author.*

brachial plexus. The remainder of the examination, however, is critical to diagnose other medical problems whose presence may simulate the symptoms of brachial plexus compression. These are given in Table 18.5. In particular, the shoulder joint should be carefully examined, as suggested by Levin and Dellon (1992) and illustrated in Figure 18.6.

It has been traditional to do a series of tests during the physical examination that relate to obliteration of the radial pulse when the arm is put into certain positions with respect to the neck and shoulder. Loss or diminution of the pulse was said to indicate the presence of a problem in the thoracic outlet. It is now well accepted from careful studies on normal subjects that these same pulse changes exist in between 30% to 50% of the population, and there is no need to record them for diagnostic purposes. A thorough evaluation of these patients must include electrodiagnostic studies for the purpose of demonstrating the presence of any peripheral nerve entrapments or systemic neuropathy, or the presence of the true neurogenic form of brachial plexus compression (compression of the lower trunk of the plexus), and not to document the presence of brachial plexus compression.

There is widespread agreement now among neurologists that neither the conduction velocity through the ulnar nerve, through the lower trunk of the plexus, or the F-wave, can demonstrate brachial plexus compression.

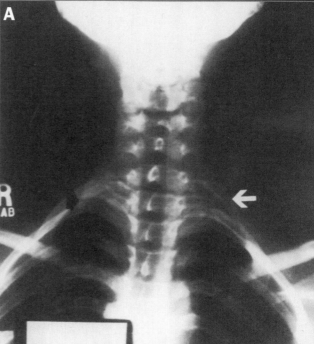

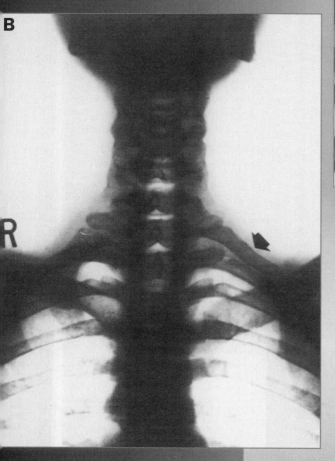

FIGURE 18.5
Osseous anomalies can cause compression of the brachial plexus, such as a cervical rib (A), or irregular formation of the first thoracic rib (B). It is also critical to determine that the symptoms are not being caused by a tumor at the apex of the lung, compressing the brachial plexus, such as is noted by the whitish area at the right upper lobe of the lung in (C). (A) and (B) from Thoracic Outlet Syndrome: A Common Sequela of Neck Injuries, *by R. J. Sanders, 1991, Philadelphia: J. B. Lippincott Company. (C) From* "Thoracic Outlet Syndromes," *by R. D. Leffert, 1992,* Hand Clinics 8:285-291. *Reprinted with permission of the authors.*

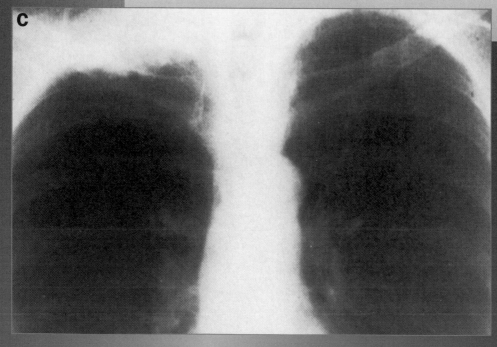

As discussed in Chapter 8, appropriately designed somatosensory evoked potential studies can demonstrate brachial plexus compression, and are worth obtaining. It is critical to obtain a chest X ray to demonstrate that there is no pulmonary pathology that might be causing the problem, and to look for the presence of either a cervical rib or first thoracic rib anomaly (see Figure 18.5). If there is any history of neck pain, or a positive Spurling sign (i.e., pain with vertical pressure applied to the top of the head), then an MRI of the cervical spine is indicated, along with appropriate neurologic or neurosurgical consultation.

If more than one diagnosis is present, the order of treatment almost always is to treat the brachial plexus last (at least surgically). Cervical spine disease demands first concern, and if a four-poster brace must be worn, then expect the brachial plexus compression symptoms to worsen. Next, orthopedic treatment for the shoulder and/or peripheral nerve decompressions must be done. However, the nonoperative treatment of the brachial plexus compression can almost always be done simultaneously with the treatment of the coexisting problems. A patient information brochure is available and it is helpful to give it to the patient (NeuroRegen, LLC, 2328 West

TABLE 18.5 MEDICAL PROBLEMS WHOSE PRESENCE MAY SIMULATE SYMPTOMS OF BRACHIAL PLEXUS COMPRESSION

Cervical disc disease

Carpal tunnel syndrome

Cubital tunnel syndrome

Shoulder joint pathology

Temporomandibular joint pathology

Tumor at apex of lung

FIGURE 18.6

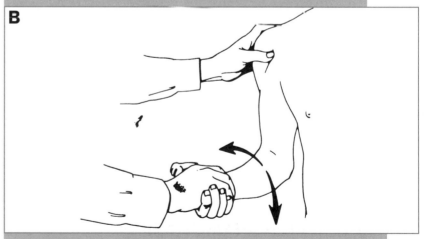

Evaluation of the shoulder to eliminate intrinsic shoulder pathology as the source of symptoms that may overlap with those from brachial plexus compression in the thoracic inlet. From "Pathology of the Shoulder as it Relates to the Differential Diagnosis of Thoracic Outlet Syndrome," by L. S. Levin & A. L. Dellon, 1992, Journal of Reconstructive Microsurgery 8:313-317. Reprinted with permission of the authors.

Joppa Road, Suite 325, Lutherville, MD 21093).

Ideally, treatment is based on an understanding of the pathophysiology of the problem. When it was widely believed (as it still is) that the cause of thoracic outlet syndrome is compression of either the vascular structures or the brachial plexus between the clavicle and the first rib, it was appropriate to direct treatment at removing the first rib. Certainly, if there were symptoms and there was a cervical rib, the treatment seemed to be removal of the cervical rib. If, however, there was direct trauma to the neck and shoulder region but without bone injury, or if the patient was being seen as the result of a cumulative trauma disorder, it remains unclear what the treatment should be.

The hypotheses put forth by Edwards (1988) and by Mackinnon and Novak (1994) for cumulative trauma disorders target muscle abnormalities as being directly related to the patient's symptoms. Edwards's muscle biopsies in fact demonstrate fibrosis. Biopsies of anterior scalene muscles from patients with thoracic outlet syndrome, when compared to those of patients without thoracic outlet syndrome, demonstrate a shift in the muscle typing pattern (see Figure 18.7) consistent with alteration of muscle function. This emphasis on muscle problems, and particularly the strong argument that can be made for abnormal posturing resulting in muscle abnormalities about the shoulder girdle (see Figures 18.1 and 18.2) suggest that treatment should first be nonoperative and directed at the muscles of the region.

The most important form of treatment is nonoperative. Peet, Hendrickson, Anderson, and Martin (1956) from the Mayo Clinic described their regimen for nonopera-

FIGURE 18.7

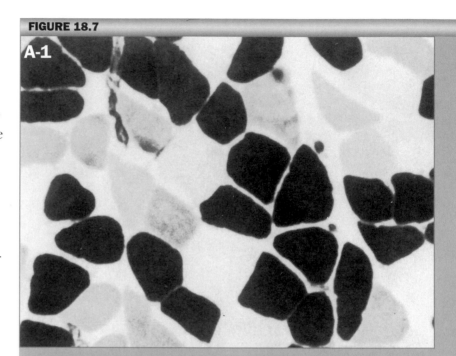

A-1

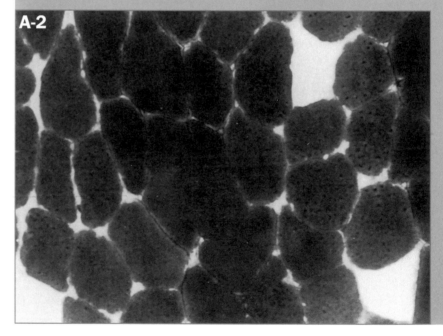

A-2

Histopathology related to brachial plexus compression in the thoracic inlet. Muscle fiber tying done on fresh frozen specimens of anterior scalene muscle. (A-1, A-2) ATPase staining at pH 4.6 at 120x demonstrates the Type I (slow-twitch, anti-gravity muscles) fibers to be dark, and Type II (fast-twitch, voluntary quick movements) to be white or intermediate in staining characteristics. Note that in the bottom photomicrograph of anterior scalene muscle from a patient with brachial plexus compression, there is an apparent loss of Type II fibers. (B-1, B-2) Histograms of Type I and II muscle fibers corresponding to the photomicrographs in (A-1, A-2) demonstrate that the Type II fibers in both males and females with brachial plexus compression are significantly smaller (p < .001) in cross-sectional area than are those fibers in normal anterior scalene muscles. From Thoracic Outlet Syndrome: A Common Sequela of Neck Injuries, by R. J. Sanders, 1991, Philadelphia: J. B. Lippincott Company. Reprinted with permission of the author.

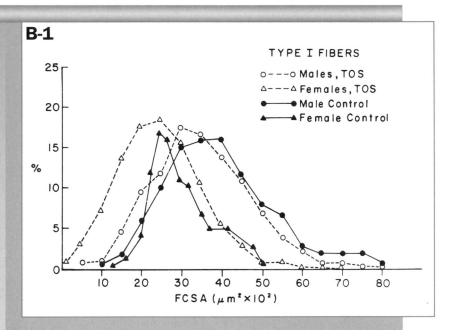

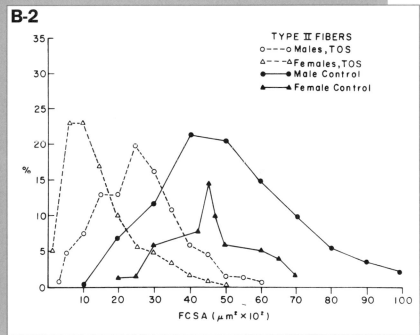

tive management of patients with symptoms of *thoracic outlet syndrome*, in the process coining the term thoracic outlet syndrome. Their approach has since become incorporated into the mainstream of medical care for this clinical problem, and their name for the problem has become accepted. This is unfortunate, since the thoracic outlet is the diaphragm!

As was reviewed by Mackinnon and Dellon (1988), as early as 1906 J. B. Murphy suggested that cervical ribs might cause neurologic symptoms besides the vascular symptoms that had first been described by Astly Cooper in 1821. By 1910, T. Murphy described "brachial neuritis" caused by pressure of the first rib, perhaps leading to Todd's 1912 description of "costal anomalies of the *thoracic inlet*," and the role of shoulder descent after birth in causing stretching of the plexus across the first rib. The term thoracic inlet appears one more time, in 1952, when Edwards uses it in the title of his case report of a man with recurrent vascular compression symptoms after a scalenotomy. However, despite their misnomer, Peet et al.'s report (1956) has become the paradigm for the nonoperative management of this clinical entity. Of 55 patients treated by Peet's team, 71% improved.

The nonoperative approach was elaborated on, thereafter, by Britt (1967). Subsequently, McGough, Pearce, and Byrne (1979), and Dunant (1987), each reported on their results in the nonoperative management of 1,200 patients in each of their series. Only 185 (15%) of McGough et al.'s patients, and only 375 (30%) of Dunant's patients, failed to improve with exercises and went on to have surgery. This clearly established that all patients with symptoms of brachial plexus compression in the thoracic inlet should have at least 6 months of nonoperative management. That regimen should include exercises to strengthen the middle and lower trapezius, the serratus anterior, and the levator scapulae, while at the same time stretching (relaxing) the pectoralis minor, the scalenes, and the upper trapezius, sternocleidomastoid, and suboccipitalis. Muscle relaxants may be appropriate, as well as trigger point injections, moist warm heat, stretching, and massage. The most recent reaffirmation of this approach is by Walsh (1994).

Diagrams of the modified Peet et al. (1956) program are given in Figure 18.19. An outcome assessment of this approach by Novak, Collins, and Mackinnon (1995) demonstrated that when 42 patients, whose pretreatment symptom duration was a mean of 38 months, were given such a 6-month course of therapy, 38 patients (90%) had improvement in neck and shoulder symptoms. Overall, 25 patients reported symptomatic improvement, 10 were the same, and 7 had worse problems. Sixteen patients reported full work and recreational activities, and 8 patients reported restriction in both work and recreational activities. Poor overall outcome was related to obesity ($p < .04$), worker's compensation ($p < .04$), and peripheral nerve compressions at the carpal and cubital tunnel ($p < .04$). Improvement in hand and arm pain was significantly better in those without distal nerve compression ($p < .006$).

The 10% or so of patients with symptoms of brachial plexus compression in the thoracic inlet that do not improve with nonoperative management should be offered surgery. What is the basis of their persistent symptoms that surgery should attempt to correct? Another reason for the dispute among neurologists and surgeons is the absence of proven pathology within the brachial plexus. The presence of the many types of fibrous bands that Roos (1990) has identified are not something the pathologist has been able to examine, and certainly the neurologist has not seen them. Indeed, the neurologist is more likely to have seen patients with nerve deficits following some surgical procedure directed toward the thoracic outlet.

I became aware of an anatomical situation that gave meaning to the supraclavicular approach to plexus neurolysis. I would see patients with persistent symptoms after transaxillary first rib resection, and after scalenotomy. It was reasonable to suppose that there were anatomic variations in and around the plexus that prevented it from gliding normally and, therefore, predisposed it to entrapment and compression after injury. I hypothesized that the scalene muscles released from the first rib after a transaxillary dissection had come to lie on, and become adherent to, the upper trunk of the plexus, and that there would be scarring within the plexus.

FIGURE 18.8

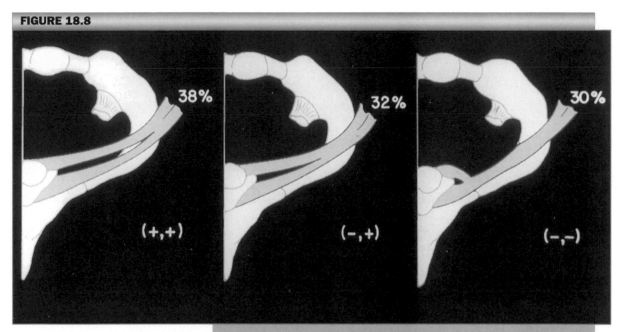

Anomalous formation of the lower trunk of the brachial plexus can contribute to compression of the C8 and T1 roots. (A) The formation of the lower trunk is usually depicted as occurring over the first rib. However, dissection demonstrates that this occurs only about one-third of the time, with the trunk forming medial or inside the curve of the first rib in the rest of the population. When the juncture of the C8 and T1 roots is very medial, excursion of the plexus is limited. While this situation is noted in about one-third of cadavers, it is present in more than 80% of patients upon whom supraclavicular brachial plexus compression has been performed. From unpublished observations of A. L. Dellon, presented to the American Association of Plastic Surgery, 1993.

In previously unoperated patients the spasms or tightness in the scalene could pull the first rib up against structures, and resecting the anterior scalene could release this pressure without the need to resect the first rib. The clavicle is concave over the plexus, and I had always found enough room for my finger between the plexus and the clavicle. Indeed, it was posterior, between the C8 and T1 roots, that compression should be occurring.

During most of the supraclavicular plexus explorations that I did, the neural structure first encountered over the posterior aspect of the first rib was not the C8 root, but the lower trunk. The T1 root had joined it very medially, or proximally, often near the transverse process of the vertebra (Dellon, 1993). In this area,

bands from the suprapleural fascia or the scalenus minimis would be present, compressing these roots against the posterior border of the first rib. Two research endeavors were, therefore, prompted. One required dissection of the C8-T1 roots in 25 cadavers to determine the usual location of the formation of the lower trunk of the plexus. These results are depicted in Figure 18.8.

About 30% of the cadavers had this formation, demonstrating a group of people at risk for brachial plexus compression problems due to reduced gliding ability.

The second project involved examining the brachial plexus under the microscope to look for possible changes within the nerve consistent with subclinical nerve compression. Examples from this cadaver, given in Figure

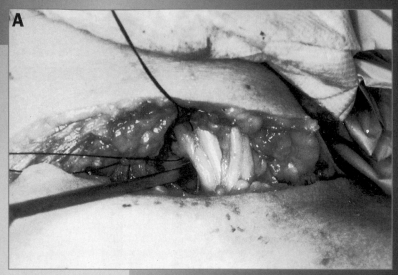

A

FIGURE 18.9

Histopathology related to brachial plexus compression in the thoracic inlet. (A) Brachial plexus specimen harvested at 48 hours from a cadaver of a 40-year-old woman, with portions of the plexus marked for histologic examination. (B) Photomicrograph of upper trunk of plexus from beneath the lateral border of the anterior scalene, and (C) of lower trunk of plexus from adjacent to the first rib's posterior border. (D) Lower trunk of brachial plexus (left) with adjacent fat cells, blood vessels, and fat droplets (right). Note the Renaut bodies (white areas, devoid of myelinated fibers) present in the lower trunk at the sites of known anatomic compression. These sites represent areas of stretch/traction injury to that nerve. From unpublished observations of A. L. Dellon, presented to the American Association of Plastic Surgery, 1993.

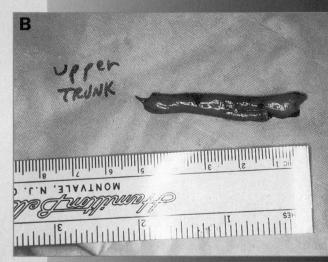

B

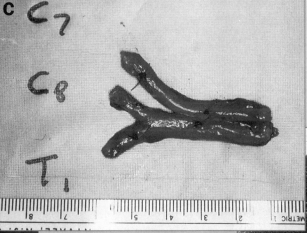

C

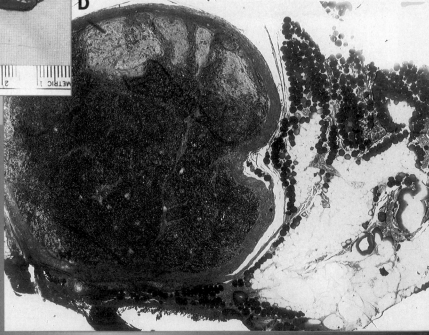

D

18.9, demonstrate that within the plexus adjacent to the edge of the anterior scalene muscle and at the border of the first rib posteriorly, there are *Renaut bodies* and *intraneural fibrosis* not present at sites such as C7, which are away from these usual stress-inducing sites. Hopefully, these observations will lend credence among our nonsurgical colleagues and skeptics for our supraclavicular decompression of the brachial plexus in those individuals who do not respond to nonoperative management of their symptoms.

The most appropriate surgical treatment for the symptoms of brachial plexus compression in the thoracic inlet remains controversial. The commonest approach is to remove the first rib through a transaxillary approach. This was popularized by Roos in 1966. I do not like this approach because (a) the exposure is difficult, necessitating special rigging to suspend the arm and dissection across the path of the second intercostobrachial nerve; (b) there is poor visualization of the plexus and subclavian vessels; (c) these combine to produce among the highest complication rates for surgery; and (d) it is impossible to do a neurolysis of the plexus itself in which there may be significant scarring and anomalous bands that cannot be removed through the axillary approach.

Sanders (1991), who has meticulously recorded every complication in his 113 of these procedures, has a combined incidence of complications of about 84% (see Table 18.6). He has compared statistically the results of his own different surgical approaches to this problem

TABLE 18.6 COMPLICATIONS OF SURGERY FOR BRACHIAL PLEXUS COMPRESSION IN THE THORACIC INLET

Complication	Transaxillary First Rib Resection (n=113)	Anterior & Middle Scalenectomy (n=301)	Rib Resection & Scalenectomy (n=326)
Plexus injury; temporary	0.9%	0.0%	2.3%
Plexus injury; permanent	1.8%	0.0%	0.6%
Phrenic nerve inj; temp.	1.0%	6.0%	2.2%
Phrenic nerve inj; perm.	0.0%	0.3%	0.3%
Long thoracic n. inj; temp.	1.8%	0.0%	0.3%
Intercostobrach n. inj.	35.0%	0.0%	0.0%
Subclavian arter. injury	0.0%	0.0%	0.3%
Subclavian vein injury2.	0.0%	0.3%	1.2%
Pluera opened; no tap	30.0%	1.3%	12.0%
Pleura opened; tap	9.0%	0.4%	2.1%
Bleeding > 500 cc	2.7%	0.3%	1.5%
Total*	84.2%	8.6%	12.8%

Note:

*Some patients probably had more than one complication.

From *Thoracic Outlet Syndrome: A Common Sequela of Neck Injuries,* by R. J. Sanders, 1991, Philadelphia: J. B. Lippincott Company. Adapted with permission of the author.

FIGURE 18.10

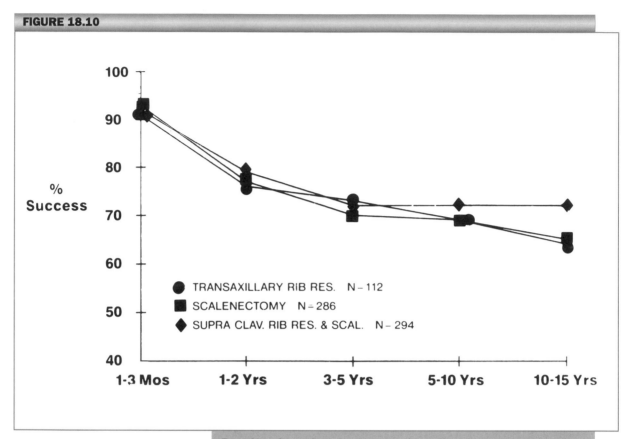

Results of surgical decompression of the brachial plexus from the personal series of Sanders. The results of three different types of surgery for this problem are analyzed by the life-table method. There was no statistically significant difference in the results by either technique. (There is, however, a significant difference in the complication rate for the different procedures; see Table 18.6). It should be noted that percent of success includes excellent, good, and fair results, with only those who failed to improve at all being excluded. Excellent results comprise up to about 25% of the total percent success at any give point. From Thoracic Outlet Syndrome: A Common Sequela of Neck Injuries, *by R. J. Sanders, 1991, Philadelphia: J. B. Lippincott Company. Reprinted with permission of the author.*

and found no differences in the overall success rates, whether he did or did not remove the first rib (see Figure 18.10). However, his complication rate for supra-clavicular anterior and middle scalenectomy without rib resection was just 8.6%.

I prefer a supraclavicular plexus neurolysis during which an anterior, and often a partial medial scalenectomy, is done. Rarely have I removed the first rib (see Figure 18.11). Many of my workmen's compensation patients have obtained excellent relief, but I still will not permit them to return to work where they must work with their arms in an overhead position, and I restrict lifting to below the shoulder level. When nonoperative management has not been helpful, surgery for patients with persistent symptoms of brachial plexus compression in the thoracic inlet can be done relatively safely by an experienced surgeon, yielding satisfying results to both the patient and the surgeon.

FIGURE 18.11

Supraclavicular brachial plexus neurolysis and scalenectomy for treatment of brachial plexus compression when nonoperative management has been unsuccessful. (A) Patient is oriented with head to left, folded towel beneath shoulder. At completion of scalenectomy and neurolysis, (B) the five numbered roots and the upper (U), middle (M), and lower (L) trunk of the plexus are identified and completely free of any compressive structures. (C) Without the vessel loupes, the trunks lie naturally but demonstrate the notch across them where the fibrous bands within the anterior scalene muscle caused compression. The supraclavicular (cutaneous) nerve (SC) crosses the plexus to the right, while the scalene fat pad (S) lies superficially to the left. From "The Results of Supraclavicular Brachial Plexus Neurolysis (Without First Rib Resection) in the Management of Post-traumatic 'Thoracic Outlet Syndrome'," by A. L. Dellon, 1993, Journal of Reconstructive Microsurgery 9:11-17.

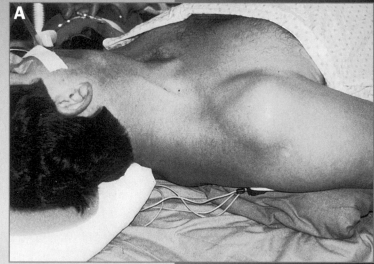

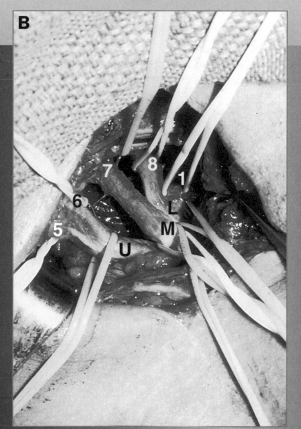

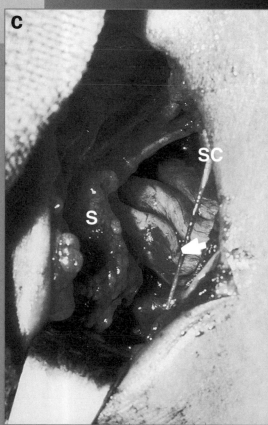

• • •

N̄o sort of exercise is so healthful or harmless that it does not cause serious disorders . . . when overdone.

Dr. Bernardino Ramazzini, 1713

• • •

• MUSICIANS •

Amadio and Russotti (1990) have summarized the literature regarding the extent of the problems related to upper extremity disorders in performing artists. They note that there are about 130,000 people who earn their living as instrumental musicians, while many more play as part-time professionals, in amateur groups, or just for fun. Among pianists and string players, the incidence of hand and wrist disorders approaches 80%. Between 10% and 15% of musicians have some hand or wrist disorder at any given time. The greatest proportion of musicians develop their problem between 20 and 40 years of age, but all ages may be affected, with a slightly greater occurrence in women than in men.

While musicians have always had problems related to extensive use of their musculoskeletal systems, there has been an increased willingness on their part to share their problems openly, and an increased realization by the medical profession that musicians deserve specialized care and attention. Toward this end, there has been a relatively recent deluge of information available. For example, a journal, *Medical Problems of the Performing Artist*, is now published by Hanley & Belfus (Philadelphia). An issue of *Hand Clinics* in 1990, and of the *Journal of Hand Therapy* in 1992 (see Tables 18.7 and 18.8 for their tables of contents) were devoted to musicians' problems and are excellent resources for more specific information than is possible to include here.

Johnson (1992), in her preface to the issue of the *Journal of Hand Therapy* she guest edited, enumerated some of the reasons why musicians make special patients. She noted that musicians wish to return to work as soon as possible, and that they are able to follow very specific hand exercise treatment plans, yet they are not interested in general body conditioning programs (which they frequently need to help their posture). They are interested in the anatomy of their bodies and can do isolated muscle strengthening exercises. They are very serious about their problem and very con-

cerned about their prognosis. In my personal, though limited, experience with musicians, I find they are very compulsive, inquisitive and, as a consequence, demanding and time-consuming patients. So, if you are going to treat musicians, be prepared to make both a time and an emotional commitment. Their care is also generally frustrated by the fact they are so "tuned in" to their body's functioning that they present almost invariably before most of our diagnostic tests become positive.

As computerized sensorimotor testing becomes more widely available, it will be of interest to learn if its sensitivity is able to demonstrate the presence of early peripheral nerve problems in musicians. Furthermore, because this testing is noninvasive and not painful, it permits the clinician to do stress testing of musicians. That is, they can be tested before and after 1 hour of playing, during which their wrist, elbow, and shoulder will be in the provocative position that is necessary for them to develop their symptoms.

The Pressure-Specified Sensory Device™ (see Chapter 7) is an example of equipment that could provide this information. With this equipment becoming available, it will be possible for normative data to be developed that will demonstrate that the cutaneous pressure threshold in the lit-

TABLE 18.7 TABLE OF CONTENTS OF *HAND CLINICS,* **AUGUST 1990**

tle finger pulp for moving touch increases a certain percentage after 1 hour of playing the violin in asymptomatic violinists. It will also be possible to demonstrate that the pressure required in the little finger to discriminate one from two points that are two millimeters apart and in static contact with the fingertip, increases a certain percentage after 1 hour of playing the violin.

Then, when a violinist complains of problems playing certain concert pieces and the physical examination and electrodiagnostic testing are (of course) normal, and when stress-testing demonstrates that the thresholds increase to twice the expected amount, it would be apparent that there is ulnar nerve compression at the wrist, elbow, or lower trunk of the brachial plexus, or perhaps there is multiple crush syndrome, or that two or three of these are present as the cause of the symptoms. The Force-Defined Vi-

TABLE 18.8 TABLE OF CONTENTS *JOURNAL OF HAND THERAPY 5:(APRIL/JUNE) 1992*

brometer™ has the same potential to generate this type of information. Obtaining this information will require help from the community of musicians to obtain the normative data.

Richard Norris, a physiatrist with the National Rehabilitation Center in Bethesda, MD, has a special interest in the problems of musicians and has compiled a list of a dozen reasons why musicians develop overuse problems (Norris, 1993). This list is given in Table 18.9.

The rehabilitation of musicians with cumulative trauma disorders is considered under the section below on rehabilitation.

TABLE 18.9 MUSICIANS: FACTORS THAT PREDISPOSE TO OVERUSE INJURY

1. Inadequate physical conditioning
2. Sudden increase in the amount of playing time
3. Errors in practice habits
4. Errors of technique
5. Change in instrument
6. Inadequate rehabilitation of previous injuries
7. Improper body mechanics and posture
8. Stressful nonmusical activities
9. Anatomical variations
10. Gender
11. Quality of instrument
12. Environmental factors

Note: From *The Musicians Survival Manual: A Guide to Preventing and Treating Injuries in Instrumentalists,* by R. Norris, 1993, International Conference of Symphony and Opera Musicians, St. Louis. Reprinted with permission of the author.

• • •

The hand therapist combines comprehensive knowledge of the upper extremity with specialized skills in assessment and treatment to prevent dysfunction, restore function, or reverse the advancement of pathology in the upper extremity.

Scope and Practice, American
Society of Hand Therapy, 1989

• • •

Increasingly, this knowledge and these skills allow hand therapists to provide more nontraditional services, such as consultation with companies for the prevention of injury. The hand therapist then becomes a member of a team of individuals working to minimize the effects of industrial injuries . . . Occupational therapists have training and knowledge in activity analysis and man's interaction with his environment. The hand therapist who combines the traditional skills of these two subjects is suitably qualified to perform specialized evaluations of injured workers and their work sites in order to better match workers with their jobs.

J. W. King, 1990

• • •

• INDUSTRIAL SCREENING •

The Occupational Safety and Health Administration (OSHA) was created by law in 1970 to protect over 50 million employees working in over 4 million establishments. The law establishes health and safety standards and provides an enforcement mechanism. OSHA's initial work was primarily related to direct or impact trauma. In response to public awareness that injury rates approached 80% in some meat packing plants, OSHA published its Safety and Health Program Management Guidelines (*Federal Register*, Volume 54, Number 16, January 26, 1989.)

These guidelines have been instrumental in devising criteria to screen workers for cumulative trauma disorders. This has been done through questionnaires, through suggesting screening and surveillance by health care professionals of cumulative trauma disorders, and through suggesting a system of interventions both in the work place and with the health care institution. There has been greater imple-

mentation of these guidelines in certain areas, such as exposure to toxins. The National Institute of Occupational Health (NIOSH) has set limits for work place exposure to noise, fumes, and low back compression forces. For example, the level at which incidence and severity rates increase moderately in exposed populations has been called the action limit, and when exposure exceeds the *action limit*, engineering or administrative action by the industry is required.

There are jobs in which the injury rate or injury severity is unacceptable for workers, and these rates are called the *maximum permissible limit*. NIOSH will require these jobs be changed. Ear plugs, preemployment testing, and break-in periods with instructions are outgrowths of these programs. At present, the "red meat" (beef, pork) component of the industry is making strides to measure sensory impairment and tendinitis in workers. This trend will need to be extended to the "white meat" (poultry) component of the industry, as well. OSHA has not been enforcing its guidelines and employers are making voluntary efforts in this regard, possibly motivated more by the high costs of their workmen's compensation insurance premiums. It is the application of these guidelines to upper extremity cumulative trauma disorders that will be considered here and, in particular, pre-employment testing or screening, and subsequent retesting, or surveillance, and the measurements required for impairment ratings.

The availability of computer-assisted sensorimotor measuring systems (see Figure 18.12) will permit occupational medicine to proceed with screening and surveillance in industry for cumulative trauma disorders. A series of 125 patients with carpal tunnel syndrome, and 75 patients with cubital tunnel syndrome, were measured with this equipment in a population of patients that was comprised almost entirely of workers with cumulative trauma disorders. The cutaneous pressure thresholds of these populations are given in Tables 18.10 and 18.11 (Dellon & Kress, 1995).

The values for clinically symptomatic problems of nerve compression have been compared to normative age-related data for which the 99% upper confidence interval is available. With this information, screening or cutoff values can be derived that permit the Pressure-Specified Sensory Device™ and the NK Digit-Grip and Pinch Device to be used in industry. These screening/surveillance values are given in Table 18.12. These values have now been incorporated into the "E-Z Way" software of the NK Industrial Testing Kit so that a worker may be screened in

FIGURE 18.12

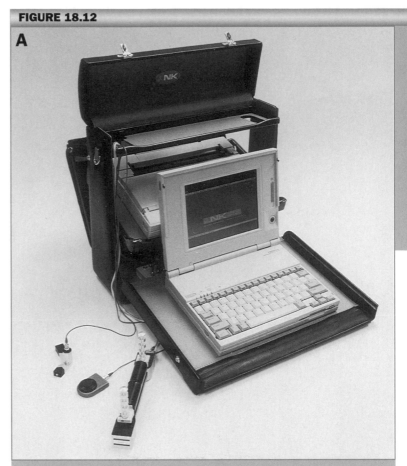

A

Industrial Screening/Surveillance using computerized sensorimotor testing equipment. (A) The NKB Industrial Testing Kit includes a laptop computer, a printer, and the Pressure-Specified Sensory Device™, the Digit-Grip, and the Pinch device. Everything comes completely connected. Testing time per employee is 15 minutes. (B) Example of a printout of two sequential measurements on an employee who at the time of initial screening was found to have elevated pressure thresholds for both index fingers, consistent with bilateral carpal tunnel syndrome. Appropriate treatment with wrist splints and alteration of job activity during the break-in period was initiated, with the result that at the second testing period, the first surveillance period, there was a decrease in thresholds, indicating that the medical and ergonomic rehabilitation was progressing successfully. Illustrations copyright A. Lee Dellon. Reprinted with permission.

about 15 minutes for the presence of carpal tunnel syndrome, cubital tunnel syndrome, or tendinitis.

The information from

computerized sensorimotor testing can be used to evaluate impairment in the industrial injury setting. As King (1990) has pointed out, "dis-

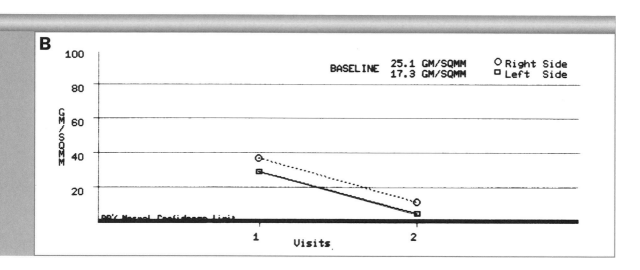

TABLE 18.10   INDUSTRIAL SCREENING: CARPAL TUNNEL SYNDROME

≤ 45 years of age (n = 79, mean age = 37.2)

	(g/mm²)		(mm)	(g/mm²)		(mm)
	1PS	2PS	2PS	1PM	2PM	2PM
mean	8.3	15.9	3.6	4.3	6.8	3.3
s.d.	18.6	19.3	1.1	13.0	9.4	0.9
95%	12.4	20.3	3.8	7.2	9.0	3.5
99%	13.8	21.8	3.9	8.1	9.6	3.6
min	0.1	1.1	2.5	0.1	0.3	2.5
max	97.0	69.0	66.0	97.0	51.0	5.7

Mean pinch 118% and mean grasp 80% of predicted

≤ 45 years of age (n = 79, mean age = 37.2)

	(g/mm²)		(mm)	(g/mm²)		(mm)
	1PS	2PS	2PS	1PM	2PM	2PM
mean	5.5	14.8	4.3	2.1	7.8	3.9
s.d.	9.0	14.0	1.0	3.0	8.6	0.9
95%	8.2	19.0	4.6	3.0	10.3	4.2
99%	9.1	20.4	4.7	3.31	1.2	4.3
min	0.4	3.0	2.5	0.2	1.0	2.5
max	39.0	66.0	7.1	95.0	37.0	6.2

Mean pinch 146% and mean grasp 90% of predicted

Note: From "Computerized Sensorimotor Testing in Patients with Carpal and Cubital Tunnel Syndrome: Comparison with Age-adjusted Normative Data," by A. L. Dellon & K. Keller, *Annals of Plastic Surgery, 38:* 493-502. 1997. Reprinted with permission of the authors.

ability is defined as the social consequence of impairment; disability is a legal issue." The quantitative measurements obtained by the therapist are assumed to represent an honest effort by the patient, but in the determination of a financial reward, or in the case of a patient who wishes to be rated for a job that does not require as much physical effort, how

may we know that the patient is truly giving the best effort, and not malingering?

Again, as King has noted, therapists are most often the evaluators who must assure all parties involved that a reasonable effort has been made by the injured worker during evaluation for the result to be accepted as true. This requires methods of testing that are fair, yet which

clearly delineate the individual into appropriate classifications of having given or not given maximum effort. This difficult subject has been approached in the past (Gilbert & Knowlton, 1983; Stokes, 1983), but an approach described by Hildreth, Briedenbach, and Lister (1989) has been modified and is in common use. These authors used the Jamar dynamometer set

TABLE 18.11   INDUSTRIAL SCREENING: CUBITAL TUNNEL SYNDROME

≤ 45 years of age (n =45, mean age = 37.2)

| | (g/mm²) | | (mm) | | (g/mm²) | (mm) | | | (g/mm²) | |
	1PS	2PS	2PS		1PM	2PM	2PM	dorsal	1PS	1PM
mean	13.7	18.4	4.6		7.5	10.4	4.2		26.9	15.1
s.d.	24.8	18.9	1.6		20.6	12.4	1.5		35.0	33.0
95%	21.0	24.4	5.1		10.5	14.3	4.7			
99%	23.6	26.4	5.3		13.5	15.8	4.8			
min	0.4	1.5	2.5		0.2	0.6	2.5			
max	97.0	70.0	8.6		97.0	49.0	8.6			

Mean pinch 69.6% and mean grasp 48.8% of predicted

> 45 years of age (n =26, mean age = 51.5)

| | (g/mm²) | | (mm) | | (g/mm²) | (mm) | | | (g/mm²) | |
	1PS	2PS	2PS		1PM	2PM	2PM	dorsal	1PS	1PM
mean	8.5	18.8	4.8		2.4	10.9	4.5		5.6	1.2
s.d.	14.6	16.8	1.3		2.8	10.7	1.1		9.0	1.3
95%	13.1	25.7	5.3		3.5	15.2	4.9			
99%	16.2	28.2	5.5		3.9	16.8	5.1			
min	0.6	3.3	3.0		0.5	1.8	2.5			
max	59.0	58.0	7.7		11.5	48.0	7.4			

Mean pinch 71.1% and mean grasp 45.6% of predicted

Note: From "Computerized Sensorimotor Testing in Patients with Carpal and Cubital Tunnel Syndrome: Comparison with Age-adjusted Normative Data," by A. L. Dellon & K. Keller, *Annals of Plastic Surgery, 38:* 493-502. 1997. Reprinted with permission of the authors.

TABLE 18.12 SUGGESTED SCREENING/SURVEILLANCE VALUES FOR NERVE COMPRESSION SYNDROMES IN INDUSTRY

	Two-Point Static Pressure Perception Threshold*	
	(g/mm²)	(mm)
Carpal Tunnel Syndrome		
≤ 45 years old	1.0	3.0
> 45 years old	2.2	4.0
Cubital Tunnel Syndrome		
≤ 45 years old	1.0	3.0
> 45 years old	1.9	4.0

Note:
* Values greater than these are considered abnormal.
From "Computerized Sensorimotor Testing in Patients with Carpal and Cubital Tunnel Syndrome: Comparison with Age-adjusted Normative Data," by A. L. Dellon & K. Keller, *Annals of Plastic Surgery, 38:* 493-502. 1997. Reprinted with permission of the authors.

of 5 different grip handle sizes and compared the curve that resulted. The assumption was that the maximum effort always generated a curve the height of which was about the strength value obtained at the second or third grip position. The curve's height, overall, might be lowered in the presence of pain or motor problems, but in the presence of voluntary effort to mislead the examiner the malingerer would generate a curve that was more or less flat.

Unfortunately, Hildreth et al.'s statistical analysis was overly complicated and its rationalization counterintuitive. The computerized motor testing systems now permit a comparison of the variation between individual grip strength trial and the interrelationship between the strength generated on the radial versus the ulnar side of the hand to identify a less than honest effort (see Chapter 7). A more complicated scheme is that of the rapid-exchange grip, during which the patient must move the grip device from the left hand to the right hand and then back to the left hand over and over again, while giving a grip effort in each hand. The printout in real time can identify a less than honest effort.

King's (1990) encouragement to therapists is an appropriate quote to end this section:

Communication is the key to bridging the gap and providing valuable services to physicians, industry, attorneys, rehabilitation nurses, insurance companies, and, of course, the injured worker. Therapists can be the ambassadors of change in the return-to-work process with all its adversarial relationships. Take a chance! Get involved by asking a company representative if it would be possible to evaluate an injured worker's job to assure he or she is capable of performing it before returning to work. Listen carefully to the needs of the employer and relate the capabilities of the worker. Offer expertise without intimidating the employer through the use of jargon. Be a liaison for the medical fields and an advocate for the patient.

• • •

● REHABILITATION ●

While there can be no question that the clinician will encounter claimants in the guise of patients—those who are clearly abusing workmen's compensation or some other part of the legal system related to some perceived injury—there is also no question that musculoskeletal strain and secondary sensorimotor complaints will result from repetitive activity, especially if the body is in some awkward posture or is enduring physical loads that exceed its capacity. For example, the incidence of carpal tunnel syndrome is possibly 10 times higher in workers than in nonworkers. The ratio of female to male workers with carpal tunnel syndrome is reversed (1:2.1) compared to nonworkers (3:1), the mean age of the population is younger in workers (34 years) compared to nonworkers (51 years), and the incidence of carpal tunnel syndrome in about 47% of all patients may be related to a work etiology (Cummings, Maizlish, Rudolph, Devlin, & Erwin, 1989; Liss, Armstrong, Kusiak, & Gailitis, 1992).

This recognition is essential for the clinician concerned with diagnosis, treatment, and prognosis because it implies that the entire care plan will be very different from that for an isolated carpal tunnel syndrome or tendinitis. The numbness in the thumb and index finger must be perceived as existing along an axis that may include problems in the forearm (pronator syndrome) and the thoracic inlet (brachial plexus compression beneath the anterior scalene), and perhaps even at the cervical disc (C5/6, C6/7 level).

The clinician must be aware that even if the patient's symptoms can be relieved, the patient may still be unable to return to his or her previous job. For example, at the 1994 meeting of the American Society for Surgery of the Hand in Cincinnati, Higgs, Edwards, Martin, and Weeks (1995) presented material that compared the results of carpal tunnel decompression by the open technique in 153 injured and working workers with 53 noninjured workers. They found that with a mean follow-up time of 42 months, 74% of noninjured workers compared to 47% of injured workers were back at their original job, that 4% of noninjured workers were unemployed compared to 15% of injured workers, and that 50% of noninjured workers had some residual symptoms compared to 81% of injured workers. Each of these differences was statistically significant. In this setting, then, rehabilitation must include not only work capacity evaluation programs, but work hardening programs and, most importantly, vocational rehabilitation programs. The therapist can and should be involved in every level, beginning with mea-

surements that assist in diagnosis and ending with measurements that determine future job placement or impairment ratings.

For cumulative trauma disorders, rehabilitation must begin with the recognition that there is some particular activity related to the specific job that induces a particular set of musculoskeletal or neurologic problems. Ergonomic change with respect to an industry with a cumulative trauma disorder, in contrast to rehabilitation of the particular patient, generally must start with a questionnaire survey of the types of problems facing the industry or particular company, and then proceed to an ergonomic study of the forces related to the types of jobs within the plant that account for the most complaints related to the musculoskeletal or neurologic system. Armstrong (1992) has been a leader in attempting to quantitate these forces, or *ergonomic stressors*. Examples from his research on meat cutters (see Figure 18.13) and keyboard users (see Figure 18.14) demonstrate the steps necessary to go from observation of the presumed factor or factors, documentation of the forces involved relating the factor or factors to workers' complaints and, finally, to instituting ergonomic changes that result in, for example, redesigned knife handles or better com-

FIGURE 18.13

A

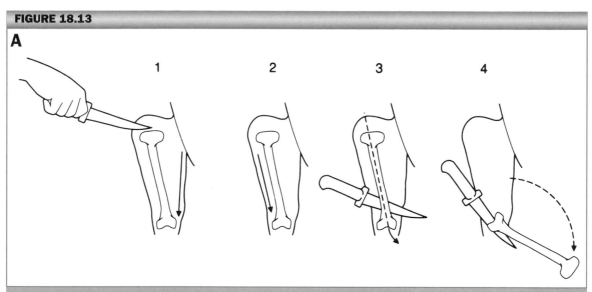

Identification of ergonomic stress factors. In the meat cutting industry, the knife must be held during various trimming activities. Among the stress factors are the shape of the knife itself and the positioning of the piece of meat being trimmed. To demonstrate the relationship between these activities, some measurement of the forces involved must be made. In this illustration, the movements of the hand/ knife during trimming of a thigh bone (A) versus simply holding the thigh bone (B) are related to the electrical activity generated by the muscles doing the work. This demonstrates that greater muscle activity is required for the trimming function. From "Investigation of Cumulative Trauma Disorders in a Poultry Processing Plant," by T. J. Armstrong, J. A. Foulke, B. A. Joseph, & S. A. Goldstein, 1982, American Industrial Hygiene Association Journal 43:102-116. Reprinted with permission of the authors.

B

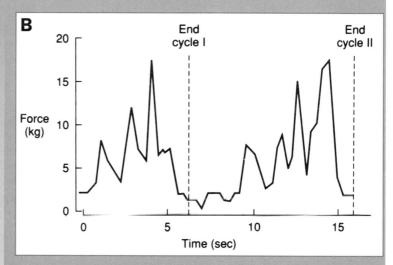

C

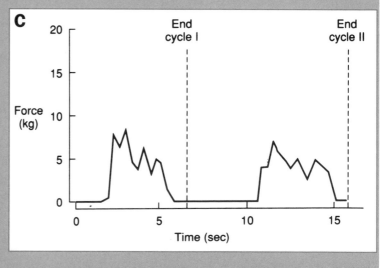

FIGURE 18.14

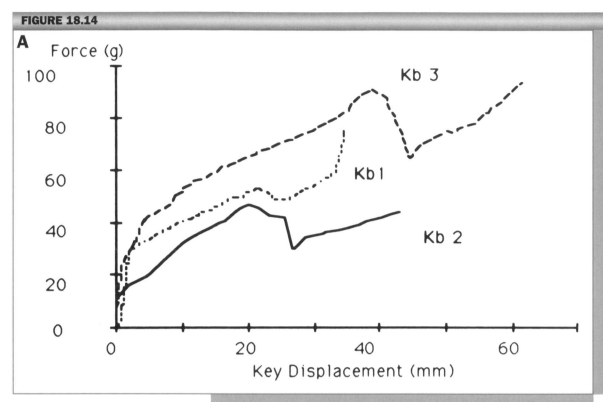

puter keyboards.

To move toward the more global concept of devising a scheme to quantify exposure, there are models that attempt to pair number of repetitions to degree of force, estimates of tendon loads and movement, frictional work done, muscle activation using electromyography, and the relationship of body posture to workload (Moore, Wells, & Ranney, 1991; McAtamney & Corlett, 1993). These global concepts produce scoring systems that can be applied to different jobs in different industries, that can be correlated with workers' subjective complaints, and that then can be used to measure change after intro-

Identification of ergonomic stress factors. In the computer data entry professions, it is hypothesized that there are problems related to both the keyboard itself and to the posture adapted during keying. (A) An attempt has been made to measure the force required for displacement of the typewriter key "E" by 10 subjects on three different keyboards. (B) An attempt has been made to measure the force required to move a typist's chair. Certainly many other measurements are possible, but these illustrate the steps required to provide data on which rehabilitation in industry, that is, ergonomic interventions, can be supported. From "Cumulative Trauma Disorders of the Upper Limb and Identification of Work-related Factors," by T. J. Armstrong, 1992, in Occupational Disorders of the Upper Extremity, *L. H. Millender, D. S. Louis, & B. P. Simmonds, Editors, New York: Churchill Livingstone. Reprinted with permission of the author.*

duction of different ergonomic strategies. The therapist may become involved in on-site evaluation and testing, outpatient muscle strengthening programs, and the design of new tools

for the work place. Examples of such tool design changes to facilitate rehabilitation of the worker with a cumulative trauma disorder are given in Figures 18.15 through 18.18.

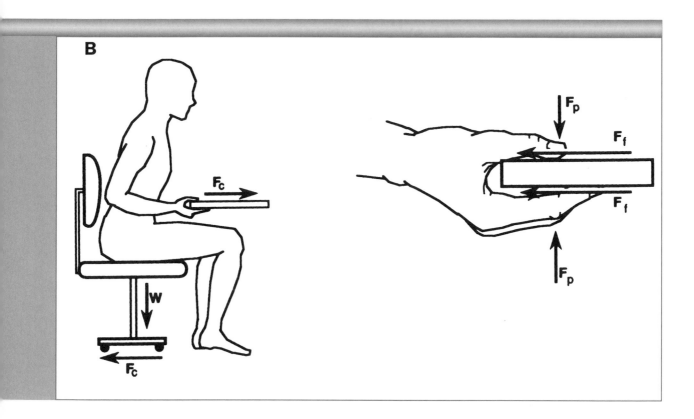

Rehabilitation for symptoms of brachial plexus compression in the thoracic inlet (traditionally called thoracic outlet syndrome) is discussed above. Illustrations of the rehabilitation exercises from Britt (1967) are given in Figure 18.19.

Work hardening for the musician, or conditioning, is discussed by Norris (1993). The process of gradually building up to normal activity for the injured industrial worker is usually guided or supervised by a physical or occupational therapist. For the injured musician this may be a problem because playing in an orchestra before the hand is truly ready may be a mistake. In industry, a worker

needs a physician's note to return to work, along with a description of the limitations on the injured extremity. However, this is not usually required for musicians, set-

ting up a situation for premature return to work and relapse, as the musician again overuses the extremity. Norris quotes from Poore in 1887:

Treatment: The most important point in treatment is rest. The excessive use of the hand must be discontinued, and it is often necessary to insist on this rather forcibly. Piano playing, if not prohibited altogether, must only be practiced to a degree short of that which causes pain or annoyance. It is often difficult to restrain the ardor of these patients in the matter of playing. Directly they feel in a small degree better, they fly to the piano; and I have known the progress of more than one case very seriously retarded by the undoing, as it were, of the good effect of rest by an hour's injudicious and prohibited "practicing."

• • •

TABLE 18.13 MUSICIAN: RETURNING TO PLAY SCHEDULE

Time Periods*	(Activity in Minutes) Play	Rest	Play	Rest	Play	Rest	Play	Rest	Play
1	5	60	5						
2	10	50	10						
3	15	40	15	60	5				
4	20	30	20	50	10				
5	30	20	25	40	15	45	5		
6	35	15	35	30	20	35	10		
7	40	10	40	20	25	25	15	50	10
8	50	10	45	15	30	15	25	40	15
9	50	10	50	10	40	10	35	30	20
10	50	10	50	10	50	10	45	20	30

Note:

*Each time period should be varied from 3 to 7 days depending on severity of injury and progress.

Warm up first, and start with slow, easy pieces; gradually progress to faster and more difficult pieces.

From *The Musicians Survival Manual: A Guide to Preventing and Treating Injuries in Instrumentalists,* by R. Norris, 1993, International Conference of Symphony and Opera Musicians, St. Louis. Reprinted with permission of the author.

Norris (1993) specifically notes that it is not always necessary to stop playing completely. The intensity can be reduced by choosing pieces easier to play, by just doing finger exercises if the wrist is hurt, or just using the right hand if the left hand is injured. Work hardening can begin before complete pain relief is achieved through resting, if a careful and guided schedule is followed. A sample of a return to play schedule is given in Table 18.13. Of course, it will need to be modified slightly for the individual musician. Norris's final recommendation is reminiscent of my experience with the rehabilitation of patients with reflex dystrophy:

To avoid discouragement, the musician should be advised from the start that setbacks are to be expected . . . Following a graduated program minimizes the risk of overdoing: if the load is too much, it will be only a little too much and the setback will be small and recovery swift. To sum it up with [an] aphorism: Hasten slowly and you shall soon arrive!

• • •

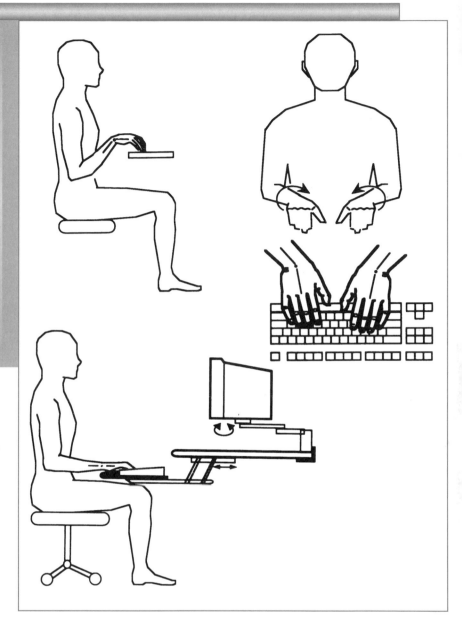

FIGURE 18.15

Ergonomic change in the work place based on analysis of stress factors. In the top of this illustration, the position of flexed wrist can be corrected, as in the bottom, by having an adjustable work station. From "Cumulative Trauma Disorders of the Upper Limb and Identification of Work-related Factors," by T. J. Armstrong, 1992, in Occupational Disorders of the Upper Extremity, L. H. Millender, D. S. Louis, & B. P. Simmonds, Editors, New York: Churchill Livingstone. Reprinted with permission of the author.

Another consideration for rehabilitation of the musician is the combination of conditioning and orthotics suggested by Prokop (1990), and attention to myofascial problems suggested by Moran (1992). Prokop says that the essence of rehabilitation is restoration of the patient to optimal functioning. In athletes and musicians, whose optimal functioning exceeds that of the general population, the goal of rehabilitation must match the needs of the sport or performance. Prokop's regimen begins with pain reduction, application of heat through many different modalities, including diathermy at varying wave-lengths, then stretching and, on return of full range of motion, strengthening. Moran looks for trigger points of referred pain, and especially observes postural abnormalities. Strengthening exercises to improve posture, as well as trigger-point injections or massage, have often solved difficult rehabil-itation problems.

The ultimate example of considering a musician's complaints as being related to cumulative trauma is to apply the ergonomic approach. Taken to its extreme, this would lead to redesigning musical instruments. Norris has begun this approach, and his example

FIGURE 18.16

Ergonomic change in the work place based on analysis of stress factors. Automotive assembly requires use of a hand-held screwdriver as well as other tools that may be used at varying vertical heights. The comfort level of these instruments was analyzed (A) and it was determined that the most comfortable level was between 100 and 150 cm in vertical height above the waist. (B) This information may then be used to redesign the work station. From "Cumulative Trauma Disorders of the Upper Limb and Identification of Work-related Factors," by T. J. Armstrong, 1992, in Occupational Disorders of the Upper Extremity, *L. H. Millender, D. S. Louis, & B. P. Simmonds, Editors, New York: Churchill Livingstone. Reprinted with permission of the author.*

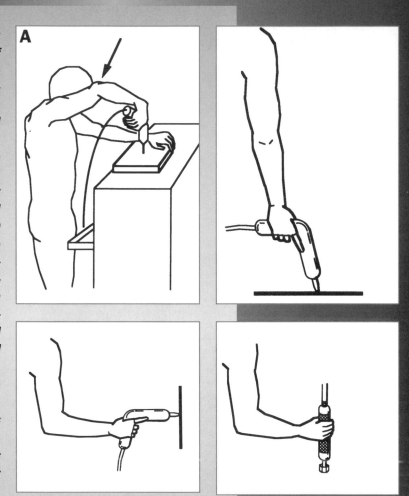

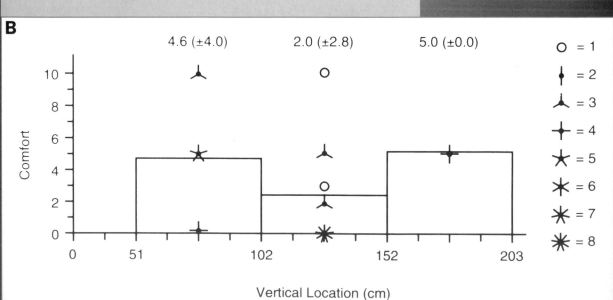

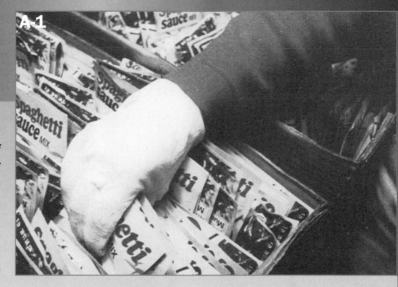

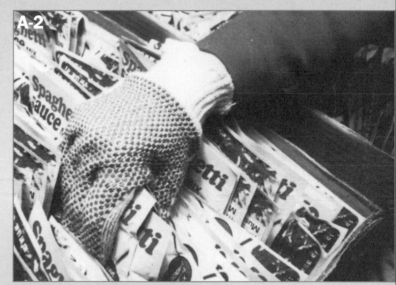

FIGURE 18.17

Ergonomic changes in work place based on analysis of stress factors. (A) Wearing a glove that increases friction makes picking up slippery objects easier. Handles of objects place the wrist into undesirable angles, such as that demonstrated by holding the iron (B), whereas a differently designed handle would be better. Similarly, (C) redesigning handles cut into the sides of a box allows for a power grasp to be substituted for a pinch. From "Neuropathy in the Workplace," by N. B. Zimmerman, S. I. Zimmerman, & G. L. Clark, 1992, Hand Clinics 8:255-262. Reprinted with permission of the authors.

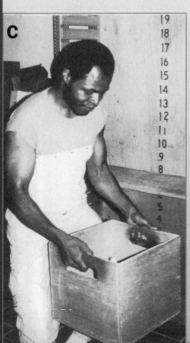

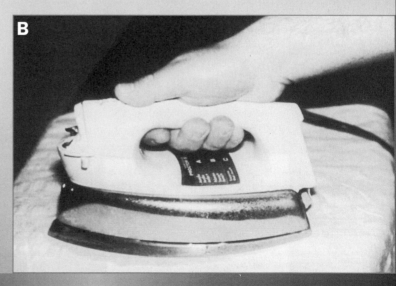

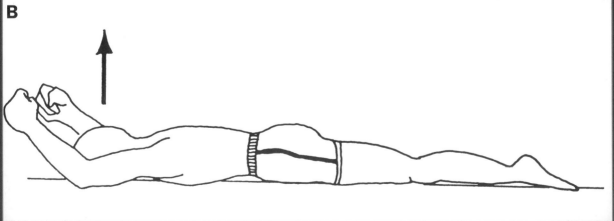

FIGURE 18.18

A series of exercises to strengthen the shoulder girdle muscles and relax and stretch other muscles comprise the nonoperative treatment of brachial plexus compression in the thoracic inlet. These are modified from Britt. (A) Shoulder shrugs strengthen the upper trapezius, while (B) lying prone and lifting the elbows and shoulders from the floor strengthens the lower trapezius. (C) The mid-trapezius and the rhomboids are strengthened by lying prone on a table holding a light weight, about 5 pounds, in the hands, and then lifting the weights while keeping the elbows bent, attempting to get the elbows to touch behind the back. (D) The pectoralis minor is stretched while the serratus is strengthened by doing push-ups in the corner of a room, while standing. The arms should be placed a little further apart than shown in the diagram. (See Figure 18.2 for exercises that stretch the scalenes and the suboccipitalis muscle.) From "Nonoperative Treatment of the Thoracic Outlet Syndrome Symptoms," by L. P. Britt, 1967, Clinical Orthopaedics and Related Research 51:45-48. *Reprinted with permission of the author.*

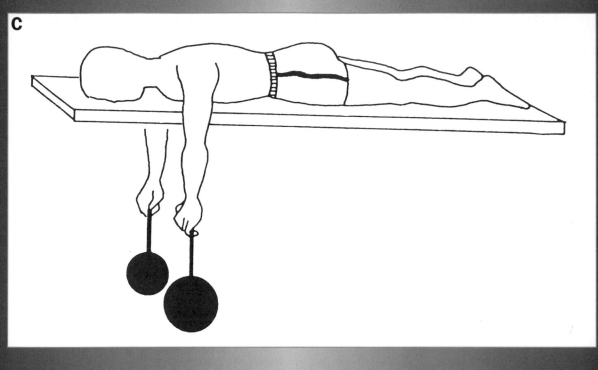

C

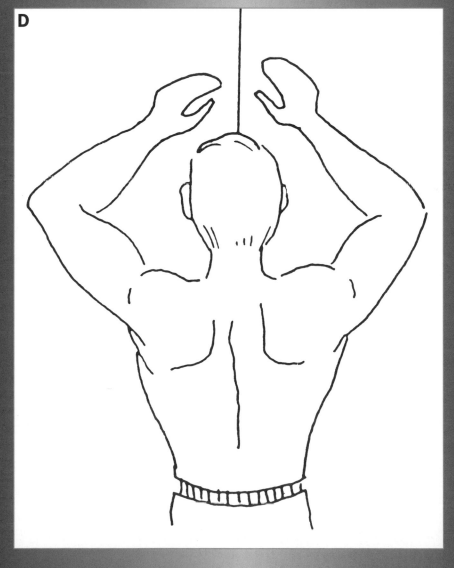

D

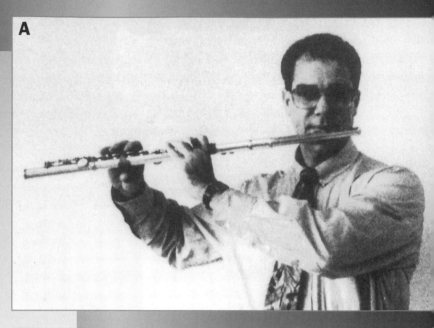

A

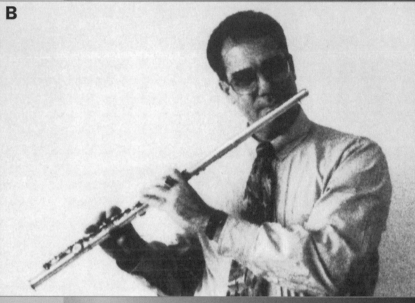

B

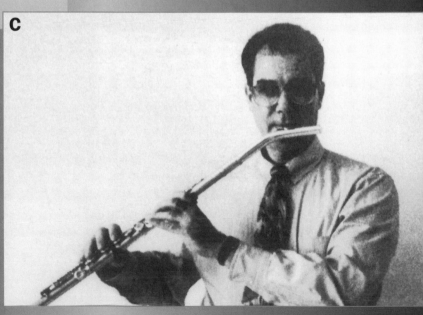

C

FIGURE 18.19

Applying the ergonomic approach to musicians leads to recognizing that the instrument was not designed with human body mechanics in mind. An analysis of the flute (A) demonstrates that if the best position for the shoulders, hands, and wrist is considered, the neck would need to be held at an awkward angle (B). The solution is to alter the instrument. With regard to the thumb position in holding the flute, it is noted that the usual position requires the thumb to be fully rotated to bring the pulp into contact with the flute (C). The solution is to alter the instrument by adding a small strut that allows the thumb to still apply the necessary force for support, but to do so from a more neutral, less stressful position. From The Musicians Survival Manual: A Guide to Preventing and Treating Injuries in Instrumentalists, *by R. Norris, 1993, St. Louis: International Conference of Symphony and Opera Musicians.*

for modification of the flute is given in Figure 18.20. Finally, it should be noted that just as the best way to understand the hand of the worker is to observe him or her doing a specific job in industry, it is most appropriate for the clinician to not only observe the musician playing his or her instrument in a room, but also in the concert hall.

• • •

• REFERENCES •

Amadio, P. C., & Rusotti, G. M. Evaluation and treatment of hand and wrist disorders in musicians. *Hand Clinics* 6:405-416, 1990.

Armstrong, T. J. Cumulative trauma disorders of the upper limb and identification of work-related factors. In *Occupational Disorders of the Upper Extremity*, L. H. Millender, D. S. Louis, & B. P. Simmonds, Editors. New York: Churchill Livingstone, 1992.

Armstrong, T. J., Foulke, J. A., Joseph, B. A., & Goldstein, S. A. Investigation of cumulative trauma disorders in a poultry processing plant. *American Industrial Hygiene Association Journal* 43:102-116, 1982.

Bleecker, M. L., & Hansen, J. A. *Occupational Neurology and Clinical Neurotoxicology*. Baltimore: Williams & Wilkins, 1994.

Britt, L. P. Non-operative treatment of the thoracic outlet syndrome symptoms. *Clinical Orthopaedics and Related Research 51*:45-48, 1967.

Cherington, M., & Cherington, C. Thoracic outlet syndrome reimbursement patterns and patient profiles. *Neurology 42*:493-495, 1992.

Cummings, K., Maizlish, N., Rudolph, L., Devlin, K., & Erwin, A. Occupational disease surveillance: Carpal tunnel syndrome. *Morbidity and Mortality Weekly Report 38:*485-489, 1989.

Dellon, A. L. The results of supraclavicular brachial plexus neurolysis without first rib resection in management of post-traumatic "thoracic outlet syndrome." *Journal of Reconstructive Microsurgery 9*:11-17, 1993.

Dellon, A. L., & Keller, K. M. Computerized sensorimotor testing in patients with carpal and cubital tunnel syndrome: *Annals of Plastic Surgery, 38:* 493-502. 1997.

Dunant, J. H. Diagnosis of thoracic outlet syndrome. *VASA 16*:345-348, 1987.

Edwards, R. H. Hypothesis of peripheral and central mechanisms underlying occupational muscle pain and injury. *European Journal of Applied Physiology and Occupational Physiology* 57:275-281, 1988.

Federal Register, Volume 54, Number 16, January 26, 1989.

Gilbert, J. C., & Knowlton, R. G. Simple method to determine sincerity of effort during a maximal isometric test of grip strength. *American Journal of Physical Medicine 62*: 35-144, 1983.

Hadler, N. M. Cumulative trauma disorders: An iatrogenic concept. *Journal of Occupational Medicine 32*:38-41, 1990.

Hadler, N. M. *Occupational Musculoskeletal Disorders*. New York: Raven Press, 1993.

Higgs, P. E., Edwards, D., Martin, D. S., & Weeks, P. M. Carpal tunnel surgery outcome in workers. *Journal of Hand Surgery*, in press: 1995.

Hildreth, D. H., Briedenbach, W. C., Lister, G. D., & Hodges, A. D. Detection of submaximal effort by use of the rapid exchange grip. *Journal of Hand Surgery 14A*:742-745, 1989.

Johnson, C. Treating the hands that make music. *Journal of Hand Therapy 5*:58-60, 1992.

Kasdan, M. *Occupational Hand and Upper Extremity Injuries and Diseases*. Philadelphia: Hanley & Belfus, 1991.

King, J. W. An integration of medicine and industry. *Journal of Hand Therapy* April-

June:45-50, 1990.

Leffert, R. D. Thoracic outlet syndromes. *Hand Clinics* 8:285-291, 1992.

Levin, L. S., & Dellon, A. L. Pathology of the shoulder as it relates to the differential diagnosis of thoracic outlet compression. *Journal of Reconstructive Microsurgery* 8:313-317, 1992.

Liss, G. M., Armstrong, C., Kusiak, R. A., & Gailitis, M. M. Use of provincial health insurance plan billing data to estimate carpal tunnel syndrome morbidity and surgery rates. *American Journal of Industrial Medicine* 22:395-409, 1992.

Louis, D. S. A historical perspective of workers and the work place. In *Occupational Disorders of the Upper Extremity*, L. H. Millender, D. S. Louis, & B. P. Simmonds, Editors. New York: Churchill Livingstone, 1992.

Mackinnon, S. E., & Dellon, A. L. Chapter 14, Multiple Crush Syndrome. In *Surgery of the Peripheral Nerve*. New York: Thieme, 1988.

Mackinnon, S.E., & Novak, C.B. Clinical commentary: Pathogenesis of cumulative trauma disorder. *Journal of Hand Surgery* 19A:873-883, 1994.

Masear, V. R., Hayes, J. M., & Hyde, A. G. An industrial cause of carpal tunnel syndrome. *Journal of Hand Surgery* 11:222-227, 1986.

McAtamney, L., & Corlett, E. N. RULA: A survey method for the investigation of work-related upper limb disorders. *Applied Ergonomics* 24:91-99, 1993.

McGough, E. C., Pearce, M. B., & Byrne, J. P. Management of thoracic outlet syndrome. *Journal of Therapeutics & Cardiovascular Medicine* 77:169-174, 1979.

Medical Problems of the Performing Arts (a journal). Philadelphia: Hanley & Belfus, Inc., 1993.

Millender, L. H., Louis, D. S., & Simmonds, B. P. *Occupational Disorders of the Upper Extremity*. New York: Churchill Livingstone, 1992.

Moore, A., Wells, R., & Ranney, D. Quantifying exposure in occupational manual tasks with cumulative trauma disorder potential. *Ergonomics* 34:1433-1453, 1991.

Moran, C. A. Using myofascial techniques to treat musicians. *Journal of Hand Therapy* 5:97-101, 1992.

Nathan, P. A., Keniston, R. C., Myers, L. D., & Meadows, K. D. Longitudinal study of median nerve sensory conduction in industry: Relationship to age, gender, hand dominance, occupational hand use, and clinical diagnosis. *Journal of Hand Surgery* 17A:850-857, 1992.

Neelam, S. R. Using torque arms to reduce CTDs. *Ergonomics in Design* October:25-28, 1994.

Norris, R. *TheMusiciansSsurvival Manual: A Guide to Preventing and Treating Injuries in Instrumentalists*. St. Louis: International Conference of Symphony and Opera Musicians, 1993.

Novak, C. B., Collins, E. D., & Mackinnon, S. E. Outcome following conservative management of thoracic outlet syndrome. *Journal of Hand Surgery, 20A:* 542-548, 1995.

Peet, R. M., Hendrickson, J. D., Anderson, T. P., & Martin, G. M. Thoracic outlet syndrome: Evaluation of a therapeutic exercise program. *Mayo Clinic Proceedings* 31:281-287, 1956.

Prokop, L. L. Upper-extremity rehabilitation: Conditioning and orthotics for the athlete and performing artist. *Hand Clinics* 6:517-524, 1990.

Roos, D., & Wilbourn, A. J. Thoracic outlet syndrome is underrated/overdiagnosed. *Archives of Neurology* 47:228-230, 1990.

Sanders, R. J. *Thoracic Outlet Syndrome: A Common Sequela of Neck Injuries*. Philadelphia: J. B. Lippincott Company, 1991.

Scope of Practice. *American Society of Hand Therapy*, 1989.

Silverstein, B. A., Fine, L. J., & Armstrong, T. J. Occupational factors and carpal tunnel syndrome. *American Journal of Industrial Medicine* 11:343-358, 1987.

Stokes, H. M. The seriously uninjured hand - Weakness of grip. *Journal of Occupational Medicine* 25:683-684, 1983.

Walsh, M. T. Therapist management of thoracic outlet syndrome. *Journal of Hand Therapy* April-June:131-144, 1994.

Wilbourn, A. J., & Urschel, H. C. Evidence for conduction delay in thoracic outlet syndrome is challenged. *New England Journal of Medicine 310*:1052-1053, 1984.

Zimmerman, N. B., Zimmerman, S. I., & Clark, G. L. Neuropathy in the workplace. *Hand Clinics 8*:255-262, 1992.

• ADDITIONAL READINGS •

Anthony, M. S. Thoracic outlet syndrome. *In Hand Rehabilitation: A Practical Guide*, G. L. Clark, E. F. S. Wilgis, B. Aiellon, D. Eckhaus, & L. V. Eddington, Editors. New York: Churchill Livingstone, 1993, pp. 171-185.

Armstrong, T. J., Punnett, L., & Ketner, P. Subjective worker assessments of hand tools used in automobile assembly. *American Industrial Hygiene Association Journal 51*:639-642, 1989.

Arndt, R. Work place, stress, and cumulative trauma disorders. *Journal of Hand Surgery 12A*:866-869, 1987.

Brammer, A. J., Piercy, J. E., Auger, P. L., & Nohara, S. Tactile perception in hands occupationally exposed to vibration. *Journal of Hand Surgery 12A*:870-875, 1987.

Campbell, C. S. Gamekeeper's thumb. *Journal of Bone and Joint Surgery 37B*:143-146, 1955.

Cannon, L. J., Bernacki, E. J., & Walter, S. D. Personal and occupational factors associated with carpal tunnel syndrome. *Journal of Occupational Medicine 23*:255-258, 1981.

Cherniak, M. G., Letz, R., Gerr, F., Brammer, A., & Pace, P. Detailed clinical assessment of neurological function in symptomatic shipyard workers. *British Journal of Industrial Medicine 46*:566-572, 1990.

Dawson, W. J. Reed-maker's elbow. *Medical Problems in the Performing Arts 1*:24-26, 1986.

Felderman, R. G., Goldman, R., & Kyeserling, W. M. Peripheral nerve entrapment syndromes and ergonomic factors. *American Journal of Industrial Medicine 4*:661-681, 1983.

Feldman, R. G., Travers, P. H., Chirico-Post, J., & Keyserling, W. M. Risk assessment in electronic assembly workers: Carpal tunnel syndrome. *Journal of Hand Surgery 12A*:849-855, 1987.

Gilliatt, R. W., LeQuesne, P. M., Logue, V., & Sumner, A. J. Wasting of the hand associated with cervical rib or band. *Journal of Neurology, Neurosurgery and Psychiatry 33*:615-618, 1970.

Hagberg, M., & Wegman, D. H. Prevalence rates and odds ratios of shoulder neck diseases in different occupational groups. *British Journal of Industrial Medicine 44*:602-610, 1987.

Hjortsberg, U., Rosen, I., & Orbaek, P. Finger receptor dysfunction in dental technicians exposed to high-frequency vibration. *Scandinavian Journal of Work, Environment and Health 15*:339-343, 1989.

Howell, A. E., & Leach, R. E. Bowler's thumb. *Journal of Bone and Joint Surgery 52A*:379-382, 1970.

Hymovich, L., & Lindholm, M. Hand, wrist, and forearm injuries. *Journal of Occupational Medicine 8*:573-577, 1966.

Jarvinen, T., & Kuorinka, I. Prevalence of tenosynovitis and other occupational injuries of upper extremities in repetitive work. *Arh Hig Rada Toksikol 30*:1281-1284, 1979.

Johnson, S. L. Ergonomic design of hand-held tools to prevent trauma to the hand and upper extremity. *Journal of Hand Therapy* April-June:86-92, 1990.

Kilbom, A., Persson, I., & Jonsson, B. G. Disorders of the cervicobrachial region among female workers in the electronics industry. *International Journal of Ergonomics 1*:37-47, 1986.

Margolis, W., & Kraus, J. F. The prevalence of carpal tunnel syndrome symptoms in female supermarket checkers. *Journal of*

Occupational Medicine 29:952-955, 1987.

Narini, P., Novak, C. B., Mackinnon, S. E., & Coulson-Ross, C. Occupational exposure to hand vibration in northern Ontario gold miners. *Journal of Hand Surgery 18A*:1051-1058, 1993.

Nathan, P. A., Keniston, R. C., Meadows, K. D., & Lockwood, R.S. Predictive value of nerve conduction measurement at the carpal tunnel. *Muscle and Nerve 16*:1377-1382, 1993.

Parsons, J. S. Tobacco-primer's wrist. *New England Journal of Medicine 305*:768, 1981.

Ramazzini, B. *DeMorbis artificum diatriba. Diseases of Workers* (W. C. Wright, Trans.). New York: Hafner Publishing Company, 1964.

Silverstein, B., Fine, L., & Stetson, D. Hand-wrist disorders among investment casting plant workers. *Journal of Hand Surgery 12A*:838-844, 1987.

Spaans, F. Occupational nerve injuries. In *Handbook of Clinical Neurology*, P. J. Vinken, & G. W. Bruyn, Editors. New York: Elsevier, 1970.

Steib, E. W., & Sun, S. F. Distal ulnar neuropathy in meat packers. *Journal of Occupational Medicine 26*:842-845, 1984.

Tadano, P. A safety/prevention program for VDT operators: One company's approach. *Journal of Hand Therapy* April-June:64-70, 1990.

Vihma, T., Nurminen, M., & Mutanen, P. Sewing machine operators' work and musculoskeletal complaints. *Ergonomics 25*:295-298, 1982.

• • •

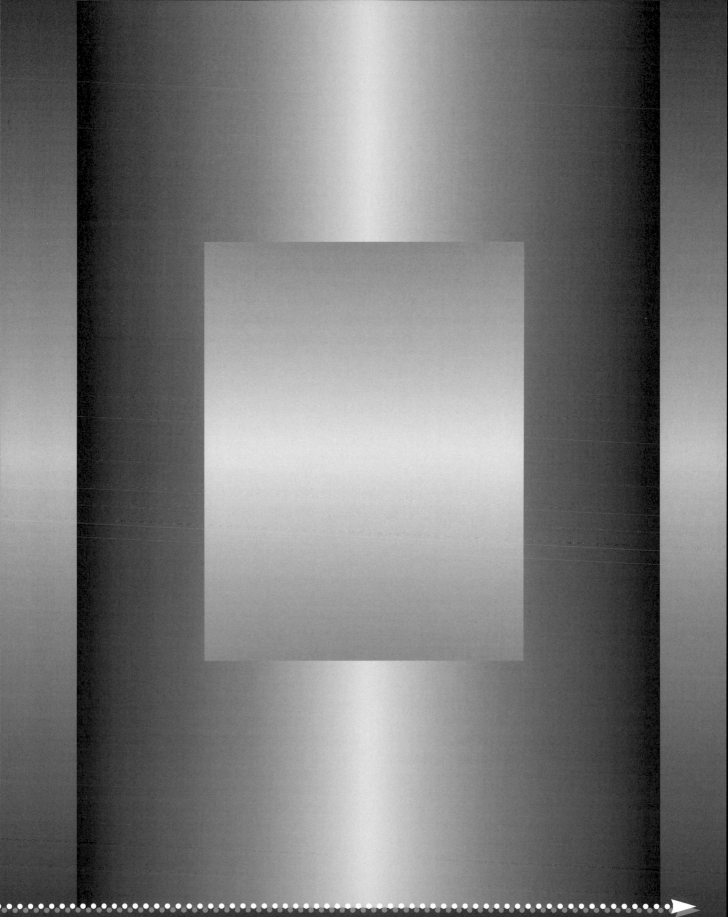

plegia

The plegias comprise a diverse group of disorders, having in common sensory disturbance. The sensory disturbance can be primary, that is, directly as a result of the disorder. For example, in spinal cord injury, sensation is lost to varying degrees at levels below the exact site of the injury. Thus, a C5/6 level spinal cord injury gives rise to *quadriplegia*, with motor and sensory loss below the C5/6 level to all four extremities. Such a patient might have sensation remaining only along the shoulders, down along the radial side of the forearm, and into the thumb and index finger. Sensory loss is also primary for a patient with *paraplegia*, in whom the spinal cord level is usually at T12 or lower, leaving both upper extremities normal, but resulting in motor and sensory loss to both legs, which may be visualized as being parallel to one another in their loss.

In contrast, *hemiplegia* refers to a condition in which just one extremity, usually by convention the upper extremity, is involved, so just half of the upper extremity limbs may be spastic. In *spastic hemiplegia* the cause is a brain injury; thus, the limb that is involved is contralateral to the injury. Sensory disturbance in spastic hemiplegia may be the direct result of injury to some portion of the brain, but it may also be due to secondary involvement of peripheral nerves from muscle tightness and flexion contractures.

A paraplegic may develop secondary sensory problems in his or her (nonplegic) upper extremities due to repetitive trauma.

Most of the attention concerning the care of patients with a plegia has been directed to the motor system. An exception to this has been the attention to decubitus ulcers, which result from sensory loss, in areas such as the lower back, buttocks, and sometimes the feet. This chapter will focus on the sensibility testing and sensory rehabilitation that patients with a plegia require. It will be clear from this chapter that the degree of sensory problems in this group of patients is considerable, and that any degree of improved function that can be restored to these severely impaired people is greatly appreciated and worthwhile. This chapter will also illustrate some techniques to transfer sensation from one area of the body into the anesthetic area in an attempt to restore protective sensibility. The unusual spinal cord condition, syringomyelia, will also be described, as its diagnosis relies on the sensory examination.

proved hygiene and overall appearance of the hand and arm, and most often also improved motor function. Therapists were almost always involved in stretching and strengthening muscles, teaching the use of the transferred muscles, splinting, and activities of daily living. Attention to sensory problems took only one form, and that was by way of a caution to the reconstructive surgeon: Do not attempt to reconstruct the hand if there is a sensory impairment!

This message was brought home forcefully to me one day in 1977, when I was doing my Hand Surgery Fellowship. I was presenting a 16-year-old boy to one of the country's leading experts on spastic hemiplegia, someone renown for his combination of reconstructive techniques. This boy had fallen 6 years before, suffering a brain injury and leaving him with a spastic hemiplegia, with the wrist flexed, the fingers all curled into the palm, the thumb clasped by the fingers, the forearm pronated, and the elbow flexed to about 30° (see Figures 19.1 & 19.2). He had not used his hand for those 6 years, but had kept his joints mobile with a range-of-motion program at home.

I had carefully worked out a plan for tendon transfers, but was cut short before ever getting to present the plan

• SPASTIC HEMIPLEGIA •

Spastic hemiplegia, as used in this chapter, will refer to a group of upper extremity disorders which may involve both the motor and sensory systems, and which are central in origin. When this disorder is present at birth, it is most commonly called cerebral palsy. While it most commonly is present at birth and is, therefore, congenital, it is not a hereditary disorder. However, it is considered to have its origin in a period of cerebral hypoxia at some time prior to birth. Spastic hemiplegia, however, can be acquired at any time of life, for example, after a head injury or after a cerebrovascular accident such as a stroke. The limb is almost always maintained in some abnormal posture, calling it to immediate attention, and focusing the medical community, the patient, and their family on the motor aspects of this disorder.

Appropriately, the medical community, and primarily orthopedic surgeons, developed techniques to relieve muscle spasticity, to transfer muscles to restore balance, to release contractures, and sometimes to fuse involved joints. Nerves were only considered as the source of innervation to the spastic muscles; therefore, in spastic hemiplegia they were objects to destroy, either by direct resection or injection of alcohol or phenol. The combination of these techniques, in skillful and experienced surgeons' hands, always im-

FIGURE 19.1

(A) Typical appearance of a hand with spastic hemiplegia. In this case, a 16-year-old boy who had fallen 6 years before, sustaining an intracranial hemorrhage, resulting in this posttraumatic problem. (B) and (C) Note the thumb clasped into the palm due to spasticity of the ulnar innervated intrinsics, and the fingers curled into the palm due to spasticity of the sublimus muscles. The spastic finger flexors draw the wrist into flexion. Spasticity of the flexor/pronator muscle group draws the elbow into flexion and pronates the forearm.

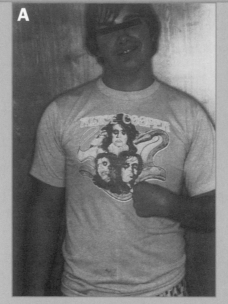

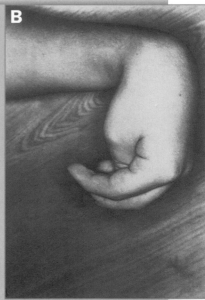

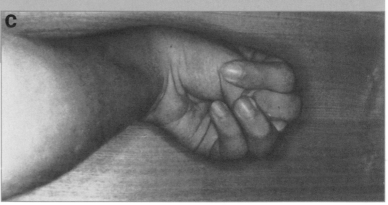

by a question from the professor: "What is his sensation like?" I had not tested it! The professor proceeded to do so, taking a pocket knife from his pocket, prying open the boy's fingers, placing the closed knife into the boy's palm, and asking the boy to identify what was within his grasp. The boy could not. The professor then indicated that this boy was not a candidate for tendon transfers because he had such poor sensation, but that we might go on and discuss the transfers for academic interest. That episode had a profound effect on me not only be- cause I had not evaluated his sensibility, but also be- cause it raised a series of questions which challenge traditional dogma. The questions follow.

• QUESTIONS REGARDING SENSATION IN SPASTIC HEMIPLEGIA •

What is the most appropriate test of sensation in a patient who has kept his fingers generally clasped into his palm, depriving his somatosensory cortex of any significant stimulation? In a patient with posttraumatic spastic hemiplegia, there is presumed to be at least a pretrauma period in which sensory stimuli built images of recognition in the cortex that later could be used to associate a new,

FIGURE 19.2

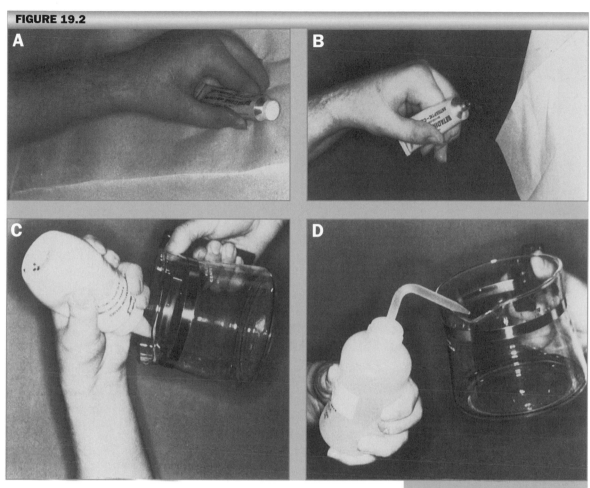

posttraumatic sensory experience with a former memory. But what about the child born with spastic hemiplegia, whose clasped fingers have generated little, if any, stimulus to the sensory cortex?

If the initial event causing the sensory disturbance or sensory loss is due to a cerebral ischemic event, then neural stimuli from the fingers may not be able to be perceived. If this were the case, then the sensation in the patient with spastic hemiplegia could not be im-

proved either with sensory reeducation or with surgery designed to improve the function of the peripheral nerve. But, if the cause of the sensory disturbance is only or partly peripheral, in the hand, wrist, and forearm, due to flexion contractures and chronic nerve compression, then there is hope that surgery on the peripheral nerve may improve sensation in the hand, and that sensory reeducation will be of value.

What would the effect on sensibility and sensation be

After tendon transfers to correct deformities, the hand of the patient in Figure 19.1 can pinch (A & B) and grasp (C & D). Removing the pressure on the median nerve by correcting wrist flexion, and by increasing sensory input as the hand becomes more functional, sensory reeducation is accomplished. Two-point discrimination was recovered in the thumb and index finger. From Evaluation of Sensibility and Re-education of Sensation of the Hand, *by A. L. Dellon, 1981. Baltimore: Williams & Wilkins. Reprinted with permission of the author.*

if a normal young child, or a normal adult, were to have the wrist held in 80° of flexion, the forearm held in full pronation, and the elbow held in 40° to 60° of flexion? What would be the effect on the development of the sensory cortex and on perception of touch if a normal young child were to have a hand covered with a snug glove, preventing other stimuli except the constant touch of the glove against the skin from reaching the sensory cortex?

This chapter will seek the answers to these questions, and will provide a basis for diagnosis of sensory impairment in a patient with spastic hemiplegia, recommend surgical procedures that will correct problems with the peripheral nerves as well as with the spastic muscles, and give guidelines for sensory and motor rehabilitation.

RELEVANT NEUROANATOMY OF SPASTIC HEMIPLEGIA

The classic finding with an upper motor neuron disorder is spasticity of the muscles in the extremity. The classic explanation is that the region of the brain that is injured has two different effects on the muscles in the extremity. The first effect is the loss of voluntary control over the muscles. This also occurs if there is a spinal cord injury of loss of the motor neurons in the ventral horn of the spinal cord. The second effect is the loss of inhibitory or negative feedback impulses. In the absence of this negative feedback, the lower motor neuron fires without regard to any voluntary control.

It is this intermittent, yet continuous, firing of the lower motor neuron that is responsible for the increased tone in the muscle, if not for the contractions. Depending on the widespread and uncoordinated sequence of contractions in the limb, there may be the appearance of a movement disorder rather than a constant spastic condition, giving rise to the term *athetoid form of cerebral palsy*, in contrast to spastic hemiplegia. This difference is important with regard to sensory disturbances, since varying types of movements will not be as likely to result in prolonged compression of a peripheral nerve. This is in contrast to the increased pressure experienced by a peripheral nerve lying beneath a contracted muscle or across a flexed or hyperextended joint. It is, therefore, the loss of inhibitory impulses that permits the muscles to be so active, giving rise to a series of therapeutic possibilities.

To diminish spasticity, direct muscle-inhibiting drugs can be given. The most commonly used muscle relaxant for spasticity is Baclofen (Lioresal). Or, the nerve may be totally or partially destroyed. This can be done chemically by injecting the nerve with alcohol or phenol, or surgically by resecting portions of the motor nerve branches going into the muscle. Cutting the tendon from the spastic muscle can also achieve the same objective. Each of these techniques has in common the fact that muscle force will be lost. While this is the desired goal of the intervention and is, therefore, good, many of these patients have actual weakness as part of their imbalance. Therefore, another strategy is to transfer the spastic muscle into the tendon of a weak muscle whose function you wish to augment. While the spastic muscle usually is not within voluntary control, its continually acting tonic force can rebalance the flexed wrist or hyperpronated forearm.

Anatomy is relevant also with regard to locations in the forearm and wrist that are potential sites of chronic nerve compression. The median nerve in the carpal tunnel, the ulnar nerve in Guyon's canal, the ulnar nerve in the cubital tunnel, the radial sensory nerve in the forearm, and the median nerve in the forearm are all potential sites of chronic nerve compression. Clear descriptions of each of these nerve compressions and procedures for their decompression are available in textbooks such as *Surgery of the Peripheral Nerve* (Mackinnon & Dellon, 1988). The usual posture of the upper extremity in spastic hemiplegia puts the peripheral nerve at risk for compression at each of these sites.

SENSORY DISTURBANCES IN CHILDREN WITH SPASTIC HEMIPLEGIA

The first detailed description of sensory disturbances in children was reported in 1954 by Tizard in London in conjunction with Paine and Crothers from the Children's Medical Center at Harvard (Tizard & Crothers, 1954). They found that 54% of 106 children had a sensory impairment and that the distribution and incidence of these types of impairments was about the same, regardless of whether the child had a congenital or an acquired hemiplegia. Another study, by Hoffman, Baker, and Reed (1958), found sensory impairment in 72% of 47 children. A third study, reported by Tachdjian and Minear (1958), was done on 96 children selected from over 800 with cerebral palsy seen at the Hospital for Crippled Children in Truth or Consequences, New Mexico.

The results of that study, which are representative of the findings of the first two, are given in Table 19.1. Many of the tests Tachdjian and Minear chose to do were supposed to test cortical activity requiring higher degrees of data processing. These were tests like stereognosis (recognizing an object when placed in the hand); number writing, in which numbers are traced on the finger's surface and the person must correctly identify the number; and two-point discrimination. Other tests were supposed to test the ability to perceive stimuli like sharp or dull, temperature, different weights, and position sense, but not requiring such a high degree of cortical processing. Of particular interest is their observation that the 8 patients they tested with the athetoid form of cerebral palsy, a form in which there are continuous movements rather than

TABLE 19.1 SENSORY DISTURBANCES IN CHILDREN WITH SPASTIC HEMIPLEGIA

Type of Sensation Impaired	Percentage of Children Impaired
Stereognosis	42%
Two-point discrimination	32%
Position sense	17%
Number writing	8%
Weighing perception	4%
Touch localization	4%
Sharp/dull discrimination	3%
Temperature	1%

Note: From "Sensory Disturbances in the Hands of Children with Cerebral Palsy," by M. O. Tachdjian & W. L. Minear, 1958, *Journal of Bone and Joint Surgery 40A:*85-90. Reprinted with permission of the authors.

spastic muscles and constant flexion contractures, had essentially no sensory impairment, thus raising the percentage of sensory disturbance to 40 of 88 patients, or 45%.

Tachdjian and Minear also noted an excellent correlation between degree of sensory impairment and degree of hand function (see Table 19.2), with those children with poor hand function having the highest percentage of sensory impairment. These observations were confirmed by Yekutiel, Jariwala, and Stretch (1994) in 55 children evaluated in Israel. Fifty-one percent of the children showed abnormalities in stereognosis and/or two-point discrimination.

By 1982, it was accepted that there was a degree of sensory impairment that accompanied spastic hemiplegia, but that it should not contraindicate tendon transfers. For example, Richard Smith, who at the time was Chief of the Hand Surgery Service at Harvard, described a tendon lengthening procedure for the flexor pollicis longus, to be done for patients with the thumb-in-palm deformity (Smith, 1982). He noted that none of the 7 patients in his series had normal sensation, but that each did well following the transfer, and that sensory impairment should not be an absolute contraindication for surgery in spastic hemiplegia.

TABLE 19.2 CORRELATION OF HAND FUNCTION WITH SENSORY IMPAIRMENT IN SPASTIC HEMIPLEGIA

Functional Status of Hand	Percentage with Sensory Impairment
No function	88%
Poor	69%
Fair	30%
Good	7%
Normal	0%

Note: From "Sensory Disturbances in the Hands of Children with Cerebral Palsy," by M. O. Tachdjian & W. L. Minear, 1958, *Journal of Bone and Joint Surgery 40A:*85-90. Reprinted with permission of the authors.

HYPOTHESES REGARDING SENSORY LOSS IN SPASTIC HEMIPLEGIA

In 1938, in classic studies drawing parallels between cortical lesions in subhuman primates and in humans, Ruch, Fulton, and German, of the Physiology Department at Yale, drew the following conclusion: Discrimination of object weight and roughness is a function of the parietal lobe. This is generally the function that neurologists have called stereognosis.

The classic concept of spastic hemiplegia is that the motor and the presumed sensory disturbances are due to deficits in the parietal lobe. The parietal lobe is supposed to be responsible for the cortical processing of spatial neural events that permit such discriminative activities as stereognosis, two-point discrimination, and identification of numbers traced on the hand. In contrast, perception of sensory temporal patterns, like vibration, are less affected by cortical lesions unless they extend deeper into the nerve fiber tracts. Finally, basic sensations related to protective responses, such as temperature, pain, and touch are not affected by cortical lesions. Rather, their absence suggests damage at a subcortical level. The sensory disturbances identified by the early clinical researchers suggested that there was a central mechanism responsible for sensory loss. Tachdjian and Minear (1958) admitted that "in some cases...inexperience in using the hand...might be a major factor." However, the succeeding four decades have essentially ignored the possibility that sensory impairment might be coming from the peripheral nerves, and might be related to chronic nerve compression combined with diminished sensory stimulation of the sensory cortex.

Moberg (1958) tried to turn attention to sensory function in the hand and coined the term *tactilegnosis* for object recognition, which he believed was related to function of the peripheral nerves. (He wished to get away from the emphasis on the central nervous system.) The earlier chapters in this text have convincingly demonstrated that hand function, as measured by object recognition, is best correlated with two-point discrimination. Today, it is considered most likely to be true that the ability to recognize an object in space requires both the parietal lobe function and the peripheral mechanisms of sensibility that provide the impulse to the parietal lobe. There can be neither stereognosis nor tactilegnosis without peripheral nerve function.

It is my suggestion that the observed decreased stereognosis in patients with spastic hemiplegia is due to impaired peripheral nerve function, as is the impaired two-point discrimination observed in these patients. If the sensory impairments were due to some cortical ischemic event, the incidence of sensory impairment would be more universal in spastic

hemiplegia, as is the motor deficit. The varying incidence and varying extent of severity of sensory impairment is more likely to be related to the varying extent to which the peripheral nerves in these patients are compressed by the primary muscle imbalances, and the extent to which the child has been deprived, or conversely, has compensated for, the motor problems and allowed sensory stimuli to reach the sensory cortex. Support for this hypothesis comes from the case studies given above, in which tendon transfers

and muscle rebalancing decompress peripheral nerves, with demonstrable improvement in sensory recovery.

Support for this hypothesis also comes from the observation by Ruch, Fulton, and German (1938) that "the degree of recovery of discriminatory ability possible after partial lesions of the parietal lobe is a striking feature of the observations on both chimpanzee and man. Retraining is an important factor in this recovery." If patients with spastic hemiplegia could use their hand and stimulate the sensory endings, they could retrain.

• PARAPLEGIA •

Paraplegia is fundamentally different from spastic hemiplegia. Whereas the upper extremities are affected in spastic hemiplegia, it is the lower extremities that are affected in paraplegia. It is because the patient has paralyzed legs that he or she must rely so heavily on the upper extremities for transportation and transfer. Thus, the upper extremities of a paraplegic receive increased use, which in and of itself can cause chronic compression of peripheral nerves (see Figure 19.3). Furthermore, the upper extremity in the paraplegic must carry out many functions in unusual positions. For example, when transferring from bed to wheelchair, or wheelchair to some other chair, or simply changing positions on the wheelchair seat every 20 to 30 minutes, the wrist is brought into extreme dorsiflexion. Then, in that position, with the median nerve maximally stretched, it is pressed upon with the patient's full weight. This activity has been termed the "raise maneuver."

In the absence of a motorized wheelchair, which may cost up to $6,000, the patient must also rely on the palm of the hand as the propulsion system for the wheelchair, adding repetitive trauma to the median and ulnar nerves at the wrist. Theoretically, there should be an increased incidence of both median and ulnar nerve compression at the wrist in paraplegics. This has been evaluated for median nerve compression at the wrist, and an incidence of carpal tunnel syn-

FIGURE 19.3

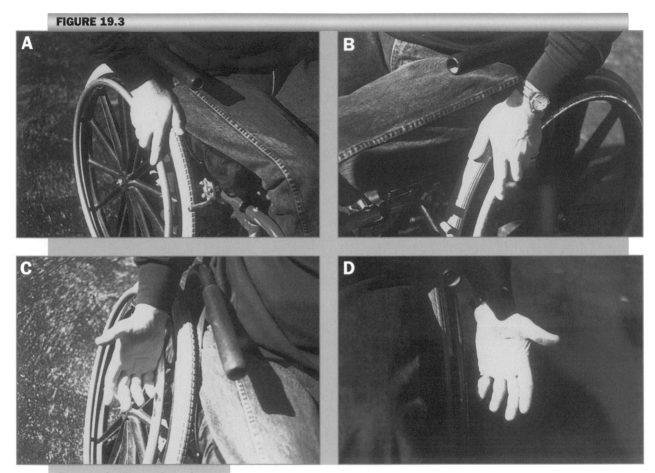

Paraplegia. Examples of pressure on the median nerve as the hand contacts the wheel of the chair. Illustrations copyright A. Lee Dellon. Reprinted with permission.

drome in paraplegics has been found of 49%, 63%, and 75% in three different studies (Aljure, Ibrahim, Bradley, Lin, & Bonnie, 1985; Gellman et al., 1988; Upton & Tun, unpublished observations, 1988).

Regardless of which study is chosen, it is clear that upper extremity nerve problems should be considered part of the evaluation of every patient with paraplegia. I have cared for just four

patients with paraplegia, none of whom was referred primarily for carpal tunnel syndrome. (Two were referred for abdominoplasty, one for decubitus ulcer of the sacrum, and one for lower leg amputation stump pain.) All four had symptomatic carpal tunnel syndromes that responded well to surgical decompression.

The classic research in this area was done in 1988 by two different groups of researchers. The first group, Gellman et al., were from the Orthopedic Surgery Department at the University of Southern California. They

evaluated 77 paraplegics at the Rancho Los Amigos Hospital spinal cord injury clinic. The diagnosis of carpal tunnel syndrome was determined by patient history of symptoms of sensory disturbance in the median nerve distribution. Gellman et al. found that the incidence of symptomatic carpal tunnel syndrome increased in relationship to the length of time the patient had been a paraplegic, increasing from an incidence of 20% at 5 years of wheelchair use to a high of 49% at more than 10 years of wheelchair use (see Table 19.3). The incidence found by these authors is less than that found in an earlier study by Aljure, Ibrahim, Bradley, Lin, & Bonnie (1985) (see Table 19.3), probably because they used patients' symptoms as their diagnostic criteria. Many patients with paraplegia become accustomed to their various discomforts and are unaware of their chronic nerve compressions. Based on the difference between these studies, and the one to follow, it is likely that about 25% of paraplegics have a subclinical median nerve compression at the wrist. This would be detected with quantitative sensory testing.

The pressure within the carpal tunnel in paraplegics has been documented by Gellman et al. (1988). Compared to a group of nonpara-plegics who have carpal tunnel syndrome (as measured by Gelberman, Hergenroeder, Hargens, Lundborg, & Akeson, 1981), it is clear that the carpal tunnel pressures in paraplegics is significantly worse. For example, with the wrist in neutral flexion, the pressures within the carpal tunnel of paraplegics is essentially the same as in non-paraplegics with carpal tunnel symptoms. However, probably because of the increased synovitis within the carpal tunnel of paraplegics from the repetitive trauma of using their wheelchair, the carpal tunnel pressures are higher for the paraplegic with the wrist in extension (110 for nonparaplegics versus 160 for paraplegics), and during the position of the raise maneuver (220 for the paraplegic, unavailable for the nonparaplegic) (see Table 19.4).

Gellman et al. (1988) did sensibility testing on their 77 patients. Of these, 34% had an abnormal Semmes-Weinstein nylon monofilament test, that is, a marking of > 2.83, and 8% had an abnormal two-point discrimination (done with a bent paper clip), that is, > 6 mm. This led to the conclusion that threshold testing was abnormal more often than innervation density testing.

The second group to evaluate this problem was from the Department of Surgery, Division of Plastic Surgery at Harvard, and the Peter Bent Brigham Hospital in Boston. Upton and Tun (1988) evaluated both hands of 30 paraplegics at the Veterans' Ad-

TABLE 19.3 INCIDENCE OF CARPAL TUNNEL SYNDROME IN PARAPLEGICS RELATED TO DURATION OF PARAPLEGIA

Time Since Injury	Symptoms of Carpal Tunnel Syndrome	
	Aljure, et al.[+]	Gellman, et al.[*]
0-5 years	25%	20%
6-10 years	60%	42%
>10 years	80%	76%
Total:	63%	49%

Note:
[+] From "Carpel Tunnel Syndrome in Paraplegic Patients," by J. Aljure, E. Ibrahim, W. E. Bradley, J. E. Lin, & J. Bonnie, 1985, *Paraplegia 23:*182-186.
[*] From "Carpal Tunnel Syndrome in Paraplegic Patients," by H. Gellman, D. R. Chandler, J. Petrasek, J. Sie, R. Adkins, & R. L. Waters, 1988, *Journal of Bone and Joint Surgery 70A:*517-519. Reprinted with permission of the authors.

TABLE 19.4 CARPAL TUNNEL PRESSURES IN PARAPLEGICS DURING ACTIVITIES OF DAILY LIVING

Position of the Wrist	Carpal Tunnel Syndrome	
	With (n=8)	Without (n=10)
Neutral	12 mm Hg	8 mm Hg
Flexion	95 mm Hg	42 mm Hg
Extension	160 mm Hg	200 mm Hg
Raise Maneuver	220 mm Hg	180 mm Hg

Note: From "Carpal Tunnel Syndrome in Paraplegic Patients," by H. Gellman, D. R. Chandler, J. Petrasek, J. Sie, R. Adkins, & R. L. Waters, 1988, *Journal of Bone and Joint Surgery 70A:*517-519. Reprinted with permission of the authors.

ministration spinal cord injury service. They relied on abnormal electrodiagnostic testing, the median sensory distal latency, for the diagnosis of carpal tunnel syndrome. With these criteria, they found that 45 hands of the 60 hands in paraplegics (75%) were abnormal, and consistent with carpal tunnel syndrome. They did quantitative sensory testing on this group of 45 hands, using the Semmes-Weinstein nylon monofilaments and static two-point discrimination with the Disk-Criminator.™ They compared their data from these paraplegic hands to that obtained from both hands of 10 normal control hands, matched for age and sex with the paraplegics (see Table 19.5). Using the criteria from their own normal population, in whom just 1 of the 20 had a Semmes-Weinstein nylon filament marking of 2.44, all the rest being either 1.65 or 2.36, 25 of the 45 (55%) paraplegics had abnormal cutaneous pressure thresholds, ranging up to the 3.84 nylon filament marking. Using the criteria from their own normal control population, in whom all 20 hands had a two-point

TABLE 19.5 SENSIBILITY TESTING IN PARAPLEGICS WITH CARPAL TUNNEL SYNDROME DIAGNOSED BY ABNORMAL NERVE CONDUCTION TESTING

		Static Two-point Discrimination (Disk-Criminator™)		Pressure Threshold (Semmes-Weinstein Monofilaments)	
		< 4mm	≥ 4mm	< 2.44	≥ marking 2.44
Paraplegic Hands	(45)	20	25	20	25[+]
Normal Hands	(20)	20	0	1	19[+]

Note:
[+] By Chi-Square analysis, p < .001.
Data from "Pressure Sensibility of Paraplegic Hands with Abnormal Nerve Conduction Associated with Carpal Tunnel Syndrome," by J. Upton & C. Tun, 1988, unpublished observations.

discrimination of 3 mm or less, 25 of the 45 (55%) paraplegics had abnormal two-point discrimination, ranging from 4 mm to 6 mm. These different proportions can be compared with the Chi-Square test, using the Yates correction for small groups. Such analysis demonstrates that paraplegics with carpal tunnel syndrome diagnosed by abnormal nerve conduction testing have a statistically significantly greater chance of having abnormal quantitative sensory testing than do the normal, non-paraplegic controls, with the p value being < .001 for both the Semmes-Weinstein and two-point discrimination tests. However, while both these tests of sensibility are specific in identifying the problem as related to median nerve compression, they were not very sensitive as screening tests. That is, they identified only 55% of those paraplegics as having the problem, whereas the electrodiagnostic test identified, by definition, the whole 100% of the population with carpal tunnel syndrome.

Many of these patients probably interpret abnormal sensibility as part of their paraplegia, or simply the result of using their hands so much. Therefore, they accept the sensory abnormalities as the inevitable consequence of their paraplegia, without being aware that peripheral nerve decompression is available to them. The therapist's role is to do quantitative sensory testing to define the extent to which this problem exists, to develop baseline values that can be followed for the paraplegic, and to indicate when these become sufficiently abnormal that surgical decompression is indicated (see Chapter 12).

• QUADRIPLEGIA •

The quadriplegic requires attention to sensory testing to evaluate the advisability of doing bilateral tendon transfers. Erik Moberg, who in his retirement began intensive study of the hand of patients with tetraplegia (Moberg, 1978), noted that if sensation was absent from the hand of such a patient, then it was not advisable to do tendon transfers. He found that quadriplegics who had little if any sensation in their hand only used the hand when it could be under direct visualization. He devised a classification scheme to describe the remaining intact motor function in the hand that also included a subclassification if the patient was visually impaired. This classification replaced the traditional classification based on the level of the spinal cord thought to be transected. The new system coded for the muscles that still worked and that were capable of voluntary control.

• SYRINGOMYELIA •

Syringomyelia is not a plegia, but a condition of the spinal cord that creates a sensory disturbance, and it usually presents a difficult diagnostic dilemma. A syrinx is a cyst in the spinal cord due to an enlargement of the spinal canal. As the spinal canal enlarges it creates pressure on the tracts of nerve fibers that are closest to the cyst. These tracts are almost always the anterior spinothalamic tracts, which carry the sensory fibers that mediate the perception of hot, cold, and pain. The spinal cord grey matter, containing cell bodies of the ventral horn, lies next to the cyst in almost all cases and, therefore, motor problems are present as well. The most common motor problem is intrinsic muscle weakness, which progresses to muscle wasting.

Note that the posterior pyramidal tracts, which carry the sensory fibers for touch and vibration, are not compressed by the cyst, which lies anterior. The patient will, therefore, present with wasting of all intrinsic muscles, and usually bilaterally symmetrical, but will not complain of numbness or paresthesias. Electromyography is critical here because a cervical disc lesion at C8/T1 could do this, as could bilateral

FIGURE 19.4

Syringomyelia. Clinical photographs of patient with a syrinx, a cyst in the spinal canal, at the C8 and T1 spinal root region of spine. This causes pressure on the motor nuclei, giving intrinsic muscle wasting noted in (A) and (B) that includes all intrinsics. This is, therefore, neither an ulnar nor a median nerve compression. In (A), note excoriations and injuries to tips of fingers, compatible with loss of perception of pain and temperature, as the cyst bulges anteriorly, destroying the anterior sensory tracts. The posterior tracts of the spinal cord, carrying perception of touch, are preserved.

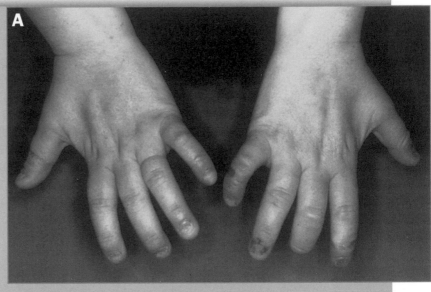

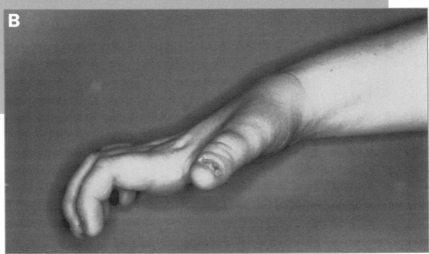

ulnar and median nerve compressions. However, both of these possibilities are rare, especially in the absence of sensory complaints. The examiner may get a clue from inspection of the patient's fingertips, which often will be reddish, ulcerated, or scarred (see Figure 19.4). Careful sensory testing in this setting is critical, as it will demonstrate normal cutaneous pressure thresholds and normal two-point discrimination, but will demonstrate abnormal perception of pain and temperature. This is one of the few instances in which sticking a patient with a sterile 25-gauge needle is indicated.

With the realization that touch sensation is preserved but pain and temperature sensation is abnormal, the diagnosis is made clinically. Confirmatory radiographic imaging with a CAT scan or MRI of the cervical spine will demonstrate the location of the syrinx (see Figure 19.5). The treatment takes two forms, first, shunting of the cyst by the neurosurgeon and, then, after determining

to what extent motor function will return, tendon transfers to restore intrinsic function. The therapist will, therefore, be involved in the initial diagnosis with quantitative sensory testing, in the initial care with teaching protective mechanisms for sensory loss, and in motor rehabilitation with splinting and muscle reeducation.

• • •

FIGURE 19.5

Syringomyelia: Radiologic imaging. In (A), a transverse view of the spinal cord, with one type of "weighting." The magnetic resonance shows the cyst as a white circle, while in (B), a sagittal section of the spinal cord, with a different "weighting," the MRI shows the cyst as a dark circle (arrows) at the C7 and T1 vertebra level.

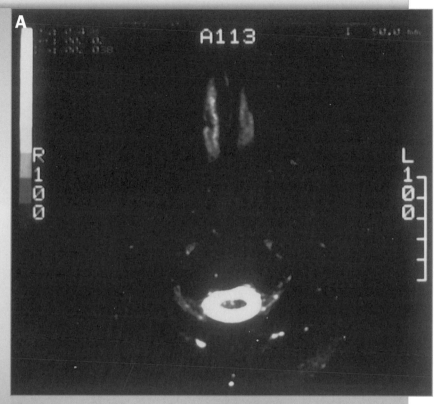

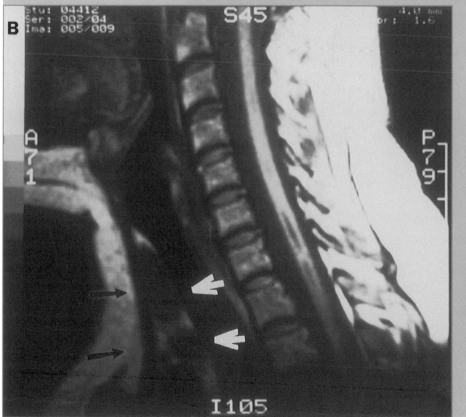

• REFERENCES •

Aljure, J., Ibrahim, E., Bradley, W. E., Lin, J. E., & Bonnie, J. Carpal tunnel syndrome in paraplegic patients. *Paraplegia 23*:182-186, 1985.

Dellon, A. L. *Evaluation of Sensibility and Re-education of Sensation in the Hand.* Baltimore: Williams & Wilkins, 1981.

Gelberman, R. H., Hergenroeder, P. T., Hargens, A. R., Lundborg, G. N., & Akeson, W. H. The carpal tunnel syndrome: A study of carpal canal pressures. *Journal of Bone and Joint Surgery 63A*:380-383, 1981.

Gellman, H., Chandler, D. R., Petrasek, J., Sie, J., Adkins, R., & Waters, R. L. Carpal tunnel syndrome in paraplegic patients. *Journal of Bone and Joint Surgery 70A*:517-519, 1988.

Hoffman, L. B., Baker, L., & Reed, R. Sensory disturbances in children with infantile hemiplegia, triplegia, and quadriplegia. *American Journal of Physical Medicine 38*:1-8, 1958.

Mackinnon, S. E., & Dellon, A. L. *Surgery of the Peripheral Nerve.* New York: Thieme Publishing, 1988, Chapters 6,7, & 8.

Moberg, E. Objective methods for determining the functional value of sensibility in the skin. *Journal of Bone and Joint Surgery 40B*:454-466, 1958.

Moberg, E. *The Upper Limb in Tetraplegia.* London: Churchill Livingstone, 1978.

Ruch, T. C., Fulton, J. F., & German, W. J. Sensory discrimination in monkey, chimpanzee, and man after lesions of the parietal lobe. *Archives of Neurology and Psychology 39*:919-938, 1938.

Smith, R. J. Flexor pollicis longus abductorplasty for spastic thumb-in-palm deformity. *Journal of Hand Surgery 7*:327-334, 1982.

Tachdjian, M. O., & Minear, W. L. Sensory disturbances in the hands of children with cerebral palsy. *Journal of Bone and Joint Surgery 40A*:85-90, 1958.

Tizard, J. P. M., & Crothers, B. Disturbances of sensation in children with hemiplegia. *Journal of the American Medical Association 155*:628-632, 1954.

Yekutiel, M., Jariwala, M., & Stretch, P. Sensory deficit in the hands of children with cerebral palsy: A new look at assessment and prevalence. *Developmental Medicine and Child Neurology 36*:619-624, 1994.

• ADDITIONAL READINGS •

Dellon, A. L. Interruption of nerve function. In *Current Therapy in Plastic and Reconstructive Surgery*, J. Marsh, Editor. Toronto: B. C. Beck, 1988.

Goldner, J. L. *Upper Extremity Reconstructive Surgery in Cerebral Palsy or Similar Conditions.* American Academy of Orthopedic Surgery Instruction Course Lecture 18:169-177, 1961.

• • •

therapist as researcher & teacher

CHAPTER 20

therapist as researcher

• WHO IS A RESEARCHER? •

There is something of a myth or stereotype that a researcher is a PhD, (or beyond!), works in a laboratory funded by the NIH (don't we all wish!), is surrounded by test tubes and little animals, or else is sandwiched between an electron microscope and an automated DNA-synthesizer (see Figure 20.1). Certainly, it is helpful to have a PhD, but it is most important to have a question to answer. Training at the doctoral level focuses your ability to define questions, interpret data, know a body of material in exquisite detail, and apply for research grants. There are actually no laws and no guidelines outlining who can do research; however, there are extensive laws and guidelines regarding how the research is to be conducted, especially if it involves the use of humans and other animals. Individual institutions may define, usually for their own protection, who is in charge of, or responsible for, research, but under that person, the people actually participating in research will range from high-school to postdoctoral students.

First and foremost, a researcher is a person with a question who is seeking an answer. Second, a researcher is a person with creativity and imagination who can identify the resources within their environment that will permit the question to be answered. Third, a researcher is a person with commitment and perseverance who will see a project through to its completion, despite the daily hurdles of personal responsibilities, academic obligations, and administrative obstructions. Fourth, a researcher is a person with integrity, pride, and a desire to increase our basic fund of knowledge to help humankind. Fifth, and unfortunately, a researcher must also be a person who, especially if the research is nontraditional, innovative, and successful, must be able to deal with distrust, misperception, and jealousy of colleagues. The therapist, working in the environment known best, the clinic, and with the patient population known best, and inspired to seek answers to questions posed by everyday problems, has every possibility of fulfilling these criteria.

Among the strategies of successful research is to align oneself with colleagues who share research interests and who can collaborate with you. For example, there will often be a physician with a special interest in surgery or rehabilitation of the area, part, or technique about which the therapist has a specific question. The research may often require special equipment, outside of what is traditionally available in the therapy department. Finding someone who already owns such

FIGURE 20.1

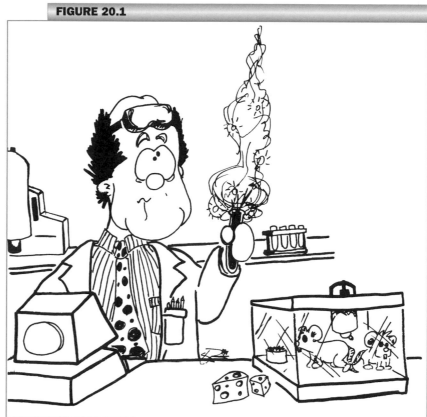

The therapist as a researcher. The therapist is inspired by the clinical problems seen every day to pose questions suitable for investigation. Drawn by Glenn George Dellon. Reprinted with permission.

equipment and with whom the therapist can collaborate goes a long way toward helping with funding a research project. If the patient population for the question in point is relatively small at the therapist's institution, including another therapist and their patients from another institution is a good strategy to pursue. Finding a basic scientist or statistician with whom to collaborate often can greatly enhance a research project's design and data analysis.

The therapist should ex-

pect to be included in any research project in which he or she contributes to some or all of the following aspects of the research: the original idea, patient evaluations, literature search, data compilation, data analysis, manuscript preparation, and so on. Therapists should consider themselves as integral members of the research team and, in addition to publishing the results of their work, they should consider presenting the results of their research at local and national meetings.

• RESEARCH THERAPISTS •

The most well-known therapist/researcher in the United States today is Judith Bell-Krotoski. She is an Occupational Therapist, a Certified Hand Therapist, and has a masters degree in public health. Her position in the Public Health Service at Carlise, Louisiana, the Unites States Leprosarium, gave her the opportunity to extend her natural curiosity into the area of peripheral nerve problems. Clearly, the nerve problems associated with leprosy gave rise to questions which led to her association with Paul Brand, MD, renown for rehabilitation and tendon transfers, as well as descriptions of problems associated with the insensitive hand and foot. Judy's training at the Hand Rehabilitation Center in Philadelphia with Evelyn Mackin and James Hunter gave her a strong background in the use of Semmes-Weinstein monofilaments for sensory testing. She found this invaluable in mapping the patchy neuropathy that can be associated with the leprosy bacteria's scattered invasion of the peripheral nerve. Her association with Bill Buford, PhD, a biomedical engineer, gave her research an added dimension needed for the evaluation of hand movements during sensibility testing. Based on her research ability, writing, and teaching, Judy Bell-Krotoski was appointed in 1993 as the Chief Therapist of the United States for the Public Health Service.

While many therapists have contributed greatly through their research and writing efforts, it is instructive to give two more vignettes. Evelyn Mackin, PT, CHT, is a founding partner, along with James Hunter, MD, of the Hand Rehabilitation Center in Philadelphia, and has been its Director of Rehabilitation since 1973. She is a founding member of the American Society for Hand Therapy, and in 1981-1982 was its president. She is also the founding editor of the Journal of Hand Therapy (1987). She continues in her role as coeditor of the book, *Rehabilitation of the Hand*, which first appeared in 1978 and is now in its 4th edition. Her research has been primarily involved with the development and evaluation of both the active and passive Hunter tendon prosthesis.

Similarly, the association since 1983 of Christine B. Novak, PT, CHT, MSc, with Susan E. Mackinnon, MD, at Sunnybrook Medical Centre in Toronto, Canada, and since June 1992 with the Division of Plastic Surgery at Washington University School of Medicine, led Christine to an interest in sensibility testing techniques. Her current academic appointment is Research Assistant Professor of Surgery in the Department of Surgery, and Research Assistant Professor of Occupational Therapy at Washington University School of Medicine. She has applied research techniques to evaluate results of nerve repair and nerve grafting. Her master's thesis led her to new insights into evaluating sensibility in the blind. Her careful statistical analysis of hand-held devices for sensibility testing has documented their validity. Her current research extends into the diagnosis and nonoperative management of thoracic outlet syndrome and cumulative trauma disorders.

I have been fortunate to do research with many talented therapists. Beginning in medical school at Johns Hopkins in 1968, I worked with Janice Maynard, OTR, who was then Senior Occupational Therapist in the Rehabilitation Department. It was with Janice that I first evaluated the pattern of recovery of sensibility in patients recovering from nerve injury and nerve repair. This work led to the introduction of tuning forks of 30 Hz and 256 Hz, and the use of the terms *constant touch* and *moving touch*, all of which appeared in the Johns Hopkins Medical Journal in 1972. My first sensory reeducation study was also done in Janice's department. Janice worked with Rod Schlegel, PT, to cofound the Rehabilitation Units of the Raymond M. Curtis Hand Center at Union Memorial Hospital in Baltimore where, in 1977, I was the first Hand Surgery Fellow. Janice eventually returned to her home in England. I still use a slide of hers in my Sensory Reeducation lecture (see Figure 20.2).

Rod Schlegel, PT was of

FIGURE 20.2

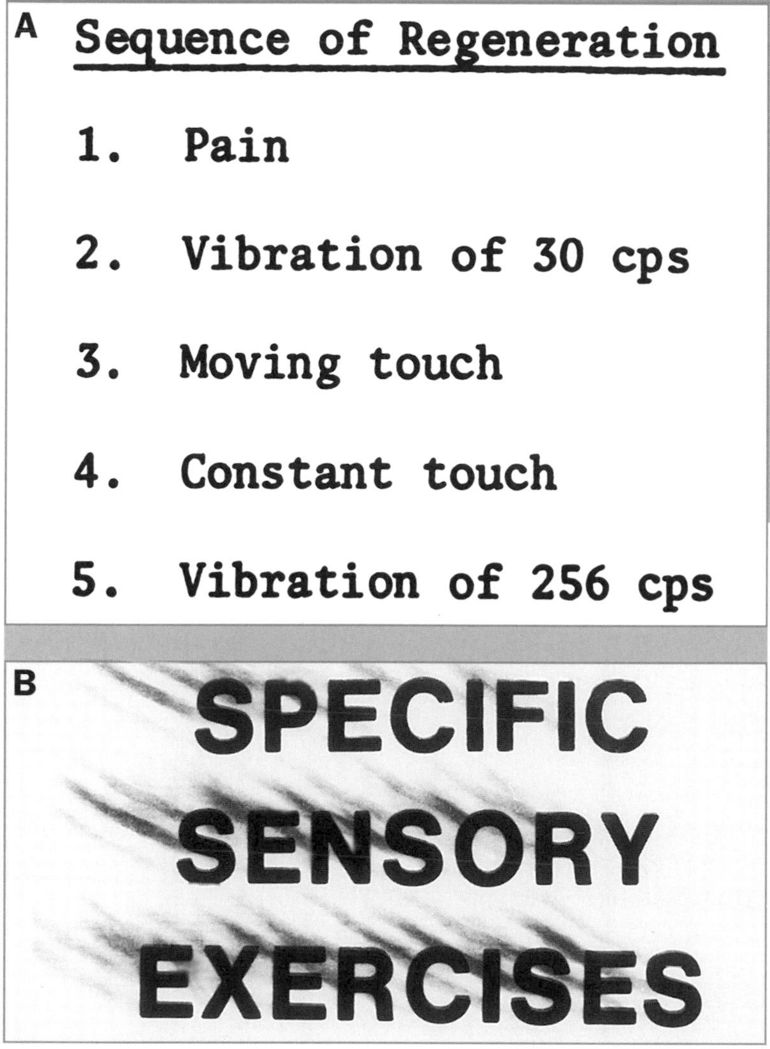

A

Sequence of Regeneration

1. Pain

2. Vibration of 30 cps

3. Moving touch

4. Constant touch

5. Vibration of 256 cps

B

SPECIFIC SENSORY EXERCISES

Slides of historic signifcance. (A) The sequence of recovery of recovery of sensation after nerve reconstruction. (Courtesy of Janice Maynard, OTR, circa 1970.) (B) The concept of applying specific sensory exercises at the appropriate time during nerve recovery to permit the most effective sensory reeducation. (Courtesy of Pegge Carter, circa 1974.)

invaluable help both in the laboratory and in the operating room, carrying out electrodiagnostic evaluation of nerve grafts in monkeys, silicone tube compression of the rat sciatic nerve, and conduction across the ulnar nerve at the elbow during different stages of intraoperative transposition in humans, with the elbow in different degrees of extension.

Probably the most enthusiastic and energetic therapist with whom I've had the privilege to work is Pegge Carter, OT, CHT, from Phoenix, Arizona. Pegge is a founding member of the American Society of Hand Therapists and was its president during 1982-1983. For the past two decades she has been Director of Hand Rehabilitation for Hand Surgery Associates in Phoenix. At the beginning of my teaching about sensory reeducation in 1971, at the annual meeting of the American Society for Surgery of the Hand, Pegge took up the challenge of helping to introduce this concept to her colleagues. Through her writing and lecturing she has been a great force in the dissemination of these techniques. I still also use some slides she was kind enough to let me borrow (see Figure 20.2). It must have been fate, for Pegge has had available to her the patient population of her husband, hand surgeon Robert (Bob) Wilson, MD. They make a unique team.

Other therapists from Baltimore with whom I have done research are Page Crosby and Robin Mourey, OTR. Robin was the senior therapist at Johns Hopkins in 1991, when the Pressure-Specified Sensory Device™ was first introduced. She, along with my son Evan

Samuel Dellon, did the first study using this computer-assisted sensory testing. Results of that study were published in 1992 (E. S. Dellon, Mourey, & A. L. Dellon). Thus, my testing of sensibility came full circle, at least in geographic location. At the Children's Hospital in Baltimore, where I have operated since 1978, when I went into practice, the Chief of Occupational Therapy there, Virginia Moratz, OTR, and Kelly Kress Keller, OTR, were the first to use the NK Biotechnical Corporation computer-assisted sensorimotor devices on a regular, full-time basis to provide patient care. This began in 1991, and still continues. The patient evaluations they have done provide the critical information needed for much of the understanding of the clinical use of this equipment.

It is also appropriate for therapists to describe their improvements for splinting, which can be for research as well as patient care. In that regard, therapists Carol Gwinn, Janice Kofkin, and Barbara Rose were helpful in both spheres of activity.

Internationally, it has been a privilege to work with therapists in Japan and Taiwan in the field of sensibility evaluation. Mayumi Nakada, Chief Therapist at the Tokyo Metropolitan College of Allied Medical Sciences, and Teruko Iwasaki, Chief Therapist at the Tokyo National Hospital School of Rehabili-

tation from Tokyo, both came to Baltimore to visit and study, and then extended our work to the patient population with stroke and leprosy in their own country. Their interest led to the founding of the Japanese Association for Sensory Rehabilitation, which had its fourth national meeting in 1995. They translated my first book, *Evaluation of Sensibility and Re-education of Sensation in the Hand* (1981) into Japanese in 1994, and this translation will serve as a textbook in their university. They also have introduced tuning fork examination and the Disk-Criminator™ into their country.

I met Helena Ma, OTR, through Fu-Chan Wei, MD, Chief of Hand Surgery and Microsurgery at Chang Gung School of Medicine in

Taipei, Taiwan. Helena is the Director of Rehabilitation at Chang Gung, and as such she visited with us in Baltimore. Subsequently she introduced sensory reeducation techniques to Taiwan, especially for the rehabilitation of the toe-to-hand transfer (see Chapter 11), making a remarkable difference in the degree of recovery of sensation for these patients and their overall hand function. The results from that unit are now the unrivaled best in the world at reconstruction of the hand by toe transfer.

Some of the published research and teaching from these therapist researchers are given in the Additional Readings section at the end of this chapter as models for future research writing by therapists.

• GETTING STARTED •

Congratulations! You have already gotten started with your research—you are reading this chapter.

Research begins in an orderly fashion. There may be many detours along the way—sudden stops, false starts—but research begins in an orderly way. The sequence of ordered events is the same sequence usually required to fill out a research grant request (see Table 20.1); therefore, a brief review of these thought processes is indicated.

The title should usually be simple, but catchy, and be perfectly clear. For example, a title might be "The Recovery of Sensorimotor Function After Ulnar Nerve Transposition at the Elbow."

The purpose should be stated as a hypothesis. For example, the purpose for the above titled research might be, "The purpose of this study is to evaluate the hypothesis that transposition of the ulnar nerve into an anterior submuscular location will give the patient improvement in sensorimotor function."

TABLE 20.1 CATEGORIES TO CONSIDER FOR INITIATING RESEARCH AND BUDGET REQUESTING

Title
Purpose
Background
Method
Collaborators
Facilities
Budget

The background should review the historical information and clinical experience that have led to the initiation of the study. For example, the background for the above study might be "The results of the surgical treatment for ulnar nerve compression at the elbow have been demonstrated in a review article by Dellon (1989) to vary with the degree of nerve compression. For a severe degree of nerve compression, in which the patient has not responded to nonoperative management, the percent of recurrence rate following traditional Learmonth (1942) submuscular transposition is about 30%. However, the number of published studies evaluating this technique are few (state the number of studies and their dates), and the number of patients included in those studies is relatively small (state the number). The experience in our clinic with this procedure has been documented over the past 6 years by preoperative sensorimotor testing."

The method should include a detailed description of each aspect of the study design. The patient population should be described. The clinical testing procedures and/or the laboratory procedures should be described in sufficient detail that another investigator could repeat your work. The data analysis should be described, including the names and rationale for use of the statistical tests that will be used.

Possible collaborators with whom you might work should be listed. A common such person might be a biostatistician. List collaborators, especially if in basic science or allied fields. For example, for the present ulnar nerve study, it might be indicated that "staging of the degree of ulnar nerve compression will be done using a numerical grading scale (Dellon, 1994), and a biostatistician will advise as to the appropriate nonparametric analysis required for comparison of post-op with pre-op grading."

The facility in which the research will be carried out will be of no importance to the ulnar nerve study being used as an example. However, should basic research using animals be required, the location of the approved facility for such a study will be needed, and the costs for the use of this facility must be reflected in the budget.

The budget should be outlined in detail to the fullest extent that can be determined. It is appropriate to include all costs legitimately attributable to this research project.

• POTENTIAL PROJECTS •

Disclaimer: This section will list some areas that would be interesting to research. To the best of my knowledge at the time of publication of this book, these projects have not appeared in the literature, and may not have even been begun. However, they involve ideas that over the last decade I have mentioned or described to individual researchers or at public lectures around the world. It is, therefore, possible that someone is already working on one of these projects. Indeed, I hope someone is! Choose your project, and get started.

• PROJECTS WITH THE PRESSURE-SPECIFIED SENSORY DEVICE™ •

1. IS HEEL PAIN DUE TO A BONE SPUR, PLANTAR FASCITIS, OR CALCANEAL NERVE ENTRAPMENT?

Many patients over 40 years of age have a calcaneal bone spur on their X ray. Does this mean that their heel pain is from a spur that should be removed? Many athletes complain of pain in the heel but have a normal X ray. Do they have plantar fascitis? The symptoms these patients experience could be due to calcaneal nerve entrapment related either to a tarsal tunnel syndrome or to separate calcaneal nerve entrapment. Electrodiagnostic testing is very difficult for the calcaneal nerve because it is a small and distal sensory nerve. Quantitative sensory testing can determine the cutaneous pressure threshold for one- and two-point static touch, looking for nerve entrapment.

Seek out a foot and ankle surgeon, whether in podiatry or orthopedic surgery. Do quantitative sensory testing on the next group of patients he or she evaluates for these problems. Compare your results to published norms, or obtain your own laboratory normative data, perhaps from the patient's asymptomatic contralateral foot. If the surgeon has no experience decompressing the calcaneal nerve, then let him or her perform the procedure he or she normally would, uninfluenced by the findings of the sensory testing. Correlate the success at relieving heel pain in each patient with the abnormality of the sensory testing. If the surgeon has experience with decompression of the calcaneal nerve, devise a protocol in which if the X rays are normal and there is not a tarsal tunnel syndrome present based on the patient's complaints, the surgeon will consider either a neurolysis of the calcaneal nerve instead of a bone spur resection or a release of the plantar fascia. Get the patients back for fol-

lowup, regardless of which of the above two choices you have pursued. Repeat the sensory measurements.

2. WHAT IS THE INCIDENCE OF STRETCH-TRACTION INJURIES TO LOWER EXTREMITY NERVES ASSOCIATED WITH KNEE OR ANKLE INJURY?

The force required to dislocate the knee, tear knee ligaments, or do the same damage to the ankle, or the force required to fracture the tibia or fibula, is sufficient to cause stretch/traction injuries to the nerves of the leg. There is no report of the incidence of these problems. This information may lead to the nerves being released or decompressed at the time of open treatment of the orthopedic problems. The Pressure-Specified Sensory Device™ is ideal to study the incidence of these nerve problems.

This study should be done in collaboration with an orthopedic surgeon, who would refer patients for quantitative sensory testing at the time they are seen for their injury, or they could be tested the week after the injury. If the initial quantitative sensory testing were normal, they should be tested again at 3 months to determine the incidence of delayed appearance of nerve compression, perhaps related to swelling from the injury, operation, or casting. If the testing is initially abnormal, they should be followed up in 3 months to determine the incidence of spontaneous resolution, or improvement with nonoperative management. The nerves to be tested are the posterior tibial nerve (big toe plantar aspect), the peroneal nerve (dorsum of the foot), and the sural nerve (calf and lateral aspect of the foot).

3. WHAT IS INCIDENCE OF SENSORY CHANGE IN THE LIP AND CHIN FOLLOWING JAW AND CHIN ADVANCEMENT SURGERY?

The advancement of the mandible and chin to improve appearance and dental occlusion requires a sagittal split of the mandible. In and of itself this may cause injury to the inferior alveolar nerve. The stretching of the nerve with the actual advancement causes sensory changes in the majority of the patients. There have been some studies to quantitate this with traditional sensory tests. This should be repeated with the Pressure-Specified Sensory Device™, which should detect a much higher incidence of this problem. Direct injury to this nerve can be corrected by nerve grafting. One report of this with the patients quantitated with this device was reported in the August 1994 issue of *Annals of Plastic Surgery* by Evans, Crawley, and Dellon.

4. WHAT IS THE EFFECT OF LIMB LENGTHENING WITH THE ILLIZAROV TECHNIQUE ON SENSORY FUNCTION OF THE NERVES OF THE LEG?

This is the same type of study as the one described in 2, above. Here, however, the hypothesis is that the common peroneal nerve, being relatively constrained at the fibular head, will have a greater change in sensory nerve function than will the posterior tibial nerve. Quantitative sensory testing with the Pressure-Specified Sensory Device™ has the potential to monitor the elongation, controlling the potential for nerve injury. Furthermore, these limbs may have preexisting nerve injury due to the initial fracture. Documentation of this preexisting nerve damage will protect the surgeon from claims that this arose during limb lengthening.

5. DOCUMENTATION OF COLLATERAL SPROUTING.

It is within the experience of all peripheral nerve surgeons that when a nerve is harvested for a nerve graft, leaving a donor site with sensory loss, the size or area of the sensory loss diminishes over time. This phenomenon has been documented in animals, primarily through the work of Jack Diamond at McMaster University, in Hamilton, Ontario, Canada, but has not been clinically documented (see Chapter 4). For example, after sural nerve harvesting, the size of the area could be mapped and thresholds obtained, then this area mapped again by sensory testing with the Pressure-Specified Sensory Device™ at 3-month intervals. At the end of 1 year, the hypothesis that the decrease in sensory loss is due to collateral sprouting from the superficial peroneal nerve can be tested by doing a xylocaine anesthetic block of that nerve at the ankle level.

6. WHAT IS THE RELATIONSHIP BETWEEN COMPRESSION OR DYSFUNCTION OF THE INTERNAL PUDENDAL NERVE AND IMPOTENCE?

The internal pudendal nerve supplies the penis with sensibility. It is possible that one group of men with impotence have this on a neurogenic basis that includes decreased function of this nerve. Such a dysfunction, due to diabetes or compression of the nerve against a bicycle seat during long-distance cycling, would interfere with the normal reflex for erection. Collaboration with a urologist would be a prerequisite. Men without impotence, as well as those coming to an impotence clinic, would have to be tested according to an institutionally-approved research protocol. This documentation would be helpful for diagnosis, and possibly lead to the acceptance of an operative procedure to decompress this nerve in Alcock's canal.

• PROJECT WITH THE DIGIT-GRIP™ •

VALIDATION OF THE CONCEPT THAT MALINGERING CAN BE DETECTED USING THE COMPUTER-ASSISTED DIGIT-GRIP™.

The Digit-Grip™ records both the index/middle finger pair and the ring/little finger pair components of grip strength. During a series of attempts at maximum grip, there is a relationship between these two components. It is hypothesized that a group of injured workers being tested at their first visit to the surgeon will be giving their most honest attempt to demonstrate their problem. In contrast, it is hypothesized that a group of injured workers being tested at the conclusion of their treatment, at the time of an impairment rating, will have the most likelihood of giving less than their maximum effort. The study would compare the variation between the index/middle finger pair and the ring/little finger pair, between the injured and the noninjured hand in these two groups of workers. The collaboration of a statistician is suggested.

PROJECTS SUITABLE • FOR SKIN COMPLIANCE • DEVICE

1. CORRELATION OF SKIN COMPLIANCE WITH NATURAL HISTORY AND TREATMENT OF SCLERODERMA.

It is known that systemic sclerosis, or scleroderma, causes changes in skin tightness. This has been difficult to document. The skin compliance device is ideal for this. Collaboration with a dermatologist is suggested.

2. DOCUMENTATION OF REHABILITATION EFFORTS FOR EDEMA CONTROL.

The traditional volumetric measurement for hand edema gives a global measurement. Often, just localized areas of the hand are edematous. Skin compliance could measure these areas during treatment, and could measure sites on the hand that might correlate with overall edema during the rehabilitation session.

3. DOCUMENTATION OF IMPROVEMENT IN HAND STIFFNESS DUE TO REFLEX SYMPATHETIC DYSTROPHY.

This has a rationale similar to 1 and 2 above.

4. DOCUMENTATION OF RESPONSE OF ARTHRITIS TO ANTI-INFLAMMATORY MEDICATIONS.

A rheumatologist will be the necessary collaborator for this study with the Skin Compliance Device™. The swelling of individual joints with gout or rheumatoid arthritis has not been clinically measured, other than by the physician making a qualitative note about progress.

5. CORRELATION OF SOFT TISSUE PRESSURE FOR COMPARTMENT SYNDROME DURING FLUID RESUSCITATION OF THE BURN PATIENT.

The burn patient is at risk for compartment syndromes. Often the patient is intubated or in sufficient pain that the symptoms of the compartment syndrome cannot be expressed. The invasive wick catheter technique requires a significant effort and runs the risk of infection. Diminished perception of vibratory stimuli has been shown to correlate with a compartment pressure within 30 mm Hg of diastolic pressure, and is an indication of decompression. This test is also difficult to do in the poorly responsive patient. Measurement of skin compliance should be evaluated prospectively to determine its correlation with vibratory perception and direct measurement of compartment pressures. Depending on the results of this study, measurement of skin compliance may become an important adjunct in the care of these patients. Collaborate with a local burn unit.

• • •

• REFERENCES •

Dellon, A. L. *Evaluation of Sensibility and Reeducation of Sensation in the Hand*. Baltimore: Williams & Wilkins, 1981.

Dellon, E. S., Mourey, R., & Dellon, A. L. Human pressure perception values for constant and moving one- and two-point discrimination. *Plastic and Reconstructive*

Surgery 90:112-117, 1992.

Evans, G. R. D., Crawley, W., & Dellon, A. L. Inferior alveolar nerve grafting: An approach without intermaxillary fixation. *Annals of Plastic Surgery 33*:221-224, 1994.

• ADDITIONAL READINGS •

Bell, J. A. Sensibility evaluation. In *Rehabilitation of the Hand: Surgery and Therapy*, J. M. Hunter, L. H. Schneider, E. J. Mackin, & A. D. Callahan, Editors. St. Louis: C. V. Mosby Company, 1978.

Bell-Krotoski, J. A. Light touch-deep pressure testing using Semmes-Weinstein monofilaments. In *Rehabilitation of the Hand: Surgery and Therapy*, J. M. Hunter, L. H. Schneider, E. J. Mackin, & A. D. Callahan, Editors. St. Louis: C. V. Mosby Company, 1990.

Bell-Krotoski, J. A., & Buford, W. L. The force/time relationships of clinically used sensory testing instruments. *Journal of Hand Therapy 1*:76-81, 1988.

Bell-Krotoski, J. A., & Tomancik, E. The repeatability of testing with Semmes-Weinstein monofilaments. *Journal of Hand Surgery 12A*:155-161, 1987.

Carter, M. S. Re-education of sensation. Hand Rehabilitation Symposium. *Journal of Hand Surgery 4*:501-507, 1978.

Carter-Wilson, M. Sensory re-education. In *Operative Nerve Repair and Reconstruction*, R. H. Gelberman, Editor. Philadelphia: J. B. Lippincott Company, 1991.

Crosby, P. M., & Dellon, A. L. A comparison of two-point discrimination test devices. *Microsurgery 10*:134-137, 1989.

Dellon, A. L., & Keller, K. M. Computer-assisted quantitative sensorimotor testing in patients with carpal and cubital tunnel syndromes. *Annals of Plastic Surgery, 38:* 493-502. 1997.

Dellon, A. L., Mackinnon, S. E., & Crosby, P. M. Reliability of two-point discrimination measurements. *Journal of Hand Surgery 12*:693-696, 1987.

Dellon, A. L., Mackinnon, S. E., & Schlegel, R. Validity of electrodiagnostic studies following anterior transposition of the ulnar nerve. *Journal of Hand Surgery 12*:700-703, 1987.

Dellon, E. S., Crone, S., Mourey, R., & Dellon, A. L. Comparison of the Semmes-Weinstein monofilaments with the Pressure-Specified Sensory Device. *Restorative Neurology Neuroscience 5*:323-326, 1993.

Dellon, E. S., Keller, K. M., Moratz, V., & Dellon, A. L. Relationship between skin hardness and human touch perception. *Journal of Hand Surgery, 20B: 44-48, 1995.*

Dellon, E. S., Keller, K. M., Moratz, V., & Dellon, A. L. Validation of cutaneous pressure threshold measurement with the Pressure-Specified Sensory Device. *Annals of Plastic Surgery, 38: 485-492, 1997.*

Fess, E. E., Harmon, K. S., & Strickland, J. W. Evaluation of the hand by objective measurement. In *Rehabilitation of the Hand: Surgery and Therapy*, J. M. Hunter, L. H. Schneider, E. J. Mackin, & A. D. Callahan, Editors. St. Louis: C. V. Mosby Company, 1978.

Kofkin, J., Tobin, M., & Dellon, A. L. Dynamic elbow splint following tendon transfer to restore triceps function. *American Journal of Occupational Therapy 34*:680-681, 1980.

Maynard, J. Sensory re-education after peripheral nerve injury. In *Rehabilitation of the Hand: Surgery and Therapy*, J. M. Hunter, E. J. Mackin, L. H. Schneider, & A. D. Callahan, Editors. Baltimore: Williams & Wilkins, 1977.

Mackinnon, S. E., & Novak, C. B. Hypothesis: Pathogenesis of cumulative trauma disorder. *Journal of Hand Surgery*, in press: 1994.

Novak, C. B., Kelly, L., & Mackinnon, S. E. Sensory recovery after median nerve grafting. *Journal of Hand Surgery 17A*:59-66, 1992.

Novak, C. B., Mackinnon, S. E., & Kelly, L. Correlation of two-point discrimination and hand function following median nerve injury. *Annals of Plastic Surgery* *31*:495-498, 1993.

Novak, C. B., Mackinnon, S. E., & Patterson, G. A. Evaluation of patients with thoracic outlet syndrome. *Journal of Hand Surgery* *18A*:292-299, 1993.

Novak, C. B., Mackinnon, S. E., Williams, J. I., & Kelly, L. Development of a new measure of fine sensory function. *Plastic and Reconstructive Surgery* 92:301-311, 1993.

Novak, C. B., Mackinnon, S. E., Williams, J. I., & Kelly, L. Establishment of reliability in the evaluation of hand sensibility. *Plastic and Reconstructive Surgery* 92:312-322, 1993.

Rose, B. W., Mackinnon, S. E., Dellon, A. L., & Snyder, R. A. Design of a protective splint for the non-human primate extremity. *Laboratory Animal Science 33*:306-308, 1983.

Seiler, W. A., Schlegel, R., Mackinnon, S. E., & Dellon, A. L. The double crush syndrome: Development of a model. *Surgical Forum 34*:596-598, 1983.

Sunderland, S. *Nerves and Nerve Injuries.* Edinburgh: Churchill Livingstone, 1968.

van Vliet, D., Novak, C. B., & Mackinnon, S. E. Duration of contact time alters cutaneous pressure threshold measurements. *Annals of Plastic Surgery 31*:335-339, 1993.

Wei, F. C., Chien, Y. Y., Ma, H. S., & Dellon, A. L. The myelinated nerve fiber population of digital nerves in the fingers and toes. *Plastic and Reconstructive Surgery*, submitted: 1997.

Wei, F. C., & Ma, H. S. Results of sensory re-education in toe to hand transfer. *Journal of Hand Surgery*: in press, 1997.

Wei, F. C., Ma, H. S., Chien, Y. Y., & Dellon, A. L. Effect of neurotization upon degree of sensory recovery in toe-to-finger transfer. *Plastic and Reconstructive Surgery*, submitted: 1997.

● ● ●

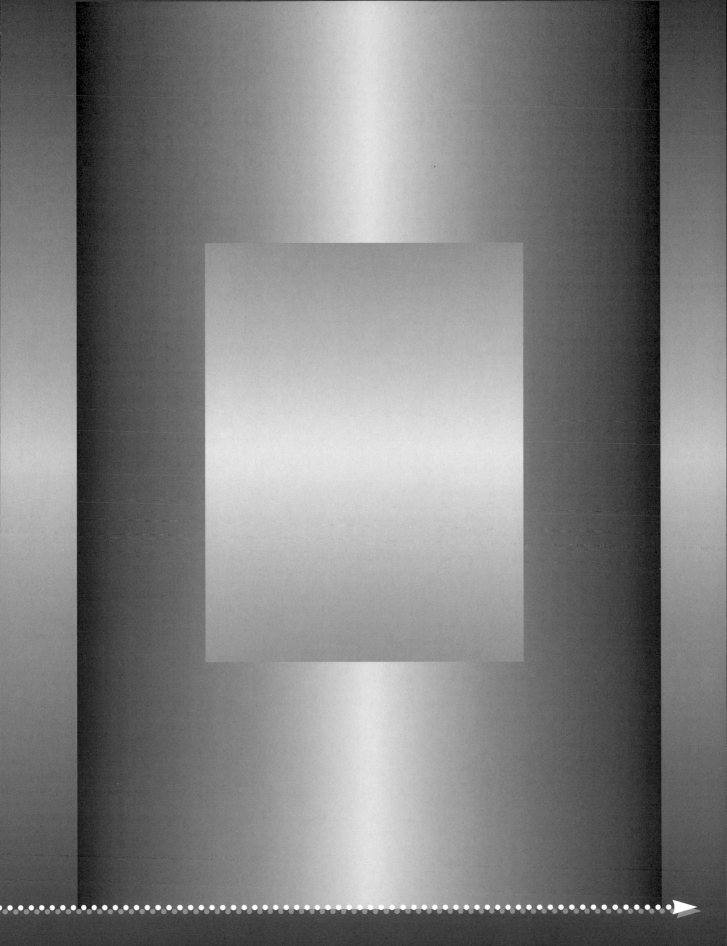

21

questions & answers

● SELF-ADMINISTERED ●
DIAGNOSTIC TESTING

The purpose of this section is to provide the student with a series of multiple choice questions that will serve as a self-administered diagnostic test to determine your knowledge of the material presented in this textbook. Thus, the questions are grouped parallel to the Table of Contents. This section of questions will also provide the teacher with possible material for examinations.

Circle one or more than one of the multiple choice answers that is correct.

The correct answers for each question are given at the end, grouped according to the corresponding chapter in the book which contains the material on which the questions are based.

● ● ●

● QUESTIONS ●

CHAPTER 1. THE NEURON

1.1   A neuron is
(a) the basic unit of the motor system
(b) the basic unit of the nervous system
(c) the basic unit of the solar system
(d) the basic unit of the urinary system

1.2 The cell body of a motor neuron is located in the
(a) intermediate grey of the spinal cord
(b) dorsal horn of the spinal cord
(c) ventral horn of the spinal cord
(d) dorsal root ganglion

1.3 The cell body of a sensory neuron is located in the
(a) intermediate grey of the spinal cord
(b) dorsal horn of the spinal cord
(c) ventral horn of the spinal cord
(d) dorsal root ganglion

1.4 The cell body of a neuron of the autonomic nervous system is located in the
(a) intermediate grey of the spinal cord
(b) dorsal horn of the spinal cord
(c) ventral horn of the spinal cord
(d) paraspinal ganglia

1.5 The supporting cell(s) for the neuron are
(a) oligodendrocytes
(b) astrocytes
(c) astroturf
(d) Schwann cells

1.6 The cell(s) that make nerve growth factor are
(a) oligodendrocytes
(b) astrocytes
(c) astroturf
(d) Schwann cells

1.7 The cell(s) that make myelin are
(a) oligodendrocytes
(b) astrocytes
(c) astroturf
(d) Schwann cells

1.8 A peripheral nerve regenerates at a rate of
(a) 1 cm/day
(b) 1 mm/day
(c) 1 inch/month
(d) 1 inch/day

1.9 The perception of a vibratory stimulus is possible due to
(a) pallesthesia
(b) A-delta fibers
(c) bone conduction
(d) A-beta touch fibers

1.10 The perception of pressure is possible due to
(a) large myelinated A-beta fibers, slowly-adapting
(b) large myelinated A-beta fibers, quickly-adapting
(c) small myelinated A-delta fibers
(d) unmyelinated C-fibers

1.11 The perception of moving-touch is due primarily to
(a) large myelinated A-beta fibers, slowly-adapting
(b) large myelinated A-beta fibers, quickly-adapting
(c) small myelinated A-delta fibers
(d) unmyelinated C-fibers

1.12 The perception of constant-touch is due primarily to
(a) large myelinated A-beta fibers, slowly-adapting
(b) large myelinated A-beta fibers, quickly-adapting
(c) small myelinated A-delta fibers
(d) unmyelinated C-fibers

1.13 Tuning forks of 30 Hz and 256 Hz are best used to test
(a) large myelinated A-beta fibers, slowly-adapting
(b) large myelinated A-beta fibers, quickly-adapting
(c) small myelinated A-delta fibers
(d) unmyelinated C-fibers

1.14 Meissner and Pacinian corpuscles are receptors for
(a) large myelinated A-beta fibers, slowly-adapting
(b) large myelinated A-beta fibers, quickly-adapting
(c) small myelinated A-delta fibers
(d) unmyelinated C-fibers

1.15 The Merkel cell neurite complex mediates perception of
(a) static touch
(b) movement
(c) vibration
(d) pressure

CHAPTER 2. CUTANEOUS SENSORY RECEPTORS

2.1 The perception of pain is mediated through which of the following
(a) free nerve endings
(b) Meissner corpuscles
(c) Pacinian corpuscles
(d) Merkel cell neurite complex

2.2 The perception of pressure is mediated through which of the following
(a) free nerve endings
(b) Meissner corpuscles
(c) Pacinian corpuscles
(d) Merkel cell neurite complex

2.3 The perception of hot and cold is mediated through which of the following
(a) free nerve endings
(b) Krause's end-bulb
(c) Ruffini end-organ
(d) Golgi apparatus

2.4 The perception of vibration is mediated through which of the following
(a) free nerve endings
(b) Meissner corpuscles
(c) Pacinian corpuscles
(d) Merkel cell neurite complex

2.5 It is possible to recover sensation after a nerve repair because
(a) sensory nerves regenerate
(b) sensory receptors can be reinnervated
(c) sensory receptors do not change after nerve transection
(d) Wallerian degeneration does not occur

2.6 The degree of recovery of sensation may be decreased if repair is delayed beyond
(a) 48 hours
(b) 3 weeks
(c) 3 months
(d) 6 months

2.7 Sensory reeducation will be of help after sensory nerve repair because
(a) quickly-adapting fibers may reinnervate a Merkel cell neurite complex
(b) slowly-adapting fibers may reinnervate a Merkel cell neurite complex
(c) less than the normal number of fibers may reinnervate the skin
(d) quickly-adapting fibers may reinnervate a Meissner corpuscle

CHAPTER 3. PROPRIOCEPTION

3.1 Proprioception is
(a) vibratory sense
(b) muscle sense
(c) nonsense
(d) position sense

3.2 Proprioception has been traditionally viewed as coming from
(a) joint receptors
(b) muscle receptors
(c) skin receptors
(d) the cerebellum

3.3 Sensory receptors within muscle report primarily to the
(a) cerebral cortex
(b) cerebellum
(c) pons
(d) frontal lobe

3.4　Proprioception is information that reaches the
(a) cerebral cortex
(b) cerebellum
(c) pons
(d) frontal lobe

3.5　Joint receptors include
(a) Ruffini end-organs
(b) Pacinian corpuscles
(c) Golgi tendon-organs
(d) spindles

3.6　Muscle sensory receptors include
(a) Ruffini end-organs
(b) Pacinian corpuscles
(c) Golgi tendon-organs
(d) spindles

3.7　Cutaneous sensory receptors are capable of mediating perception of
(a) touch
(b) vibration
(c) proprioception
(d) muscle tension

3.8　A person who has had a total hip replacement, and therefore has no hip joint receptors
(a) has proprioception maintained through the opposite, normal hip
(b) has no proprioception in the replaced hip
(c) walks well, but must visualize the ground to prevent falling
(d) uses information from the skin of the leg and hip to be aware of hip position

CHAPTER 4. NERVE RECONSTRUCTION

4.1　The peripheral nerve regenerates
(a) at 1 mm/day or about 1 inch/month
(b) up to 3 cm without the need for a Schwann cell
(c) at 1 cm/day or about 1 m/month
(d) up to 30 cm without the need for a Schwann cell

4.2　Peripheral nerve regeneration is directed by
(a) a growth cone
(b) an ice cream cone
(c) the organ of Eimer
(d) target end-organs

4.3　To guide its movement, the growth cone is able to utilize
(a) laminin
(b) basement membrane
(c) Type IV collagen
(d) Type I collagen

4.4　Neural regeneration across a suture or repair site is inhibited by
(a) residual injured tissue at either end of the nerve repair
(b) tension across the suture line
(c) nonabsorbable entubulation or wrapping material, like silicon
(d) poor vascularization of the surrounding tissues

4.5　Reconstruction of a nerve defect may be accomplished by
(a) a trunk graft
(b) a cable graft
(c) cable TV
(d) an interfascicular graft

4.6　Reconstruction of a human nerve defect may be accomplished today by
(a) an allograft
(b) an autograft
(c) an autobahn
(d) a xenograft

4.7　Avoidance of tension across a nerve defect is best accomplished by
(a) flexing adjacent joints
(b) shortening adjacent bone
(c) interposing a conduit
(d) fibrin glue

4.8   Acceptable techniques for achieving a
       nerve repair after a clean transection
       are
(a) fibrin glue
(b) a nonabsorbable suture
(c) laser
(d) an absorbable conduit

4.9   Thwarted neural regeneration may
       result in
(a) a painful neuroma
(b) RSD
(c) an incontinuity neuroma
(d) a painless neuroma

4.10   Reflex sympathetic dystrophy is
       manifested by
(a) pain in the distribution of a peripheral
    nerve
(b) diffuse pain, not in the distribution of
    a peripheral nerve
(c) swelling and stiffness of the affected part
(d) a knee-jerk response when the painful
    part is touched

4.11   Reflex sympathetic dystrophy may be
(a) diagnosed with a bone scan
(b) treated with a stellate ganglion block
(c) treated with a Bier block
(d) caused by a cinder block

4.12   Selective denervation may be used
       to treat pain, providing that
(a) reconstruction of the nerve function is
    not possible or desirable
(b) desensitization techniques have not
    been successful
(c) the patient is willing to accept loss of
    sensation related to that nerve
(d) diagnostic blocks identify the nerve
    causing the pain

4.13   Selective denervation, used to treat
       dorsoradial wrist pain, may cause
(a) loss of sensibility in the distribution of
    the resected nerve
(b) loss of both the radial sensory and
    the lateral antebrachial cutaneous nerve
(c) collateral sprouting
(d) alfalfa sprouting

4.14   Conduits used to reconstruct a nerve
       defect include
(a) muscle
(b) vein
(c) silicone
(d) polyglycolic acid

4.15   Distinction of a painful neuroma from
       a nonpainful one is based on
(a) histologic examination of the resected
    specimen
(b) ultrasound
(c) magnetic resonance imaging
(d) the patient's complaints of pain

CHAPTER 5. GOALS

5.1   Metrology is the
(a) science of weather forecasting
(b) science of predicting appearance
    of meteors
(c) science of measurement
(d) science of city planning

5.2   A measurement device is valid if
(a) its a measurement that correlates with
    function
(b) it has established norms
(c) its measurement can be duplicated by
    another examiner
(d) its measurement can be duplicated by
    the same examiner at another testing

5.3 A measurement device is reliable if
(a) it's a measurement that correlates with function
(b) it has established norms
(c) its measurement can be duplicated by another examiner
(d) its measurement can be duplicated by the same examiner at another testing

5.4 A malingerer is
(a) a hysteric
(b) an exaggerator
(c) a worker
(d) an injured person

5.5 A hysteric is
(a) a malingerer
(b) an exaggerator
(c) a liar (falsifier)
(d) not to be trusted

5.6 Objective testing of a person suspected of being a malingerer would include
(a) a lie detector test
(b) a ninhydrin test
(c) a ninja test
(d) an electrodiagnostic test

5.7 The wrinkling test is
(a) employed by plastic surgeons
(b) employed by the tailor
(c) related to rain
(d) positive in the presence of denervation

5.8 The rapid exchange grip test can demonstrate
(a) the detection of heat
(b) frostbite
(c) malingering
(d) ulnar motor function

5.9 Impairment rating is
(a) a disability rating
(b) a hand function evaluation
(c) an anatomic loss measurement
(d) a mental aptitude test

5.10 A guitarist who is unable to play the guitar due to an absent distal phalanx of the index finger is an example of
(a) 90 % partial impairment of the hand
(b) 90 % partial impairment of the entire upper extremity
(c) 90 % partial impairment of the entire body
(d) minimal impairment

CHAPTER 6. THRESHOLD VERSUS INNERVATION DENSITY

6.1 A threshold measurement
(a) is a numerical value
(b) is part of quantitative sensory testing
(c) is applicable to perception of vibration
(d) is applicable to perception of touch

6.2 A threshold measurement requires a device
(a) whose stimulus contains just one variable
(b) that is electrical
(c) that is computer assisted
(d) that is hand held

6.3 The device for evaluating pressure perception that uses two different stimulus variables (force and probe contact area) is the
(a) Two-Point Disk-Criminator™
(b) Semmes-Weinstein nylon monofilaments
(c) WEST™
(d) Pressure-Specified Sensory Device™

6.4 The device(s) that estimates a threshold is (are)
(a) Two-Point Disk-Criminator™
(b) Semmes-Weinstein nylon monofilaments
(c) WEST™
(d) Pressure-Specified Sensory Device™

6.5 The device that measures both the distance and pressure thresholds for two-point discrimination is the
(a) Two-Point Disk-Criminator™
(b) Semmes-Weinstein nylon monofilaments
(c) WEST™
(d) Pressure-Specified Sensory Device™

6.6 The distance at which two points may be distinguished as two is best considered
(a) an illusion
(b) a hoax
(c) a threshold
(d) innervation density

6.7 The distance at which two points may be distinguished as two is best described by
(a) a measurement of distance alone
(b) a measurement of pressure alone
(c) a measurement of both distance and pressure
(d) morphometric assessment of number of nerve fibers in the dermis

6.8 The Pressure-Specified Sensory Device™ enables
(a) a measurement of distance alone
(b) a measurement of pressure alone
(c) a measurement of both distance and pressure
(d) morphometric assessment of number of nerve fibers in the dermis

6.9 Unification is a
(a) World Health Organization research program
(b) theory regarding sensibility testing
(c) software program for Unisys computers
(d) program to convert horses to unicorns

6.10 Threshold testing is useful in
(a) staging nerve compression
(b) evaluating neural regeneration
(c) providing world peace
(d) measuring all skin surfaces

CHAPTER 7. INSTRUMENTATION

7.1 Instruments to measure pain include the
(a) iron maiden
(b) visual analog scale
(c) McGill pain questionnaire
(d) fish scale

7.2 Indications for clinical pain testing include
(a) malingering
(b) earliest detection of sensory recovery
(c) syringomyelia
(d) carpal tunnel syndrome

7.3 Indications for clinical testing of temperature detection threshold include
(a) malingering
(b) earliest detection of sensory recovery
(c) syringomyelia
(d) carpal tunnel syndrome

7.4 Detection of pain and temperature threshold abnormality may be most useful for screening for
(a) neuropathy
(b) myopathy
(c) mosquitos
(d) myelopathy

7.5 The most valid and reliable instrument to quantitate pain level is a
(a) #25 gauge needle at various pressures
(b) #25 gauge needle at various forces
(c) #18 gauge needle at various pressures
(d) visual analog scale

7.6 Instrumentation available to determine cutaneous pressure thresholds include the
(a) WEST™ device
(b) Optacon™
(c) Semmes-Weinstein nylon monofilaments
(d) Pressure-Specified Sensory Device™

7.7 Instrumentation available to measure (not estimate) the pressure threshold include the
(a) CASE IV system™
(b) Automated Tactile Tester™
(c) Pressure-Specified Sensory Device™
(d) nylon monofilaments

7.8 Instrumentation that is traceable to the National Institute of Standards and Technology includes the
(a) CASE IV system™
(b) Automated Tactile Tester™
(c) Pressure-Specified Sensory Device™
(d) Semmes-Weinstein nylon monofila-ments

7.9 Instrumentation that is traceable to the National Institute of Standards and Technology include the
(a) Jamar dynamometer
(b) Preston pinch meter
(c) NK Digit-Grip™
(d) NK pinch device

7.10 Instrumentation that is capable of measuring more than one type of nerve fiber includes the
(a) Neurometer™ (current perception threshold)
(b) Neurometer (Nerve Pace™)
(c) CASE IV system™
(d) Automated Tactile Tester™

7.11 The best standardized instrument to measure the pressure threshold, for any body surface area is the
(a) Semmes-Weinstein nylon monofilaments
(b) CASE IV system™
(c) Universal Tactometer™ (computer-assisted)
(d) Pressure-Specified Sensory Device™

7.12 The best standardized instrument to measure the pressure threshold at which two points can be distinguished from one, for any body surface area is the
(a) Semmes-Weinstein nylon monofilaments
(b) CASE IV system™
(c) Universal Tactometer™ (computer-assisted)
(d) Pressure-Specified Sensory Device™

7.13 Disadvantages of the hydraulic-type dynamometers are
(a) frequent need for calibration
(b) fluid leakage
(c) friction between post and handle
(d) measured force is from the center of the curved handle

7.14 Advantages of the electromechanical computer-assisted NK strength instruments are
(a) self-contained diagnostic software to indicate need for recalibration
(b) recalibration is needed only every 3 years
(c) accuracy of + 1%
(d) reliable measurement at any point along the handle

7.15 Advantages of computer-assisted sensorimotor testing include
(a) expense of equipment
(b) reliable measurements
(c) valid measurements
(d) report formats

CHAPTER 8. ELECTRODIAGNOSTIC TESTING

8.1 Compared with quantitative sensory testing, such as measurement of cutaneous pressure or vibratory thresholds, electodiagnostic testing is
(a) subjective
(b) objective
(c) painful
(d) nonpainful

8.2　Compared with quantitative sensory testing, such as measurement of cutaneous pressure or vibratory thresholds, electrodiagnostic testing, such as electromyography, is

(a) more expensive
(b) less expensive
(c) invasive
(d) noninvasive

8.3　Compared with quantitative sensory testing, such as measurement of cutaneous pressure thresholds, electrodiagnostic testing is

(a) more specific for radiculopathy
(b) more specific for myopathy
(c) more specific for neuromuscular disease
(d) more specific for muscle denervation

8.4　Electrodiagnostic testing is best able to identify which of the following sites of chronic nerve compression

(a) median nerve in the forearm
(b) median nerve at the wrist
(c) ulnar nerve at the elbow
(d) radial nerve in the radial tunnel

8.5　Electrodiagnostic testing has the following inherent errors

(a) temperature dependence
(b) requires cooperation of the patient
(c) only tests large diameter nerve fibers
(d) only tests small diameter nerve fibers

8.6　Electrodiagnostic testing in the patient with symptoms of carpal tunnel syndrome may result in false negative (normal) reports because

(a) the patient was nervous at the time of testing
(b) there is such a severe systemic neuropathy present that the electrodiagnostic testing cannot demonstrate the superimposed nerve compression site
(c) the temperature of the extremity is too high
(d) only a portion of the fascicles of the peripheral nerve may be affected by the

nerve compression

8.7　A normal electrodiagnostic test result in a patient who has symptoms consistent with median nerve compression at the wrist, that is, carpal tunnel syndrome, means

(a) surgery is contraindicated
(b) the patient is malingering
(c) the patient may be tested again when the symptoms get worse
(d) the patient's history and physical exam should remain the guide to treatment

8.8　Somatosensory evoked potentials may be most helpful in the diagnosis of

(a) carpal tunnel syndrome
(b) Schwanoma
(c) thoracic outlet syndrome
(d) diffuse sensorimotor polyneuropathy

8.9　Intraoperative electrodiagnostic testing is useful for the management of

(a) carpal tunnel syndrome
(b) neuroma-in-continuity
(c) sensorimotor fascicular identification for nerve grafting
(d) denervation procedures for spasticity or for pain

8.10　The most cost-effective testing technique for monitoring peripheral nerve function that is also most acceptable to the patient is

(a) electrodiagnostic testing with needle electrodes
(b) electrodiagnostic testing with surface electrodes
(c) quantitative sensory testing
(d) electromyography

CHAPTER 9. GRADING PERIPHERAL NERVE FUNCTION

9.1   Currently accepted grading scales for peripheral nerve function include the
(a) International Grading Scale of the World Health Organization
(b) British System
(c) Hand Society Functionality Score
(d) Neuropathy Scoring System

9.2   Disadvantages of the British System include
(a) the need for two different scores to represent the level of nerve function
(b) the categories are not well defined
(c) it is difficult to analyze statistically
(d) it is not metric

9.3   An ideal numerical grading system should feature
(a) mutually exclusive categories
(b) rank ordering of the scale
(c) uniform intervals of the scale
(d) a valid scale

9.4   A grading system that does not have uniform intervals requires
(a) unconventional analysis
(b) parametric statistical analysis
(c) nonparametric statistical analysis
(d) conventional analysis only if data is to be used at a convention

9.5   An ideal numerical grading system should
(a) be applicable to any peripheral nerve
(b) be based on the pathophysiology of peripheral nerve problems
(c) require validation by a panel of experts
(d) demonstrate differences in results with clinical conditions

CHAPTER 10. CORTICAL PLASTICITY

10.1   Maps of the cerebral cortex may refer to
(a) gyrus and sulcus
(b) gyro and baklava
(c) Brodman's areas
(d) no-fly zones

10.2   Cortical plasticity refers to
(a) the movement of the precentral gyrus to a postcentral location
(b) the shift of Brodman's area 3b into area 1
(c) the shift of Brodman's area 1 into 3b
(d) a change in functional properties within area 3b

10.3   Cortical plasticity occurs in response to
(a) a decrease in peripheral neural inputs
(b) a loss of peripheral neural inputs
(c) an increase in peripheral neural inputs
(d) wishful thinking

10.4   Cortical plasticity occurs in
(a) racoons
(b) cats
(c) monkeys
(d) man

10.5   Cortical plasticity is the basis for
(a) columnar organization of area 3b
(b) sensory reeducation
(c) cranial base reconstruction
(d) use of plastic instead of titanium

10.6   Rehabilitation strategies that follow from cortical plasticity might include
(a) sensory stimulation of an area of skin during neural regeneration
(b) sensory stimulation of an area of transplanted skin
(c) simultaneous stimulation of an innervated flap and adjacent innervated skin
(d) simultaneous audio and sensory stimulation during neural regeneration

10.7 Rehabilitation strategies that follow from cortical plasticity might include
(a) moving-touch stimuli
(b) vibrating stimuli
(c) constant-touch stimuli
(d) any touch stimuli

10.8 Cortical plasticity can be accomplished
(a) at any time
(b) by the patient
(c) only by the therapist
(d) by both the patient and the therapist

CHAPTER 11. TECHNIQUES FOR SENSORY REEDUCATION

11.1 Sensory reeducation
(a) is not necessary
(b) should be an integral part of rehabilitation of the patient with a nerve injury
(c) increases the rate of neural regeneration
(d) applies only to the hand

11.2 Sensory reeducation can
(a) correct mislocalization
(b) help achieve the potential for recovery given at surgery
(c) redirect a regenerating axon into the correct finger
(d) redirect a sensory axon away from reinnervating muscle

11.3 Sensory reeducation is done
(a) by the patient
(b) by the therapist
(c) as often as possible
(d) only to relieve pain

11.4 Sensory reeducation is effective because
(a) a motivated patient always gets a better result
(b) increased sensory stimulation causes cortical plasticity
(c) increased sensory stimulation causes increased axonal sprouting
(d) a motivated patient increases axonal sprouting

11.5 Early phase sensory reeducation should begin as soon as
(a) constant-touch perception occurs in the target area
(b) 30 Hz stimuli are perceived in the target area
(c) 256 Hz stimuli are perceived in the target area
(d) psuedomotor function is recovered in the target area

11.6 Late phase sensory reeducation should begin as soon as
(a) moving-touch perception occurs in the target area
(b) 30 Hz stimuli are perceived in the target area
(c) 256 Hz stimuli are perceived in the target area
(d) pseudomotor function is recovered in the target area

11.7 Two-point discrimination testing is
(a) a form of sensory reeducation
(b) the goal of sensory reeducation
(c) a method of following the results of sensory reeducation
(d) a method of documenting the results of sensory reeducation

11.8 Sensory reeducation can improve the sensory function of
(a) a nerve repair
(b) a nerve graft
(c) an innervated free-tissue transfer
(d) replanted fingers

11.9 Sensory reeducation protocols are
(a) standardized across the United States
(b) based on universal principles
(c) accepted worldwide
(d) reimbursed by third-party insurance payers

11.10 The ideal sensory reeducation protocol to return a worker to work is
(a) intensive two-point discrimination testing
(b) repetitive Semmes-Weinstein monofilament testing
(c) late phase reeducation that incorporates the patient's work activities
(d) desensitization

11.11 Techniques that achieve sensory reeducation include
(a) desensitization
(b) identifying objects within a bowl of coffee beans
(c) identifying objects within a paper bag
(d) contrast baths

11.12 Techniques that achieve sensory reeducation require
(a) an I.Q. greater than 98
(b) repetitive sensory stimuli to the area being reeducated
(c) linkage of interest in the activity and attention to the stimuli
(d) avoidance of distracting sensory inputs during therapy

CHAPTER 12. UPPER EXTREMITY

12.1 The upper extremity nerve(s) related to the lateral cord of the brachial plexus is/are the
(a) musculocutaneous
(b) median
(c) lateral antebrachial cutaneous
(d) radial sensory

12.2 The upper extremity nerve(s) related to the medial cord of the brachial plexus is/are the
(a) ulnar
(b) median
(c) medial antebrachial cutaneous
(d) radial sensory

12.3 The upper extremity nerve(s) related to the posterior cord of the brachial plexus is/are the
(a) radial
(b) median
(c) posterior interosseous
(d) radial sensory

12.4 The upper extremity nerve(s) related to the C6 root is/are the
(a) palmar cutaneous branch of median
(b) radial sensory
(c) lateral antebrachial cutaneous
(d) palmar digital nerves to index finger

12.5 The cutaneous nerve territory involved with proximal median nerve compression that is not involved in the carpal tunnel syndrome is the
(a) dorsal surface of the thumb
(b) hypothenar eminence
(c) thenar eminence
(d) anatomic snuff box

12.6 The cutaneous nerve territory involved with proximal ulnar nerve compression that is not involved with compression of the ulnar nerve in Guyon's canal is the
(a) dorsal surface of the little finger
(b) hypothenar eminence
(c) thenar eminence
(d) dorsal anatomic snuff box

12.7 The sensory nerve territory involved with posterior interosseous nerve compression that is not involved with radial sensory nerve compression in the forearm is/are the
(a) dorsal surface of the thumb
(b) dorsal wrist capsule
(c) thenar eminence
(d) dorsal anatomic snuff box

12.8 Radial tunnel syndrome may be caused by the splinting employed to treat
(a) cubital tunnel syndrome
(b) carpal tunnel syndrome
(c) medial humeral epicondylitis
(d) lateral humeral epicondylitis

12.9 The ideal wrist position for splinting to treat carpal tunnel syndrome is
(a) 20° dorsiflexion
(b) 20° flexion
(c) neutral
(d) 30° dorsiflexion

12.10 The ideal elbow position for splinting to treat cubital tunnel syndrome is
(a) 0° to 30° of flexion
(b) 30° to 60° of flexion
(c) 60° to 90° of flexion
(d) 120° of flexion

12.11 After nerve reconstruction by a nerve graft, the first touch perception to recover is
(a) 256 Hz
(b) 30 Hz
(c) constant touch
(d) moving touch

12.12 After nerve reconstruction by a nerve conduit, the first touch perception to recover is
(a) 256 Hz
(b) 30 Hz
(c) constant touch
(d) moving touch

12.13 After nerve reconstruction by a nerve repair, the first touch perception to recover is
(a) 256 Hz
(b) 30 Hz
(c) constant touch
(d) moving touch

12.14 The test of sensibility that correlates best with hand function, and is, therefore the best test to measure the end result of nerve reconstruction is
(a) vibratory threshold
(b) cutaneous pressure threshold
(c) two-point discrimination threshold in millimeters
(d) two-point discrimination threshold in g/mm^2

12.15 The first test of sensibility to become abnormal during chronic nerve compression is the one for
(a) vibratory threshold
(b) cutaneous pressure threshold
(c) two-point discrimination threshold in millimeters
(d) two-point discrimination threshold in g/mm^2

CHAPTER 13. LOWER EXTREMITY

13.1 Appropriate sensory tests to evaluate sensibility in the lower extremity are
(a) nylon monofilaments
(b) two-point discrimination
(c) vibrometry
(d) computer-assisted pressure threshold

13.2 The commonest nerve compression syndrome in the lower extremity is
(a) anterior tarsal tunnel syndrome
(b) common plantar digital nerve syndrome
(c) tarsal tunnel syndrome
(d) common peroneal nerve at fibular head

13.3 The tarsal tunnel is homologous to the
(a) carpal tunnel
(b) Holland tunnel
(c) distal forearm
(d) Guyon's canal

13.4   If the medial plantar nerve were in the hand, it would innervate the
(a) ring and little fingers
(b) middle, ring, and little fingers
(c) thumb, index, and middle fingers
(d) all fingers

13.5   Clawing of the toes suggests compression of the
(a) medial plantar nerve
(b) calcaneal nerve
(c) lateral plantar nerve
(d) posterior tibial nerve

13.6   The Pressure-Specified Sensory Device™
(a) measures pressure perception on any surface of the foot
(b) reports pressure threshold in g
(c) reports pressure threshold in g/mm²
(d) must be zeroed for gravity between testing sites

13.7   The Pressure-Specified Sensory Device™
(a) is more sensitive than electrodiagnostic testing in the diagnosis of chronic nerve compression
(b) assists in differentiating neuropathy from a localized nerve compression, such as tarsal tunnel syndrome
(c) makes a measurement that is traceable to the National Institute of Standards and Technology
(d) uses an electrical stimulus

13.8   A severe knee injury may result in
(a) sensory loss over the dorsum of the foot
(b) sensory loss over the plantar aspect of the foot
(c) tarsal tunnel syndrome
(d) common peroneal nerve entrapment

13.9   A severe ankle injury may result in
(a) sensory loss over the dorsum of the foot
(b) sensory loss over the plantar aspect of the foot
(c) tarsal tunnel syndrome
(d) common peroncal nerve entrapment

13.10 Plantar fascitis may give symptoms that resemble
(a) anterior tarsal tunnel syndrome
(b) calcaneal nerve entrapment
(c) common peroneal nerve entrapment
(d) Morton's metatarsalgia

CHAPTER 14. NEUROPATHY

14.1   Symptoms of neuropathy may be related to the
(a) pain part of the sensory system
(b) motor system
(c) touch part of the sensory system
(d) autonomic system

14.2   Etiologies of neuropathy include
(a) diabetes
(b) thyroid dysfunction
(c) alcoholism
(d) lead poisoning

14.3   Symptoms of neuropathy usually occur in the
(a) head and neck
(b) trunk
(c) extremities
(d) cortex

14.4   Diabetic neuropathy usually occurs
(a) at the onset of Type I
(b) at the onset of Type II
(c) after 5 to 10 years of Type I
(d) after 5 to 10 years of Type II

14.5   Diabetic neuropathy is most often
(a) in a single arm
(b) carpal tunnel syndrome
(c) in both arms
(d) in both feet

14.6   Diabetic neuropathy is most commonly a
(a) distal axonopathy
(b) mononeuritis multiplex
(c) cranial monopathy
(d) bilateral symmetrical neuropathy

14.7   Alcoholic neuropathy is most commonly a
(a) distal axonopathy
(b) mononeuritis multiplex
(c) cranial monopathy
(d) bilateral symmetrical neuropathy

14.8   The neuropathy that accompanies
        lead poisoning is a
(a) distal axonopathy
(b) mononeuritis multiplex
(c) cranial monopathy
(d) bilateral symmetrical neuropathy

14.9   The double crush hypothesis
        suggests that
(a) two nerves are involved in a
       given extremity
(b) two nerves are involved in two extremities
(c) a single nerve is involved in two
       different locations
(d) a single nerve is involved twice in
       the same location

14.10 The stocking and glove distribution is
(a) a social service program for the wintertime
(b) a program to protect extremities
       with neuropathy
(c) the source of fungal infections
(d) the skin territories commonly involved
       by neuropathy

14.11 The glove distribution may be
        comprised of
(a) multiple peripheral nerve involvements
(b) a brachial plexus injury
(c) median nerve compression at the wrist
       and elbow, ulnar nerve compression at
       the wrist and elbow, and radial sensory
       nerve compression in the forearm
(d) median and ulnar nerve compression at
       the wrist level and radial sensory nerve
       compression in the forearm

14.12 Mechanisms that render the
        peripheral nerve susceptible to
        compression are
(a) increased endoneurial water content
       due to hydrophilic molecules
(b) decreased axoplasmic transport; slow
       component, anterograde
(c) increased endoneurial water due to
       blood-nerve barrier breakdown
(d) microtubule dysfunction

14.13 The surgeon can
(a) correct a metabolic neuropathy
(b) improve the symptoms of a metabolic
       neuropathy
(c) decompress entrapped peripheral
       nerves
(d) decrease endoneurial water content

14.14 Measurement of sensory neuropathy
        can be done with
(a) electrodiagnostic testing
(b) testing of temperature perception
(c) testing of vibratory perception
(d) testing of touch perception

14.15 Quantitative sensory testing, endorsed
        by the American Diabetes Association
        and the American Peripheral
        Neuropathy Association includes
(a) electrodiagnostic testing
(b) testing of temperature perception
(c) testing of vibratory perception
(d) testing of touch perception

CHAPTER 15. THE HEAD AND NECK

15.1   The nerves that supply sensibility to
        the head and neck region include the
(a) trigeminal nerve
(b) cervical plexus
(c) brachial plexus
(d) hypoglossal nerve

15.2 The nerves that supply sensibility to the oral cavity include the
(a) buckle nerve
(b) mental nerve
(c) lingual nerve
(d) buccal nerve

15.3 The nerves that supply taste sensation include the
(a) lingual nerve
(b) inferior alveolar nerve
(c) glossopharyngeal nerve
(d) tasteticular nerve

15.4 The most commonly injured nerves during dental extraction are the
(a) lingual nerve
(b) inferior alveolar nerve
(c) glossopharyngeal nerve
(d) testiticular nerve

15.5 During reconstruction of the tongue and anterior oral cavity, the ideal nerve to which the free-flap's nerve should be connected is the
(a) lingual nerve
(b) inferior alveolar nerve
(c) glossopharyngeal nerve
(d) tasteticular nerve

15.6 The theoretical advantage of sensory reconstruction of the oral cavity include rehabilitation of
(a) speech
(b) deglutition
(c) drooling
(d) eructation

15.7 Appropriate sensory testing for the oral cavity includes measurement of
(a) taste
(b) two-point discrimination
(c) stereognosis
(d) pain

15.8 Appropriate sensory testing for the face includes measurement of
(a) pressure perception
(b) two-point discrimination
(c) vibratory perception
(d) stereognosis

15.9 During orthognathic surgery, the most commonly injured nerve is the
(a) lingual nerve
(b) inferior alveolar nerve
(c) glossopharyngeal nerve
(d) testiticular nerve

15.10 The sensory loss from injury to the mental nerve includes the
(a) mind
(b) upper lip
(c) lower lip
(d) chin

15.11 Facial nerve injury results in sensory loss to the
(a) ipsilateral forehead
(b) ipsilateral cheek
(c) contralateral forehead and cheek
(d) nowhere

15.12 The congenital anomaly, cleft lip, results in sensory abnormalities of
(a) the upper lip
(b) the lower lip
(c) the nose
(d) nowhere

15.13 Facial blunt trauma that results in facial fractures may result in
(a) elevated sensory thresholds
(b) damage to branches of the trigeminal nerve
(c) damage to branches of the facial nerve
(d) no nerve injury

15.14 Pain due to neuroma of branches of the trigeminal nerve is
(a) rare
(b) treatable by neuroma resection
(c) treatable by nerve grafting
(d) best approached by ablation of the trigeminal nucleus

15.15 Absence of sensibility to the lower lip is
(a) of no functional consequence
(b) causes drooling
(c) causes injury to the lower lip
(d) unpleasant

CHAPTER 16. THE BREAST

16.1 Nerves that innervate the breast are the
(a) supraclavicular nerve
(b) internal mammary nerve
(c) intercostal nerves 2-6
(d) intercostal nerves 7-10

16.2 The nerve most likely to innervate the nipple/areolar complex is the
(a) supraclavicular nerve
(b) internal mammary nerve
(c) 4th intercostal nerve
(d) 7th intercostal nerve

16.3 The most likely structure(s) to permit the nipple/areolar complex to perceive vibratory stimuli is (are)
(a) Pacinian corpuscles
(b) Meissner corpuscles
(c) innervated hair follicles
(d) milk ducts

16.4 It is now clear that appropriate sensibility testing of the breast may include perception of
(a) vibration
(b) pain
(c) pressure
(d) two-point discrimination

16.5 The most appropriate choice for the normal value of static two-point discrimination of the nipple/areolar complex is
(a) 2 mm
(b) 4 mm
(c) 6 mm
(d) none

16.6 Vibratory and pressure threshold testing demonstrate that the nipple/areolar complex is
(a) more sensitive than the index fingertip
(b) less sensitive than the index fingertip
(c) more sensitive than the thumb
(d) less sensitive than the thumb

16.7 Normative data for the breast exists for the following testing instruments
(a) Semmes-Weinstein monofilaments
(b) Biothesiometer™
(c) Pressure-Specified Sensory Device™
(d) Aesthesiometer™

16.8 A theoretical objection to using the hand-held Biothesiometer™ to measure breast vibratory thresholds is
(a) hand-held testing is invalid
(b) the entire breast vibrates
(c) pressure against the breast damps the vibrating probe
(d) it tests just one frequency, 120 Hz

16.9 Sensory testing with which Pressure-Specified Sensory Device™ modalities are most likely to give equivalent meaning to vibratory testing of the breast is
(a) one-point static touch
(b) two-point static touch
(c) one-point moving touch
(d) two-point moving touch

16.10 Breast sensation is least likely to change following
(a) breast augmentation
(b) breast reduction
(c) breast reconstruction
(d) breast mammography

16.11 Breast sensation is not likely to be altered by a breast augmentation that uses
(a) an inframammary incision
(b) a periareolar incision
(c) an axillary incision
(d) an umbilical incision

16.12 The pressure and vibratory perception thresholds of a breast that overflows a D-size bra cup
(a) are the same as that of a breast that just fills an A- size bra
(b) are higher(less sensitive) than that of a breast that just fills an A-size bra
(c) are lower(more sensitive) than that of a breast that just fills an A-size bra
(d) are not comparable for breasts of different sizes

16.13 Breast reduction by the amputation and free nipple/areola grafting technique must inevitably produce a reconstructed breast that is
(a) less sensitive because the graft must become reinnervated
(b) less sensitive because the graft is located close to the supraclavicular nerve region
(c) usually without change in sensation because the breast was less sensitive than normal initially
(d) even more sensitive due to psychological reasons and nipple/areola reinnervation by normal nerves

16.14 The breast reconstructed by which of the following is likely to recover sensation
(a) a TRAM pedicled flap
(b) a free TRAM flap
(c) a free gluteal flap
(d) a silicone implant placed subpectorally

CHAPTER 17. THE PENIS

17.1 Impotence is common in which disorder(s)?
(a) arthritis
(b) renal failure
(c) diabetes
(d) gout

17.2 The nerve(s) responsible for inability to ejaculate is/are the
(a) parasympathetic
(b) sympathetic
(c) pudendal
(d) perineal

17.3 The nerve(s) responsible for the inability to have an erection is/are the
(a) parasympathetic
(b) sympathetic
(c) pudendal
(d) perineal

17.4 The nerve(s) responsible for decreased penile sensation is/are the
(a) parasympathetic
(b) sympathetic
(c) pudendal
(d) perineal

17.5 The nerve(s) that may be responsible for neurogenic impotence is/are the
(a) parasympathetic
(b) sympathetic
(c) pudendal
(d) perineal

17.6 The nerve(s) that may be responsible for psychogenic impotence is/are the
(a) parasympathetic
(b) sympathetic
(c) pudendal
(d) none of the above

17.7 Phalloplasty should include connection of a donor nerve to which recipient nerve
(a) the parasympathetic
(b) the sympathetic
(c) the pudendal
(d) the genitofemoral

17.8 Vasculogenic impotence is characterized by abnormal
(a) brachiopenile index
(b) nocturnal penile tumescence
(c) vibration threshold
(d) bulbocavernosus reflex

17.9 Neurogenic impotence is characterized by abnormal
(a) brachiopenile index
(b) nocturnal penile tumescence
(c) vibration threshold
(d) bulbocavernosus reflex

17.10 Psychogenic impotence is characterized by normal
(a) brachiopenile index
(b) nocturnal penile tumescence
(c) vibration threshold
(d) bulbocavernosus reflex

17.11 Penile sensibility is least effectively assessed by
(a) cutaneous pressure threshold
(b) cutaneous vibratory threshold
(c) current perception threshold
(d) two-point discrimination

17.12 Neurogenic impotence may be commonly associated with
(a) carpal tunnel syndrome
(b) phantom limb syndrome
(c) diabetic neuropathy
(d) neurogenic bladder

17.13 Sensory rehabilitation of the reconstructed penis is best accomplished through
(a) biofeedback
(b) masturbation
(c) sexual intercourse
(d) ultrasound

CHAPTER 18. CUMULATIVE TRAUMA DISORDERS

18.1 A worker on the assembly line whose glove becomes stuck in the conveyer belt while at work, sustaining a broken wrist has a
(a) cumulative trauma disorder
(b) repetitive motion disease
(c) workmen's compensation claim
(d) compensable injury

18.2 A worker on the assembly line who develops numbness and tingling of the fingers associated with weakness, which worsens toward the end of the shift and becomes improved over the weekend, has a
(a) cumulative trauma disorder
(b) repetitive motion disease
(c) workmen's compensation claim
(d) compensable injury

18.3 The initial approach to a worker who may have a cumulative trauma disorder is
(a) surgical decompression of the carpal tunnel
(b) ergonomic restructuring of the work environment
(c) taking a careful history and physical examination
(d) referral for electrodiagnostic testing

18.4 The initial treatment for a worker with symptoms and signs of carpal tunnel syndrome caused by job-related repetitive motion includes
(a) surgical decompression of the carpal tunnel
(b) ergonomic restructuring of the work environment
(c) nonsteroidal antiinflammatory medication
(d) appropriate wrist splinting

18.5 Continued treatment for a work-related carpal tunnel syndrome that does not respond to initial treatment efforts includes
(a) surgical decompression of the carpal tunnel
(b) applying for social security disability benefits
(c) taking time off from work
(d) cortisone injection into the carpal tunnel

18.6 Thoracic outlet syndrome is a diagnosis that
(a) remains controversial
(b) is not correctly named anatomically
(c) is best treated by first rib removal
(d) does not exist

18.7 Thoracic outlet syndrome is a diagnosis that
(a) is difficult to demonstrate objectively
(b) is definitively made with traditional electrodiagnostic testing
(c) may be made with somatosensory-evoked potential testing
(d) is always associated with a cervical rib

18.8 Thoracic outlet syndrome may include
(a) numbness in all fingers
(b) headaches
(c) neck and shoulder pain
(d) swelling in the hand and forearm

18.9 Thoracic outlet syndrome may include
(a) worsening of symptoms when the arm is elevated
(b) nighttime awakening
(c) color changes in the hand
(d) intrinsic muscle wasting

18.10 Important diagnostic possibilities to exclude before treating thoracic outlet syndrome include
(a) carpal tunnel syndrome
(b) cervical disc disease
(c) intrinsic shoulder pathology
(d) pulmonary disease

18.11 Thoracic outlet syndrome should be treated first by
(a) relaxation of the scalenes, levator scapulae, and upper trapezius
(b) strengthening of the rhomboids, serratus anterior, and mid-trapezius
(c) relaxation of the rhomboids, serratus anterior, and mid-trapezius
(d) strengthening of the scalenes, levator scapulae, and upper trapezius

18.12 Thoracic outlet syndrome may be treated by
(a) a scalenectomy
(b) a transaxillary first rib resection
(c) a supraclavicular first rib resection
(d) neurolysis of the supraclavicular brachial plexus

18.13 Prior to surgically treating thoracic outlet syndrome
(a) there should be at least a 6-month course of nonoperative management
(b) peripheral nerve entrapments should be treated
(c) cervical disc disease should be treated
(d) shoulder pathology should be treated

18.14 Musicians with aching, pain, or numbness in the hands
(a) may have a cumulative trauma disorder
(b) are best approached by early surgical intervention
(c) should be observed while playing before instituting treatment
(d) have stage fright

18.15 OSHA is an acronym for
(a) the Ohio Hand Surgery Association
(b) the Official Society for the Healing Arts
(c) the government agency concerned with cumulative trauma
(d) multiple trauma, "Oh Shucks, Hurt Again"

CHAPTER 19. PLEGIAS

19.1 Upper extremity paralysis, flaccid or spastic, that is unilateral is called
(a) uniplegia
(b) hemiplegia
(c) paraplegia
(d) quadriplegia

19.2 Lower extremity paralysis may be found in
(a) uniplegia
(b) hemiplegia
(c) paraplegia
(d) quadriplegia

19.3 Chronic nerve compression may be found in the plegic limb in
(a) uniplegia
(b) hemiplegia
(c) paraplegia
(d) quadriplegia

19.4   Chronic nerve compression may be found in a nonplegic limb in
(a) uniplegia
(b) hemiplegia
(c) paraplegia
(d) quadriplegia

19.5   Cerebral palsy most commonly is
(a) spastic
(b) congenital
(c) reversible
(d) athetoid

19.6   Cerebral palsy is most likely due to a developmental problem in the
(a) limbic system
(b) hypothalamus
(c) parietal lobe
(d) occipital lobe

19.7   Tendon reconstruction for spastic hemiplegia is indicated despite the presence of
(a) thumb-in-palm deformity
(b) no two-point discrimination
(c) poor stereognosis
(d) visual impairment

19.8   Sensory impairment in spastic hemiplegia may be due to
(a) postcentral gyrus ischemic injury
(b) lack of cortical stimulation
(c) chronic nerve compression at the wrist level
(d) chronic nerve compression at the forearm/elbow level

19.9   Sensory rehabilitation will improve hand function in
(a) syringomyelia
(b) hemiplegia
(c) paraplegia
(d) quadriplegia

19.10 Quantitative sensory testing is indicated for the patient with
(a) syringomyelia
(b) hemiplegia
(c) paraplegia
(d) quadriplegia

19.11 Neurosurgical consultation for shunting is indicated with
(a) syringomyelia
(b) hemiplegia
(c) paraplegia
(d) quadriplegia

19.12 Touch perception will be normal most of the time with
(a) syringomyelia
(b) hemiplegia
(c) paraplegia
(d) quadriplegia

19.13 Pain perception will be abnormal most of the time with
(a) syringomyelia
(b) hemiplegia
(c) paraplegia
(d) quadriplegia

19.14 Reassessment of sensibility will be useful for patients with
(a) syringomyelia
(b) hemiplegia
(c) paraplegia
(d) quadriplegia

19.15 Bilateral tendon transfers may be altered by sensibility in
(a) syringomyelia
(b) hemiplegia
(c) paraplegia
(d) quadriplegia

CHAPTER 20. THERAPIST AS RESEARCHER

There are no questions for this chapter.

● ANSWERS ●

CHAPTER 1. THE NEURON

1) B
2) C
3) D
4) A,D
5) A,B,D
6) D
7) A,D
8) B,C
9) D
10) A
11) B
12) A
13) B
14) B
15) A,D

CHAPTER 2. CUTANEOUS SENSORY RECEPTORS

1) A
2) C
3) A
4) B,C
5) A,B
6) D
7) A,C

CHAPTER 3. PROPRIOCEPTION

1) D
2) A
3) B
4) A
5) A,B
6) C,D
7) A,B
8) D

CHAPTER 4. NERVE RECONSTRUCTION

1) A,B
2) A,D

3) A,B,C
4) A,B,C,D
5) D
6) A,B
7) C
8) A,B,C,D
9) A,B,C,D
10) A,B,C
11) A,B,C,D
12) A,B,C,D
13) A,B,C
14) A,B,C,D
15) D

CHAPTER 5. GOALS

1) C
2) A,B
3) C,D
4) B,D
5) B
6) B,D
7) D
8) C
9) C
10) D

CHAPTER 6. THRESHOLD VERSUS INNERVATION DENSITY

1) A,B,C,D
2) A
3) B
4) B,C
5) D
6) C
7) C
8) A,B,C
9) B
10) A,B,D

CHAPTER 7. INSTRUMENTATION

1) B,C
2) A,B,C
3) A,B,C
4) A
5) D
6) A,C,D
7) A,B,C
8) C
9) C,D
10) A,C,D
11) D
12) D
13) A,B,C,D
14) A,B,C,D
15) B,C,D

CHAPTER 8. ELECTRODIAG-NOSTIC TESTING

1) B,C
2) A,C
3) A,B,C,D
4) B
5) A,B,C
6) B,C,D
7) C,D
8) C
9) A,B,C,D
10) C

CHAPTER 9. GRADING PERIPHERAL NERVE FUNCTION

1) B
2) A,B,C
3) A,B,C,D
4) C
5) A,B,C,D

CHAPTER 10. CORTICAL PLASTICITY

1) A, C
2) D
3) A,B,C

4) A,B,C,D
5) B
6.) A,B,C
7) A,B,C,D
8) A,B,D

CHAPTER 11. SENSORY REEDUCATION

1) B
2) A,B
3) A,B,C
4) A,B
5) B
6) A
7) A,C,D
8) A,B,C,D
9) A,B,C,D
10) C
11) A, B,C
12) B,C,D

CHAPTER 12. UPPER EXTREMITY

1) A,B,C
2) A,B,C
3) A,C, D
4) B,C,D
5) C
6) A
7) B
8) D
9) C
10) A
11) B
12) B
13) B
14) C
15) D

CHAPTER 13. LOWER EXTREMITY

1) A,B,C,D
2) C
3) C

4) C
5) C,D
6) A,C,D
7) A,B,C
8) A,D
9) B,C
10) B

CHAPTER 14. NEUROPATHY

1) A,B,C,D
2) A,B,C,D
3) A,B,C
4) C,D
5) D
6) A,D
7) A,D
8) A,D
9) C
10) D
11) C
12) A,B,C,D
13) B,C
14) A,B,C,D
15) B,C,D

CHAPTER 15. HEAD AND NECK

1) A,B,C
2) B,C,D
3) A,C
4) A,B
5) A
6) A,B,C
7) A,B,C,D
8) A,B,C,D
9) B
10) C,D
11) D
12) D
13) A,B,C,D
14) A

CHAPTER 16. THE BREAST

1) A,C
2) C
3) C
4) A,B,C
5) D
6) B,D
7) A,B
8) C
9) C
10) D
11) C,D
12) B
13) C,D
14) A,B,C,D

CHAPTER 17. THE PENIS

1) C
2) B
3) A
4) C
5) A,B,C
6) D
7) C
8) A,B
9) B,C,D
10) A,B,C,D
11) D
12) C,D
13) B,C

CHAPTER 18. CUMULATIVE TRAUMA DISORDERS

1) C,D
2) A,C
3) C
4) B,C,D
5) A,C,D
6) A,B
7) A,C
8) A,B,C,D
9) A,C,D
10) A,B,C,D
11) A,B
12) A,B,C,D
13) A,B,C,D

14) A,C
15) C

CHAPTER 19. PLEGIAS

1) B
2) C,D
3) B
4) C
5) A,B
6) C
7) A,B,C,D
8) A,B,C,D
9) B
10) A,B,C
11) A
12) A
13) A
14) A,B,C
15) D

CHAPTER 20. THERAPIST AS RESEARCHER

There are no questions for this chapter.

• • •

combined
bibliography
& index

• A •

AAEM Quality Assurance Committee, Literature review of the usefulness of nerve conduction studies and electromyography for the evaluation of patients with carpal tunnel syndrome. *Muscle and Nerve* 16:1392-1414, 1993.

Adrian, E. D. Afferent discharges to the cerebral cortex from peripheral sense organs. *Journal of Physiology 100:*159-191, 1941.

Aljure, J., Ibrahim, E., Bradley, W. E., Lin, J. E., & Bonnie, J. Carpal tunnel syndrome in paraplegic patients. *Paraplegia 23*:182-186, 1985.

Allard, T. A., Clark, S. A., Jenkins, W. M., & Merzenich, M. M. Reorganization of somatosensory area 3b representations in adult owl monkeys after digital syndactyly. *Journal of Neurophysiology 66*:1048-1058, 1991.

Almli, C. R. Early brain damage and time course of behavioral dysfunction: Parallels with neural maturation. In *Early Brain Damage: Volume 2, Neurobiology and Behavior*, S. Finger & C. R. Almli, Editors. New York: Academic Press, Inc., 1984.

—— Influence of perinatal risk factors (preterm birth, low birth weight, and oxygen deficiency) on movement patterns: An animal model and premature human infants. In *At-risk Infants: Interventions, Families and Research*, N. J. Anastasiow & S. Harel, Editors. Baltimore: Paul H. Brookes Publishing Company, 1993.

Almli, C. R., & Mohr, N. M. Born too soon: Intervention theory and research with premature infants in the NICU. In *Foundations for Practice in the Neonatal Intensive Care Unit and Early Intervention: A Self-Guided Practice Manual*, E. Vergara, Editor. Rockville: American Occupational Therapy Association, Inc., 1993.

Altissimi, M., Mancini, G. B., & Azzara, A. Results of primary repair of digital nerves. *Journal of Hand Surgery 16B*:546-547, 1991.

Amadio, P. C., & Rusotti, G. M. Evaluation and treatment of hand and wrist disorders in musicians. *Hand Clinics 6*:405-416, 1990.

Anthony, M. S. Desensitization. In *Hand Rehabilitation: A Practical Guide*, G. L. Clark, E. F. S. Wilgis, B. Aiello, D. Eckhaus, & L. V. Eddington, Editors. New York: Churchill Livingstone, 1993.

—— Sensory re-education helps patients regain function of hands. *Advances in Physical Therapy 21*:19-21, March 1994.

—— Sensory Re-education. In *Hand Rehabilitation: A Practical Guide*, G. L. Clark, E. F. S. Wilgis, B. Aiello, D. Eckhaus, & L. V. Eddington, Editors. New York: Churchill Livingstone, 1993.

—— Thoracic outlet syndrome. In *Hand Rehabilitation: A Practical Guide*, G. L. Clark, E. F. S. Wilgis, B. Aiello, D. Eckhaus, & L. V. Eddington, Editors. New York: Churchill Livingstone, 1993.

Antonini, G., Palmieri, G., Spagnoli, L. G., Millefiorini, M. Lead brachial neuropathy in heroin addiction: A case report. *Clinical Neurology and Neurosurgery 91*:167-170, 1989.

Arezzo, J. C., Bolton, C. F., Boulton, A., & Dyck, P. J. Quantitative sensory testing: A consensus report from the Peripheral Neuropathy Association. *Neurology 43*:1050-1052, 1993.

Arezzo, J. C., & Schaumberg, H. H. The use of the Optacon as a screening device: A new technique for detecting sensory loss in individuals exposed to neurotoxins. *Journal of Occupational Medicine 22*:461-464, 1980.

Arezzo, J. C., Schaumberg, H. H., & Laudadio, C. Thermal sensitivity tester: Device for quantitative assessment of thermal sense in diabetic neuropathy. *Diabetes 35*:590-592, 1986.

Arezzo, J. C., Schaumberg, H. H., & Petersen, C. A. Rapid screening for peripheral neuropathy: A field study with the Optacon. *Neurology 33*:626-629, 1983.

Armstrong, T. J. Cumulative trauma disorders of the upper limb and identification of work-related factors. In *Occupational Disorders of the Upper Extremity*, L. H. Millender, D. S. Louis, & B. P. Simmonds, Editors. New York: Churchill Livingstone, 1992.

Armstrong, T. J., Foulke, J. A., Joseph, B. A., & Goldstein, S. A. Investigation of cumulative trauma disorders in a poultry processing plant. *American Industrial Hygiene Association Journal 43*:102-116, 1982.

Armstrong, T. J., Punnett, L., & Ketner, P. Subjective worker assessments of hand tools used in automobile assembly. *American Industrial Hygiene Association Journal 51*:639-642, 1989.

Arndt, R. Work place, stress, and cumulative trauma disorders. *Journal of Hand Surgery 12A*:866-869, 1987.

Asbury, A. K. Pain in generalized neuropathies. In *Pain Syndromes in Neurology*, H. L. Fields, Editor. London: Butterworths, 1990.

Asbury, A. K., & Porte, D., Jr. Consensus statement of the American Diabetes Association: Standard measures in diabetic neuropathy. *Diabetes Care 16*:2:82-92, 1993.

—— Diabetic neuropathy: Consensus statement. *Diabetes 37*:1000-1010, 1988.

—— Standardized measures in diabetic neuropathy. *Diabetes Care 18*:59-82, 1995.

Aviv, J. E., Hecht, C., Wineberg, H., Dalton, J. F., & Urken, M. L. Surface sensibility of the floor of the mouth and tongue in healthy controls and in radiated patients. *Otolaryngology and Head and Neck Surgery 107*:418-422, 1992.

Azman, O., Dellon, A. L., Birely, B., McFarlane, E. Clinical implications of innervation of the human shoulder joint. *Clinical Orthopedics and Related Research*, submitted: 1995.

Azman, O., Muse, V., & Dellon, A. L. Evidence in support of collateral sprouting in the human. *Annals of Plastic Surgery*, in press: 1996.

• **B** •

Bain, J. R., Mackinnon, S. E., Hudson, A. R., Wade, J., Evans, P., Mackin, A., & Hunter, D. Peripheral nerve allograft in primate immunosuppressed with Cyclosporin A: I. Histologic and electrophysiologic assessment. *Plastic and Reconstructive Surgery 90*:1036-1046, 1992.

Barber, L. M. Desensitization of the traumatized hand. In *Rehabilitation of the Hand: Surgery and Therapy*, J. M. Hunter, L. H. Schneider, E. J. Mackin, & A. D. Callahan, Editors. St. Louis: C. V. Mosby Company, 1984.

Baum, C. M., & Edwards, D. F. *From ICV to community: A model for determining effectiveness*. Presented at the American Occupational Therapy Association Annual Meeting, Denver, 1995.

Beale, S., Hambert, G., & Lisper, H. O. Augmentation mammaplasty: The surgical and psychological effects of the operation and prediction of the results. *Annals of Plastic Surgery 14*:473-493, 1985.

Bechtol, C. D. Grip test: Use of a dynamometer with adjustable handle spacing. *Journal of Bone and Joint Surgery 36A*:820-823, 1954.

Bell, J. A. Sensibility evaluation. *In Rehabilitation of the Hand: Surgery and Therapy*, J. M. Hunter, L. H. Schneider, E. J. Mackin & A. D. Callahan, Editors. St. Louis: C. V. Mosby Company, 1978.

—— Light touch-deep pressure testing using Semmes-Weinstein monofilaments. In *Rehabilitation of the Hand: Surgery and Therapy*, 2nd edition, J. M. Hunter, L. H. Schneider, E. J. Mackin, & A. D. Callahan, Editors. St. Louis: C. V. Mosby Company, Chapter 35, 1984.

Bell-Krotoski, J. A. Light touch-deep pressure testing using Semmes-Weinstein monofilaments. In *Rehabilitation of the Hand: Surgery and Therapy*, J. M. Hunter, L. H. Schneider, E. J. Mackin & A. D. Callahan, Editors. St. Louis: C. V. Mosby Company, 1990.

Bell-Krotoski, J. A., & Buford, W. L. The force/time relationships of clinically used sensory testing instruments. *Journal of Hand Therapy 1*:76-81, 1988.

Bell-Krotoski, J. A., & Tomancik, E. The repeatability of testing with Semmes-Weinstein monofilaments. *Journal of Hand Surgery 12A*:155-161, 1987.

Bemelmans, B. L. H., Hendrikx, L. B. P. M., Koldewijn, E. L., Lemmens, W. A. J. G., Debruyne, F. M. J., & Meueleman, E. J. H. Comparison of biothesiometry and neuro-urophysiological investigations for the clinical evaluation of patients with erectile dysfunction. *Journal of Urology 153*:1483-1486, 1995.

Bemelmans, B. L. H., Meueleman, E. J. H., Antem, B. W. M., Doesburg, W. H., Van Kerrebroeck, P. W. V., & Debruyne, F. M. J. Penile sensory disorders in erectile dysfunction: Results of a comprehensive neuro-urophysiological diagnostic evaluation in 123 patients. *Journal of Urology 146*:777-783, 1991.

Biemesderfer, D., Munger, B. L., & Binck, J. The Pilo-Ruffini complex: A non-sinus hair and associated slowly-adapting mechanoreceptor in primate facial skin. *Experimental Brain Research 142*:197-222, 1978.

Birke, J. A., & Sims, D. S. Plantar sensory threshold in the ulcerative foot. *Leprosy Review 57*:261-267, 1986.

Black, D. L. Somatosensory evoked potential monitoring during total hip arthroplasty. *Clinical Orthopedics 262*:170-177, 1991.

Bleecker, M. L. Vibration perception thresholds in entrapment and toxic neuropathies. *Journal of Occupational Medicine 28*:991-994, 1986.

Bleecker, M. L., & Hansen, J. A. *Occupational Neurology and Clinical Neurotoxicology*. Baltimore: Williams & Wilkins, 1994.

Borg, K., & Lindblom, U. Increase of vibration threshold during wrist flexion in patients with carpal tunnel syndrome. *Pain 26*:211-219, 1986.

Borges, L. F., Hallett, M., Selkoe, D. J., &

Welch, K. The anterior tarsal tunnel syndrome. *Journal of Neurosurgery 54*:89-92, 1981.

Bosma, J. F. *Symposium on Oral Sensation and Perception*. Springfield, IL: Charles C. Thomas, Publisher, 1967.

Boulton A. J. M., Kubrusly, D. B., & Bowker, J. G. Impaired vibratory perception and diabetic foot ulceration. *Diabetes Medicine 3*:192, 1986.

Boyd, B., Mulholland, S., Gullane, P., & Kelly, L. Reinnervated lateral antebrachial cutaneous neurosome flaps in oral reconstruction: Are we making sense? *Plastic and Reconstructive Surgery 93*:1350-1359, 1994.

Boyd, I. A., & Smith, R. S. The muscle spindle. In *Peripheral Neuropathy,* 2nd edition, P. J. Dyck, P. K. Thomas, E. H. Lambert, & R. Bunge, Editors. Philadelphia: Saunders, 1984.

Brammer, A. J., Piercy, J. E., Auger, P. L., & Nohara, S. Tactile perception in hands occupationally exposed to vibration. *Journal of Hand Surgery 12A*:870-875, 1987.

Brandenberg, A., & Mann, D. Sensory nerve crush and regeneration and the receptive fields and response properties of neurons in the primary somatosensory cerebral cortex of cats. *Experimental Neurology 103*:256-266, 1989.

Braun, R. M., & Jackson, W. J. Electrical studies as a prognostic factor in the surgical treatment of carpal tunnel syndrome. *Journal of Hand Surgery 19A*:893-900, 1994.

Britt, L. P. Non-operative treatment of the thoracic outlet syndrome symptoms. *Clinical Orthopaedics and Related Research 51*:45-48, 1967.

Brodman, K. *Vergleichende Lokalisationlehre der Grosshimrinde in ihren Prinzipien dargestellt auf Grund des Zellenbaues*. Leipzig: J. A. Barth, 1909.

Brown, C. J., Mackinnon, S. E., Dellon, A. L., & Bain, J.R. The sensory potential of free flap donor sites. *Annals of Plastic Surgery 23*:135-140, 1989.

Brown, W. F., & Bolton, C. F. *Clinical electromyography*. Boston: Butterworth-Heinemann, 1993.

Brunelli, G. Neurotization of avulsed roots of the brachial plexus by means of anterior nerves of the cervical plexus. In *Microreconstruction of Nerve Injuries*. Philadelphia: W. B. Saunders Company, 1987.

Brushart, T. M., & Seiler, W. A. Selective reinnervation of distal motor stumps by peripheral motor axons. *Experimental Neurology 97*:289-300, 1987.

Buch-Jaeger, N., & Foucher, G. Correlation of clinical signs with nerve conduction tests in the diagnosis of carpal tunnel syndrome. *Journal of Hand Surgery 19B*:720-724, 1994.

Burgess, P. R., & Horch, K. W. Specific regeneration of cutaneous fibers in the cat. *Journal of Neurophysiology 36*:101-114, 1973.

• C •

Caffee, H. H. Measurement of implant capsules. *Annals of Plastic Surgery 11*:412-415, 1983.

Caine, D. B., & Pallis, C. A. Vibratory sense: A critical review. *Brain 89*:723-733, 1966.

Callahan, A. D. Methods of compensation and reeducation of sensory dysfunction. In *Rehabilitation of the Hand: Surgery and Therapy*, J. M. Hunter, L. H. Schneider, E. J. Mackin, & A. D. Callahan, Editors. St. Louis: C. V. Mosby Company, 1984.

—— Sensibility testing: Clinical methods. In *Rehabilitation of the Hand: Surgery and Therapy*, 2nd Edition, J. M. Hunter, L. H. Schneider, E. J. Mackin, & A. D. Callahan, Editors. St. Louis: C. V. Mosby Company, Chapter 36, 1984.

Campbell, C. S. Gamekeeper's thumb. *Journal of Bone and Joint Surgery 37B*:143-146, 1955.

Campbell, J. N., Meyer, R. A., & La Motte, R. H. Sensitization of myelinated nociceptive afferents that innervate the monkey's

hand. *Journal of Neurophysiology 42*:1669-1679, 1979.

Campbell, J. N., Raja, S. N., Meyer, R. A., & Mackinnon, S. E. Myelinated fibers in peripheral nerves signal hyperalgesia that follows nerve injury. *Pain 32*:89-94, 1988.

Cannon, L. J., Bernacki, E. J., & Walter, S. D. Personal and occupational factors associated with carpal tunnel syndrome. *Journal of Occupational Medicine 23*:255-258, 1981.

Carter, M. S. Re-education of sensation. Hand Rehabilitation Symposium. *Journal of Hand Surgery 4*:501- 507, 1978.

Carter-Wilson, M. Sensory Re-Education. In *Operative Nerve* Repair and Reconstruction, R. H. Gelberman, Editor. Philadelphia: J. B. Lippincott Company, 1991.

Catton, M. J., Harrison, M. J. G., Fullerton, P. M., & Kazantzis, G. Subclinical neuropathy in lead workers. *British Medical Journal 2*:80-82, 1970.

Cauna, N. Nature and functions of the papillary ridges of the digital skin. *Anatomical Record 119*:449-468, 1954.

—— Nerve supply and nerve endings in Meissner's corpuscles. *American Journal of Anatomy 99*:315-350, 1956.

Chaise, F., & Roger, B. Neurolysis of the common peroneal nerve in leprosy. *Journal of Bone and Joint Surgery 67B*:426-429, 1985.

Chambers, M. R., Andres, K. H., & von Duering, M. The structure and function of the slowly-adapting type II mechanoreceptors in hairy skin. *Quarterly Journal of Experimental Physiology 57*:417-445, 1972.

Chang, B., & Dellon, A. L. Surgical management of recurrent carpal tunnel syndrome. *Journal of Hand Surgery 18B*:467-470, 1993.

Chang, K. N., DeArmond, S. J., & Buncke, H. J., Jr. Sensory reinnervation in microsurgical reconstruction of the heel. *Plastic and Reconstructive Surgery 78*:652-663, 1986.

Chapelle, P. A., Roby-Brami, A., Yakovleff, A., & Bussel, B. *Journal of Neurology, Neu-*

rosurgery and Psychiatry 51:197-202, 1988.

Chapman, C. E. Active versus passive touch: Factors influencing the transmission of somatosensory signals to primary somatosensory cortex. *Canadian Journal of Physiologic Pharmacology 72*:558-570, 1994.

Chassard, M., Pham, E., & Comtet, J. J. Two-point discrimination tests versus functional sensory recovery in both median and ulnar nerve complete transections. *Journal of Hand Surgery 18B*:790-796, 1993.

Cheng, K-X., Hwang, W-Y., Eid, A. E., Wang, S-L., Chang, T-S., & Fu, K-D. Analysis of 136 cases of reconstructed penis using various methods. *Plastic and Reconstructive Surgery 95*:94-98, 1995.

Cherington, M., & Cherington, C. Thoracic outlet syndrome reimbursement patterns and patient profiles. *Neurology 42*:493-495, 1992.

Cherniak, M. G., Letz, R., Gerr, F., Brammer, A., & Pace, P. Detailed clinical assessment of neurological function in symptomatic shipyard workers. *British Journal of Industrial Medicine 47*:566-572, 1990.

Cherniak, M. G., Moalli, D., & Viscolli, C. A comparison of digital neurometry, tactometry, and nerve conduction studies in the diagnosis of carpal tunnel syndrome. *Journal of Hand Surgery*, in press: 1995.

Clark, C. M., Jr., & Lee, A. Prevention and treatment of the complications of diabetes mellitus. *New England Journal of Medicine 332*:1210-1217, 1995.

Clark, F. J., & Burgess, P. R. Slowly-adapting receptors in cat knee joint: Can they signal joint angle? *Journal of Neurophysiology 38*:1448-1463, 1975.

Clark, F. J., Horch, K. W., & Bach, S. M. Contributions of cutaneous and joint receptors to static knee-position sense in man. *Journal of Neurophysiology 42*:877-888, 1979.

Clark, G. L., Wilgis, E. F. S., Aiello, B., Eckhaus, D., & Eddington, L. V. *Rehabilitation of the Hand: A Practical Guide.* New York: Churchill Livingstone, Inc., 1993.

Clark, S. A., Allard, T., Jenkins, W. M., & Merzenich, M. M. Syndactyly results in the emergence of double digit receptive fields in somatosensory cortex in adult owl monkeys. *Nature 332*:444-445, 1988.

Coert, H. J., & Dellon, A. L. Clinical implications of the anatomy of the sural nerve. *Plastic and Reconstructive Surgery 94*:850-855, 1994.

Cornblath, D. R., Kuncl, R. W., & Mellits, E. D. Nerve conduction studies in amyotrophic lateral sclerosis. *Muscle and Nerve 15*:1111-1115, 1992.

Cosh, J. A. Studies on the nature of vibration sense. *Clinical Science 12*:131-151, 1953.

Costas, P. D., Heatley, G., & Seckel, B. R. Normal sensation of the human face and neck. *Plastic and Reconstructive Surgery 93*:1141-1145, 1994.

Courtiss, E. H., & Goldwyn, R. M. Breast sensation before and after plastic surgery. *Plastic and Reconstructive Surgery 58*:1-10, 1976.

Craig, J. Anomalous responses following prolonged tactile simulation. *Neuropsychology 31*:277-291, 1993.

Craig, R. D. P., & Sykes, P. A. Nipple sensitivity following reduction mammoplasty. *British Journal of Plastic Surgery 23*:165-168, 1970.

Crosby, C. A., & Wehbe, M. A. Hand strength: Normative values. *Journal of Hand Surgery 19A*:665-670, 1994.

Crosby, P. M., & Dellon, A. L. A comparison of two-point discrimination test devices. *Microsurgery 10:* 134-137, 1989.

Cummings, K., Maizlish, N., Rudolph, L., Devlin, K., & Erwin, A. Occupational disease surveillance: Carpal tunnel syndrome. *Morbidity and Mortality Weekly Report 38*:485-489, 1989.

Curtis, R. M., & Dellon, A. L. Sensory re-education after peripheral nerve injury. In *Management of Peripheral Nerve Injuries*, M. Spinner & G. Omer, Editors. Philadelphia: W. B. Saunders Company, 1980.

Curtis, R. M., & Eversmann, W. W., Jr. Internal neurolysis as an adjunct to the treatment of the carpal tunnel syndrome. *Journal of Bone and Joint Surgery 55A*:733-740, 1973.

• D •

Daniel, C. R., Bower, J. D., Pearson, J. E., & Holbert, R. D. Vibrometry and neuropathy. *Journal of the Mississippi State Medical Association 18*:30-34, 1977.

Dannenbaum, R.M., & Dykes, R.W. Sensory loss in the hand after sensory stroke: Therapeutic rationale. *Archives of Physical Medicine and Rehabilitation 69*:833-839, 1988.

Dannenbaum, R. M., & Jones, L. A. The assessment and treatment of patients who have sensory loss following cortical lesions. *Journal of Hand Therapy 6*:130-138, 1993.

Dawson, D. M. Entrapment neuropathies of the upper extremities. *New England Journal of Medicine 329*:2013-2017, 1993.

Dawson, W. J. Reed-maker's elbow. *Medical Problems in the Performing Arts 1*:24-26, 1986.

DeLisa, J. A., Lee, H. J., Baran, E. M., Lai, K-S. & Spielholz, N. *Manual of Nerve Conduction Velocity and Clinical Neurophysiology,* 3rd edition. New York: Raven Press, 1994.

Dellon, A. L. A cause for optimism in diabetic neuropathy. *Annals of Plastic Surgery 20*:103-105, 1988.

—— A numerical grading scale for peripheral nerve function. *Journal of Hand Therapy 6*:152-160, 1993.

—— Clinical use of vibratory stimuli to evaluate peripheral nerve injury and compression neuropathy. *Plastic and Reconstructive Surgery 65*:466-476, 1980.

—— Electrodiagnosis in the management of focal neuropathies: The "WOG" Syndrome. *Muscle and Nerve 17*:1336-1342, 1994.

—— Entrapment of the deep peroneal nerve on the dorsum of the foot. *Foot and Ankle 11*:73-80, 1990.

—— *Evaluation of Sensibility and Re-education of Sensation in the Hand*. Baltimore: Williams & Wilkins, 1981.

—— Interruption of nerve function. In *Current Therapy in Plastic and Reconstructive Surgery*, J. Marsh, Editor. Toronto: B. C. Beck, 1988.

—— Management of peripheral nerve injuries: Basic principles of microneurosurgical repair. *Oral Maxillofacial Surgery Clinics - North America 4*:393-403, 1992.

—— Muscle sense or non-sense. *Annals of Plastic Surgery 26*:444-448, 1991.

—— Operative technique for submuscular transposition of the ulnar nerve. *Contemporary Orthopedics 16*:17-24, 1988.

—— Partial dorsal wrist denervation; Resection of distal posterior interosseous nerve. *Journal of Hand Surgery 10A*:527-533, 1985.

—— Pitfalls in electrodiagnosis. In *Operative Nerve Repair and Reconstruction*, R. H. Gelberman, Editor. Philadelphia: J.B. Lippincott, Company, 1991.

—— Recurrent ulnar nerve compression at the elbow treated by the musculofascial lengthening technique. Presented at the American Society of Surgery of the Hand meeting, Phoenix, AZ, 1992. *Journal of Hand Surgery*, submitted: 1997.

—— Reinnervation of denervated Meissner corpuscles: A sequential histologic study in primates following interfascicular nerve repair. *Journal of Hand Surgery 1*:98-109, 1976.

—— Reoperative peripheral nerve surgery. In *Reoperative Surgery*, J. Grotting, Editor. St. Louis: Quarterly Medical Publishers, 1995.

—— Sensory recovery in replanted digits and transplanted toes; A review. *Journal of Reconstructive Microsurgery 2*:123-129, 1986.

—— Techniques for successful management of ulnar nerve entrapment at the elbow. *Neurosurgical Clinics-North America 2*:227-234, 1991.

—— Testing for facial sensibility. *Plastic and*

Reconstructive Surgery 87:1140-1141, 1991.

—— The results of supraclavicular brachial plexus neurolysis without first rib resection in management of post-traumatic "thoracic outlet syndrome." *Journal of Reconstructive Microsurgery 9*:11-17, 1993.

—— The vibrometer. *Plastic and Reconstructive Surgery 71*:427-431, 1983.

—— Tinel or not Tinel? *Journal of Hand Surgery (British) 9*:216, 1984.

—— Treatment of symptoms of diabetic neuropathy by peripheral nerve decompression. *Plastic and Reconstructive Surgery 89*:689-697, 1992.

—— Tube, or not tube.... (Editorial) *Journal of Hand Surgery 19B*:271-272, 1994.

—— Wound healing in nerve. *Clinics in Plastic Surgery 17*:545-570, 1990.

Dellon, A. L., Chang, E., Coert, H. J., & Campbell, K. R. Intraneural ulnar pressure changes related to operative techniques for cubital tunnel decompression. *Journal of Hand Surgery 19A*:923-930, 1994.

Dellon, A. L., & Coert, H. Results of the treatment of ulnar nerve compression at the elbow by the musculofascial lengthening technique. *Journal of Bone and Joint Surgery*, submitted: 1996.

Dellon, A. L., & Crawley, W. A. Nerve reconstruction with alloplastic material in the head and neck region. *Oral Maxillofacial Surgery Clinics - North America 4*:527-533, 1992.

Dellon, A. L., Curtis, R. M., & Edgerton, M. T. Re-education of sensation in the hand following nerve injury. *Journal of Bone and Joint Surgery 53A*:813, 1971.

—— Evaluating recovery of sensation in the hand following nerve injury. *Johns Hopkins Medical Journal 130*:235-243, 1972.

—— Re-education of sensation in the hand following nerve injury. *Plastic and Reconstructive Surgery 53*:297-305, 1974.

Dellon, A. L., Dellon, E. S., & Seiler, W. A., IV. The effect of tarsal tunnel decompression in the streptozotocin-induced diabetic rat. *Microsurgery 15*:265-268, 1994.

Dellon, A. L., Dellon, E. S., Tassler, P. L., Ellefson, R. E., Hendrickson, M., & Francel, T. G. Experimental model of pyridoxine (B6) deficiency-induced neuropathy. *Annals of Plastic Surgery*, submitted: 1997.

Dellon A. L., Hament, W., & Gittelsohn, A. Nonoperative management of cubital tunnel syndrome: Results of an eight-year prospective study. *Neurology 43*:1673-1677, 1993.

Dellon, A. L., & Horner, G. Partial wrist denervation. In *Problems in Plastic and Reconstruction Surgery: The Wrist*, S. Levin, Editor. Philadelphia: Lippincott, 1993.

Dellon, A. L., & Kallman, C. H. Evaluation of functional sensation in the hand. *Journal of Hand Surgery 8*:865-870, 1983.

Dellon, A. L., Keller, K. M., Computer-assisted quantitative sensorimotor testing in patients with carpal and cubital tunnel syndrome. *Annals of Plastic Surgery 38*:493-502, 1997

Dellon, A. L., & Mackinnon, S. E. An alternative to the classical nerve graft for the management of the short nerve gap, *Plastic and Reconstructive Surgery 82*:849-856, 1988.

—— Human ulnar nerve compression at the elbow: Clinical, histologic and electrodiagnostic correlations. *Journal of Reconstructive Microsurgery 4*:179-187, 1988.

—— Injury to the medial antebrachial cutaneous nerve during cubital tunnel surgery. *Journal of Hand Surgery 10B*:33-36, 1985.

—— Radial sensory nerve entrapment. *Archives of Neurology 43*:833-837, 1986.

—— Treatment of the painful neuroma by neuroma resection and muscle implantation. *Plastic and Reconstructive Surgery 77*:427-436, 1986.

Dellon, A. L., Mackinnon, S. E., & Brandt, K. E. The markings of the Semmes-Weinstein nylon monofilaments. *Journal of Hand Surgery 18A*:756-757, 1993.

Dellon, A. L., Mackinnon, S. E., & Crosby, P. M. Reliability of two-point discrimination measurements. *Journal of Hand Surgery 12A*:693-696, 1987.

Dellon, A. L., Mackinnon, S. E., & Schlegel, R. Validity of electrodiagnostic studies following anterior transposition of the ulnar nerve. *Journal of Hand Surgery 12*:700-703, 1987.

Dellon, A. L., Mackinnon, S. E., & Seiler, W. A., IV. Susceptibility of the diabetic nerve to chronic compression. *Annals of Plastic Surgery 20*:117-119, 1988.

Dellon, A. L., & Munger, B. L. Correlation of histology and sensibility after nerve repair. *Journal of Hand Surgery 8*:871-878, 1983.

Dellon, A. L. Computer-assisted sensibility evaluation and surgical treatment of tarsal tunnel syndrome. *Adv. Podiatry, 2:* 17-40, 1996.

Dellon, A. L., Tassler, P. L., & Keller, K. Compensatory contralateral change; abnormal pressure perception in the non-injured foot. *Journal of Podiatric Medicine and Surgery*, submitted 1997.

Dellon, A. L., Witebsky, F. G., & Terrill, R. E. The denervated Meissner corpuscle: A sequential histologic study following nerve division in the Rhesus monkey. *Plastic and Reconstructive Surgery 56*:182-193, 1975.

Dellon, E. S., Cronc, S., Mourey, R., & Dellon, A. L. Comparison of the Semmes-Weinstein monofilaments with the Pressure-Specified Sensory Device. *Restorative Neurology Neuroscience 5*:323-326, 1993.

Dellon, E. S., & Dellon, A. L. Quantitative sensory testing with the force-defined vibrometer. *Journal of Reconstructive Microsurgery*, submitted 1997.

———- The first nerve graft, Vulpian and the 19th Century neural regeneration controversy. *Journal of Hand Surgery 4*:1993.

Dellon, E. S., Keller, K. M., Moratz, V., & Dellon, A. L. Relationship between skin hardness and human touch perception. *Journal of Hand Surgery 20B:* 44-48, 1995.

Dellon, E. S., Keller, K. M., Moratz, V., & Dellon, A. L. Validation of cutaneous pressure threshold measurements for the evaluation of hand function. *Annals of Plastic Surgery, 38:*485-492, 1997.

Dellon, E. S., Mourey, R., & Dellon, A. L. Human pressure perception values for constant and moving one- and two-point discrimination. *Plastic and Reconstructive Surgery 90*:112-117, 1992.

DeMedinacelli, L., Wyatt, R. J., & Freed, W. J. Peripheral nerve reconnection: Mechanical, thermal and ionic conditions that promote the return of function. *Experimental Neurology 81*:469-474, 1983.

DeSantis, M., & Norman, W. P. An ultrastructural study of nerve terminal degeneration in muscle spindles of the tenuissimus muscle of the cat. *Journal of Neurocytology 8*:67-71, 1979.

Deutinger, M., Girsh, W., & Burgasser, G. Clinical application of motorsensory differentiated nerve repair. *Microsurgery 14*:297-303, 1993.

Devor, M., Schonfeld, D., Seltzer, Z., & Wall, P. D. Two models of cutaneous reinnervation following peripheral nerve injury. *Journal of Comparative Neurology 185*:211-220, 1979.

Diao, E., & Peimer, C. A. Sutureless methods of nerve repair. In *Operative Nerve Repair and Reconstruction*, R. H. Gelberman, Editor. Philadelphia: Lippincott, 1991.

Dijkstra, R., & Box, K. E. Functional results of thumb reconstruction. *Hand 14*:120-128, 1982.

Dubner, S., & Heller, K. S. Re-innervated radial forearm free flaps in head and neck reconstruction. *Journal of Reconstructive Microsurgery 8*:467-468, 1992.

Dunant, J. H. Diagnosis of thoracic outlet syndrome. *VASA 16*:345-348, 1987.

Duncan, G. J., Yospur, G., Gomez-Garcia, A., & Lesavay, M. A. Entrapment of the palmar cutaneous branch of the median nerve by a normal palmaris longus tendon. *Annals of Plastic Surgery 35*:534-536, 1995.

Dyck, P. J., Curtis, D.J., Bushek, W., & Litchy, W. J. Description of "Minnesota thermal disks" and normal values of cutaneous thermal discrimination in man. *Neurology 24*:325-330, 1974.

Dyck, P. J., Karnes, J. L., Gillen, D. A.,

O'Brien, P. C., Zimmerman, I. R., & Johnson, D. M. Comparison of algorithms of testing for use in automated evaluation of sensation. *Neurology 40*:1607-1613, 1990.

Dyck, P. J., Karnes, J. L., O'Brien, P. C., & Zimmerman, I. R. Detection thresholds of cutaneous sensation in humans. In *Peripheral Neuropathy*, 3rd edition, P. J. Dyck, P. K. Thomas, J. W. Griffin, P. A. Low, & J. F. Poduslo, Editors. Philadelphia: W. B. Saunders Company, 1993.

Dyck, P. J., Thomas, P. K., Asbury, A. K., Winegrad, A. I., & Porte, D. J., Jr. *Diabetic Neuropathy.* Philadelphia: W. B. Saunders Company, 1987.

Dyck, P. J., Thomas, P. K., Lambert, E. H., Bunge, R., Editors, *Peripheral Neuropathy*, Second Edition. Philadelphia: W. B. Saunders Company, 1984.

Dyck, P. J., Zimmerman, I. R., Gillen, D. A., Johnson, D., Karnes, J. L., & O'Brien, P. C. Warm, and heat-pain detection thresholds: Testing methods and inferences about anatomic distribution of receptors. *Neurology 43*:1500-1508, 1993.

Dyck, P. J., Zimmerman, I. R., O'Brien, P. C., Ness, A., Caskey, P. E., Karnes, J., & Bushek, W. Introduction of automated systems to evaluate touch-pressure, vibration, and thermal cutaneous sensation in man. *Annals of Neurology 4*:502-510, 1978.

Dykes, R. W., & Terzis, J. K. Reinnervation of glabrous skin in baboons: Properties of cutaneous mechanoreceptors subsequent to nerve crush. *Journal of Neurophysiology 42*:1461-1478, 1979.

• E •

Ebeling, P., Gilliatt, R. W., & Thomas, D. K. A clinical and electrical study of ulnar nerve lesions in the hand. *Journal of Neurology, Neurosurgery, and Psychiatry 23*:1-9, 1960.

Edwards, E. A. Surgical anatomy of the breast. In *Plastic and Reconstructive Surgery of the Breast*, R. M. Goldwyn, Editor. Boston: Little, Brown & Company, Inc., 1976.

Edwards, R. H. Hypothesis of peripheral and central mechanisms underlying occupational muscle pain and injury. *European Journal of Applied Physiology and Occupational Physiology 57*:275-281, 1988.

Eisen, A., & Danen, J. The mild cubital tunnel syndrome. *Neurology 24*:608-613, 1974.

Ellenberg, M. Impotence in diabetes: The neurologic factor. *Annals of Internal Medicine 75*:213-219, 1971.

Enna, C. D. Neurolysis and transposition of the ulnar nerve in leprosy. *Journal of Neurosurgery 40*:734-737, 1974.

Erlanger, J., & Gasser, H. S. *Electrical Signs of Nervous Activity.* Philadelphia: University of Pennsylvania Press, 1937.

Evans, G. R. D., Crawley, W., & Dellon, A. L. Inferior alveolar nerve grafting: An approach without intermaxillary fixation. *Annals of Plastic Surgery 33*:221-224, 1994.

Evans, G. R. D., & Dellon, A. L. Implantation of palmar cutaneous branch of the median nerve into the pronator quadratus for treatment of painful neuroma. *Journal of Hand Surgery 19A*:203-206, 1944.

• F •

Farina, M. A., Newby, B. G., & Alani, H. M. Innervation of the nipple-areola complex. *Plastic and Reconstructive Surgery 66*:497-501, 1980.

Federal Register, Volume 54, Number 16, January 26, 1989.

Feierstein, M. S. The performance and usefulness of nerve conduction studies in the orthopedic office. *Orthopedic Clinics of North America 19*:859-866, 1989.

Felderman, R. G., Goldman, R., & Kyeserling, W. M. Peripheral nerve entrapment syndromes and ergonomic factors. *American Journal of Industrial Medicine 4*:661-681, 1983.

Feldman, R. G., Travers, P. H., Chirico-Post, J., & Keyserling, W. M. Risk assessment in electronic assembly workers: Carpal tunnel syndrome. *Journal of Hand Surgery 12A*:849-855, 1987.

Fess, E. E. Documentation: essential elements of an upper extremity assessment battery. In *Rehabilitation of the Hand: Surgery and Therapy*, J. M. Hunter, L. H. Schneider, E. J. Mackin, & A. D. Callahan, Editors. St. Louis: Mosby, 1985.

Fess, E. E., Harmon, K. S., & Strickland, J. W. Evaluation of the hand by objective measurement. In *Rehabilitation of the Hand: Surgery and Therapy*, J. M. Hunter, L. H. Schneider, E. J. Mackin, & A. D. Callahan, Editors. St. Louis: C. V. Mosby Company, 1978.

Fiala, T. G. S., Lee, W. P. A., & May, J. W., Jr. Augmentation mammoplasty: Results of a patient survey. *Annals of Plastic Surgery 30*:503-509, 1993.

Fine, E. J., & Wongjirad, C. The ulnar flexion maneuver. *Muscle and Nerve 8*:612, 1985.

Finger, S., & Almli, C. R. Brain damage and neuroplasticity: Mechanisms of recovery or development? *Brain Research Review 10*:177-186, 1985.

Fish, J. S., Bain, J. R., McKee, N., & Mackinnon, S. E. The peripheral nerve allograft in the primate immunosuppressed with cyclosporin A: II. Functional evaluation of reinnervated muscle. *Plastic and Reconstructive Surgery 90*:1047-1052, 1992.

Foucher, G., Merle, M., Maneaud, M., & Michon, J. Microsurgical free partial toe transfer in hand construction: A report of 12 cases. *Plastic and Reconstructive Surgery*

65:616-626, 1980.

Fox, J. C., & Klemperer, W. W. Vibratory sensibility. *Archives of Neurology and Psychology 48*:622-645, 1942.

Francel, T. J., Dellon, A. L., & Campbell, J. N. Quadrilateral space syndrome. *Plastic and Reconstructive Surgery 87*:911-916, 1991.

Franzblau, A., Werner, R. A., Johnston, E., & Torrey, S. Evaluation of current perception threshold testing as a screening procedure for carpal tunnel syndrome among industrial workers. *Journal of Occupational Medicine 36*:1015-1021, 1994.

Friedman, R. M., Rohrich, R. J., & Finn, S. S. Management of traumatic supraorbital neuroma. *Annals of Plastic Surgery 28*:573-574, 1992.

Freilinger, G., Holle, J., & Sulzgruber, S. C. Distribution of motor and sensory fibers in the intercostal nerves: Significance in reconstructive surgery. *Plastic and Reconstructive Surgery 62*:240-244, 1978.

Frykman, G. K., O'Brien, B. McC., Morrison, W. A., & MacLeod, A. M. Functional evaluation of the hand and foot after one-stage toe-to-hand transfer. *Journal of Hand Surgery 11A*:9-17, 1986.

Fucci, D., Harris, D., & Petrosino, L. Sensation magnitude scales for vibrotactile stimulation of the tongue and thenar eminence. *Perception and Motor Skills 58*:843-848, 1984.

• G •

Gaul, J. S., Jr. Electrical fascicle identification as an adjunct to nerve repair. *Hand Clinics 2*:709-722, 1986.

Gelberman, R. H. *Operative Nerve Repair and Reconstruction*. Philadelphia: J. B. Lippincott Company, 1991.

Gelberman, R. H., Hergenroeder, P. T., Hargens, A. R., Lundborg, G. N., & Akeson, W. H. The carpal tunnel syndrome: A study of carpal canal pressures. *Journal of Bone and Joint Surgery 63A*:380-383, 1981.

Gelberman, R. H., Urbaniak, J. R., & Bright, D. S. Digital sensibility following replantation. *Journal of Hand Surgery* 3:313-319, 1978.

Gelfan, S., & Carter, S. Muscle sense in man. *Experimental Neurology* 18:469-473, 1967.

Gellman, H., Chandler, D. R., Petrasek, J., Sie, J., Adkins, R., & Waters, R. L. Carpal tunnel syndrome in paraplegic patients. *Journal of Bone and Joint Surgery* 70A:517-519, 1988.

Gerr, F. E., Hershman, D., & Letz, R. Vibrotactile threshold measurement for detecting neurotoxicity: Reliability and determination of age- and height-standardized normative values. *Archives of Environmental Health* 45:148-154, 1990.

Gerr, F. E., & Letz, R. Reliability of a widely used test of peripheral cutaneous vibration sensitivity and a comparison of two testing protocols. *British Journal of Industrial Medicine* 45:635-639, 1988.

Gerstenberg, T. C., & Bradley, W. E. Nerve conduction velocity measurement of dorsal nerve of penis in normal and impotent males. *Journal of Urology* 21:90-92, 1983.

Gilbert, D. A., Williams, M. W., & Horton, C. E., Terzis, J. P., & Devine, A. Phallic reinnervation via the pudendal nerve. *Journal of Urology* 140:295-299, 1988.

Gilbert, J. C., & Knowlton, R. G. Simple method to determine sincerity of effort during a maximal isometric test of grip strength. *American Journal of Physical Medicine* 62:135-144, 1983.

Gilliatt, R. W., LeQuesne, P. M., Logue, V., & Sumner, A. J. Wasting of the hand associated with cervical rib or band. *Journal of Neurology, Neurosurgery and Psychiatry* 33:615-618, 1970.

Gilliatt, R. W., & Thomas, P. K. Changes in nerve conduction with ulnar nerve lesions at the elbow. *Journal of Neurology, Neurosurgery, and Psychiatry* 23:312-320, 1960.

Gilliatt, R. W., & Wilson, R. G. Peripheral nerve conduction in diabetic neuropathy. *Journal of Neurology, Neurosurgery, and Psychiatry* 25:11-16, 1962.

Gilmore, J. E., Allen J. A., & Hayes, J. R. Autonomic function in neuropathic diabetic patients with foot ulceration. *Diabetes Care* 16:61, 1993.

Glasby, M. A., Gschmeissner, S. E., Hitchcock, R. J. I., & Huang, C. L. H. The dependence of nerve regeneration through muscle grafts in the rat on the availability and orientation of basement membrane. *Journal of Neurocytology* 15:497-510, 1986.

Glickman, L. T., & Mackinnon, S. E. Sensory recovery following digital replantation. *Microsurgery* 11:236-240, 1990.

Goldie, B. S., Coates, C. J., Birch, R. The long-term results of digital nerve repair in no-man's land. *Journal of Hand Surgery* 17B:75-77, 1992.

Goldner, J. L. *Upper Extremity Reconstructive Surgery in Cerebral Palsy or Similar Conditions*. American Academy of Orthopedic Surgery Instruction Course Lecture, 18:169-177, 1961.

Gombault, A. Contribution á l'étude anatomique de la névrite parenchymateuse subaigue et chronique-névrite segmentaire peri-axile. *Archives of Neurology (Paris)* 1:11, 1880.

Gonzalez, F., Brown, F. E., Gold, M. E., Walton, R. L., & Schafer, B. Pre-operative and post-operative nipple-areola sensibility in patients undergoing reduction mammoplasty. *Plastic and Reconstructive Surgery* 92:809-814, 1993.

Gonzalez, F., Schafer, B., Walton, R. L., & Bora, G. Reduction mammoplasty improves the symptoms of macromastia. *Plastic and Reconstructive Surgery* 91:1265-1270, 1993.

Goodgold, J., Koeppel, H. P., & Sprelholz, N. I. The tarsal tunnel syndrome: Objective diagnostic criteria. *New England Journal of Medicine* 173:742-745, 1965.

Goodman, H. V., & Gilliatt, R. W. The effect of treatment on median nerve conduction in patients with the carpal tunnel syndrome. *Annals of Physical Medicine* 6:137-155, 1961.

Gottschalk, P. G., Dyck, P. J., & Kiely, J. M.

Vinca alkaloid neuropathy: Nerve biopsy studies in rats and in man. *Neurology 18*:875-882, 1968.

Grafin, S. R., Botte, M. J., & Waters, R. L. Complications associated with the use of the halo fixation device. *Journal of Bone and Joint Surgery 68*:320-325, 1986.

Graham, B., & Dellon, A. L. Sensory recovery in innervated free-tissue transfers. *Journal of Reconstructive Microsurgery 11*:157-166, 1995.

Gregg, E. C., Jr. Absolute measurement of the vibratory threshold. *Archives of Neurology and Psychology 66*:403-411, 1951.

Grigg, P., Finerman, G. A., & Riley, L. H. Joint-position sense after total hip replacement. *Journal of Bone and Joint Surgery 5 5A*:1061-1025, 1973.

Grigg, P., & Greenspan, B. J. Response of primate joint afferent neurons to mechanical stimulation of knee joint. *Journal of Neurophysiology 40*:1-8, 1977.

Grunert, B. K., Wertsch, J. J., Matloub, H. S., & McCallum-Burke, S. Reliability of sensory threshold measurement using a digital vibrogram. *Journal of Occupational Medicine 32*:100-102, 1990.

Guide to Impairment, 3rd edition, American Medical Association, Chicago, 1990.

Guy, R. J. C., Clark, C. A., Malcolm, P. N., & Watkins, P. J. Evaluation of thermal and vibration sensation in diabetic neuropathy. *Diabetologia 38*:131-137, 1985.

● **H** ●

Hadler, N. M. Cumulative trauma disorders: An iatrogenic concept. *Journal of Occupational Medicine 32*:38-41, 1990.

—— *Occupational Musculoskeletal Disorders.* New York: Raven Press, 1993.

Hagberg, M., & Wegman, D. H. Prevalence rates and odds ratios of shoulder neck diseases in different occupational groups. *British Journal of Industrial Medicine 44*:602-610, 1987.

Halata, Z. The sensory innervation of the glans penis and the prepuce in man (an ultrastructural study). In *Sensory Receptor Mechanisms*, W. Hamann & A. Iggo, Editors. Singapore: World Scientific Publishing Co., 1984.

Halata, Z., & Munger, B. L. The neuroanatomical basis for the protopathic sensibility of the human glans penis. *Brain Research 371*:205-230, 1986.

Hammarback, J. A., Palm, S. L., Furct, L. T., & Letourneau, P. C. Guidance of neurite growth by pathways of substra absorbed lamini. *Journal of Neuroscience Research 13*:213-222, 1985.

Hardy, M. A., Jimenez, S., Jabaley, M., & Horch, K. Evaluation of nerve compression with the automated tactile tester. *Journal of Hand Surgery 17A*:838-842, 1992.

Hardy, M. A., Moran, C. A., & Merritt, W. H. Desensitization of the traumatized hand. *Virginia Medicine 109*:134-140, 1982.

Hendler, N., & Fenton, J. A. *Coping with Chronic Pain.* New York: Clarkson N. Potter Publishers, 1979.

Hendler, N., Mollett, A., Talo, S., & Levin, S. A comparison between the Minnesota Multiphasic Personality Inventory and the Mensana Clinic Back Pain Test for validating the complaint of chronic back pain. *Journal of Occupational Medicine 30*:98-102, 1988.

Hetter, G. P. Satisfactions and dissatisfactions of patients with augmentation mammaplasty. *Plastic and Reconstructive Surgery 64*:151-154, 1979.

Higgs, P. E., Edwards, D., Martin, D. S., & Weeks, P. M. Carpal tunnel surgery outcome in workers. *Journal of Hand Surgery,* in press: 1995.

Hildreth, D. H., Briedenbach, W. C., Lister, G. D., & Hodges, A. D. Detection of submaximal effort by use of the rapid exchange grip. *Journal of Hand Surgery 14A*:742-745, 1989.

Hjortsberg, U., Rosen, I., & Orbaek, P. Finger receptor dysfunction in dental technicians exposed to high-frequency vibration. *Scandinavian Journal of Work, Environment and Health 15*:339-343, 1989.

Hoffman, L. B., Baker, L., & Reed, R. Sensory disturbances in children with infantile hemiplegia, triplegia, and quadriplegia. *American Journal of Physical Medicine 38*:1-8, 1958.

Holewski, J. Aesthesiometry: Quantification of cutaneous pressure sensation in diabetic peripheral neuropathy. *Journal of Rehabilitation Research and Development 25*:1, 1988.

Holewski, J., Stess, R. M., Graff, P. M., & Grunfeld, C. Aesthesiometry: Quantification of cutaneous pressure sensation in diabetic peripheral neuropathy. *Journal of Rehabilitation Research and Development 25*:1-10, 1988.

Horch, K., Hardy, M., Jimenez, S., & Jabaley, M. An automated tactile tester for evaluation of cutaneous sensibility. *Journal of Hand Surgery 17A*:829-837, 1992.

Houpt, P., Dikstra, R., & van Leeuwen, J. B. S. The result of breast reconstruction after mastectomy for breast cancer in 109 patients. *Annals of Plastic Surgery 21*:517-525, 1988.

Howell, A. E., & Leach, R. E. Bowler's thumb. *Journal of Bone and Joint Surgery 52A*:379-382, 1970.

Hulliger, M., Nordh, E., & Thelin, A. E. The response of afferent fibers from the glabrous skin of the hand during voluntary finger movements in man. *Journal of Physiology 291*:233-249, 1979.

Hunter, J. M., Schneider, L. H., Mackin, E. J., & Callahan, A. *Rehabilitation of the Hand,* 1st Edition. Philadelphia: C. V. Mosby, 1978.

—— *Rehabilitation of the Hand,* 4th Edition, 1994.

Hymovich, L., & Lindholm, M. Hand, wrist, and forearm injuries. *Journal of Occupational Medicine 8*:573-577, 1966.

• **I** •

Ide, C. Nerve regeneration through the basal lamina scaffold of the skeletal muscle. *Journal of Neuroscience Research 1*:379-391, 1984.

Iggo, A. New specific sensory structures in hairy skin. *Acta Neurosurgery 24*:175-180, 1963.

Iggo, A., & Muir, A. R. The structure and function of a slowly adapting touch corpuscle in hairy skin. *Journal of Physiology 200*:763-796, 1969.

Imai, H., Tajima, T., & Natsuma, Y. Interpretation of cutaneous pressure threshold (Semmes-Weinstein monofilament measurement) following median nerve repair and sensory re-education. *Microsurgery 10*:142-145, 1989.

—— Successful re-education of functional sensibility after median nerve repair at the wrist. *Journal of Hand Surgery 16A*:60-65, 1991.

• **J** •

Jackson, P., & Diamond, J. Colchicine block of cholinesterase transport in rabbit sensory nerves without interference with the long-term viability of the axons. *Brain 130*:579-584, 1977.

Jakobsen, J. Peripheral nerves in early experimental diabetes: Expansion of the endoneurial space as a cause of increased water content. *Diabetologia 14*:113-119, 1978.

Jakobsen, J., & Sidenius, P. Decrease in axonal transport of structural proteins in streptozotocin diabetic rats. *Journal of Clinical Investigation 66*:292-296, 1980.

Jarvinen, T., & Kuorinka, I. Prevalence of tenosynovitis and other occupational injuries of upper extremities in repetitive work. *Arh Hig Rada Toksikol 30*:1281-1284, 1979.

Jenkins, W. M., Merzenich, M. M., Ochs, M., Allard, T. T., & Guic-Robles, E. Functional reorganization of primary somatosensory cortex in adult owl monkeys after behaviorally controlled tactile stimulation. *Journal of Neurophysiology 63*:82-104, 1990.

Jetzer, T. C. Use of vibration testing in the early evaluation of workers with carpal tunnel syndrome. *Journal of Occupational Medicine 33*:117-120, 1991.

Jiang, W., Chapman, C. E., & Lamarre, Y. Modulation of the cutaneous responsiveness of neurones in the primary somatosensory cortex during conditioned arm movements in the monkey. *Experimental Brain Research 84*:342-354, 1991.

Johnson, C. Treating the hands that make music. *Journal of Hand Therapy 5*:58-60, 1992.

Johnson, M. E., Chao, E. Y. S., & Cooney, W. P. III. Computer-assisted pinch and grip strength measurements; Normative values using a non-hydraulic system. *Journal of Hand Therapy*, submitted: 1994.

Johnson, S. L. Ergonomic design of hand-held tools to prevent trauma to the hand and upper extremity. *Journal of Hand Therapy* April-June:86-92, 1990.

Joughin, K., Gulati, P. Mackinnon, S. E., McCabe, S., Murray, J. F., Griffiths, S., & Richards, R. An evaluation of rapid exchange and simultaneous grip tests. *Journal of Hand Surgery 18A*:245-252, 1993.

• K •

Kaas, J. H. Plasticity of sensory and motor maps in adult mammals. *Annual Review of Neuroscience 14*:137-161, 1991.

Kallio, P. K. The results of secondary repair of 254 digital nerves. *Journal of Hand Surgery 18B*:327-330, 1993.

Kallio, P. K., & Vastamaki, M. An analysis of the results of late reconstruction of 132 median nerves. *Journal of Hand Surgery 18B*:97-105, 1993.

Kaplan, M., Dellon, A. L., Mullick, T., & Hendler, N. Somatosensory evoked potentials in diagnosis of brachial plexus compression in the thoracic inlet. Presented at the American Society of Peripheral Nerve, October 1995, Montreal. *Journal of Hand Surgery*, submitted: 1995.

Kaplan, M., Mullick, T., Dellon, A. L., & Hendler, N. Value of somatosensory evoked potentials in the diagnosis of brachial plexus compression in the thoracic inlet (thoracic outlet syndrome). *Journal of Hand Surgery*, submitted: 1995.

Kaplan, P. E., & Kernahan, W. T. Tarsal tunnel syndrome: An electrodiagnostic and surgical correlation. *Journal of Bone and Joint Surgery 63A*:96-99, 1981.

Kasdan, M. *Occupational Hand and Upper Extremity Injuries and Diseases*. Philadelphia: Hanley & Belfus, 1991.

Katims, J. J., Naviasky, E., Ng, L. K. Y., Bleecker, M. L., & Rendell, M. New screening device for the assessment of peripheral neuropathy. *Journal of Occupational Medicine 28*:1219-1221, 1986.

Katims, J. J., Naviasky, E. H., Rendell, M. S., Ng, L. K. Y., & Bleecker, M. I. Constant current sine wave transcutaneous nerve stimulation for the evaluation of peripheral neuropathy. *Archives of Physical Medicine and Rehabilitation 68*:210-213, 1987.

Katims, J. J., Patil, A. S., Rendell, M., Rouvelas, P., Sadler, B., Weseley, S. A., & Bleecker, M. L. Current perception threshold screening for carpal tunnel syndrome. *Archives of Environmental Health 46*:207-212, 1991.

Kaye, B. L. Neurologic changes associated with macromastia. *Southern Medical Journal 65*:177-180, 1972.

Kendall, H. O., & Kendall, F. P. *Muscles: Testing and Function*. Baltimore: Williams & Wilkins, 1949.

Kennard, M. A. Age and other factors in motor recovery from precentral lesions in the monkey. *American Journal of Physiology 115*:138-146, 1936.

Kesarwani, A., Antonyshyn, O., Mackinnon, S. E., Gruss, J. S., Novak, C., & Kelly, L. Facial sensibility testing in the normal and posttraumatic population. *Annals of Plastic Surgery 22*:416-421, 1989.

Kilbom, A., Persson, I., & Jonsson, B. G. Disorders of the cervicobrachial region among female workers in the electronics industry. *International Journal of Ergonomics 1:*37-47, 1986.

Kimura, J. A method for determining median nerve conduction velocity across the carpal tunnel. *Journal of Neurological Sciences 38:*1-10, 1978.

—— *Electrodiagnosis in diseases of nerve and muscle.* Philadelphia: F. A. Davis Company, 1983.

King, J. W. An integration of medicine and industry. *Journal of Hand Therapy April-June:*45-50, 1990.

Kirkpatrick, J. Evaluation of grip loss: A factor of permanent partial disability in California. *Industrial Medicine and Surgery 26:*285-289, 1957.

Kline, D. G., Hackett, E. R., & May, P. Evaluation of nerve injuries by evoked potentials and electromyography. *Journal of Neurosurgery 31:*136-138, 1969.

Kline, D. G., & Judice, D. J. Operative management
of selected brachial plexus lesions. *Journal of Neurosurgery 58:*631-649, 1983.

Kofkin, J., Tobin, M., &
Dellon, A. L. Dynamic
elbow splint following
tendon transfer to restore triceps function. *American Journal of Occupational Therapy 34:*680-681, 1980.

Krane, R. J., & Siroky, M. B. Studies on sacral evoked potentials. *Journal of Urology 124:*872-877, 1980.

Kress, K., Dellon, E. S., Moratz, V., & Dellon, A. L. Relationship between skin hardness and human touch perception. *Restorative Neurology Neuroscience,* in press: 1993.

Kroner, K., Krebs, B., Skov, J., & Jorgensen, H. S. Immediate and long-term phantom breast syndrome after mastectomy: Incidence, clinical characteristics, and relationship to pre-mastectomy breast pain. *Pain 36:*327-324, 1989.

Kuhn, R.A. Functional capacity of the isolated human spinal cord. *Brain 73:*1-6, 1950.

• **L** •

LaMotte, R. H., & Mountcastle, V. B. Disorders in somesthesia following lesions of parietal lobe. *Journal of Neurophysiology 42:*400-419, 1979.

Lampert, P. W., & Schochet, S. S., Jr. Demyelination and remyelination in lead neuropathy. *Journal of Neuropathology and Experimental Neurology 27:*527, 1968.

Laquerriere, A., Peulve, P., & Jin, O. Effect of basic fibroblast growth factor and alpha-melanocytic stimulating hormone on nerve regeneration through a collagen channel. *Microsurgery 15:*203-210, 1994.

Law, M., & Baum, C. M. *Creating the future: A joint effort.* Health Care Brochure, 1994.

Lebedev, L. V., Bogomolov, M. S., Vavylov, V. N., Slomin, V. V., Tokavetich, K. K., Yustaev, E. A., Garbunov, G. N., Dadalov, M. I. Long-term results of hand function after digital replantation. *Annals of Plastic Surgery 31:*322-326, 1993.

Leffert, R. D. Thoracic outlet syndromes. *Hand Clinics 8:*285-291, 1992.

Letourneau, P. C. Neurite extension by peripheral and central nervous system neurons in response to substratum bound fibronectin and laminin. *Developmental Biology 98:*212-215, 1983.

Levin, L. S., & Dellon, A. L. Pathology of the shoulder as it relates to the differential diagnosis of thoracic outlet compression. *Journal of Reconstructive Microsurgery 8:*313-317, 1992.

Levin, S., Pearsall, G., Ruderman, R. J. von Frey's method of measuring pressure sensibility in the hand: An engineering analysis of the Weinstein-Semmes pressure aesthesiometer. *Journal of Hand Surgery 3:*211-216, 1978.

Lin, J. T., & Bradley, W. E. Penile neuropathy in insulin-dependent diabetes mellitus. *Journal of Urology 133:*213-215, 1985.

Lindquist, C. C., & Obeid, G. Complications of genioplasty done alone or in combination with sagittal split ramus osteotomy. *Journal of Oral Surgery 66:*13-17, 1988.

Liss, G. M., Armstrong, C., Kusiak, R. A., & Gailitis, M. M. Use of provincial health insurance plan billing data to estimate carpal tunnel syndrome morbidity and surgery rates. *American Journal of Industrial Medicine 22*:395-409, 1992.

Lister, G. *The Hand: Diagnosis and Indications*. Edinburgh: Churchill Livingstone, 1977.

—— *The Hand: Diagnosis and Indications*. 3rd edition. Edinburgh: Churchill Livingstone, Inc., 1993.

Lister, G. D., Belsoe, R. B., & Kleinert, H. E. The radial tunnel syndrome. *Journal of Hand Surgery 4*:52-59, 1979.

Liu, S., Kopacz, D. J., & Carpenter, R. L. Quantitative assessment of differential sensory nerve block after lidocaine spinal anesthesia. *Anesthesiology 82*:60-63, 1995.

Loi, F., Battista, G., & Malentacchi, G. M. Familial lead poisoning from contaminated wine. *Italian Journal of Neurological Sciences 3*:283-290, 1981.

Louis, D. S. A historical perspective of workers and the work place. In *Occupational Disorders of the Upper Extremity*, L. H. Millender, D. S. Louis, & B. P. Simmonds, Editors. New York: Churchill Livingstone, 1992.

Lowe, M. A., Chapman, W., & Berger, R. E. Repair of a traumatically amputated penis with return of erectile function. *Journal of Urology 145*:1267-1270, 1991.

Lowenthal, L. M., & Hockaday, T. D. R. Vibration sensory thresholds depend on pressure of applied stimulus. *Diabetes Care 10*:100-102, 1987.

Lue, T. F., Zeineh, S. J., Schmidt, R. A., & Tanagho, E. A. Neuroanatomy of penile erection: Its relevance to iatrogenic impotence. *Journal of Urology 131*:273-280, 1984.

Lundborg, G. *Nerve Injury and Repair*. Edinburgh: Churchill Livingstone, 1988.

—— Structure and function of the intraneural microvessels as related to trauma, edema formation and nerve function. *Journal of Bone Joint Surgery 57A*:938-948, 1975.

Lundborg, G., Dahlin, L. B., Lundstrom, R., Necking, L. E. & Stromberg, T. Vibrotactile function of the hand in compression and vibration-induced neuropathy. Sensibility index — A new measure. *Scandinavian Journal of Plastic Reconstructive Surgery and Hand Surgery 26*:275-281, 1992.

Lundborg, G., Lie-Stenstrom, A. K., Sollerman, C., Stromberg, T., & Pyykko, L. Digital vibrogram: A new diagnostic tool for sensory testing in compression neuropathy. *Journal of Neurology, Neurosurgery and Psychiatry 11A*:693-699, 1986.

• M •

Ma, H. S., El-Gammal, T. A., & Wei, F. C. Current concepts of toe-to-hand transfer: Surgery and Rehabilitation. *Journal of Hand Therapy*, in press: 1996.

MacDermid, J. C., Kramer, J. F., Woodbury, M. G., McFarlane, R. M., & Roth, J. H. Interrater reliability of pinch and grip strength measurements in patients with cumulative trauma disorders. *Journal of Hand Therapy 7*:10-14, 1994.

Mackinnon, S. E. Double and multiple "crush" syndromes. *Hand Clinics 8*:369-390, 1992.

—— Invited discussion on nerve allografting. *Annals of Plastic Surgery 33*:516-517, 1994.

Mackinnon, S. E., & Dellon, A. L. Clinical nerve reconstruction with a bioabsorbable polyglycolic acid tube. *Plastic and Reconstructive Surgery 85*:419-424, 1990.

—— Experimental study of chronic nerve compression: Clinical implications. *Clinics of Hand Surgery 2*:639-650, 1986.

—— Homologies between the tarsal and carpal tunnels: Implications for surgical treatment in the tarsal tunnel syndrome. *Contemporary Orthopedics 14*:75-78, 1987.

—— Multiple Crush Syndrome. In *Surgery of the Peripheral Nerve*. New York: Thieme, 1988.

—— Overlap of lateral antebrachial cutaneous nerve and superficial sensory radial nerve. *Journal of Hand Surgery 10A*:522-526, 1985.

—— Results of treatment of recurrent dorso-radial wrist neuromas. *Annals of Plastic Surgery 19*:54-61, 1987.

—— *Surgery of the Peripheral Nerve*. New York: Thieme, 1988.

—— Tarsal Tunnel Syndrome. In *Surgery of the Peripheral Nerve*, New York: Thieme, 1988.

—— Terminal branch of anterior interosseous nerve as source of wrist pain. *Journal of Hand Surgery 9B*:316-322, 1984.

—— Tibial nerve branching in the tarsal tunnel. *Archives of Neurology 41*:645-646, 1984.

—— Two-point discrimination tester. *Journal of Hand Surgery 10*:906-907, 1985.

Mackinnon, S. E., Dellon, A. L., Hudson, A. R., & Hunter, D. A. A primate model for chronic nerve compression. *Journal of Reconstructive Microsurgery 1*:185-194, 1985.

—— Alteration of neuroma formation by manipulation of neural microenvironment. *Plastic and Reconstructive Surgery 76*:345-352, 1985.

—— Chronic nerve compression: An experimental model in the rat. *Annals of Plastic Surgery 13*:112-120, 1984.

Mackinnon, S. E., Dellon, A. L., Lundborg, G., Hudson, A. R. & Hunter, D. A. A study of neurotropism in a primate model. *Journal of Hand Surgery 11*:888-894, 1986.

Mackinnon, S. E., & Holder, L. E. Use of three-phase radionuclide bone scanning in the diagnosis of reflex sympathetic dystrophy. *Journal of Hand Surgery 9*:556-563, 1984.

Mackinnon, S. E., & Hudson, A. R. Clinical application of peripheral nerve transplantation. *Plastic and Reconstructive Surgery 90*:695-699, 1992.

Mackinnon, S.E., & Novak, C.B. Clinical commentary: Pathogenesis of cumulative trauma disorder. *Journal of Hand Surgery 19A*:873-883, 1994.

—— Hypothesis: Pathogenesis of cumulative trauma disorder. *Journal of Hand Surgery*, in press: 1994.

Margolis, W., & Kraus, J. F. The prevalence of carpal tunnel syndrome symptoms in female supermarket checkers. *Journal of Occupational Medicine 29*:952-955, 1987.

Markowski, J., Wilcox, J. P., & Helm, P. A. Lymphedema incidence after specific postmastectomy therapy. *Archives of Physical Medicine and Rehabilitation 62*:449-452, 1981.

Marshall, W. H., Woolsey, C. N., & Bard, P. Observations on cortical somatic sensory mechanisms of cat and monkey. *Journal of Neurophysiology 4*:1-24, 1941.

Masear, V. R., Hayes, J. M., & Hyde, A. G. An industrial cause of carpal tunnel syndrome. *Journal of Hand Surgery 11*:222-227, 1986.

Masson, D. A. Lingual nerve damage following lower third molar surgery. *International Journal of Oral Maxillofacial Surgery 17*:290-294, 1988.

Masson, E. A., & Boulton, A. J. M. The neurometer: Validation and comparison with conventional tests for diabetic neuropathy. *Diabetes Medicine 8*:63-366, 1991.

Masson, V. E., Veves, A., Fernando, D. J. S., & Boulton, A. J. M. Current perception thresholds: A new, quick, and reproducible method for the assessment of peripheral neuropathy in diabetes mellitus. *Diabetologia 32*:724-728, 1989.

Mathiowetz, V. Grip-strength measurement: A comparison of three Jamar Dynamometers. *Occupational Therapy Journal of Research 7*:235-243, 1987.

Mathiowetz, V., Rennels, C., & Donahoe, L. Effect of elbow position on grip and key pinch strength. *Journal of Hand Surgery 10A*:694-697, 1985.

Mathiowetz, V., Weber, K., & Volland, G. Reliability and validity of grip and pinch strength evaluations. *Journal of Hand Surgery 9*:222-226, 1984.

Maxwell, G. P., & Tornambe, R. Second- and third-degree burns as a complication in breast reconstruction. *Annals of Plastic*

Surgery 22:386-390, 1989.

May, J. W., Halls, M. J., & Simon, S. R. Free microvascular muscle flaps with skin graft reconstruction of extensive defects of the foot: A clinical and gait analysis study. *Plastic and Reconstructive Surgery* 75:627-632, 1985.

Maynard, J. Sensory re-education after peripheral nerve injury. In *Rehabilitation of the Hand: Surgery and Therapy*, J. M. Hunter, E. J. Mackin, L. H. Schneider, & A. D. Callahan, Editors. Baltimore: Williams & Wilkins, 1977.

McAtamney, L., & Corlett, E. N. RULA: A survey method for the investigation of work-related upper limb disorders. *Applied Ergonomics* 24:91-99, 1993.

McCroskey, R. L., Jr. The relative contribution of auditory and tactile cues to certain aspects of speech. *Southern Speech Journal* 24:84-90, 1958.

McFarlane, R. M., & Moyer, J. R. Digital nerve grafts with the lateral antebrachial cutaneous nerve. *Journal of Hand Surgery* 1:169-173, 1976.

McGough, E. C., Pearce, M. B., & Byrne, J. P. Management of thoracic outlet syndrome. *Journal of Therapeutics & Cardiovascular Medicine* 77:169-174, 1979.

McGowan, A. J. Results of transposition of the ulnar nerve for traumatic ulnar neuritis. *Journal of Bone and Joint Surgery* 32B:293-301, 1950.

McLeod, J. G., Hargrave, J. C., Gye, R. S., & Sedal, L. Nerve grafting in leprosy. *Brain* 98:203-212, 1975.

Meals, R. A., Rob, C. A., & Nelissen, G. H. H. The origin and meaning of "neurotization." *Journal of Hand Surgery* 20A:144-146, 1995.

Medical Problems of the Performing Arts (a journal). Philadelphia: Hanley & Belfus, Inc., 1993.

Melzak, R. The McGill Pain Questionnaire: Major properties and scoring methods. *Pain* 1:277-299, 1975.

Merrill, R. G. Prevention, treatment and prognosis for nerve injury related to the difficult impaction. *Dental Clinics - North America* 23:471-488, 1979.

Merzenich, M. M., & Harrington, T. The sense of flutter-vibration evoked by stimulation of the hairy skin of primates: Comparison of human sensory capacity with the responses of mechanoreceptive afferents innervating the hairy skin of monkeys. *Experimental Brain Research* 9:236-260, 1969.

Merzenich, M. M., & Jenkins, W. M. Reorganization of cortical representations of the hand following alterations of skin inputs induced by nerve injury, skin island transfers, and experience. *Journal of Hand Therapy* 6:89-104, 1993.

Merzenich, M. M., Kaas, J. H., Sur, M., & Lin, C. S. Double representation of the body surface within cytoarchitectonic areas 3b and 1 in "S1" in the owl monkey (*Aortus trivirgatus*). *Journal of Comparative Neurology* 181:41-74, 1978.

Merzenich, M. M., Kaas, J. H., Wall, J. T., Sur, M., Nelson, R. J., & Fellerman, D. J. Progression of change following median nerve section in the cortical representation of the hand in areas 3b and 1 in adult owl and squirrel monkeys. *Neuroscience* 10:639-665, 1983.

Merzenich, M. M., Nelson, R. J., & Kaas, J. H. Variability in hand surface representations in areas 3b and 1 in adult owl and squirrel monkeys. *Journal of Comparative Neurology* 258:281-297, 1987.

Merzenich, M. M., Nelson, R. J., Stryker, M. P., Cyndaer, M. S., Schoppmann, A., & Zook, J. M. Somatosensory cortical map changes following digit amputation in adult monkeys. *Journal of Comparative Neurology* 224:591-605, 1984.

Meyer, R. A., & Campbell, J. N. Peripheral neural coding of pain sensation. *Johns Hopkins APL Technical Digest* 2:164-171, 1981.

Meyer, R. A., Raja, S. N., Campbell, J. N., Mackinnon, S. E., & Dellon, A. L. Neural activity originating from a neuroma in the baboon. *Brain Research* 325:255-260, 1985.

Millender, L. H., Louis, D. S., & Simmonds, B. P. *Occupational Disorders of the Upper Extremity*. New York: Churchill Livingstone, 1992.

Millesi, H. Nerve grafting. *Clinics in Plastic Surgery 11*:105-120, 1984.

Millesi, H., Meisse, G., & Berger, A. The interfascicular nerve grafting of the median and ulnar nerves. *Journal of Bone and Joint Surgery 54A*:727-750, 1972.

Millesi, H., & Terzis, J. K. Nomenclature in peripheral nerve surgery. *Clinics in Plastic Surgery 11*:3-8, 1984.

Minami, A., Masamichi, V., Hiroyuki, K., & Seiichi, J. Thumb reconstruction by free sensory flaps from the foot using microsurgical techniques. *Journal of Hand Surgery (British) 9*:239-244, 1984.

Mitchell, S. W. *Injuries of Nerves and their Consequences*. American Academy of Neurology Reprint Series. New York: Dover, 1965.

Mitterhauser, M. D., Muse, V. L., Dellon, A. L., Jetzer, T. C. Detection of submaximal effort with computer-assisted grip strength measurements. *Journal of Occupational Medicine*, submitted: 1996.

Moberg, E. Aspects of sensation in reconstructive surgery of the upper extremity. *Journal of Bone and Joint Surgery 46A*:817-825, 1964.

—— Criticism in study of methods for examining sensibility in the hand. *Neurology (Minneapolis) 12*:8-19, 1962.

—— Fingers were made before forks. *Hand 4*:201-206, 1972.

——- Methods for examining sensibility of the hand. In *Hand Surgery*, J. E. Flynn, Editor. Baltimore: Williams & Wilkins, 1966.

—— Objective methods of determining functional value of sensibility in the skin. *Journal of Bone and Joint Surgery (British) 40B*:454-466, 1958.

—— Reconstructive hand surgery in tetraplegia, stroke and cerebral palsy: Some basic concepts on physiology and neurology. *Journal of Hand Surgery 1*:29-34, 1976.

—— The role of cutaneous afferents in position sense, kinaesthesia and motor function of the hand. *Brain 106*:1-12, 1984.

—— *The Upper Limb in Tetraplegia*. London: Churchill Livingstone, 1978.

—— Two-point discrimination test. *Scandinavian Journal of Rehabilitation Medicine 22*:127-134, 1990.

Mokken, R. J., & Lewis, C. A. Nonparametric approach to the analysis of dichotomous item responses. *Applied Psychology Measures 6*:417-430, 1982.

Molenaar, I. W., & Sijtsma, K. Mokkern's approach to reliability estimation extended to multicategory items. *Quantitative Methods 9*:115-126, 1988.

Mollman, J. E. Cisplatin neurotoxicity. *New England Journal of Medicine 322*:126-127, 1990.

Mondelli, M., Rossi, A., Passero, S., & Guazzi, G. C. Involvement of peripheral sensory fibers in amyotrophic lateral sclerosis: Electrophysiological study of 64 cases. *Muscle and Nerve 16*:166-172, 1993.

Montague, D. K. *Disorders of Male Sexual Function*. Chicago: Year Book Medical Publishers, 1988.

Moore, A., Wells, R., & Ranney, D. Quantifying exposure in occupational manual tasks with cumulative trauma disorder potential. *Ergonomics 34*:1433-1453, 1991.

Moran, C. A. Using myofascial techniques to treat musicians. *Journal of Hand Therapy 5*:97-101, 1992.

Mori, A., Hanashima, N., Tsuboi, Y., Hiraba, H., Goto, R., Sumino, R. Fifth somatosensory cortex (SV) representation of the whole body surface in the medial bank of the anterior suprasylvian sulcus of the cat. *Neuroscience Research 11*:198-208, 1991.

Mori, A., Yamaguchi, Y., Kikuta, R., Furukawa, T., & Sumino, R. Low threshold motor effects produced by stimulation of the facial area of the fifth somatosensory cortex in the cat. *Brain Research 602*:143-147, 1993.

Mountcastle, V. B. *Medical Physiology* 12th

edition. St. Louis: Mosby, 1968.
—— Modality and topographic properties of single neurons of cat's somatic sensory cortex. *Journal of Neurophysiology 20*:408-434, 1957.

Mountcastle, V. B., & Powell, T. P. S. Neural mechanisms subserving cutaneous sensibility with special reference to the role of afferent inhibition in sensory perception and discrimination. *Bulletin of Johns Hopkins Hospital 105*:201-232, 1959.

Mountcastle, V. B., Talbot, W. H., Darian-Smith, I., & Kornhuber, H. H. Neural basis for the sense of flutter-vibration. *Science 155*:597-600, 1967.

Munger, B. L., & Pubols, L. M. The sensorineural organization of the digital skin of the raccoon. *Brain, Behavior and Evolution 5*:367-393, 1972.

Munger, B. L., Pubols, L. M., & Pubols, B. H., Jr. The Merkel rete papilla - A slowly-adapting sensory receptor in mammalian glabrous skin. *Brain Research 29*:47-61, 1971.

• **N** •

Naff, N., Dellon, A. L., & Mackinnon, S. E. The anatomic source of the palmar cutaneous branch of the median nerve, including a description of its own unique tunnel. *Journal of Hand Surgery 18B*:316-317, 1993.

Nakada, M. Localization of a constant-touch and moving-touch stimulus in the hand: A preliminary study. *Journal of Hand Therapy 6*:23-28, 1993.

Nakada, M., & Dellon, A. L. Relationship between sensibility and ability to read braille in diabetics. *Microsurgery 10*:138-141, 1989.

Narini, P., Novak, C. B., Mackinnon, S. E., & Coulson-Ross, C. Occupational exposure to hand vibration in northern Ontario gold miners. *Journal of Hand Surgery 18A*:1051-1058, 1993.

Narita, M., & Aoki, M. Clinical study on sensory disturbance of the hand in leprosy. *Japanese Journal of Leprosy 55*:1-12, 1986.

Nathan, P. A., Keniston, R. C., Meadows, K. D., & Lockwood, R.S. Predictive value of nerve conduction measurement at the carpal tunnel. *Muscle and Nerve 16*:1377-1382, 1993.

Nathan, P. A., Keniston, R. C., Myers, L. D., & Meadows, K. D. Longitudinal study of median nerve sensory conduction in industry: Relationship to age, gender, hand dominance, occupational hand use, and clinical diagnosis. *Journal of Hand Surgery 17A*:850-857, 1992.

Neelam, S. R. Using torque arms to reduce CTDs. *Ergonomics in Design* October:25-28, 1994.

Nelson, R. J., Sur, M., Fellerman, D. J., & Kaas, J. H. Representation of the body surface in postcentral parietal cortex of Macaca fascicularis. *Journal of Comparative Neurology 192*:611-643, 1981.

Nettor, F. H. *The CIBA Collection of Medical Illustrations, Volume 1.* New Jersey: Donnelly & Sons, 1983.

Newman, H. F. Vibratory sensitivity of the penis. *Fertility and Sterility 21*:791-793, 1970.

Nishioka, G. J., Zysset, M. K., & VanSickels, J. E. Neurosensory disturbances with rigid fixation of the bilateral sagittal split osteotomy. *Journal of Oral Maxillofacial Surgery 45*:20-24, 1987.

Norris, R. *The musicians survival manual: A guide to preventing and treating injuries in instrumentalists.* St Louis: International Conference of Symphony and Opera Musicians, 1993.

Novak, C. B., Collins, E. D., & Mackinnon, S. E. Outcome following conservative management of thoracic outlet syndrome. *Journal of Hand Surgery,* 20A: 542-548, 1995.

Novak, C. B., Kelly, L., & Mackinnon, S. E. Sensory recovery after median nerve grafting. *Journal of Hand Surgery 17A*:59-66, 1992.

Novak, C. B., Mackinnon, S. E., & Kelly, L. Correlation of two-point discrimination and hand function following median nerve injury. *Annals of Plastic Surgery 31*:495-498, 1993.

Novak, C. B., Mackinnon, S. E., & Patterson, G. A. Evaluation of patients with thoracic outlet syndrome. *Journal of Hand Surgery 18A*:292-299, 1993.

Novak, C. B., Mackinnon, S. E., Williams, J. I., & Kelly, L. Development of a new measure of fine sensory function. *Plastic and Reconstructive Surgery 92*:301-311, 1993.

—— Establishment of reliability in the evaluation of hand sensibility. *Plastic and Reconstructive Surgery 92*:312-322, 1993.

● **O** ●

O'Brien Cofelice, M., Lumpkin, D., & Kerstein, M. D. Penile waveform analysis: Its usefulness in evaluating vasculogenic impotence. *Bruit 10*:242-243, 1986.

Ochoa, J., & Torebork, E. Sensations evoked by intraneural microstimulation of single mechanoreceptor units innervating the human hand. *Journal of Physiology 342*:633-654, 1983.

Ohnishi, A., Schilling, K., Brimijoin, W. S., Lambert, E. H., Fairbanks, V. F., & Dyck, P.J. Lead neuropathy. 1. Morphometry, nerve conduction and choline acetyltransferase transport: New finding of endoneurial edema associated with segmental demyelination. *Journal of Neuropathology and Experimental Neurology 36*:499, 1977.

Olmstead, C. E., & Villablanca, J. R. Effects of caudate or frontal cortex ablation in cats and kittens: Passible avoidance. *Experimental Neurology 68*:335-345, 1980.

Olmstead, C. E., Villablanca, J. R., Sonnier, B. J., McAllister, J. P., & Gomez, F. Reorganization of cerebellorubral terminal fields following hemispherectomy in adult cats. *Brain Research 274*:336-340, 1983.

Önne, L. Recovery of sensibility and submotor activity in the hand after nerve suture. *Acta Chirugia (Scandinavia) (Supplement)* *300*:1-70, 1962.

Osterman, A. L., Aversa, B. A., & Greenstein, D. Use of the Nerve Pace Electroneurometer as an affective screening tool in the diagnosis of carpal tunnel syndrome. *Journal of Hand Surgery*, in press: 1995.

● **P** ●

Padma-Nathan, H., & Levine, F. Vibration testing of the penis. *Journal of Urology 4*:201-206, 1987.

Pandya, J. N. Surgical decompression of nerves in leprosy. An attempt at prevention of deformity: A clinical, electrophysiologic, histopathologic and surgical study. *International Journal of Leprosy 46*:47-55, 1976.

Papakostopoulos, D., Cooper, R., & Crow, H. J. Inhibition of cortical evoked potentials and sensation by self-initiated movement in man. *Nature 258*:321-324, 1975.

Parsons, J. S. Tobacco-primer's wrist. *New England Journal of Medicine 305*:768, 1981.

Peet, R. M., Hendrickson, J. D., Anderson, T. P., & Martin, G. M. Thoracic outlet syndrome: Evaluation of a therapeutic exercise program. *Mayo Clinic Proceedings 31*:281-287, 1956.

Penfield, W., & Boldrey, E. Somatic motor and sensory representation in the cerebral cortex of man as studied by electrical stimulation. *Brain 60*:389-443, 1937.

Penfield, W., & Rasmussen, A. T. *The Cerebral Cortex of Man: A Clinical Study of Localization of Function.* New York: Macmillan Publishing Company, 1950.

Pennisi, E., Cruccu, G., Manfredi, M., & Palladini, G. Histometric study of myelinated fibers in the human trigeminal nerve. *Journal of Neurological Sciences 105*:22-28, 1991.

Pernkopf, Eduard. *Eduard Pernkopf's Atlas of Topographical and Applied Human Anatomy,* Helmut Ferner, Editor. Philadelphia: W. B. Saunders Company, 1963.

Peterson, R. D., Bowen, D., Netscher, D. T., & Wigoda, P. Capsular compliance: A measure of a "hard" prosthesis. *Annals of Plastic Surgery 32*:237-341, 1994.

Phalen, G. S. The carpal tunnel syndrome: Seventeen years experience in diagnosis and treatment of 654 hands. *Journal of Bone and Joint Surgery 48A*:211-228, 1966.

Poppen, N. K., McCarroll, H. K., Jr., & Doyle, J. Recovery of sensibility after suture of digital nerves. *Journal of Hand Surgery 4*:212-226, 1979.

Posnick, J. C., Al-Qattan, M. M., & Pron, G. Facial sensibility in adolescents with and without clefts one year after undergoing LeForte I osteotomy. *Plastic and Reconstructive Surgery 94*:431-435, 1994.

Posnick, J. C., Al-Qattan, M. M., Pron, G. E., & Grossman, J. A. I. Facial sensibility in adolescents born with cleft lip after undergoing repair in infancy. *Plastic and Reconstructive Surgery 93*:682-689, 1994.

Posnick, J. C., Al-Qattan, M. M., & Stepner, N. M. Facial sensibility in adolescents one year after undergoing sagittal split and chin osteotomies of the mandible. *Plastic and Reconstructive Surgery*, in press: 1996.

Posnick, J. C., Zimbler, A. G., & Grossman, J. A. I. Normal cutaneous sensibility of the face. *Plastic and Reconstructive Surgery 86*:429-433, 1990.

Powell, T. P. S., & Mountcastle, V. B. The cytoarchitecture of the post-central gyrus of the monkey *Macaca mulatta*. *Bulletin of Johns Hopkins Hospital 105*:108-131, 1959.

Pradas, J., Finison, L., Andres, P. L., Thornell, B., Hollander, D., & Munsant, T. L. Natural history of amyotrophic lateral sclerosis. *Neurology 43*:751-755, 1993.

Price, D. D., McGrath, P. A., Rafii, A., & Buckingham, B. The validation of visual analogue scales as ratio scales measures for chronic and experimental pain. *Pain 83*:45-56, 1974.

Prokop, L. L. Upper-extremity rehabilitation: Conditioning and orthotics for the athlete and performing artist. *Hand Clinics 6*:517-524, 1990.

Pubols, L. M., Pubols, B. H., Jr., & Munger, B. L. Functional properties of mechanoreceptors in glabrous skin of the raccoon's forepaw. *Experimental Neurology 31*:165-182, 1971.

• R •

Raja, S. N., Davis, K., & Campbell, J. N. Alpha-adranertic pharmacology in sympathetically-maintained pain. *Journal of Reconstructive Microsurgery 8*:63-69, 1992.

Raja, S. N., Meyer, R. A., & Campbell, J. N. Hyperalgesia and sensitization of primary afferent fibers. In *Pain Syndromes in Neurology*, H. L. Fields, Editor. London: Butterworths, 1990.

Raja, S. N., Treede, R., Davis, K. D., & Campbell, J. N. Systemic alpha-adrenergic blockade with phentolamine: A diagnostic test for sympathetically maintained pain. *Anesthesiology 74*:691-698, 1991.

Ramachandran, V. S., Rogers-Ramachandran, D., & Stewart, M. Perceptual correlates of massive cortical reorganization. *Science 258*:1159-1160, 1992.

Ramazzini, B. *DeMorbis artificum diatriba. Diseases of Workers* (W. C. Wright, Trans.). New York: Hafner Publishing Company, 1964.

Rasmussen, D. D. Reorganization of raccoon somatosensory cortex following removal of the fifth digit. *Journal of Comparative Neurology 205*:313-326, 1982.

Rautio, J., Kekoni, J., Hamalainen, H., Harma, M., & Asko-Seljavaara, S. Mechanical sensibility in free and island flaps of the foot. *Journal of Reconstructive Microsurgery 5*:119-125, 1989.

Recanzone, G. H., Jenkins, W. M., Hradek, G. M., & Merzenich, M. M. Progressive improvement in discriminative abilities in adult owl monkeys performing a tactile frequency discrimination task. *Journal of Neurophysiology 67*:1015-1030, 1992.

Recanzone, G. H., Merzenich, M. M., Jenkins, W. M., Grajski, K. A., & Dinse, H. A. Topographic reorganization of the hand representational zone in cortical area 3b paralleling improvements in frequency discrimination performance. *Journal of Neurophysiology 67*:1031-1056, 1992.

Recanzone, G. H., Merzenich, M. M., & Schreiner, C. S. Changes in the distributed temporal response properties of SI cortical neurons reflect improvements in performance on a temporally-based tactile discrimination task. *Journal of Neurophysiology 67*:1071-1091, 1992.

Research Plan for the National Center for Medical Rehabilitation on Research. National Institutes of Health Publication #93-3509, 1993.

Revill, S. I., Robinson, J. O., Rosen, M., & Hogg, M. I. J. The reliability of a linear analogue scale for evaluating pain. *Anaesthesiology 31*:1191-1198, 1976.

Riggs, J. E., Ashraf, M., Snyder, R. D., & Gutmann, L. Prospective nerve conduction studies in cisplatin therapy. *Annals of Neurology 23*:92-94, 1988.

Ringel, R. L., & Steer, M. D. Some effects of tactile and auditory alterations on speech output. *Journal of Speech and Hearing Research 6*:369-378, 1963.

Robertson, S. L., & Jones, L. A. Tactile sensory impairments and prehensile function in subjects with left-hemisphere cerebral lesions. *Archives of Physical Medicine and Rehabilitation 75*:1108-1117, 1994.

Robinson, P. P., Smith, K. G., Johnson, F. P., & Coppins, D. A. Equipment and methods for simple sensory testing. *British Journal of Oral Maxillofacial Surgery 30*:387-389, 1992.

Roelofs, R. I., Hrushessky, W., & Roghn, J. Peripheral sensory neuropathy and cisplatin chemotherapy. *Neurology 34*:934-938, 1984.

Rood, J. P. Degrees of injury to the inferior alveolar nerve sustained during the removal of impacted mandibular third molars by the lingual split technique. *British Journal of Oral Surgery 21*:103-116, 1983.

Roos, D. B., & Owens, J. C. Thoracic outlet syndrome. *Archives of Surgery 93*:71-74, 1966.

Roos, D. B., & Wilbourn, A. J. Thoracic outlet syndrome is underrated/overdiagnosed. *Archives of Neurology 47*:228-230, 1990.

Rose, B. W., Mackinnon, S. E., Dellon, A. L., & Snyder, R. A. Design of a protective splint for the non-human primate extremity. *Laboratory Animal Science 33*:306-308, 1983.

Rose, E. H., Kowalski, T. A., & Norris, M. S. The reversed venous arterialized nerve graft in digital nerve reconstruction across scarred beds. *Plastic and Reconstructive Surgery 83*:593-602, 1989.

Rosen, B., Lundborg, G., Dahlin, L. B., Holmberg, J., & Karlson, B. Nerve repair: Correlation of restitution of functional sensibility with specific cognitive capacities. *Journal of Hand Surgery 19B*:452-458, 1994.

Rowinsky, E. K., & Donnehower, E. C. Paclitaxel (Taxol). *New England Journal of Medicine 332*:1004-1014, 1995.

Rowntree, T. Anomalous innervation of hand muscles. *Journal of Bone and Joint Surgery 31B*:505-510, 1949.

Ruch, T. C., Fulton, J. F., & German, W. J. Sensory discrimination in monkey, chimpanzee, and man after lesions of the parietal lobe. *Archives of Neurology and Psychology 39*:919-938, 1938.

Rydevik, B., & Lundborg, G. Permeability of intraneural microvessels in perineurium following acute graded experimental nerve compression. *Plastic Reconstructive Surgery (Scandinavia) 11*:179, 1977.

• S •

Sachs, B. D., & Liu, Y-C. Maintenance of erection of penile glans, but not penile body, after transection of rat cavernous nerves. *Journal of Urology 146*:900-905, 1991.

Sanders, R. J. *Thoracic Outlet Syndrome: A Common Sequela of Neck Injuries*. Philadelphia: J. B. Lippincott Company, 1991.

Saplys, R., Mackinnon, S. E., & Dellon, A. L.

The relationship between nerve entrapment versus neuroma complications and the misdiagnosis of DeQuervain's Disease. *Contemporary Orthopedics 15*:51-57, 1987.

Schoumburg, H. H., Spencer, P. S., & Thomas, P. K. Toxic neuropathy: Occupational biological and environmental agents. In *Disorders of Peripheral Nerves*, H. H. Schoumburg, P. S. Spencer, & P. K. Thomas, Editors. Philadelphia: F. A. Davis Company, 1983.

Schusterman, M. A., Miller, M. J., Reece, G. P., Kroll, S. S., Marchi, M., & Goepfert, H. A single center's experience with 308 free flaps for repair of head and neck cancer defects. *Plastic and Reconstructive Surgery 93*:472-478, 1994.

Schwartzman, R. J., & McLellan, T. L. Reflex sympathetic dystrophy: A review. *Archives of Neurology 44*:554-561, 1987.

Scope of Practice. *American Society of Hand Therapy,* 1989.

Seddon, H. J. Peripheral nerve injuries. *Medical Research Council, Special Report Series 282.* London: Her Majesty's Stationery Office, 1954.

—— *Surgical Disorders of the Peripheral Nerves*. Edinburgh: Churchill Livingstone, 1975.

—— Three types of nerve injury. *Brain 66*:237, 1943.

Seiler, W. A., Schlegel, R., Mackinnon, S. E., & Dellon, A. L. The double crush syndrome: Development of a model. *Surgical Forum 34*:596-598, 1983.

Semmes, J., Weinstein, S., Ghent, L., & Teuber, H. L. *Somatosensory Changes After Penetrating Brain Wounds in Man*. Cambridge, MA: Harvard University Press, 1960.

Seror, P. Sensitivity of the various tests for the diagnosis of carpal tunnel syndrome. *Journal of Hand Surgery 19B*:725-728, 1994.

Shaw, W. W., Orringer, J. S., Ratto, L. L., & Mersmann, C. A. Data presented at the 68th annual meeting of the American Association of Plastic Surgeons, Scottsdale, AZ, May 10, 1989.

Shrout, P. E., & Fleiss, J. L. Intraclass correlation coefficient: Uses in assessing rater reliability. *Psychology Bulletin 86*:420-428, 1979.

Siegal, T., & Haim, N. Cisplatin-Induced Peripheral Neuropathy. *Cancer 66*:1117-1123, 1990.

Siitonen, O. I., Niskanen L. K., Laakso, M. Lower extremity amputations in diabetic and nondiabetic patients. *Diabetes Care 16*:16, 1993.

Silverstein, B. A., Fine, L. J., & Armstrong, T. J. Occupational factors and carpal tunnel syndrome. *American Journal of Industrial Medicine 11*:343-358, 1987.

Silverstein, B. A., Fine, L. J., & Stetson, D. Hand-wrist disorders among investment casting plant workers. *Journal of Hand Surgery 124*:838-844, 1987.

Sinclair, R. J., & Burton, H. Neuronal activity in the second somatosensory cortex of monkeys (Macaca mulatta) during active touch of gratings. *Journal of Neurophysiology 70*:331-350, 1993.

Slezak, S., & Dellon, A. L. Quantitation of sensibility in gigantomastia and alteration following reduction mammaplasty. *Plastic and Reconstructive Surgery 91*:1265-1269, 1993.

Slezak, S., McGibbon, B., & Dellon, A. L. The sensational transverse rectus abdominous myocutaneous (TRAM) flap: Return of sensibility after TRAM reconstruction. *Annals of Plastic Surgery 28*:210-217, 1992.

Smith, K. G., & Robinson, P. P. Does a delay prior to lingual nerve repair prejudice the outcome? *British Journal of Oral Maxillofacial Surgery 31*:57, 1993.

Smith, R. J. Flexor pollicis longus abductorplasty for spastic thumb-in-palm deformity. *Journal of Hand Surgery 7*:327-334, 1982.

Smith, R. O., & Benge, M. W. Pinch and grasp strength: Standardization of terminology and protocol. *American Journal of Occupational Therapy 39*:531-535, 1985.

Sosenko, J. M., Kato, M., & Soto, R. Comparison of quantitative sensory threshold measures for their association with foot ulceration in diabetic patients. *Diabetes Care* 13:1057, 1990.

Soteranos, D. G., & Dellon, A. L. Chronic ulnar nerve compression caused by an implantable silastic neural stimulator. *Journal of Neurosurgery*, submitted: 1995.

Soutar, D. S., & McGregor, I. A. The radial forearm flap in intraoral reconstruction: The experience of 60 consecutive cases. *Plastic and Reconstructive Surgery 78*:1-8, 1986.

Spaans, F. Occupational nerve injuries. In *Handbook of Clinical Neurology*, P. J. Vinken, & G. W. Bruyn, Editors. New York: Elsevier, 1970.

Spinner, M. *Injuries to the Major Branches of the Peripheral Nerves of the Forearm,* 2nd edition. Philadelphia: W. B. Saunders Company, 1978.

Spindler, H. A., & Dellon, A. L. Nerve conduction studies and sensibility testing in the carpal tunnel syndrome. *Journal of Hand Surgery 7*:260-263, 1982.

—— Nerve conduction studies in the superficial radial sensory nerve entrapment syndrome. *Muscle and Nerve 13*:1-5, 1990.

Steib, E. W., & Sun, S. F. Distal ulnar neuropathy in meat packers. *Journal of Occupational Medicine 26*:842-845, 1984.

Stein, B. E., & Meredith, M. A. *The Merging of the Senses.* Cambridge, MA: MIT Press, 1993.

Steinberg, D. R., Gelberman, R. H., Rydevik, B., & Lundborg, G. The utility of portable nerve conduction testing for patients with carpal tunnel syndrome: A prospective clinical study. *Journal of Hand Surgery 17A*:77-81, 1992.

Stokes, H. M. The seriously uninjured hand— Weakness of grip. *Journal of Occupational Medicine 25*:683-684, 1983.

Sunderland, S. Capacity of reinnervated muscles to function efficiently after prolonged denervation. *Archives of Neurology and Psychology 64*:755-771, 1950.

—— *Nerves and Nerve Injuries* 1st edition. Edinburgh: Churchill Livingstone, 1968.

—— *Nerves and Nerve Injuries* 2nd edition. Edinburgh: Churchill Livingstone, 1978.

—— The connective tissues of peripheral nerves. *Brain 88*:841, 1956.

—— The internal anatomy of nerve trunks in relation to the neuronal lesions of leprosy—Observations on pathology, symptomatology and treatment. *Brain 96*:865-868, 1973.

• **T** •

Tachdjian, M. O., & Minear, W. L. Sensory disturbances in the hands of children with cerebral palsy. *Journal of Bone and Joint Surgery 40A*:85-90, 1958.

Tadano, P. A safety/prevention program for VDT operators: One company's approach. *Journal of Hand Therapy* April-June:64-70, 1990.

Talbot, W. H., Darian-Smith, I., Kornhuber, H. H., & Mountcastle, V. B. The sense of flutter-vibration: Comparison of the human capacity with response patterns of mechanoreceptive afferents from the monkey hand. *Journal of Neurophysiology 31*:301-334, 1968.

Tarlov, A. R. *Disability in America: Towards a National Agenda for Prevention*. Washington, DC: National Academy Press, 1991.

Tassler, P. L., & Dellon, A.L. A draught of historical significance. *Plastic and Reconstructive Surgery 91*:400-401, 1994.

—— Correlation of measurements of pressure perception using the Pressure-Specified Sensory Device with electrodiagnostic testing. *Journal of Occupational Medicine 37*:862-866, 1995.

—— Pressure perception in the normal lower extremity and in the tarsal tunnel syndrome. *Muscle and Nerve 19*:285-289, 1996.

Tassler, P. L., Dellon, A. L., & Canoun, C. Identification of elastic fibers in the peripheral nerve. *Journal of Hand Surgery 19B*:48-54, 1994.

Tassler, P. L., Dellon, A. L., Lesser, G., &

Grossman, S. Cisplatin neuropathy: Prevention and treatment of neuropathy by tarsal tunnel decompression in the rat model. *Annals of Plastic Surgery*, submitted: 1997.

Tassler, P. L., Dellon, A. L., & Scheffler, N. M. Cutaneous pressure threshold in diabetics with and without foot ulceration: Evaluation of sensibility with the Pressure-Specified Sensory Device. *Journal of the American Podiatric Medical Association*, 85:679-684, 1995.

Terzis, J. K., & Dykes, R. W. Reinnervation of glabrous skin in baboons: Properties of cutaneous mechanoreceptors subsequent to nerve transection. *Journal of Neurophysiology* 44:1214-1219, 1980.

Terzis, J. K., Dykes, R. W., & Hakstian, R. W. Electrophysiologic recordings in peripheral nerve surgery - A review. *Journal of Hand Surgery 1*:52-66, 1976.

Terzis, J. K., Vincent, M. P., Wilkins, L. M., Rutledge, K., & Deane, L. M. Breast sensibility: A neurophysiologic appraisal in the normal breast. *Annals of Plastic Surgery* 19:318-322, 1987.

Thompson, S. W., Davis, L. E., & Kornfeld, M. Cisplatin neuropathy, clinical, electrophysiologic, morphologic, and toxicologic studies. *Cancer* 54:1269-1275, 1984.

Tinel, J. The tingling sign in peripheral nerve lesions. Translation by Emmanuel B. Kaplan. In *Injuries to the Major Branches of Peripheral Nerves of the Forearm*, M. Spinner, Editor. Philadelphia: W. B. Saunders Company, 1978.

Tizard, J. P. M., & Crothers, B. Disturbances of sensation in children with hemiplegia. *Journal of the American Medical Association* 155:628-632, 1954.

Townsend, P. L. G. Nipple sensation following breast reduction and free nipple transplantation. *British Journal of Plastic Surgery* 27:308-310, 1974.

Turkof, E., Tambwekar, S., Mansukhani, K., Millesi, H., & Mayr, N. Intraoperative spinal root stimulation to detect most proximal site of leprous ulnar neuritis.

Lancet 343:1604-1605, 1994.

• U •

Uematsu, S., Hendler, N., Hungerford, D., Long, D., & Ono, N. Thermography and electromyography in the differential diagnosis of chronic pain syndromes and reflex sympathetic dystrophy. *Electromyography of Clinical Neurophysiology 21*:165-182, 1981.

Upton, A. R. M., & McComas, A. J. The double crush in nerve entrapment syndromes. *Lancet 2*:359-362, 1973.

Urken, M. L., & Biller, H. F. A new bilobed design for the sensate radial forearm flap to preserve tongue mobility following significant glossectomy. *Archives of Otolaryngological Head and Neck Surgery 120*:26-29, 1994.

• V •

Van Beek, A. L. Electrodiagnostic evaluation of peripheral nerve injuries. *Hand Clinics 2*:747-760, 1986.

van Brakel, W. H. Peripheral neuropathy in leprosy: The continuing challenge. *CIP-Gegevens Koninklijke Bibliotheek*. The Hague, The Netherlands, 1994.

van Brakel, W. H., Shute, J., Dixon, J. A., & Arzet, H. Evaluation of sensibility in leprosy—Comparison of various clinical methods. *Leprosy Review*, in press: 1995.

van Vliet, D., Novak, C. B., & Mackinnon, S. E. Duration of contact time alters cutaneous pressure threshold measurements. *Annals of Plastic Surgery 31*:335-339, 1993.

Vastamaki, M., Kallio, P. K., & Solonen, K. A. The results of secondary microsurgical repair of ulnar nerve injury. *Journal of Hand Surgery 18B*:323-326, 1993.

Vergara, J., Medina, L., Maulen, J., Inestrosa, N. C., & Alvarez, J. Nerve regeneration is improved by insulin-like growth factor I (IGF-I) and basic fibroblast growth factor (bFGF). *Restorative Neurology Neuroscience* 5:181-189, 1993.

Vihma, T., Nurminen, M., & Mutanen, P. Sewing machine operators' work and musculoskeletal complaints. *Ergonomics* 25:295-298, 1982.

von Fry, M. The distribution of afferent nerves in the skin. *Journal of the American Medical Association* 47:645-648, 1908.

Vriens, J. P. M., Acosta, R., Soutar, D. S., & Webster, M. H. C. Recovery of sensation in the radial forearm free flap in oral reconstruction. *Journal of Reconstructive Microsurgery*, submitted: 1995.

Vriens, J. P. M., Moos, M. B., & Scott, E. M. Evaluation of normal values for static and dynamic two-point discrimination and for static light touch sensation in the face. *Plastic and Reconstructive Surgery*, submitted: 1994.

● **W** ●

Wall, J. T., Cusik, C. G., Migani-Wall, S. A., & Wiley, R. G. Cortical organization after treatment of a peripheral nerve with ricin: An evaluation of the relationship between sensory neuron death and cortical adjustments after nerve injury. *Journal of Comparative Neurology* 277:578-592, 1988.

Wall, J. T., Fellerman, D. J., & Kaas, J. H. Recovery of normal topography in the somatosensory cortex of monkeys after nerve crush and regeneration. *Science* 221:771-773, 1983.

Wall, J. T., Kaas, J. H., Sur, M., Nelson, R. J., Fellerman, D. J., & Merzenich, M. M. Functional reorganization in somatosensory cortical areas 3b and 1 of adult monkeys after median nerve repair: Possible relationships to sensory recovery in humans. *Journal of Neuroscience* 6:218-233, 1986.

Wall, P. D., & Mclzak, R. *Textbook of Pain.* Edinburgh: Churchill Livingstone, Inc. 1984.

Waller, A. Experiments on the section of the glossopharyngeal and hypoglossal nerves

of the frog, and observations of the alterations produced thereby in the structure of their primitive fibers. *Philosophical Transactions of the Royal Society of London* 140:423-429, 1850.

Walsh, M. T. Therapist management of thoracic outlet syndrome. *Journal of Hand Therapy* April-June:131-144, 1994.

Walsh, P. C., & Donker, P. J. Impotence following radical prostatectomy: Insight into etiology and prevention. *Journal of Urology* 128:492-497, 1982.

Wasserman, J. D., Pollack, C. P., & Spielman, A. J. The differential diagnosis of impotence: The measurement of nocturnal penile tumescence. *Journal of the American Medical Association* 243:2038-2042, 1980.

Watts, D., Tassler, P. L., & Dellon, A. L. The effect of double gloving on cutaneous sensibility, skin compliance, and suture identification. *Contemporary Surgery* 44:289-292, 1994.

Weber, E. Ueber den Tatsinn. Archive fur Anatomy und Physiology. *Wissenshaft Medical Muller's Archives* 1:152-159, 1835.

Wei, F-C., Chien, Y. Y., Ma, H. S., & Dellon, A. L. The myelinated nerve fiber population of digital nerves in the fingers and toes. *Plastic and Reconstructive Surgery*, submitted: 1997.

Wei, F-C., & Ma, H. S. Delayed sensory reeducation after toe- to-hand transfer. *Journal of Reconstructive Microsurgery*, in press: 1997.

—— Results of sensory re-education in toe to hand transfer. *Journal of Hand Surgery* 19A: in press, 1994.

Wei, F-C., Ma, H. S., Chien, Y. Y., & Dellon, A. L. Effect of neurotization upon degree of sensory recovery in toe-to-finger transfer. *Plastic and Reconstructive Surgery*, submitted: 1997.

Weinstein, S. Fifty years of somatosensory research: From the Semmes-Weinstein Monofilaments to the Weinstein Enhanced Sensory Test. *Journal of Hand Therapy* 6:11-22, 1993.

Werner, G., & Mountcastle, V. B. Neural activity in mechanoreceptive afferents: Stimulus-response relations, Weber functions, and information transmission. *Journal of Neurophysiology 28*:359-397, 1965.

Wilbourn, A. J., & Urschel, H. C. Evidence for conduction delay in thoracic outlet syndrome is challenged. *New England Journal of Medicine 310:*1052-1053, 1984.

Williams, H. B., & Terzis, J. K. Single fascicular recordings - An intraoperative diagnostic tool for the management of peripheral nerve lesions. *Plastic and Reconstructive Surgery 57*:562-569, 1976.

Wilson, R. L. Management of pain following peripheral nerve injuries. *Orthopedic Clinics of North America 12*:343-353, 1981.

Windebank, A. J., & Dyck, P. J. Lead intoxication as a model of primary segmental demyelination. In *Peripheral Neuropathy*, Second Edition, P. J. Dyck, P. K. Thomas, E. H. Lambert, & E. Bunge, Editors. Philadelphia: W. B. Saunders Company, 1984.

Wingate, L., Croghan, I., Natarajan, N., & Michalek, R. Rehabilitation of the mastectomy patient: A randomized, blind, prospective study. *Archives of Physical Medicine and Rehabilitation 70*:21-24, 1989.

Winkelman, R. K. *Nerve Endings in Normal and Pathologic Skin. Contributions to the Anatomy of Sensation.* Springfield, IL: Charles C Thomas, Publishers, 1960.

Wofford, D. T., & Miller, R. I. Prospective study of dysesthesia following odontectomy of impacted mandibular third molars. *Journal of Oral Maxillofacial Surgery 45*:15-19, 1987.

Wynn Parry, C. *Rehabilitation of the Hand.* London: Butterworths, 1966.

• **Y** •

Yekutiel, M., Jariwala, M., & Stretch, P. Sensory deficit in the hands of children with cerebral palsy; A new look at assessment and prevalence. *Developmental Medicine and Child Neurology 36*:619-624, 1994.

Yoshimura, M., Nomura, S., Yamauchi, S., Umeda, S., Uneo, T. & Iwai, Y. Toe-to-hand transfer: Experience with thirty-eight digits. *Australian and New Zealand Journal of Surgery 50*:248-254, 1980.

• **Z** •

Zachary, L. S., Dellon, E. S., Nicholas, E. M., & Dellon, A. L. The structural basis of Felice Fontana's spiral bands and their relationship to nerve injury. *Journal of Reconstructive Microsurgery 9*:March, 1993.

Zachary, R. B. Results of nerve suture. In *Peripheral Nerve Injuries*, H. J. Seddon, Editor. London: Her Majesty's Stationery Office, 1954.

Zimmerman, N. B., Zimmerman, S. I., & Clark, G. L. Neuropathy in the workplace. *Hand Clinics 8*:255-262, 1992.

• • •

index